Organ Transplantation

A Clinical Guide

Organ Transplantation

A Clinical Guide

Edited by

Andrew A. Klein

Consultant, Anaesthesia and Intensive Care, Papworth Hospital, Cambridge, UK

Clive J. Lewis

Consultant Cardiologist and Transplant Physician, Papworth Hospital, Cambridge, UK

Joren C. Madsen

Director of the MGH Transplant Center, Section Chief for Cardiac Surgery, and
W. Gerald and Patricia R. Austen Distinguished Scholar in Cardiac Surgery,
Massachusetts General Hospital, Boston, MA, USA

CAMBRIDGE
UNIVERSITY PRESS

CAMBRIDGE UNIVERSITY PRESS
Cambridge, New York, Melbourne, Madrid, Cape Town,
Singapore, São Paulo, Delhi, Tokyo, Mexico City

Cambridge University Press
The Edinburg Building, Cambridge CB2 8RU, UK

Published in the United States of America by Cambridge University Press, New York

www.cambridge.org
Information on this title: www.cambridge.org/9780521197533

First published 2011

Printed in the United Kingdom at the University Press, Cambridge

A catalogue record for this publication is available from the British Library.

Library of Congress Cataloguing in Publication data
Organ transplantation : a clinical guide / edited by Andrew Klein, Clive J. Lewis, Joren C. Madsen.
p. ; cm.
Includes bibliographical references and index.
ISBN 978-0-521-19753-3 (hardback)
1. Transplantation of organs, tissues, etc.
2. Transplantation immunology. I. Klein, Andrew.
II. Lewis, Clive J., 1968– III. Madsen, Joren C., 1955–
[DNLM: 1. Organ Transplantation. 2. Transplantation Immunology. WO 660]
RD120.7.O717 2011
617.9′5 – dc22 2011002165

ISBN 978-0-521-19753-3 Hardback

Contents

Section 4 – Liver

Section 5 – Kidney

Section 6 – Other abdominal organs

Section 7 – Other

Section 8 – The transplant service

Color plate section falls between pages 181 and 182.

Contributors

Graeme J.M. Alexander, MA, MD, FRCP
Consultant Hepatologist, Addenbrooke's Hospital
Cambridge, UK

Heung Bae Kim, MD
Assistant Professor of Surgery, Harvard Medical School, and Director, Pediatric Transplant Center, Children's Hospital Boston, Boston, MA, USA

Michael Burch
Lead Transplant Consultant, Consultant Cardiologist, Great Ormond Street Hospital for Sick Children, London, UK

Andrew J. Butler, MD
Consultant, Department of Transplantation Surgery, Addenbrooke's Hospital, Cambridge, UK

Tanveer Butt, FRCS
Department of Cardiopulmonary Transplantation, The Newcastle upon Tyne Hospitals NHS Foundation Trust (NUTH), Freeman Hospital, High Heaton, Newcastle upon Tyne, UK

Roy Calne, MD
Yeah Ghim Professor of Surgery at the National University of Singapore, Singapore

Edward Cantu III, MD
Associate Surgical Director of Lung Transplantation, University of Pennsylvania, Philadelphia, PA, USA

Robert B. Colvin, MD
Department of Pathology, Massachusetts General Hospital, and Harvard Medical School, Boston, MA, USA

Paul Corris, MB, FRCP
Professor, Department of Respiratory Medicine, Freeman Hospital, Newcastle upon Tyne, UK

Charles Crawley
Consultant, Department of Hematology, Addenbrooke's Hospital, Cambridge, UK

Hiroshi Date, MD
Professor, Department of Thoracic Surgery, Kyoto University Graduate School of Medicine, Kyoto, Japan

Francis L. Delmonico, MD
Medical Director, New England Organ Bank, and Professor of Surgery, Harvard Medical School, Massachusetts General Hospital, Boston, MA, USA

Bimalangshu R. Dey, MD, PhD
Bone Marrow Transplant Program, Department of Medicine, Massachusetts General Hospital, and Harvard Medical School, Boston, MA, USA

Kate Drummond, MD
Fellow, Anaesthesia and Intensive Care, Papworth Hospital, Cambridge, UK

John Dunning, MD
Consultant Cardiothoracic Surgeon, Papworth Hospital, Cambridge, UK

John D. Firth, DM, FRCP
Consultant Physician and Nephrologist, Cambridge University Hospitals Foundation Trust, Cambridge, UK

John Forsythe, MD
Consultant Transplant Surgeon, Royal Infirmary of Edinburgh, Edinburgh, UK

Simon M. Gabe
Lennard Jones Intestinal Failure Unit, St Mark's Hospital, Northwick Park, Harrow, London, UK

Robert S. Gaston, MD, MRCP
Endowed Professor, Transplant Nephrology, and Medical Director, Kidney and Pancreas Transplantation, Division of Nephrology, University of Alabama at Birmingham, Birmingham, AL, USA

William Gelson, MD, MRCP
Consultant Surgeon, Department of Transplant Surgery, Addenbrooke's Hospital, Cambridge, UK

Paul Gibbs
Consultant Surgeon, Department of Transplant Surgery, Addenbrooke's Hospital, Cambridge, UK

Alex Gimson
Consultant Physician, Department of Hepatology, Addenbrooke's Hospital, Cambridge, UK

Leo C. Ginns, MD
Medical Director, Lung Transplantation, Massachusetts General Hospital, and Associate Professor of Medicine, Harvard Medical School, Boston, MA, USA

Samuel Goldfarb, MD
Attending Physician, Division of Pulmonary Medicine, Children's Hospital of Philadelphia; Medical Director, Lung and Heart/Lung Transplant Programs, and Assistant Professor of Pediatrics, University of Pennsylvania School of Medicine, Philadelphia, PA, USA

Ryoichi Goto, MD
Clinical Research Fellow, Nuffield Department of Surgery, University of Oxford, Oxford, UK

Walter K. Graham, JD
Executive Director, United Network for Organ Sharing, Richmond, VA, USA

Simon J.F. Harper
Clinical Lecturer in Transplantation, University of Cambridge and Addenbrooke's Hospital, Cambridge, UK

Koji Hashimoto, MD, PhD
Department of Surgery, Cleveland Clinic, Cleveland, OH, USA

David G. Healy, PhD, FRCSI (C-Th)
Honorary Fellow, Department of Cardiothoracic Surgery, Papworth Hospital, Cambridge, UK

Hassan N. Ibrahim, MD
Department of Medicine, University of Minnesota, Minneapolis, MN, USA

David Ip, MBBS, FANZCA
Anaesthesia Fellow, Toronto General Hospital, Toronto, ON, Canada

Fadi G. Issa, MA, BMBCh, MRCS
Clinical Research Fellow, Nuffield Department of Surgery, University of Oxford, Oxford, UK

Neville V. Jamieson
Consultant Transplantation and HPB Surgeon, University of Cambridge and Addenbrooke's Hospital, Cambridge, UK

David P. Jenkins, MB BS, FRCS (Eng), MS (Lond), FRCS (CTh)
Consultant Cardiothoracic Surgeon, Papworth Hospital, Cambridge, UK

Dixon B. Kaufman, MD, PhD
Professor and Chief, Division of Transplantation, Department of Surgery, University of Wisconsin, Madison, WI, USA

Kiran K. Khush, MD, MAS
Division of Cardiovascular Medicine, Department of Medicine, Stanford University, Stanford, CA, USA

Heung Bae Kim, MD
Director, Pediatric Transplant Center, Department of Surgery, Children's Hospital Boston, and Associate Professor of Surgery, Harvard Medical School, Boston, MA, USA

Andrew A. Klein, MD
Consultant, Cardiothoracic Anaesthesia and Intensive Care, Papworth Hospital, Cambridge, UK

John Klinck, MD
Consultant Anesthetist, Addenbrooke's Hospital, Cambridge, UK

Camille Nelson Kotton, MD
Clinical Director, Transplant and Immunocompromised Host Infectious Diseases, Infectious Diseases Division, Massachusetts General Hospital, Boston, MA, USA

Vineeta Kumar, MD
Assistant Professor of Medicine and Director, Transplant Nephrology Fellowship Program, Division of Nephrology, University of Alabama at Birmingham, Birmingham, AL, USA

Yael B. Kushner, MD
Department of Pathology, Massachusetts General Hospital, and Harvard Medical School, Boston, MA, USA

D. Frank. P. Larkin, MD, FRCPI, FRCOphth2
Consultant Surgeon, Moorfields Eye Hospital, London, UK

Clive J. Lewis, MB, BChir, MRCP, PhD
Consultant, Department of Cardiology, Transplant Unit, Papworth Hospital, Cambridge, UK

Yvonne H. Luo, MA, MRCOphth
Specialist Registrar, Moorfields Eye Hospital, London, UK

Richard S. Luskin
President and CEO, New England Organ Bank, Waltham, MA, USA

Ernest I. Mandel, MD
Clinical Fellow in Medicine, Brigham and Women's Hospital/Massachusetts General Hospital, Boston, MA, USA

James F. Markmann, MD, PhD
Chief, Division of Transplantation, Department of Surgery, and Clinical Director, Transplant Center, Massachusetts General Hospital, and Professor of Surgery, Harvard Medical School, Boston, MA, USA

Lorna Marson
Senior Lecturer in Transplant Surgery, University of Edinburgh, Edinburgh, UK

Arthur J. Matas, MD
Department of Surgery, University of Minnesota, Minneapolis, MN, USA

Mandeep R. Mehra, MBBS, FACP, FACC
Division of Cardiology, Department of Medicine, University of Maryland School of Medicine, Baltimore, MD, USA

Stephen J. Middleton, MA, MD, FRCP, FAHE
Consultant Physician, Department of Gastroenterology, Addenbrooke's Hospital, Cambridge University, Cambridge, UK

Giorgina Mieli-Vergani, MD, PhD, FRCP, FRCPCH
Alex Mowat Professor of Paediatric Hepatology, Institute of Liver Studies, King's College London School of Medicine, London, UK

Charles Miller
Director of Liver Transplantation, Cleveland Clinic, Cleveland, OH, USA

Sharon Mulroy, MD
Locum Consultant Nephrologist, Department of Renal Medicine, Addenbrooke's Hospital, Cambridge, UK

Faruk Özalp, MRCS
Department of Cardiopulmonary Transplantation, The Newcastle upon Tyne Hospitals NHS Foundation Trust, Freeman Hospital, High Heaton, Newcastle upon Tyne, UK

Can Ozturk, MD
Dermatology and Plastic Surgery Institute, Cleveland Clinic, Cleveland, OH, USA

Jayan Parameshwar, MD, MPhil, FRCP
Consultant Cardiologist, Advanced Heart Failure and Transplant Programme, Papworth Hospital, Cambridge, UK

J.S. Parmar, BM, PhD, FRCP
Consultant Transplant Physician (Respiratory), Transplant Unit, Papworth Hospital, Papworth Everard, Cambridge, UK

Hari K. Parthasarathy, MD, MRCP
Transplant Unit, Papworth Hospital, Cambridge, UK

Nick Pritchard, BSc, MBBS, PhD, FRCP
Consultant Physician, Department of Renal Medicine, Addenbrooke's Hospital, Cambridge, UK

Cristiano Quintini, MD
Department of General Surgery, Cleveland Clinic, Cleveland, OH, USA

Axel O. Rahmel
Medical Director, Eurotransplant International Foundation, Leiden, The Netherlands

Chris J. Rudge, FRCS
National Clinical Director for Transplantation, Department of Health, London, UK

Stephan V.B. Schueler, MD, PhD, FRCS
Consultant Surgeon, Department of Cardiopulmonary Transplantation, The Newcastle upon Tyne Hospitals NHS Foundation Trust, Freeman Hospital, High Heaton, Newcastle upon Tyne, UK

Maria Siemionow, MD, PHD, DSC
Professor of Surgery, Dermatology and Plastic Surgery Institute, Cleveland Clinic, Cleveland, OH, USA

Jacob Simmonds
Specialist Registrar, Department of Cardiothoracic Transplantation, Great Ormond Street Hospital, London, UK

Peter Slinger, MD, FRCPC
Professor of Anesthesia, Toronto General Hospital, Toronto, ON, Canada

Thomas R. Spitzer, MD
Director, Bone Marrow Transplant Program, Massachusetts General Hospital, and Professor of Medicine, Harvard Medical School, Boston, MA, USA

Stuart C. Sweet, MD, PhD
Medical Director, Pediatric Lung Transplant Program, and Associate Professor of Pediatrics, Department of Pediatrics, Washington University, St. Louis, MO, USA

Nina E. Tolkoff-Rubin, MD
Medical Director for Renal Transplantation, Massachusetts General Hospital, and Professor of Medicine, Harvard Medical School, Boston, MA, USA

Steven S.L. Tsui, MA (Cantab), MD, FRCS (Eng), FRCS (C-Th)
Consultant Surgeon and Director of Transplantation, Papworth Hospital, Cambridge, UK

Khashayar Vakili, MD
Instructor in Surgery, Harvard Medical School, and Department of Surgery, Children's Hospital Boston, Boston, MA, USA

R.V. Venkateswaran, MS, MD, FRCS-CTh
Fellow, Department of Cardiothoracic Surgery, Papworth Hospital, Papworth Everard, Cambridge, UK

Hector Vilca-Melendez, MD, PhD
Consultant Surgeon, Institute of Liver Studies, King's College Hospital, London, UK

Vladimir Vinarsky, MD
Clinical Fellow in Medicine, Massachusetts General Hospital, Boston, MA, USA

Kathryn J. Wood, DPhil
Professor of Immunology, Nuffield Department of Surgery, University of Oxford, Oxford, UK

Heidi Yeh, MD
Assistant in Surgery, Massachusetts General Hospital, and Instructor in Surgery, Harvard Medical School, Boston, MA, USA

David W. Zaas
Medical Director, Lung Transplantation, and Vice-Chair for Clinical Practice, Department of Medicine, Duke University, Durham, NC, USA

Jonathan G. Zaroff, MD
Division of Cardiology, Kaiser Permanente, San Francisco, CA, USA

Foreword

The ever expanding nature of transplantation means that a book aimed at encompassing all aspects of all transplant subspecialties would be vast. Instead, this book focuses on the *clinical* aspects of transplantation. It provides a concise yet comprehensive guide to the art and science of caring for transplant patients. It will undoubtedly provide an excellent resource for physicians, surgeons, anesthesiologists and, indeed, all transplant practitioners – medical and non-medical. It will also be of interest to patients and their families because it is written and presented in an easy-to-read format.

This text provides state-of-the-art knowledge from experts in their respective fields. As such, it will become an essential companion for anyone involved in transplantation, especially those at the beginning of their careers. It will be available as an e-book, and in the traditional print form. I am sure that you will enjoy, *Organ Transplantation – A Clinical Guide*.

Thomas E. Starzl, MD, PhD
Professor of Surgery and Distinguished Service
Professor, University of Pittsburgh

Preface

The field of solid organ transplantation has developed enormously in the last three decades and what was pioneering surgery has now become routine. Outcomes are no longer considered in terms of 1-year survival, but clinicians and patients are looking to 20 years and beyond. The current success of transplantation is based on many different factors: developments in surgical technique, better immunosuppression, improved anesthetic and intensive care, improved microbiology, and close collaboration between – all those involved in the transplant pathway have contributed.

However, there are still many problems to be overcome and success has brought its own challenges. The adverse impact of immunosuppression – such as increased risk of some cancers and infections, increased cardiovascular and cerebrovascular disease, diabetes and renal failure – have not yet been avoided by the development of more effective and specific agents; tolerance remains elusive, although inducing operational tolerance is perhaps less distant now than it was a decade ago. In many situations, recurrent disease is yet to be overcome. Most transplant recipients still have a reduced life expectancy compared with the normal population and so clinicians are now focussing on maintaining the quality and length of life.

Overcoming many of the technical barriers to transplantation has increased the number of people who could benefit from transplantation and highlighted the need for more donors. Donation rates vary between countries and many factors contribute to this variation: cultural, logistical, financial, legal, and medical. The success of initiatives to reduce premature death from road accidents and cardiovascular and cerebrovascular disease are of course hugely welcome but have resulted in a reduction in the potential donor pool, and those who are potential donors are becoming older and heavier so that the number and quality of retrieved organs is falling. The reduction in the traditional donor pool has encouraged clinicians to look at additional sources of donors, including living donors and donors after circulatory death. These approaches will go some way toward mitigating the impact of the shrinking traditional donor pool; however, the widening gap between need and supply does bring into focus the moral, ethical, and legal implications of the introduction of policies for what is, effectively, the rationing of life-saving organs.

Transplantation remains a high-risk procedure and its risks have to be balanced against those of ongoing medical management. Donated organs are not free of risks of transmission of cancer or infection and should be considered "second hand" rather than new. Recipient's expectations must be managed appropriately. An excessive focus on outcomes and avoidance of risk will encourage risk-averse behavior by clinicians and may inhibit some surgeons from remaining in this challenging field. Therefore, unless regulation is maintained at an appropriate level, over-monitoring will ultimately adversely affect the recipient.

The future of transplantation is, for the moment, secure and there is little doubt that the need for transplantation will continue to exceed the supply of organs. Although many problems have been overcome, many challenges remain. We are encouraged by the progress in immune tolerance, regenerative medicine, organ support, and even xenotransplantation. However, there is much yet to be learned and then applied to patients. The race between perfecting the process of organ transplantation-fabrication on one hand and the curing of diseases that lead to organ failure and the need for transplantation on the other, is on. Fortunately, however, no matter which side wins, it the patient who is ultimately the victor.

This book, with contributions from experts in the broad field of transplantation from all over the world, provides an authoritative account of where transplantation has come from, where it is now, and where it might go in the future. The state-of-the-art knowledge contained within this volume will help make all who read it better caregivers to recipients of organ transplants and better prepared to embrace the exciting future of our field.

Andrew A. Klein, MD
Consultant, Cardiothoracic Anaesthesia and Intensive Care, Papworth Hospital, Cambridge, UK

James Neuberger, DM, FRCP
Honorary Professor of Medicine, University of Birmingham, and Associate Medical Director, Organ Donation and Transplantation, NHS Blood and Transplant, Bristol, UK

Abbreviations

6-MP	6-mercaptopurine
A2ALL	Adult-to-Adult Living Donor Liver Transplantation Cohort Study
ABOi	ABO incompatible
ABVC	doxorubicin, bleomycin, vinblastine, and dacarbazine
ACAID	Anterior chamber–associated immune deviation
ACD	acquired cystic disease
ACE	angiotensin-converting enzyme
ACOT	Advisory Committee on Transplantation
ACR	acute cellular rejection
ACT	activated clotting time
ADCC	antibody-dependent cell-mediated cytotoxicity
ADH	anti-diuretic hormone
AHR	acute humoral rejection
aHUS	atypical HUS
aICB	atraumatic intracranial bleed
AIDS	acquired immune deficiency syndrome
AIH	autoimmune hepatitis
ALF	acute liver failure
ALG	anti-lymphocyte globulin
AMR	antibody mediated rejection
AP-1	activator protein 1
APC	antigen-presenting cell
APOLT	auxiliary partial orthotopic liver transplantation
ARB	angiotensin receptor blocker
ARDS	acute respiratory distress syndrome
ATC	anti-thymocyte globulin
ATG	antithymocyte globulin
ATN	acute tubular necrosis
ATP	adenosine triphosphate production
AV	atrioventricular
AZA	azathioprine
BASM	biliary atresia splenic malformation
BCC	basal cell carcinoma
BKV	BK virus
BLT	bilateral lung transplantation
BMD	bone mineral density
BMI	body mass index
BNP	B-type natriuretic peptide
BODE	body mass index, airflow obstruction, dyspnea, and exercise capacity
BOS	bronchiolitis obliterans syndrome
BTT	bridging to transplant
C3	complement component 3
C4d	complement component 4d
CAN	chronic allograft nephropathy
CAV	cardiac allograft vasculopathy
CAV	coronary artery vasculopathy
CBD	common bile duct
CBP	cardiopulmonary bypass
CD3	cluster of differentiation (CD) 3 molecule
CDC	complement-dependent cytotoxicity cross-match
CDR	chronic ductopenic rejection
CF	cystic fibrosis
CHOP	cyclophosphamide, doxorubicin, vincristine, and prednisone
CHR	chronic humoral rejection
CIT	cold ischemic time
CKD	chronic kidney disease
C_{max}	maximum concentration
CMV	cytomegalovirus
CNI	calcineurin inhibitor
CNS	central nervous system
CO	carbon monoxide
COPD	chronic obstructive pulmonary disease
CPB	cardiopulmonary bypass
CPEX	cardiopulmonary exercise testing
CR	complete remission
CRP	C-reactive protein
CRT	cardiac resynchronization therapy

c-SMAC	central supramolecular activation cluster
CT	computed tomography
CTA	composite tissue allotransplantation
CTL	cytotoxic T cell
CTLA-4	cytotoxic T-lymphocyte antigen 4
CTTR	Cincinnati Transplant Tumor Registry
CVP	central venous pressure
CY	cyclophosphamide
CyA	cyclosporine
D	donor
D–	no diarrhea
D+	diarrhea associated
DAG	diacylglycerol
DBD	donation after brain death
DC	dendritic cell
DCD	donation after cardiac death
DEXA	dual-energy X-ray absorptiometry
DGF	delayed graft function
DLCO	diffusing capacity of carbon monoxide
DLI	donor lymphocyte infusion
DM1	type 1 diabetes mellitus
DM2	type 2 diabetes mellitus
DSA	donor specific antibodies
DTC	donor transplant coordinator
DTH	delayed-type hypersensitivity
DVT	deep venous thrombosis
EBV	Epstein-Barr virus
ECD	extended criteria donor
ECMO	extracorporeal membrane oxygenation
EC-MPS	enteric-coated mycophenolate sodium
EF	ejection fraction
eGFR	estimated glomerular filtration rate
EHBA	extra-hepatic biliary atresia
ELITE	Efficacy Limiting Toxicity Elimination
ENT	ear, nose, and throat
ER	endoplasmic reticulum
ESC	embryonic stem cell
ESRD	end-stage renal disease
ETT	endotracheal tube
EVL	everolimus
EVLP	ex vivo lung perfusion
FasL	Fas ligand
FCXM	flow cytometry cross-match
FDA	US Food and Drug Administration
FEF	forced expiratory flow
FEF25–75%	forced expiratory flow 25–75%
FEV_1	forced expiratory volume in 1 second
FLR	future liver remnant
FRC	functional residual capacity
FSGS	focal segmental glomerulosclerosis
FVC	forced vital capacity
GBM	glomerular basement membrane
G-CSF	granulocyte colony-stimulating factor
GDA	gastroduodenal artery
GERD	gastroesophageal reflux disease
GFR	glomerular filtration rate
GI	gastrointestinal
GRWR	graft-to-recipient body weight ratio
GvHD	graft-versus-host disease
GvL	Graft versus leukemia
HAR	hyperacute rejection
HARI	hepatic artery resistance index
HAT	hepatic artery thrombosis
HBV	hepatitis B virus
HCC	hepatocellular carcinoma
HCV	hepatitis C virus
HF	heart failure
HFSS	Heart Failure Survival Score
HHS	Department of Health and Human Services
HHV	human herpes virus
HHV-8	human herpes virus type 8
HIV	human immunodeficiency virus
HLA	human leukocyte antigen
HLAi	HLA incompatible
HLT	combined heart–lung transplantation
HLT	heart–lung transplantation
HMGB-1	high-mobility group box 1 protein
HPC	human progenitor cell
HPV	human papillomavirus
HRQOL	health related quality of life
HRSA	Health Resources and Services Administration
HSC	hematopoietic stem cells
HSCT	hematopoietic stem cell transplantation
HSP	heat shock protein
HSV	herpes simplex virus
HT	heart transplant
HT	heart transplantation
HTA	Human Tissue Authority
HUS	hemolytic uremic syndrome
IBMIR	immediate blood-mediated inflammatory reaction
ICAM-1	intercellular adhesion molecule 1

ICD	implantable cardioverter-defibrillator
ICOS	inducible T-cell costimulator
ICP	intra-cranial pressure
ICU	intensive care unit
IE	islet equation
IF/TA	interstitial fibrosis and tubular atrophy
IFN	interferon
IFNγ	interferon γ
Ig	immunoglobulin
IgA	immunoglobulin A
IgG	immunoglobulin G
IHD	ischemic heart disease
IL	interleukin
IL-2	interleukin-2
IL-2R	interleukin-2 receptor
IMP	inosine monophosphate
IMV	inferior mesenteric vein
iNO	inhaled nitric oxide
INR	international normalized ratio
INTERMACS	International Registry for Mechanically Assisted Circulatory Support
IP_3	inositol triphosphate
IPAH	idiopathic pulmonary arterial hypertension
IPEX	immune dysregulation, polyendocrinopathy, enteropathy X-linked
IPF	idiopathic pulmonary fibrosis
IPTR	International Pancreas Transplant Registry
IRI	ischemia/reperfusion injury
ISHLT	International Society for Heart and Lung Transplantation
iTreg	inducible Treg
ITU	intensive treatment unit
IV	intravenous
IVC	inferior vena cava
IVIg	intravenous immunoglobulin
IVUS	intravascular ultrasound
Jak	Janus kinase
JCV	JC virus
KS	Kaposi's sarcoma
LAS	lung allocation system
LCR	late cellular rejection
LDH	lactate dehydrogenase
LDLLT	living donor lobar lung transplantation
LDLT	living donor liver transplantation
LDLT	living donor lung transplantation
LFA-1	leukocyte function-associated antigen 1
LFA-1	lymphocyte-function associated antigen-1
LT	liver transplantation
LT	lung transplantation
LV	left ventricle
LV	left ventricular
LVAD	left ventricular assist device
LVEDP	left ventricular end-diastolic pressure
LVH	left ventricular hypertrophy
MAC	membrane attack complex
MAG3	mercaptoacetyltriglycine
MAP	mitogen-activated protein
MAPK	MAP kinase
MBD	mineral bone disease
MCSD	mechanical circulatory support devices
MELD	Model for End-Stage Liver Disease
MHC	major histocompatability complex
MHV	middle hepatic vein
miH	minor histocompatibility
MMF	mycophenolate mofetil
MMR	measles, mumps, and rubella
MPA	mycophenolic acid
MPGN	membranoproliferative glomerulonephritis
MPSC	Membership and Professional Standards Committee
MRI	magnetic resonance imaging
MRR	medical record review
MRSA	methicillin-resistant *Staphylococcus aureus*
mTOR	mammalian target of rapamycin
NAPRTCS	North American Pediatric Renal Trials and Collaborative Studies
NFAT	nuclear factor of activated T cells
NF-κB	nuclear factor-κB
NHL	non-Hodgkin's lymphoma
NHS	National Health Service
NHSBT	NHS Blood and Transplant
NK	natural killer
NKT	natural killer T
NO	nitric oxide
NOD	non-obese diabetic
NODAT	new-onset diabetes after transplantation

NODAT	new-onset diabetes after transplantation
NOTA	National Organ Transplant Act
NRM	non-relapse mortality
nTreg	naturally occurring Treg
NYHA	New York Heart Association
OB	obliterative bronchiolitis
OKT3	muromonab-CD3
OLV	one-lung ventilation
OP	osteoporosis
OPO	organ procurement organization
OPTN	Organ Procurement and Transplantation Network
PA	pulmonary artery
PAK	pancreas after kidney transplant
PAP	pulmonary artery pressure
PAS	Periodic Acid-Schiff
PCA	patient-controlled analgesia
PCR	polymerase chain reaction
PCWP	pulmonary capillary wedge pressure
PDA	UK Potential Donor Audit
PDGF	platelet-derived growth factor
PEEP	positive end expiratory pressure
PGD	primary graft dysfunction
PGE2	prostaglandin E2
PGI_2	prostacyclin
PK	pharmacokinetic
PKC	protein kinase C
PML	progressive multifocal leukoencephalopathy
PMN	polymorphonuclear neutrophil
PN	parenteral nutrition
ppm	parts per million
PRA	panel-reactive antibody
PRAISE	Prospective Randomized Amlodipine Survival Evaluation
PRR	pattern recognition receptor
PSC	primary sclerosing cholangitis
p-SMAC	peripheral SMAC
PT	prothrombin time
PTA	pancreas transplant alone
PTLD	post-transplant lymphoproliferative disease
PTM	post-transplant malignancy
PUVA	psoralen and UVA therapy
PVR	pulmonary vascular resistance
PVT	portal vein thrombosis
QoL	quality of life
R	recipient
RAD	everolimus
RAS	renal artery stenosis
rATG	rabbit ATG
RBCs	red blood cells
RCC	renal cell carcinoma
RCT	randomized controlled trial
RER	respiratory exchange ratio
RIC	reduced intensity conditioning
ROS	reactive oxygen species
RR	relative risk
RSV	respiratory syncytial virus
RV	right ventricle
RV	right ventricular
RVAD	right ventricular assist device
RVI	respiratory viral infections
SA	sinoatrial
SARS	severe acute respiratory syndrome
SCC	squamous cell carcinoma
SCID	severe combined immunodeficiency
SFSS	small-for-size syndrome
SIOPEL	International Childhood Liver Tumour Strategy Group of the International Society of Paediatric Oncology
SIRS	systemic inflammatory response syndrome
SLT	single lung transplantation
SMA	smooth muscle antibody
SMA	superior mesenteric artery
SMV	superior mesenteric vein
SOT	solid organ transplant
SPK	simultaneous pancreas and kidney transplant
SRL	sirolimus
SRTR	Scientific Registry of Transplant Recipients
SRTR	US Scientific Registry of Transplant Recipients
SVC	superior vena cava
SVR	systemic vascular resistance
T3	triiodothyronine
T4	tetraiodothyronine
TA	transplant arteriopathy
TAC	tacrolimus
TAH	total artificial heart
TBBx	transbronchial biopsy
TBI	total body irradiation
TCD	T-cell depleted
TCMR	T-cell mediated rejection
TCR	T-cell receptor
TEA	thoracic epidural anesthesia

TEE	transesophageal echocardiography
TEG	thromboelastography
TG	transplant glomerulopathy
TGFβ	transforming growth factor β
Th	helper T cell
TIVA	total intravenous anesthesia
TLC	total lung capacity
TLCO	transfer coefficient for carbon monoxide
TLI	total lymphoid irradiation
TLR	Toll-like receptor
TMA	thrombotic microangiopathy
Tn	troponin
TNF	tumor necrosis factor
TNF-α	tumor necrosis factor alpha
TNFR	TNF receptor
TPEX	therapeutic plasma exchange
TPG	transpulmonary gradient
TPG	transpulmonary pressure gradient
TR	tricuspid regurgitation
Treg	regulatory T cell
TSH	thyroid-stimulating hormone
UCLA	University of California, Los Angeles
UKELD	United Kingdom Model for End-Stage Liver Disease
UNOS	United Network for Organ Sharing
UTI	urinary tract infection
VA	arteriovenous
VAD	ventricular assist device
VBDS	vanishing bile duct syndrome
VOD	veno-occlusive disease
VRE	vancomycin-resistant *Enterococcus faecalis*
VTE	venous thromboembolism
VV	venovenous
VZV	varicella zoster virus
WHO	World Health Organization
WU	Wood units

Chapter 1

Historical perspectives

John Dunning and Sir Roy Calne

Key points

- Successful techniques for vascular anastomoses developed at the end of the nineteenth century made the transplantation of internal organs possible.
- The first successful human allograft, a corneal transplant, was performed in 1905.
- The recognition that the body's reactions to foreign tissue led to the failure of allograft transplantation gave rise to the new discipline of immunology.
- The discovery that cyclosporine, a metabolite from the fungus *Tolypocladium inflatum*, is 300 times more active against the proliferation of splenic lymphocytes than against other cell lines changed the face of transplantation.
- As transplantation has become more successful in terms of survival, quality of life, and cost benefit, the demand for donor organs has increased so that it is now greater than supply.

Transplantation of organs represents the pinnacle of medical achievement in so many different ways. It epitomizes the multi-disciplinary team approach to patient care. It has a foundation in refined surgical technique, supported by an understanding of complex immunological events, and requires a complex approach to pretransplant assessment and postoperative care of multiple organ systems. Yet in some respects it also represents a failure: the inability to repair diseased organs such that the only way forward is to cast aside the worn out tissue!

The idea of organ and tissue transplantation is not new, and reference to it may be found in the ancient literature of China and India. The first description of a skin transplant is contained in the Sushrutta manuscripts dating from around 450 BC. The technique described found use in Europe during the Middle Ages in the hands of the Italian surgeon Gaspare Tagliacozzi. He used it for the reconstruction of damaged noses, frequently a result of syphilitic injury, using a skin flap from the forearm. At the time he wrote that "the singular nature of the individual entirely dissuades us from attempting this work on another person." Perhaps he had already attempted the repair using allogeneic donors (transplantation between genetically disparate individuals) prior to his successful autograft (transplant of tissue in the same individual). Although the technique was new to the people of the time, the concept of tissue transplantation was well established among Europeans following the legend of a total leg transplant by Saints Damon and Cosmos illustrated by artists such as Fra Angelico and sculpted by Donatello. Such legendary optimism was not rewarded clinically until much later, but it is certain that interest in skin grafting was revived due to the substantial need for treatment of the gross leg ulcers prevalent in the nineteenth century as a result of injury from syphilis, nutritional deficiency, and burns. Great advances were made with the observations of the French Physiologist Paul Bert, who recognized the importance of graft neovascularization and described the success of autografting in comparison with the failures of allografting.

It was the ophthalmic surgeons who really led the way to successful allografting with the transplantation of corneal grafts. Samuel Bigger reported what was probably the first successful full-thickness corneal allograft when he performed an operation on a blind pet gazelle while he was a prisoner in Egypt in 1835. He replaced the cornea, apparently with good results.

Organ Transplantation: A Clinical Guide, ed. A.A. Klein, C.J. Lewis, and J.C. Madsen. Published by Cambridge University Press.

Attempts to reproduce this success continued through the latter part of the nineteenth century, and with technical improvements and increasing frequency of trials, the results with animal corneal grafts improved steadily. Finally, in 1905, the first successful human corneal allograft was performed. Although therapeutic transplantation of the cornea became firmly established as part of ophthalmic practice from this time, there was no theoretical explanation why corneal grafting should be successful whereas the grafting of other organs and tissues was not, nor of the observation that from time to time corneal grafts were rejected.

It was not until Alexis Carrel and Mathieu Jaboulay developed successful techniques for vascular anastomoses at the end of the nineteenth century that the transplantation of internal organs became possible. Many different animal models were used with attempts to transplant almost every organ, but the kidney was the first organ to which this technique was repeatedly applied.

Carrel remained a prominent contributor to the field of transplant surgery throughout the early 1900s, moving from France to the United States, where his collaboration with Guthrie led to significant contributions to vascular surgery with the development of techniques for venous patching of arteries and the use of cold storage to protect tissue for reimplantation up to 20 hours from its procurement. The result of their labors was a series of 35 papers describing their experimental achievements in a wide variety of animal models for transplantation. However, it was not until 1908 that survival became extended when Carrel performed a kidney transplant in a dog with survival of the graft for several years. With the survival of grafts beyond a few hours, the opportunity to study tissue histologically emerged, and by 1905, parenchymal infiltration by "round cells" and arterial lesions were recognized.

Of course human donors were not available at this time, and all organs transplanted were obtained from animals so that a mixture of pig, goat, monkey, and sheep *xenografts* (transplantation between species) were undertaken in human patients with acute renal failure. Although none of these attempts were successful, the last attempt by Neuhof in 1923 was particularly encouraging, with the recipient surviving for 9 days. It demonstrated clearly that thrombosis and hemorrhage from vascular anastomoses was not inevitable. Although most attempts to perform organ transplantation were made in animals, Mathieu Jaboulay attempted the technique in man, and in 1906 he reported his observations in Lyon Medical. His attempts used a pig kidney in one patient and a goat's kidney in a second, with the organs implanted in the cubital fossa and anastomosed to the humeral artery and cephalic vein. Ultimately both attempts failed as a result of vascular thrombosis, but the kidneys did start to diurese initially.

It quickly became apparent that whereas autografts generally succeeded, allografts and xenografts mostly failed. Although the technical problems of the operation had largely been sorted out, it was clear that "from a biological standpoint … the interactions of the host and of the new organ are practically unknown." The increasing understanding that the resistance to foreign grafts was caused by systemic factors led to the repeated suggestion that an immune response of the "anaphylactoid type" was somehow responsible for graft rejection. It was recognized that research had now to be directed toward understanding the body's reactions to foreign tissue, and so from experimental transplantation in the early part of the century, the two new disciplines of vascular surgery and immunology emerged.

Other landmarks were reached throughout the early years of the twentieth century, with growing understanding of skin grafts used to treat burns, and with Voronoy transplanting the first cadaveric human kidney in 1933. His recipient was a 26-year-old woman who had attempted suicide by swallowing sublimed mercury. This led to uremic coma. The kidney was procured from a 60-year-old man who died following a fracture of the base of the skull. The operation was performed on April 3, 1933, with the renal vessels anastomosed using Carrel's technique to the femoral vessels and the kidney placed in a subcutaneous pouch, with externalization of the ureter. Local anesthetic was used. The donor was known to be blood group B, and the recipient blood group O. The grafted kidney did diurese for a while, but unfortunately the patient died 2 days later.

Despite the demonstration of second-set skin graft rejection in man as early as 1924 and the successful exchange of skin between identical twins in 1927, no useful generalizations were made to further elucidate the immunological mechanisms involved. The practice of corneal grafting continued, but it seemed to be accepted that the transplantation of other tissues and organs was impractical, and there was a lull in activity among surgeons for the next 20 years, with further interruptions to the field brought about by the Second World War.

The area of skin grafting became of greater importance for the treatment of war burns and other injuries, and the death from kidney disease also provided impetus to focus once more on kidney transplantation. Short-term success in the late 1940s was reported by a number of individuals, including Voronoy, and David Hume working in Boston. Both transplanted kidneys into patients with uremic coma that diuresed for a number of days, before stopping and being removed again. The technique was not seen as replacement therapy but a method of stimulating a recovery reflex in the native diseased kidney. However, as the immunological basis of rejection became established, scientific interest in organ transplantation waned until effective immunosuppressive regimens were found.

Abdominal organ transplantation

Transplantation of abdominal organs has been a long-term success story, with patients surviving 40 years with excellent function in their original grafted organs. The success of clinical allograft transplantation began with transplantation of kidneys between identical twins by Murray and colleagues at Peter Bent Brigham Hospital in Boston in 1956. This was an outstanding achievement and demonstrated clearly that the kidney would withstand the trauma of removal, periods of ischemia, and then the procedure of transplantation into another individual of the same species. The fact that identical twins would not be able to reject skin grafts and the experimental auto-transplantation of the kidney in the dog enabled the group in Boston to proceed with the clinical operation with reasonable optimism. Unfortunately, a twin donor would not be available for most patients dying of kidney failure, and the immunological barrier between individuals proved to be an enormous biological problem.

For more than a decade, clinical kidney transplantation was the only form of organ grafting that was seriously studied and yielded some success. The identical twin experience was reproduced, and conditioning of the recipient with total-body irradiation was applied to kidney grafting between donor and recipient who were not twins. This was based mainly on experimental work with bone marrow transplantation; however, in the clinic the results were disastrous, except in two cases of kidney grafting between non-identical twins. Patients subjected to total-body irradiation frequently succumbed to infection, aplasia, and cancer.

The introduction of chemotherapy to supplement irradiation and allow dose reduction improved the outcomes further, and in 1960, William Goodwin introduced methotrexate and cyclophosphamide to the field of living related transplantation and treated an episode of rejection with prednisolone. Then, in London in the mid 1950s, the prolongation of survival of renal allografts in dogs by the anti-leukemia drug 6-mercaptopurine (6-MP) heralded clinical immunosuppression and azathioprine (AZA), a derivative of 6-MP, was found to be slightly better experimentally. Although 6-MP was used briefly with irradiation, it was rapidly abandoned because of significant toxicity. The use of AZA in clinical kidney transplantation was originally disappointing, but when corticosteroids were added, this immunosuppressive regimen resulted in some long-term clinical renal allograft successes from the early 1960s.

Further understanding of transplant immunology was gained with insights into the human leukocyte antigen (HLA) system and histocompatibility. Cross-match techniques became established through the 1960s, and understanding of the "transfusion effect" was also gained (Opelz and Terasaki), whereby previous transfusion appeared to confer protection for the transplanted organ.

In the 1960s, experimental transplantation of the liver, pancreas, intestines, and heart led to a clarification of the technical requirements involved, and in 1963, Starzl in Denver carried out the first clinical liver transplant. Unfortunately, the results of this clinical series were dismal, and Starzl self-imposed a moratorium until 1967, when he resumed clinical liver transplantation, having in the meantime improved the surgical technique and the assessment of graft function and prevention of rejection. The first orthotopic liver transplant in Europe was performed in Cambridge by Calne in 1968. For nearly 10 years, Denver and Cambridge were the only two centers with regular programs of clinical liver transplantation. There were a few outstandingly good results, but many disappointments. Patients were referred for operation too late, and anti-rejection therapy was still in the process of development using modified regimens of AZA, steroids, and polyclonal anti-lymphocyte serum. In addition to rejection, sepsis, biliary, and vascular complications and recurrence of the patient's own disease often resulted in failure. During this uncertain and disappointing phase of development, the vascularized pancreas was also transplanted and shown to be capable of curing diabetes in a few patients. However, many patients suffered from complications of leakage of pancreatic enzymes, causing inflammation and fatal sepsis.

A watershed in organ transplantation was the discovery of the immunosuppressive properties of cyclosporine (CyA), a metabolite from the fungus *Tolypocladium inflatum*, by Jean Borel working in the Sandoz laboratories. CyA was 300 times more active against the proliferation of splenic lymphocytes than against other cell lines. Experimental and clinical application of CyA transformed the attitude of previously sceptical clinicians to organ transplantation. Calne's paper published in *The Lancet* in 1979 described its use in 32 kidney transplants, 2 liver transplants, and 2 pancreatic transplants and showed improved 1-year functional survival of kidney transplants from below 50% to approximately 80%. It was introduced to clinical immunosuppressive regimens worldwide in 1982 and radically improved the survival of heart, kidney, liver, and pancreas recipients. About 10 centers had soldiered on in the pre-CyA era, but after the introduction of CyA, there were soon more than 1000 centers. The improved results led to an expanding mismatch of numbers of available donors to potential recipients seeking a life-saving organ graft.

Unfortunately, the nephrotoxic side effects of CyA led to late renal failure in many cases. Hopes that there might be a dosage window in which rejection could be controlled and side effects avoided were only realized in a minority of cases. However, the concept was established of combining immunosuppressive drugs with the objective of obtaining added immunosuppressive effect but reducing the individual side effects. Thus AZA, CyA, and steroids became a standard immunosuppressant regimen.

The liver proved to be less susceptible to rejection than other organs. This had been anticipated by experiments in pigs and rats. In an important "patient-led clinical study," a group of patients from Denver stopped taking their maintenance immunosuppression without telling their doctors. Although lack of compliance is a common cause of organ graft failure due to rejection, a surprising number of young patients with liver transplants did well long-term. A number of patients, in whom immunosuppression was stopped for medical indications, usually infection, also did not require renewal of their immunosuppressive regimen of drugs. Confidence in the surgery and immunosuppression gradually increased.

A variety of complicated organ graft procedures were reported, including small bowel on its own (1988) and in combination with liver and other organ grafts. The first combined heart, lung, and liver transplant was performed by Wallwork and Calne in 1987 at Papworth (Cambridge, United Kingdom), with survival of the patient for more than 10 years.

There is now a move toward minimization of immunosuppression and tolerance. Alemtuzumab (Campath), an extremely powerful anti-lymphocyte antibody developed in Cambridge by Waldmann and colleagues, has induced "*prope* or almost tolerance" when used as an induction agent followed by maintenance immunosuppression with half-dose CyA, rather than a full dose of three drugs. Of the original series of kidney transplantation patients treated in Cambridge, 80% have never received steroids, and their quality of life has been excellent after more than 10 years of follow-up. This immunosuppressive regimen has reduced complications of anastomotic leakage in pancreas transplants, with encouraging results.

Pancreas grafting can never be a treatment for all diabetics, but when transplanted together with a kidney in patients with diabetic renal failure, pancreas transplantation has produced excellent long-term results. A move toward islet transplantation to avoid the major operation has had some early encouraging results. This is a field in which stem cell and/or gene therapy may well lead to fruitful developments in the future.

Cardiothoracic transplantation

While the field of kidney transplantation research and experimentation moved rapidly into the clinical arena, progress was not so rapid for the transplantation of other organs. The first heart transplant described in the literature was performed in 1905 by Carrel and Guthrie. The heart, transplanted from one dog into a heterotopic position in the neck of another dog, continued to beat for 2 hours. This model demonstrated that it was possible to transplant a heart with all four chambers pumping blood. More importantly, it demonstrated that the heart could be removed from its blood supply and sutured into the circulation of a second animal and still recover its normal organized contractile pattern. This brought into focus the concept of "preservation" of the heart during its ischemic period.

Further reference to transplantation of the mammalian heart was made in 1933 by Mann and colleagues at the Mayo clinic, who were seeking a denervated heart model. They made contributions to the area of preservation, advising that ventricular distension and coronary air embolism should be avoided; made observations on the general behavior of the transplanted heart; and made the first observations on the phenomenon of cardiac allograft rejection, noting that "histologically the heart was completely infiltrated with lymphocytes, large mononuclears and polymorphonuclears." They concluded that "the failure of the heart is not due to the technique of transplantation but to some biologic factor...."

Interest in cardiac transplantation waned until 1951, when workers at the Chicago Medical School reported their experience with a slightly modified Mann preparation. They were interested in the possibility of transplanting organs as a treatment modality for end-stage disease, but their experiments, although elaborate, were disappointing, with a maximum survival of only 48 hours. It was apparent to them that "the greatest deterrent to long survival of the heart is the biologic problem of tissue specificity" and concluded that "a transplanted heart...must be considered, at present, a fantastic dream, and does not fall within the scope of the present considerations." The Mann preparation continued to be used by various investigators to evaluate the transplanted heart, and Downie, working at the Ontario Veterinary College, reported excellent results, which he attributed to the use of penicillin and appropriate commercial suture material. Demikhov published results in 1962 in which an intrathoracic heterotopic heart continued to beat for 32 days. The long survival of this graft strengthened his belief that failure of transplanted organs was not due to immunological factors, but to simple technical problems.

The successful intrathoracic transplantation of the heart without interrupting the circulation led to the idea that a cardiac allograft might be able to assume some of the normal circulatory load. Demikhov led the way, performing 22 such auxiliary heart transplants between 1951 and 1955. The donor heart was implanted, and when fully resuscitated, the great vessels of the native heart were ligated so that the donor heart assumed the full load. One such animal recovered from anesthetic, stood up, and drank, but died 15 hours later, an event attributed to superior vena caval thrombosis. Other workers were pursuing the same goal but were less successful.

By the early 1950s, it was well established that cardiac transplantation was technically feasible, and studies were undertaken to clarify the physiology of cardiac transplantation. However, the move to orthotopic transplantation had not been achieved, and this was largely due to the difficulties associated with the transfer phase, when the recipient's own heart had been removed, and the problems associated with protection of the donor heart during transfer. These problems were addressed in a report published in 1953 in which the operative technique was simplified by transplanting a heart–lung block, thus reducing the number of anastomotic connections, and the problems of recipient preservation and myocardial protection were solved as both animals were "placed in an ordinary beverage cooler for the production of hypothermia." Using these techniques and arresting the recipient circulation for up to 30 minutes, the authors reported successful transplantation in three dogs, with survival of up to 6 hours.

The recognition of the value of hypothermia as a protective medium was important, but a further step was made toward the possibility of clinical transplantation with the development of the heart–lung machine, pioneered by Gibbon and attributed largely to the technical expertise of the famous pilot Charles Lindbergh. This allowed the circulating blood to bypass completely the patient's own heart and lungs, allowing an extended operative period.

The result of these innovations was that in 1958, the first orthotopic heart transplants were performed, and further steps were taken toward clinical transplantation with the development of a simplified operative technique (Lower and Shumway), which removed the necessity of individual venous anastomoses. The recipient left atrium was circumscribed, leaving a cuff of tissue to sew to the donor left atrium, a relatively simple anastomosis compared with the complex multiple anastomoses of four pulmonary veins. The cavae were reconnected with synthetic tubes, and the arteries were simply sutured end to end. Recipient circulation was maintained with the cardiopulmonary bypass machine, but hypothermia was not required for either donor or recipient. Donor organs were ischemic for between 25 and 32 minutes, and the longest support of circulation by the allografts was 20 minutes.

Further experiments in the late 1950s established that orthotopic transplantation was technically possible, and advances in the surgical techniques used were described. An important paper published in 1960 integrated the developments of the previous decade into a single method for orthotopic transplantation, and five of eight consecutive canine transplant recipients survived for between 6 and 21 days, eating and exercising normally in the postoperative phase. This was the first description of a truly successful procedure in which the circulation was maintained by the transplanted organ.

However, technical ability to perform the transplant operation is clearly not all that is required. In Lower's series, none of the dogs received immunosuppression, and they all died as a result of rapid myocardial failure due to the massive infiltration with round cells and interstitial hemorrhage. Lower and Shumway concluded that "if the immunologic mechanisms of the host were prevented from destroying the graft, in all likelihood it would continue to function adequately for the normal lifespan of the animal."

A further significant step was taken in 1965 when Lower reported the use of the surface electrocardiograph as a marker of rejection episodes. A voltage drop was seen during rejection episodes, which was reversible with the administration of methylprednisolone and azathioprine. With this test as a guide to the intermittent administration of immunosuppressive therapy, survival of 250 days was achieved in an adult dog.

Thus there had been a step-wise progression over the years providing the solution to many of the most difficult problems faced in transplanting the heart, and in 1964, Shumway wrote that "only the immunological barrier lies between this day and a radical new era in the treatment of cardiac diseases." Others clearly felt that the time was already right to undertake cardiac transplantation in man, and a planned approach was made toward this goal at the University Hospital in Jackson, Mississippi, in 1964. Legal and logistic reasons meant that the first man to receive a heart transplant was to receive the heart of a large chimpanzee, and not that of another man. The suture technique of Lower and Shumway was used, and although the operation was technically successful, the heart was unable to maintain the circulatory load, and about 1 hour after cardiopulmonary bypass, attempts at further support were abandoned.

In 1967, the first human-to-human orthotopic heart transplant was performed by Christian Barnard in South Africa. The patient was a 54-year-old man suffering from ischemic cardiomyopathy who received the heart of a 16-year-old female donor. He recovered from the operation but on the 18th day succumbed to pseudomonas pneumonia. On the day that he died, Barnard performed a second transplant, and this recipient survived 594 days.

Following the initial efforts of Barnard in Cape Town and Kantrowitz in New York, 102 cardiac transplants had been performed in 17 countries by the end of 1968. The early results were discouraging, and by 1970, there were only a few centers persevering. Gradually the problems were dealt with, and by 1978 the 1-year survival rate had risen from 22% to 68%, with a return to normal function in 90% of these patients. This was a time of real growth for clinical heart transplantation, with many reports of the early results, infectious complications, and the hemodynamics of the transplanted heart. The indications and contraindications became clearly defined, and donor management was described.

A further great advance was made by Philip Caves, who devised the bioptome for obtaining repeated transvenous endomyocardial biopsies to detect cardiac allograft rejection, and by Margaret Billingham, who described a histological system for grading the rejection reaction seen in these specimens. Further improvements were to be seen with the introduction of rabbit antithymocyte globulin for the prevention and treatment of acute rejection. As the concept of brainstem death became accepted and methods of long-distance procurement were developed, together with donor organ-sharing networks, donor organs became more readily available, ensuring the continued practice of clinical transplantation.

Combined heart and lung transplantation

Demikhov developed a method of heart–lung transplantation in dogs in the 1940s, but it was not revisited until 1953, when Marcus and colleagues at the Chicago Medical School described a technique for heterotopic heart–lung grafting to the abdominal aorta and inferior vena cava in dogs. Disappointingly, however, failure to resume normal spontaneous respiration was noted by a number of groups. Later primates were found to develop a normal respiratory pattern following complete denervation with cardiopulmonary replacement. A Stanford series showed survival for well over 5 years after heart–lung allograft transplants in primates, allowing Reitz and colleagues to perform the first successful human heart–lung transplant in a 45-year-old woman with end-stage primary pulmonary hypertension in 1981. They utilized a technique that preserved the donor sinoatrial node and eliminated the potential for caval anastomotic stenosis. Subsequently, "domino" transplant was developed, in which the healthy heart of a heart–lung recipient is itself donated for grafting in a cardiac transplant recipient.

Lung transplantation

Experimental lung transplantation developed in parallel with heart–lung transplantation. Metras described important technical concepts, including preservation of the left atrial cuff for the pulmonary venous anastomoses and reimplantation of an aortic patch containing the origin of the bronchial arteries to prevent bronchial dehiscence in 1949. The technique was technically difficult and did not gather widespread acceptance. Transection of the transplant bronchus close to the lung parenchyma was advocated in the 1960s by Blumenstock to prevent ischemic bronchial necrosis. Further surgical modifications to prevent bronchial anastomotic complications included telescoping of the bronchial anastomosis, described by Veith in 1969, and coverage of the anastomosis with an omental flap, described by the Toronto group in 1982. The first human lung transplant was performed in 1963 by Hardy and colleagues at the University of Mississippi; however, the patient only survived for 18 days. It was only in 1986 that the first series of successful single lung transplants with long-term survival were reported from Toronto (with the first patient undergoing transplantation in 1983). En-bloc double lung transplantation was performed by Patterson in 1988 but was later superseded by sequential bilateral lung transplantation, described by Pasque and colleagues in 1990. Subsequently, Yacoub introduced live lung lobar transplantation in 1995.

Indications and refinements

There has been a steady growth in the number of transplants performed, and as transplantation has become more successful in terms of survival, quality of life, and cost benefit, the demand for donor organs has increased so that it is greater than supply. For example, there were 454 thoracic organ transplants performed in the United Kingdom in the year ending December 1992, but at the end of the same year, the number of patients on the waiting lists for cardiac and pulmonary transplantation had grown to 763. Thus even if no more patients were accepted onto the lists, it would take nearly 2 years to clear the back-log of potential recipients. The flaw in this argument is that of these potential recipients, approximately 25–30% will die on the waiting list before suitable organs become available. It is worth noting that the patients who are accepted for transplantation are the tip of the iceberg; many are not referred, and for every patient who is accepted, there are two or three who are rejected, but who might have benefited from transplantation if there were a limitless donor pool.

The annual need for kidneys in the United Kingdom is estimated at between 2500 and 4000, whereas a recent audit of intensive care units in England suggested an absolute maximum number of 1700 potential donors. Even if all these patients were consented for donation and were medically suitable, there would still be a deficit in supply compared with the demand. The demand can be expected to continue to rise, whereas the number of potential donors may be expected to fall as factors such as seat-belt legislation and better trauma care reduce the pool of patients declared brainstem dead.

The indications for transplantation are widening, and although kidney, liver, heart, and even lung transplantation is now seen as routine, the necessary skills are being developed to transplant other organs, such as the small intestine, pancreas, face, hand, and uterus. Clearly this stretches the donor pool beyond its limit.

Other solutions to the donor shortage must be sought if transplantation is to be extended to treat all those in need. Recent trends have seen increased use of living related donors for kidney transplantation, and although renal transplant surgeons have used this resource for a long time, the potential to use livers (first performed in 1989) and lungs from live related donors has only recently been explored. The potential hazards for the donor of such procedures have stimulated fierce ethical debate. Living related donation will never solve the problem entirely, and the fact that such drastic measures can be considered and indeed put into practice underlines the severity of the donor organ shortage.

Another recent development has been the use of organs procured from individuals who die without ever meeting brainstem death criteria. In these patients, once cardiac activity has ceased, kidneys, liver, and even lungs may be removed and used for transplantation as a result of advanced preservation techniques. However, despite the first successful heart transplant being performed using a donor of this nature, there has been no widespread adoption of the non–heart-beating donor for cardiac transplantation.

Organ transplantation may be supplemented or even replaced in due course using totally artificial organs. The only implantable device that finds clinical use at present is the artificial heart. The range of devices available and their apparent complexity underline the difficulties encountered in replacing a relatively simple biological organ with mechanical substitutes. Fundamental problems such as power supply, thrombosis, infection and biocompatibility of mechanical surface-blood interfaces remain, but these obstacles may be overcome in due course to allow long-term function. However, the replacement of those organs with more complex metabolic functions is more difficult, and complete replacements for the kidneys, lungs, and liver are still a long way distant.

The field of organ transplantation has grown massively over the last hundred years. It has been made possible by developments in individual disciplines, supported by growth in our knowledge and understanding of individual organ system physiology and pathology. It remains a challenging and rewarding activity. However, successful as it is, transplantation is not without problems, and it would not be possible at all it were not for the death, often in tragic circumstances, of patients who are suitable for organ donation. Frequently the donors are young people who have met an unexpected accident, or suffered a catastrophic medical event such as subarachnoid hemorrhage, and their death is always an emotionally charged event. Our reliance on the goodwill of the donor's relatives to make available their organs in order that others may live is somewhat perverse, yet it is central to the success of transplantation.

Further reading

Barnard CN. Human cardiac transplantation: an evaluation of the first two operations performed at Groote Schuur Hospital, Cape Town. *Ann Cardiol* 1968; **22**: 284–96.

Calne RY. The rejection of renal homografts. Inhibition in dogs by using 6-mercaptopurine. *Lancet* 1960; **1**: 417.

Calne RY. Inhibition of the rejection of renel homografts in dogs by purine analogues. *Transplant Bull* 1961; **28**: 445–61.

Calne RY, Friend PJ, Moffatt S, *et al.* Prope tolerance, perioperative campath IH, and low-dose cyclosporin monotherapy in renal allograft recipients. *Lancet* 1998; **351**: 1701–2.

Calne RY, Rolles K, White DJ, *et al.* Cyclosporin A initially as the only immunosuppressant in 34 recipients of cadaveric organs; 32 kidneys, 2 pancreases, and 2 livers. *Lancet* 1979; **2**: 1033–6.

Calne RY, Williams R. Liver transplantation in man. Observations on technique and organization in five cases. *BMJ* 1968; **4**: 535–50.

Hamilton D. Kidney transplantation: a history. In Morris, PJ (ed). *Kidney Transplantation.* New York: Grune & Stratton, 1988, pp. 1–13.

Medawar PB. The behaviour and fate of skin autografts and homografts in rabbits. *J Anat* 1944; **79**: 157–76.

Merrill JP, Murray JE, Harrison JH, Guld WR. Successful homotransplantations of the human kidney between identical twins. *JAMA* 1956; **160**: 277–82.

Merrill JP, Murray JE, Harrison JH, *et al.* Successful homotransplantations of the human kidney between non-identical twins. *JAMA* 1960; **262**: 1251–60.

Murray JE, Merrill JP, Harrison JH. Renal homotransplantation in identical twins. *Surg. Forum* 1955; **6**: 432–6.

Murray JE, Merrill JP, Harrison JH, Wilson RE, Dammin GJ. Prolonged survival of human kidney homografts by immunosuppressive drug therapy. *N Eng J Med* 1963; **268**: 1315–23.

Report of the Ad Hoc Committee of the Harvard Medical School to examine the definition of brain death. *JAMA* 1968; **205**: 339–40.

Roitt IM, Greaves MF, Torrigiano G, Brostroff J, Playfair JHL. The cellular basis of immunological responses. *Lancet* 1969; **ii**: 366–71.

Schwartz RS, Damashek W. Drug-induced immunological tolerance. *Nature* 1959; **183**: 1682.

Starzl TE, Marchioro TL, Von Kaulla KN, *et al.* Homotransplantation of the liver in humans. *Surgery Gynecology and Obstetrics* 1963; **117**: 659–76.

Starzl TE, Marchioro TL, Huntley RT, *et al.* Experimental and clinical homotransplantations of the liver. *NY Acad Sci* 1964; **120**: 739–65.

Wallwork J, Williams R, Calne RY. Transplantation of liver, heart, and lungs for primary biliary cirrhosis and primary pulmonary hypertension. *Lancet* 1987: 182–4.

Chapter 2 Immunological principles of acute rejection

Fadi G. Issa, Ryoichi Goto, and Kathryn J. Wood

Key points

- The immune response to a transplant is a consequence of a complex interplay between the innate and adaptive immune systems.
- The adaptive immune system mounts a highly destructive, sustained, and specific attack on the transplant through recognition of foreign antigens, activation of T cells, expansion of donor-reactive lymphocytes, and infiltration of allografts with effector lymphocytes.
- Immunosuppressive drugs are required to prevent the immune system from destroying the transplant. The majority of immunosuppressants act to inhibit T-cell responses.
- Current immunosuppressive regimens have improved the short-term but not the long-term survival of organ transplants. The broad immunosuppressive activity of these drugs is associated with serious complications, such as an increased risk of malignancies and opportunistic infections.
- An ideal solution to both rejection and the complications of immunosuppression is the induction of tolerance. Research on achieving tolerance clinically is most promising in the fields of mixed chimerism and regulatory T-cell therapy.

The immune system has evolved to clear the host of invading microorganisms and its own cells that have become altered in some way, such as infected cells or mutated tumorigenic cells. The immune system recognizes such cells as "foreign" and the molecules they express as antigens. When organs are transplanted between genetically disparate (allogeneic) individuals, the immune system recognizes and reacts with the foreign antigens of the other individual (alloantigens) on the transplant (allograft) to cause rejection. This rejection response is the result of interplay between the host innate and adaptive immune systems. The innate response is mediated by cells and molecules that include macrophages, dendritic cells (DCs), granulocytes (neutrophils, basophils, and eosinophils), natural killer (NK) cells, and the complement cascade, as well as proinflammatory cytokines and chemokines (chemoattractant cytokines). It represents a preformed defense that is immediately available until a specific response can be mounted by the adaptive immune system. The innate response is less specific than the adaptive response and will be induced even if a transplant has been performed between genetically identical individuals (isograft), simply as a result of implanting or transplanting the cells or organ. Adaptive immunity is mediated by lymphocytes (T and B cells) and displays slower kinetics than the innate response. However, the adaptive response is specific to foreign antigens (alloresponse) and is therefore not activated by isografts. Although the innate immune response is important for the initiation of the alloresponse and can initiate tissue damage, it cannot alone cause rejection (in other words, the complete destruction of the tissue). On the other hand, the adaptive immune response is more damaging and is essential to rejection. The importance of the adaptive response is reflected in the observation that animals experimentally depleted of T cells cannot reject allografts.

This chapter outlines the events involved in the adaptive and innate immune responses to a transplant and the subsequent mechanisms of rejection, concluding with current clinical and experimental strategies to protect transplants from immune-mediated damage.

Organ Transplantation: A Clinical Guide, ed. A.A. Klein, C.J. Lewis, and J.C. Madsen. Published by Cambridge University Press.

Initiation of rejection

The immune system is frequently exposed to harmless (and sometimes beneficial) foreign antigens that do not require an aggressive effector response, such as gut flora. The context in which such foreign antigens are encountered is important in dictating the magnitude of the immune response. For instance, the activation of leukocytes in an inflammatory environment augments the immune response. In transplantation, these inflammatory signals can be provided by the surgical trauma, the oxidative stress of ischemia/reperfusion injury (IRI), and brain death. Indeed, the innate immune response is mediated by cells that express invariant pattern recognition receptors (PRRs), such as Toll-like receptors (TLRs), that recognize altered endogenous molecules on the allograft produced as a result of tissue injury by reactive oxygen species (ROS), heat shock proteins (HSP), or high-mobility group box 1 protein (HMGB-1) or as a direct consequence of donor brain death. Activation of innate immune cells by TLR ligation results in the production of "danger" signals such as chemokines and preformed P-selectin (CD62P), which help recruit and direct host leukocytes into the transplant site. Macrophages release cytokines such as tumor necrosis factor (TNF) α, interleukin (IL)-1, and IL-6, which contribute to the inflammatory environment and assist in the activation of other leukocytes. On recognition of inflammatory signals, antigen-presenting cells (APCs) such as DCs in the allograft migrate to the draining lymphoid tissues, where they present antigen to host T cells, leading to an adaptive immune response.

The recognition of foreign antigens by naive host (recipient) T cells (*allorecognition*, otherwise known as *signal 1*) is a principal step in the rejection process. Allorecognition in the presence of costimulation (otherwise known as *signal 2*) results in the activation and expansion of T cells that recognize the mismatched donor alloantigens (alloreactive T cells). Alloreactive T cells orchestrate the development of T cells with effector activity that can either have direct destructive activity against the transplant or promote and amplify B-cell function and other elements of the innate and adaptive immune response that can damage the transplant.

Allorecognition is mediated by the T-cell receptor (TCR), which is associated with the cluster of differentiation (CD) 3 molecule (TCR-CD3 complex). TCRs on host T cells bind to antigens encoded by genes of the major histocompatibility complex (MHC) on donor cells and, to a lesser extent, minor histocompatibility (miH) antigens. In humans, the MHC complex is termed the *human leukocyte antigen (HLA) system*. miH antigens are peptides derived from other molecules that are mismatched between the donor and recipient and are presented by host MHC molecules to host T cells. miH antigens alone cannot cause rapid rejection. However, when multiple miH are mismatched, rejection can be as rapid as when MHC antigens are mismatched. miH mismatches alone may be present in transplants between siblings with identical MHC molecules, leading to slow rejection of these transplants.

There are two pathways by which foreign antigens are recognized by T cells. The more common or natural one is called the *indirect pathway*. Antigens, such as viral antigens, are first processed by host APCs and then presented to host T cells by self-MHC molecules on the APCs. In the transplant setting, the indirect pathway occurs when APCs process and present donor HLA antigens to host T cells within self-MHC molecules. The TCR-CD3 complex on host T cells recognizes unique features of the small processed donor HLA peptides (epitopes) in the context of self-MHC. The second pathway of allorecognition, the direct pathway, is the dominant pathway in transplantation and occurs when T cells react directly with intact donor HLA antigens. By way of comparison, T cells that react to peptides derived from a nominal antigen (indirect pathway) are estimated to be less than 0.1% of the total T-cell repertoire, whereas a much higher frequency (about 10%) of T cells react to an MHC mismatched transplant (direct pathway).

Following organ transplantation, donor-derived "passenger" APCs residing in the donor organ and expressing large amounts of donor HLA antigens migrate out of the transplant into the draining lymphoid tissue, where they interact with host T cells via the direct pathway. With time after transplantation, passenger APCs diminish in number, and the direct pathway becomes less important. In contrast, the indirect pathway of allorecognition is maintained and remains active for as long as the transplant is present. The direct pathway is therefore theoretically more active during acute allograft rejection, whereas the indirect pathway becomes more important later in chronic allograft rejection.

A newly recognized third pathway, called the semidirect pathway, may also be involved in allorecognition. It occurs when intact donor HLA antigens are

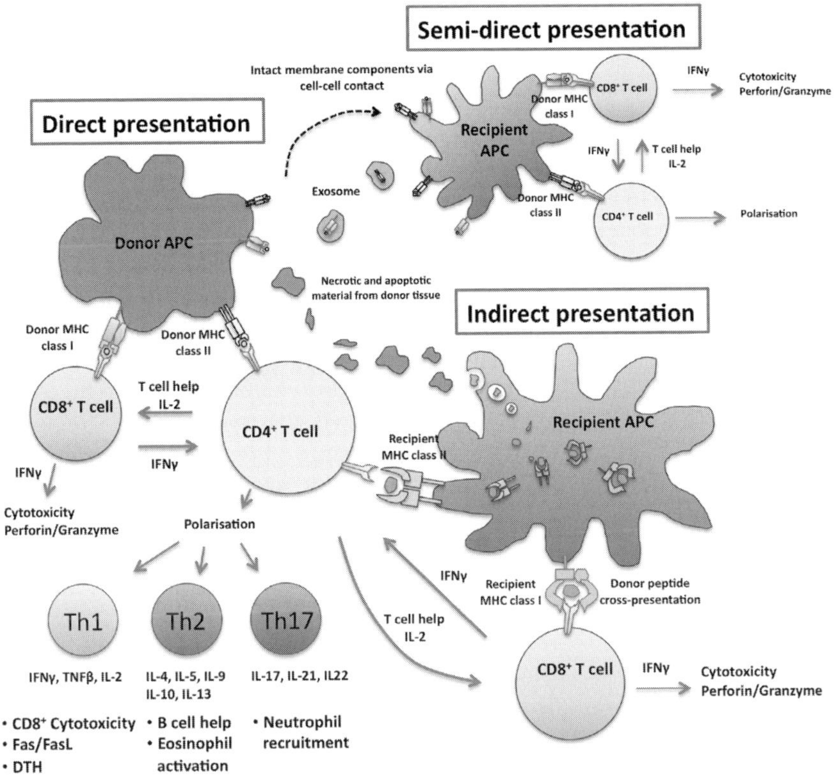

Figure 2.1 Allorecognition in transplantation occurs via the direct, indirect, and semi-direct pathways. Indirect allorecognition occurs when T-cell receptors (TCR) of T cells engage donor major histocompatibility complex (MHC) molecules that have been processed and presented by host antigen-presenting cells (APC) and presented in the context of self-MHC. Direct allorecognition is the recognition of intact MHC molecules on donor-derived passenger APCs by T host T cells. In semi-direct allorecognition, intact donor MHC molecules are transferred to recipient APCs by direct cell-to-cell contact or membrane fusion. These intact foreign molecules are then recognized by host T cells. $CD4^+$ T cells engage MHC class II, whereas $CD8^+$ T cells engage MHC class I. The effector response develops after allorecognition and T-cell costimulation by professional APCs. Activated T cells clonally expand, differentiate, and infiltrate the allograft. $CD4^+$ T cells are polarized to a T helper (Th)1, Th2, or Th17 phenotype, depending on the local cytokine environment. Each Th subtype is associated with a distinct effector response. $CD8^+$ T cells receive stimulation from activated $CD4^+$ T cells and in turn produce interferon γ (IFNγ). Both activated $CD8^+$ T cells and activated Th1 cells have the potential to become cytotoxic, predominantly employing perforin/granzyme and Fas/Fas ligand (FasL) to kill target cells, respectively. Th1 cells also produce IFNγ and promote a delayed-type hypersensitivity (DTH) response from macrophages with the ensuing production of inflammatory molecules such as nitric oxide, tumor necrosis factor (TNF)α, and reactive oxygen species. Th2 cells activate B cells to produce alloantibodies, which mediate complement activation or antibody-dependent cell-mediated cytotoxicity (ADCC). The hallmark of a Th17 response is neutrophil recruitment. See text for further details.

physically transferred to the membrane of host APCs and are then recognized by host T cells. Host APCs appear to acquire intact HLA molecules from exosomes secreted by donor APCs or through cell-to-cell contact. The relative contribution of this pathway to allograft rejection is not clear. Figure 2.1 illustrates the pathways of allorecognition and subsequent effector mechanisms.

Allorecognition alone is insufficient to promote T-cell activation. The second essential signal is costimulation, which is provided by the interaction of pairs of cell-surface molecules present on T cells and APCs. Absence or blockade of costimulatory signals typically results in T-cell unresponsiveness, or *anergy*. Costimulatory molecules are divided into two families: the B7 family, of which the prototype receptor-ligand pair are CD28 (on the T cell) and CD80/86 (B7.1/B7.2, on the APC), and the TNF and TNF receptor (TNFR) family, best characterized by CD40 (on the APC) and CD154 (CD40L, on the T cell). Other costimulatory T-cell/APC pairs include CD27/CD70, inducible T-cell costimulator (ICOS or CD278)/ICOS ligand, 4–1BB/4–1BB ligand, OX40/OX40 ligand, and CD279/CD274. Signaling via CD28 lowers the threshold for T-cell activation and increases the expression of the T-cell growth factor (leukocytotropic) IL-2 by stabilizing the mRNA species, thereby promoting T-cell proliferation and resistance to apoptosis. During an immune response, activated T cells also upregulate expression of cytotoxic T-lymphocyte antigen 4 (CTLA-4, CD152), a molecule that has close homology to CD28 but has an inhibitory effect on T-cell activation. CTLA-4 has a higher affinity for CD28 than CD80/86 and is able to attenuate immune responses by competing for CD28. CD28 signaling also upregulates expression of other costimulatory molecules, such as CD154 (CD40 ligand), which, on ligation with CD40, activates APCs, leading to increased expression of B7 family molecules and therefore a greater ability to activate further T cells. The balance of positive and negative signals transmitted through costimulatory molecules to the T cell ultimately determines whether the T cell will be activated or become anergic.

The interface of a T cell with an APC in which both the TCR-MHC and costimulatory molecule interaction occurs is termed the *immunological synapse*. This immunological synapse forms a "bull's eye" structure with a central supramolecular activation cluster (c-SMAC) containing the TCR-MHC complex, surrounded by a peripheral SMAC (p-SMAC) ring containing adhesion molecules, such as leukocyte function-associated antigen 1 (LFA-1) on the T cell bound to intercellular adhesion molecule 1 (ICAM-1, CD54) on the APC.

Within the cell membrane biphospholipid layer are cholesterol-rich regions that have been termed *lipid rafts*. Certain membrane-bound molecules are preferentially associated with lipid rafts, in particular, those with lipophilic attachments to the cell membrane. In resting T cells, the TCR-CD3 complex is not usually associated with lipid rafts and is therefore unable to interact with other signal transduction molecules found within these lipid rafts. During the formation of an immunological synapse, clustering of signaling and adhesion molecules occurs as a result of multiple TCRs binding to MHC peptide on the surface of the APC. A reorganization of the cell membrane subsequently occurs, allowing TCR-CD3 complexes to integrate into lipid rafts. This facilitates downstream signaling by placing the TCR-CD3 complex in close proximity to signal transduction molecules, which are then activated by phosphorylation. The end result is the activation of the intracellular Ras and Rac mitogen-activated protein (MAP) kinase (MAPK) pathways and hydrolysis of membrane phosphatidylinositol 4,5-biphosphate to generate the secondary messengers inositol triphosphate (IP_3) and diacylglycerol (DAG). IP_3 leads to the release of stored calcium from the endoplasmic reticulum (ER) and activation of phosphatase calcineurin, which dephosphorylates the transcription factor nuclear factor of activated T cells (NFAT), allowing it to translocate to the nucleus. Generation of DAG results in the activation of the transcription factor nuclear factor-κB (NF-κB). The MAPK cascade also leads to the generation of transcription factor activator protein 1 (AP-1). The action of these transcription factors alters the expression of many genes, and in particular leads to upregulation of IL-2 and the high-affinity IL-2 receptor (IL-2R) α-chain (CD25) required for T-cell growth. Large amounts of IL-2 and other leukocytotropic cytokines are produced and act to provide further signaling to promote cell cycle progression, clonal expansion, and differentiation of activated T cells.

Activated lymphocytes also upregulate chemokine receptor expression, allowing them to activate further leukocytes and subsequently infiltrate the allograft. The process by which leukocytes migrate into the graft is termed *leukocyte recruitment*. Leukocyte recruitment is enhanced by vasodilation and endothelial activation in the vicinity of the transplant. Chemokines that have been released from the allograft become tethered to the activated endothelium, providing a signal gradient recognized by passing leukocytes. When leukocytes bind to activated endothelium, further adhesions are made between integrin molecules on the leukocyte and endothelial adhesion molecules such as ICAM-1, which result in arrest of the leukocyte and extravasation into the transplanted organ.

Following the clearance of a pathogen by naive cells of the adaptive immune system (*the primary response*), a small number of antigen-specific T and B cells survive as memory cells that are able to mount a rapid response in the event of reintroduction of the same pathogen (*the secondary* or *memory response*). The immune response to a transplanted organ results from the stimulus of both naive and memory alloreactive T cells. Unlike naive T cells, memory T cells can survive in the absence of antigen and can be activated in the absence of costimulatory molecules essential for naive T cells. Memory T cells may be present due to prior exposure to alloantigen during pregnancy, from a previous transplant, or from a blood transfusion. However, memory cells capable of responding to alloantigen may also be present in individuals even without prior exposure to that antigen. This occurs through the operation of three mechanisms: cross-reactivity through molecular mimicry from prior infectious agents, bystander proliferation following lymphopenia, or heterologous immunity. Properties of memory cells not only include more rapid and efficient responses to previously encountered antigen, but also a resistance to apoptosis (programmed cell death) due to the upregulation of anti-apoptotic molecules such as Bcl-2 and Mcl-1. These characteristics confer an especially detrimental role for memory cells in rejection.

The effector response

The adaptive immune system

Two types of T cells, identified by the cell surface markers CD4 and CD8, are active in rejection. $CD4^+$ T cells are activated by MHC (HLA) class II molecules, which have two transmembrane domains and are expressed by APCs. Functionally, $CD4^+$ T cells are usually helper T cells (Th) and are therefore often referred to as *Th cells*. $CD4^+$ Th cells can differentiate into several subtypes, including Th1, Th2, or Th17. In contrast, $CD8^+$ T cells are activated by MHC (HLA) class I molecules, which differ structurally from MHC class II molecules in that they have only one transmembrane domain. $CD8^+$ T cells often have cytotoxic activity and are therefore known as *cytotoxic T lymphocytes* (CTLs). Class I MHC is expressed, albeit at varying levels, by all nucleated cells. As discussed in the previous section, alloreactive T cells are activated only after an immunological synapse is formed with an APC that provides the appropriate MHC and costimulation signals. APCs that are able to provide these signals are termed *immunostimulatory*, or "professional," and constitutively express MHC class II (e.g., DCs, macrophages, and B cells). TLR ligation on DCs induces upregulation of costimulatory molecules and MHC class II, thus enhancing the ability of these APCs to activate T cells. So-called non-professional APCs express MHC class II only on stimulation with a cytokine, such as interferon (IFN) γ (e.g., fibroblasts and endothelial cells).

$CD4^+$ Th cells are critical for allograft destruction. The type of Th response is determined by the cytokine microenvironment in which APC and T-cell interactions take place. Both cell-mediated immunity, driven by Th1 cells, and humoral immunity, driven by Th2 cells, are independently capable of causing allograft destruction. IL-17–producing Th17 cells have also recently been implicated in allograft rejection. Notably, although $CD4^+$ activity is triggered in an antigen-specific manner, the effector mechanisms of allograft destruction are non-specific.

Th1 cells express the transcription factor T-bet and produce IFNγ, TNFα, and IL-2, which result in the activation of $CD8^+$ cytotoxicity, macrophage-dependent delayed-type hypersensitivity (DTH), and the synthesis of immunoglobulin (Ig) G2a by B cells (which activates complement), all of which contribute to allograft rejection. Furthermore, Th1 cells express Fas-ligand (FasL), enabling them to exhibit cytotoxic activity. The Th1 DTH response is a nonspecific effector mechanism that induces the production of mediators such as nitric oxide, ROS, and inflammatory arachidonic acid derivatives such as prostaglandin E2, thromboxane, and leukotrienes from macrophages. Th1-mediated effects have been shown to directly affect graft physiology by altering cell permeability and vascular smooth muscle tone and are implicated in the early stages of rejection, otherwise known as *acute cellular rejection*.

Th2 cells express the transcription factor GATA-3 and secrete IL-4, IL-5, IL-9, IL-10, and IL-13, which activate B cells (inducing Ig class switching) and eosinophils to promote graft rejection primarily through the humoral immune response. B cells utilize surface Ig as an antigen receptor, internalizing alloantigens that are processed and presented in conjunction with class II MHC molecules. Antigen-specific recognition and costimulatory signaling from activated $CD4^+$ T cells is required for the activation and differentiation of primary and memory B-cell responses that result in plasma cell generation and the production of alloantibodies. This results in B-cell–induced antibody-mediated rejection (AMR), a phenomenon that is increasingly recognized as problematic in transplantation. AMR appears to be contributory in 20–30% of acute transplant rejection episodes and up to 60% of chronic allograft dysfunction cases. Antibodies directed against donor HLA molecules, ABO blood group antigens, or endothelial cell antigens may be generated during the immune response to the allograft, or in the case of antibodies to endothelial cells, may be pre-existing at the time of transplantation. Patients with detectable anti-HLA antibodies at the time of transplantation have significantly worse graft survival rates than patients who are not sensitized, and the development of anti-HLA antibodies in previously non-sensitized patients following transplantation is highly predictive of early graft failure. AMR may be subdivided into hyperacute, acute, and chronic. Hyperacute AMR is a rare event, occurring when recipients have preformed antibody directed against allogeneic MHC molecules or ABO isoagglutinins expressed on the graft endothelium. It is defined by rejection occurring within 24 hours of reperfusion and is characterized by immediate or near-immediate loss of graft function secondary to complement-mediated thrombosis within the allograft vascular supply. Modern cross-matching techniques have made hyperacute rejection extremely rare, whereas acute AMR and chronic AMR remain problematic. Acute AMR occurs around the same time as acute cellular rejection and is likely due to a recall response of B cells that have been sensitized by a previous antigen encounter during pregnancy, a blood transfusion, or a previous transplant. Chronic AMR is increasingly seen as a contributor to late attrition of allografts that succumb to chronic graft dysfunction. The hallmark of AMR is the activation of complement and membrane attack complex (MAC) formation, leading to target cell lysis. Positive histological staining for complement 4d (C4d) in biopsies is therefore indicative of AMR. Cell killing by antibody may also occur via a mechanism termed *antibody-dependent cell-mediated cytotoxicity* (ADCC), in which NK cells or macrophages recognize and kill target cells that have been coated in antibody.

Th17 cells express the transcription factor RORγt and produce IL-17, IL-21, and IL-22, which act alone and synergistically with other cytokines to promote neutrophil recruitment to the site of rejection. In mouse experimental models, neutralization of IL-17 has been shown to reduce the features of vascular acute rejection of aortic allografts and to significantly extend the survival of cardiac allografts. In a vessel allograft model, graft-derived IL-1 has been shown to promote IL-17 production from alloreactive T cells, enhancing the production of the proinflammatory cytokines IL-6, CXCL8, and CCL20. Further research is required to fully clarify the relative contribution of Th17 cells to rejection.

$CD8^+$ T cells can be involved in transplant destruction via cytotoxic activity leading to cell death. Activated CTLs migrate to the graft site, where they are able to identify their target cells in the graft by recognition of allogeneic class I MHC molecules. Once a target cell is located, CTLs release granules containing cytotoxic molecules such as perforin and granzyme B. In addition, CTLs are able to upregulate cell surface expression of FasL and secrete soluble mediators such as TNFα. Perforins polymerize and insert into the target cell membrane, forming a pore that facilitates the entry of granzyme B and other compounds into the cell. Granzyme B is a protease that is able to initiate apoptosis by several mechanisms, including activation of caspase cascades. Binding of FasL to Fas on the target cell surface is also able to trigger apoptosis by activating caspases.

The innate immune system

Due to the intimate relationship of the adaptive and innate immune responses, many of the aspects of the innate immune response have already been discussed. This section discusses the mechanisms of action of two innate immune system components that have not been fully covered, the complement cascade and NK cells.

The complement cascade is a proteolytic cascade that generates a range of effector molecules: C5a and C3a are chemoattractant molecules that assist leukocytes in migrating toward the allograft; C3b, C4b, and their fragments opsonize cells (thus targeting them for destruction by phagocytes, e.g., macrophages and neutrophils) and facilitate antigen presentation and T-cell activation. The terminal components of the cascade, C5b-9, result in the formation of the MAC in the target cell membrane, inducing cell lysis. Apart from being activated by immunoglobulin, complement can be activated as a result of IRI, cytomegalovirus infection (CMV), and anti-lymphocyte antibody treatment.

NK cells kill target cells in an identical manner to CTLs but do not possess antigen-specific TCRs and do not require activation. NK cells express a variety of receptors that regulate their activity. Self-cells are able to deliver an inhibitory signal to NK cells, whereas infected or malignant cells cannot deliver this signal and are subsequently killed. Allogeneic cells are also unable to deliver an inhibitory signal to NK cells and theoretically should be destroyed, which is the case in bone marrow transplantation. Until recently, NK cells have not been shown to contribute significantly to solid organ rejection. However, recent results demonstrate that NK cells can contribute to chronic rejection, at least in experimental models of heart transplantation. NK cells have also been shown to kill donor-derived APCs, in theory reducing the relative contribution of direct allorecognition to rejection and

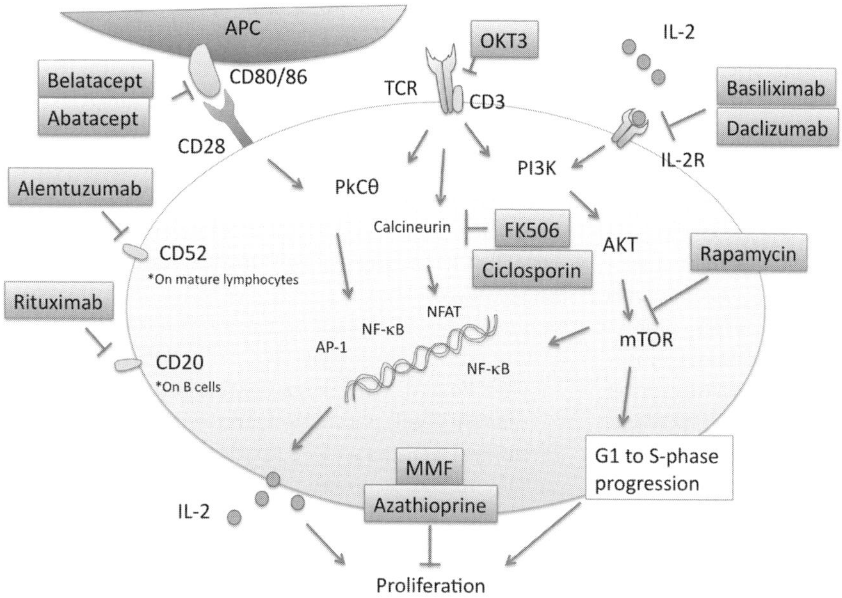

Figure 2.2 This figure illustrates the targets of some common immunosuppressants in clinical use. The majority of immunosuppressants target T cells, apart from rituximab (which targets B cells) and alemtuzumab (which targets most nucleated bone marrow–derived cells). See text for further details. AP-1: activator protein 1; APC: antigen presenting cell; CD: cluster of differentiation; FK-506: tacrolimus; IL: interleukin; IL-R: interleukin receptor; MMF: mycophenolate mofetil; mTOR: mammalian target of rapamycin; NFAT: nuclear factor of activated T cells; NFκB: nuclear factor-κB; PI3K: phosphoinositide 3-kinase; PkCθ: protein kinase-Cθ.

promoting tolerance. Further studies are needed to determine when NK cells may be harmful and when they may be beneficial to long-term graft survival.

The tempo and timing of rejection is defined in immunological terms and divided into hyperacute rejection, acute rejection, and delayed graft dysfunction. Hyperacute rejection, as discussed, is a rapid event caused by preformed antibodies against allogeneic MHC molecules or ABO blood group antigens. Acute rejection is characterized by a sudden deterioration in transplant function over days to weeks and is predominantly secondary to acute cellular rejection or acute AMR. Delayed graft dysfunction, often referred to as chronic rejection, is a term that encompasses long-term damage to the organ caused both by the immune system and toxicity of immunosuppressive agents and is often characterized by fibrointimal proliferation of intragraft arteries.

Modulating the immune system to prevent rejection

Immunosuppressive therapy can be credited with the vast improvements in transplant survival over the past 50 years. This chapter explores the underlying mechanisms of action in relation to the immunobiology, whereas clinical use is explored in the following chapter. Broadly speaking, immunosuppressants can be divided into those that act on intracellular targets affecting signal initiation (such as antimetabolites and macrolides) or signal reception (such as mammalian target of rapamycin [mTOR] inhibitors), and those acting on extracellular targets (such as antibodies and fusion proteins). Corticosteroids cannot be placed into one of these classes, as their effects are widespread.

Figure 2.2 summarizes the mechanisms of action of common immunosuppressive drugs currently in clinical use.

Corticosteroids act by binding to cytoplasmic glucocorticoid receptors, altering the expression of multiple cytokines and inflammatory mediators by targeting the transcription factors NF-κB and AP-1. Molecules affected include IL-1, IL-2, IL-3, IL-6, TNF-α, IFN-γ, leukotrienes, and prostaglandins, as well as several chemokines. Corticosteroids therefore possess both immunosuppressive and anti-inflammatory effects. At high doses, corticosteroids can have receptor-independent effects. Side effects of corticosteroid therapy include weight gain, hyperlipidemia, osteoporosis, and glucose intolerance.

Antimetabolites such as azathioprine (AZA) and mycophenolate mofetil (MMF) interfere with DNA synthesis and cell cycle progression, therefore impairing the clonal expansion of T cells. MMF is a more lymphocyte-specific drug than AZA, which also has bone marrow suppressive effects. AZA is metabolized in the liver into 6-mercaptopurine, which is then incorporated into DNA, inhibiting purine nucleotide synthesis with widespread effects on gene transcription and cell cycle progression. Sir Roy Calne originally introduced 6-mercaptopurine as an experimental immunosuppressive therapy. AZA was subsequently found to be less toxic than 6-mercaptopurine and was therefore pioneered as a clinical therapy. MMF is metabolized in the liver into mycophenolic acid, a non-competitive reversible inhibitor of inosine monophosphate (IMP) dehydrogenase, an enzyme required for purine generation. IMP dehydrogenase inhibition has downstream effects on DNA and RNA synthesis.

Calcineurin inhibitors (CNIs) are a subset of the macrolide compounds (so called because their activity depends on the structural presence of a macrolide ring) and include cyclosporine and tacrolimus (FK-506 or Fujimycin). Both drugs bind cytoplasmic immunophilins to form complexes that inhibit calcineurin, a phosphatase enzyme in the T-cell signal transduction pathway. Inhibition of calcineurin prevents the translocation of the transcription factor NFAT to the nucleus. Effects include inhibition of the production of the cytokines IL-2, IL-4, TNFα, and IFNγ, as well as the downregulation of costimulatory molecules such as CD154.

mTOR inhibitors include sirolimus (rapamycin) and everolimus. These drugs act by binding and inhibiting mTOR, which has a critical role in cytokine receptor signal transduction, specifically in relation to IL-2, IL-4, and IL-15. These cytokines act through mTOR to induce the production of proteins that are necessary for progression from the growth phase to the DNA synthesis phase of the cell cycle and are therefore critical for T-cell clonal expansion.

Antibodies can be polyclonal, such as antithymocyte globulin (ATG) directed against multiple epitopes of antigens on human lymphocytes, or monoclonal, such as OKT3 directed against human CD3ε. Both antibodies can initially activate lymphocytes, inducing the release of cytokines and leading to a "cytokine release syndrome." This may manifest as a severe systemic inflammatory response with hypotension, rigors, and pulmonary edema, although it more commonly results in milder signs such as a pyrexia and flu-like symptoms. This has led to the virtual abandonment of OKT3 for clinical use.

Newer monoclonal antibodies include alemtuzumab, rituximab, basiliximab, and daclizumab, which target specific T-cell surface proteins. Alemtuzumab is a humanized monoclonal antibody against human CD52, present on most mature nucleated bone marrow–derived cells. Alemtuzumab therefore depletes T and B cells both centrally and peripherally, monocytes, macrophages, NK cells, and some granulocytes. Evidence also suggests that it may expand the regulatory T-cell population, and it is likely to deplete memory T cells as well. A single dose exerts a depletional effect as profound and prolonged as multi-dose administration of ATG. Recovery of these cells to normal levels can take years after administration of alemtuzumab, and it is therefore reserved for special circumstances in a select group of transplant recipients for induction immunosuppression or for the treatment of rejection episodes. Rituximab is directed against CD20, present on most mature B cells, and is useful for the treatment of AMR. Basiliximab and daclizumab (which only differ slightly in structure) are humanized monoclonal antibodies directed against CD25, which is present on activated T and B cells. These antibodies bind and inhibit the high-affinity alpha chain of the IL-2 receptor (CD25), which is expressed in greater density by antigen-activated T cells. Thus they are thought to target only those T cells involved in rejection, avoiding the more generalized immunosuppression and adverse effects associated with ATGs.

The advances in immunosuppression have improved short- and medium-term graft survival rates and reduced the rates of acute rejection, but this has not been followed by a comparable reduction in long-term graft dysfunction rates. Furthermore, the immunosuppressive regimens currently used are not ideal as they are non-specific, required lifelong, and risk the development of opportunistic infections and tumors in transplant patients. There is therefore substantial research into strategies that may allow a reduction or complete withdrawal of immunosuppression with improved long-term outcomes in transplantation. Long-term graft acceptance with normal function in the complete absence of immunosuppression with otherwise normal immune responses is known as tolerance and is the "holy grail" of transplantation immunology research. The hallmark of tolerance is donor-specific immune hyporesponsiveness. Current experimental and early clinical strategies to induce tolerance center on the use of regulatory T cells (Tregs) and the induction of chimerism.

Tregs are a population of T cells with profound suppressive or regulatory capabilities. Tregs physiologically act to maintain immune tolerance against self-antigens and to provide negative feedback for immune responses that may become detrimental to the host. Patients with defects in the master transcription factor of Tregs, FoxP3, develop the devastating autoimmune disease IPEX (immune dysregulation, polyendocrinopathy, enteropathy X-linked), demonstrating the importance of Tregs in maintaining immune homeostasis. Because Tregs are able to suppress effector responses in an antigen-specific manner, there is potential for these cells to be used as a therapy to suppress immune responses to an allograft while keeping all other effector responses intact. Many types of suppressive leukocytes exist, but the most studied populations are the naturally occurring Tregs (nTregs) that develop in the thymus and express CD4, CD25, and FoxP3, and the inducible Tregs (iTregs) that are induced in the periphery under particular conditions of cytokine and antigen exposure and that express CD4 and FoxP3. Another population of regulatory T cells, the $CD4^+$ Tr1 cells, have also been described. These cells can be induced in the periphery and produce the suppressive cytokines IL-10 and transforming growth factor β (TGFβ) in a FoxP3-independent manner.

Tregs suppress effector responses at multiple levels, by directly inhibiting $CD4^+$ and $CD8^+$ T-cell activation and proliferation as well as by modulating APC function. Other targets of Tregs include B cells, NK cells, natural killer T (NKT) cells, and mast cells. Mechanisms of Treg suppression include the cytolysis of target cells by perforin and granzyme B; the secretion of the inhibitory cytokines IL-10, TGFβ, and IL-35; and the consumption of IL-2 in the surrounding environment by their high-affinity CD25 receptors, therefore depriving naive and effector T cells of this growth factor. Furthermore, Tregs express CTLA-4, which, as described previously, prevents the costimulatory interaction of CD80/86 with CD28.

Various studies have demonstrated the ability of Tregs to induce long-term graft survival experimentally, with some studies even demonstrating inhibition of transplant arteriosclerosis, a manifestation of chronic graft dysfunction. Some experimental techniques induce Tregs in vivo by employing lymphocyte depletion around the time of transplantation in conjunction with a donor-specific antigen challenge, such as a donor-specific blood transfusion. Other techniques generate Tregs for therapy ex vivo by isolation of nTregs from peripheral or cord blood and subsequent in vitro expansion, or by conversion of non-Treg cell types to iTregs under certain in vitro cytokine and antigen environments. Several clinical studies are currently running to test the safety and efficacy of Treg therapy for graft-versus-host disease (GvHD) after bone marrow transplantation. To date, no trials in solid organ transplantation have been undertaken. Early reports from bone marrow transplantation trials have demonstrated that Tregs may be efficacious at inhibiting the development of GvHD without affecting the crucial graft-versus-tumor effect of treatment.

During T-cell development in the thymus, T cells that are strongly reactive to host MHC are deleted by a process termed *negative selection*. This physiological process has been harnessed experimentally for the induction of tolerance to foreign antigens, whereby hematopoietic complete chimerism (the replacement of all host hematopoietic cells with donor-derived stem cells) through myeloablative therapy and donor-derived bone marrow transplantation results in the repopulation of the host thymus with donor-type DCs that delete donor-reactive T cells. A number of successful clinical cases have been reported whereby patients with hematological indications for bone marrow ablation who also require renal transplantation have received a bone marrow transplant and a kidney transplant from the same donor, resulting in long-term donor-specific tolerance. Nevertheless, the morbidity and mortality of myeloablative therapy and risk of GvHD in most transplant patients makes this mode of therapy unacceptable to those without a hematological indication for bone marrow ablation. On the other hand, mixed chimerism, in which donor cells represent a varying proportion (but not 100%) of the total hematopoietic pool, is a more promising area of research. Mixed chimerism can be established using non-myeloablative conditioning regimens, therefore maintaining immunocompetence and reducing the risk of GvHD.

Two promising clinical trials utilizing mixed chimerism for the induction of tolerance have been performed. An initial trial enrolled six patients with renal failure consequent to multiple myeloma, a hematological malignancy. Patients received non-myeloablative bone marrow transplants and renal transplants from an HLA-identical sibling followed by a donor leukocyte infusion as treatment for both the multiple myeloma and renal failure. These patients successfully accepted their renal transplants long-term without any immunosuppression. Following this study, a similar approach was piloted in five patients *without* a hematological malignancy. Patients received an HLA-mismatched haploidentical related donor bone marrow transplant along with a renal transplant from the same donor. Four patients in the trial currently maintain graft function after weaning from their initial immunosuppression (follow-up 2–5 years postweaning). However, one kidney transplant was lost due to acute AMR, leading to a modification in the trial protocol to include B-cell depletion with rituximab.

Although the attainment of tolerance is an ideal solution, whether this can be achieved in each and every transplant recipient is unknown. For the majority of patients, reducing immunosuppression to a minimal level would offer many advantages in terms of reduced complications of long-term drug therapy. This state, in which graft function is maintained in the presence of low doses of non-toxic immunosuppression, has been termed *prope tolerance* and may represent a more realistic goal.

Further reading

Brent L. *A History of Transplantation Immunology.* San Diego, CA: Academic Press/Elsevier, 1996.

Ginns LC, Cosimi AB, Morris PJ. *Organ Transplantation.* Oxford: Wiley-Blackwell, 1999.

Kingsley CI, Nadig SN, Wood KJ. Transplantation tolerance: lessons from experimental rodent models. *Transpl Int* 2007; **20**: 828–41.

Paul WE. *Fundamental Immunology.* Philadelphia: Lippincott Williams & Wilkins, 2008.

Warrell DA, Cox TM, Firth JD. *Oxford Textbook of Medicine.* Oxford: Oxford University Press, 2010.

Wood KJ, Sakaguchi S. Regulatory T cells in transplantation tolerance. *Nat Rev Immunol* 2003; **3**: 199–210.

Chapter 3

Immunosuppression

Past, present, and future

Vineeta Kumar and Robert S. Gaston

Key points

- The modern era of transplantation was made possible by the introduction of azathioprine and cyclosporine to prevent acute rejection.
- Modern immunosuppression regimes utilize induction therapy with polyclonal or monoclonal antibodies directed against T cells followed by maintenance therapy.
- Clinical trials suggest that tacrolimus, mycophenolate mofetil, and corticosteroid as maintenance are better at preventing acute rejection.
- New agents have the potential to provide more effective immunosuppression by targeting different immunobiological pathways.

Clinical solid organ transplantation became a reality with the serendipitous recognition that use of an isograft from a genetically identical living donor circumvented immunological responses. However, the ability to utilize solid organ transplants as therapy for large numbers of patients with end-organ failure is a direct consequence of the development of pharmacological immunosuppression. The Nobel Prizes awarded to Hitchings and Elion, Medawar, Murray, and Dausset bear witness to the interplay of surgical skill, immunological understanding, and bold therapeutics that still resides at the core of clinical transplantation. To the newly initiated struggling to understand the whys and wherefores of current immunosuppression, lessons learned in the past help simplify the process. Furthermore, future therapies are likely to evolve from equally important experience acquired in the present. This chapter focuses on current practice, as informed by past experiences and as a basis for understanding newer therapeutics on the horizon.

Immunosuppression: past

The AZA era (1962–1981)

Long-term survival of allografts in humans first occurred with the introduction of azathioprine (AZA), a modification of 6-mercaptopurine (6-MP) in the early 1960s. It was recognized that most renal recipients experienced, usually within the first month after engraftment, a rejection "crisis," comprised of graft tenderness, fever, reduced urine production, and rising blood urea. These crises could be ameliorated with high doses of corticosteroids, often requiring repeated administration. Ultimately, it was recognized that the best patient outcomes were fostered with concomitant daily or alternate-day use of smaller corticosteroid doses together with AZA, and experience in those early years defined the proper dosing regimen (1.5–3 mg/kg/day) for AZA. In the absence of ongoing rejection, renal function was well preserved. However, as many as half the allografts failed within a year of transplantation, and opportunistic infections (thought to be the consequence of high-dose steroids) were a common cause of mortality.

Production and administration of anti-lymphocyte globulin (ALG) or anti-thymocyte globulin (ATG) emerged during this same period, with source (rabbit or equine) and immunizing agent (harvested thymic tissue or cultured lymphoblasts) often dependent on resources available at individual transplant centers. Earliest use of these agents was as adjunctive treatment for rejection "crises," although by the mid 1970s, several centers were administering ATG or ALG prophylactically at the time of transplantation to either reduce

Organ Transplantation: A Clinical Guide, ed. A.A. Klein, C.J. Lewis, and J.C. Madsen. Published by Cambridge University Press.

or delay onset of rejection episodes. The first multi-center randomized, controlled trials in kidney transplantation were two studies of prophylactic ATG conducted in the late 1970s and early 1980s: the Upjohn equine ATG (Atgam) trial in the United States and the Medical Research Council trial in the United Kingdom. Both produced similar results: overall outcomes (graft and patient survival) were no better with prophylactic ATG, but treated patients tended to have fewer rejection episodes, occurring later after transplantation, and with better preservation of kidney function.

With or without prophylactic ATG, kidney transplantation during this period was challenging due to rejection on the one hand and immunosuppressive complications on the other, but with enough long-term survivors to push forward. It was during this period that chronic dialysis emerged as the "default" therapy for end-stage renal disease, with transplantation limited more by poor outcomes than any other variable. Successful transplantation of other solid organs (liver, lung, heart) was even more challenging during this era of relative ineffective immunosuppression, though surgical technique and organ preservation became ever more sophisticated.

The cyclosporine era (1982–1995)

Early use of cyclosporine (CyA) in animals and humans as monotherapy (with doses commonly ranging between 20 and 50 mg/kg/day) seemed effective in preventing acute rejection crises, but was associated with significant graft dysfunction among other disabling toxic effects. Ultimately, the drug was made available to several groups for clinical trials, some at individual centers and others multi-center, each of which modified dosing and administration in some fashion. Simply using lower doses to minimize toxicity seemed effective in some patients; others combined lower doses with long-term corticosteroids (at lower doses than previously thought necessary) or ALG to produce excellent outcomes, with rejection rates cut to 50% rather than near 100%, and 1-year renal graft survival of 70–75%. These approaches even seemed to work in extra-renal transplantation, with successful cardiac and hepatic transplantation in ever-growing numbers of patients. Some even deemed AZA "obsolete."

There remained, however, one overriding, nagging issue: nephrotoxicity. Coincident with its release in the United States was the report in a prominent journal of progressive CyA nephrotoxicity in recipients of cardiac transplants, with onset of end-stage renal disease (ESRD) in an alarming number. This resulted in two major changes in approach to CyA-based immunosuppression. The first was rediscovery of AZA, and "triple" therapy, with low-dose AZA and corticosteroids utilized to reduce the maintenance CyA requirement to 8–12 mg/kg/day, with equally effective control of rejection and better preservation of kidney function. The second was based on the realization that, unlike assumptions based on animal models, CyA could be effective when introduced late, several days or more after engraftment, under effective ALG-based alternative prophylaxis. Thus sequential or quadruple immunosuppression was born, with non-nephrotoxic ALG induction allowing delayed administration of nephrotoxic CyA (in even lower doses) until after adequate allograft function could be established. Although some remained committed to immediate CyA use in higher doses either alone or with steroids, the most effective, widely used protocols contained some or all of these modifications.

Parallel to these developments were advances in a new technology: monoclonal antibodies produced via the mouse hybridoma technique of Kohler and Milstein (recipients of yet another Nobel Prize). Muromonab-CD3 (OKT3), an early anti–T-lymphocyte monoclonal antibody, was compared with corticosteroids in a prospective, randomized trial for treatment of an initial rejection crisis, with better efficacy in reversing the episode, but little impact on recurrent rejection and only marginal improvement in graft survival at 1 year. On the basis of this trial, OKT3 was released for use in the United States in 1986 and hailed as the first of many monoclonal antibodies that would enable delivery of targeted immunosuppression to transplant recipients.

These advances in immunosuppression enabled solid organ transplantation to emerge as a major therapy for end-organ failure. In kidney transplantation, triple or quadruple immunosuppression resulted in 1-year allograft survival routinely in excess of 80%, with rejection rates of 40–50%. OKT3 became an alternative to polyclonal ALG for induction at some centers. Those who experienced rejection most often were treated initially with high-dose steroids; "steroid-resistant" rejections were treated with a second course of OKT3 or ALG. Long-term toxicities, including renal dysfunction, seemed manageable. In addition, financial profits associated with manufacture and use of CyA and OKT3 (Sandoz and Ortho Biotech, respectively) laid to rest the notion that transplantation as an enterprise was too limited in scope to justify private investment in novel therapeutics. The ensuing decade witnessed the development and approval of at least a half dozen novel agents, ushering in the era of what some have called *modern* immunosuppression.

Modern immunosuppression (1995–)

Tacrolimus (TAC), known during its developmental phase as FK506, was discovered in a soil sample from Japan in 1984. Early development occurred largely at a single center (the University of Pittsburgh), with use as a single agent or in combination with low-dose corticosteroids and primarily in liver transplantation. US Food and Drug Administration (FDA) approval of TAC (initially for liver transplantation) came in 1994 based on two large multicenter phase 3 trials (one in the United States and one in Europe) involving over a thousand liver transplant recipients. In both studies, acute rejection episodes occurred less often with TAC, though only the European study documented a survival benefit. A subsequent trial in kidney transplantation (comparing TAC versus CyA in combination with ALG induction, AZA, and prednisone) with similar results (less rejection, especially in African Americans) led to approval in kidney transplantation.

Mycophenolate mofetil (MMF) was a new modified preparation of an older agent (mycophenolic acid, MPA) that enhanced its absorption and stability. After dosing and safety were established in a small preliminary study, three large phase 3 studies (1500 patients) were conducted in North America, Europe, and Australia, each showing a 50% decline in frequency of acute rejection in kidney transplant recipients treated with several different CyA-based regimens, with efficacy documented for most patients at a 2-g daily dose. Pooling of data from the three studies documented additional benefit from MMF in improving allograft survival at 1 and 3 years. These data led to FDA approval and release in 1995, with a subsequent registration trial also documenting efficacy in cardiac transplantation.

Sirolimus (SRL) was discovered in a soil sample collected in a Pacific island, Rapa Nui. Originally developed as an anti-fungal agent, it was later found to have immunosuppressive and antiproliferative properties. In the pivotal trials that led to FDA approval, SRL was administered in fixed doses of 2 mg and 5 mg daily, in combination with CyA and corticosteroids. In these trials, although SRL reduced the risk of acute rejection compared with AZA or placebo, it was associated with significant complications (nephrotoxicity, impaired wound healing, hyperlipidemia) that have, in practice, limited its utility.

By the mid 1990s, antibody induction had become less popular due to the disappearance of locally produced polyclonal ATG/ALG, the cost and relative unreliability of the Upjohn equine polyclonal (Atgam), and the lack of effective alternatives. In 1995, OKT3 was the primary induction agent utilized, but only in a quarter of kidney transplant recipients. The second half of the decade, however, witnessed introduction of several new biologic preparations into the marketplace, including Thymoglobulin (rabbit ATG) and alemtuzumab, which was developed as an anti-tumor agent, but quickly became widely used in transplantation. Availability of these agents has coincided with novel understanding and clinical approaches to induction immunosuppression.

Thus transplant pharmacotherapeutics entered the new millennium with nearly all the tools that comprise current immunosuppressive protocols. It must be stated that use of these potent new agents would have been nearly impossible without commensurate advances in anti-infective therapies, notably antivirals (ganciclovir and valganciclovir) and anti-fungals (liposomal amphotericin, imidazoles, etc.). Current practice in immunosuppression is the product of protocols that have evolved over the last decade in an attempt to provide the most effective therapy with the least adverse impact on patients.

Immunosuppression: present

Current practice involves utilizing the agents available in combination protocols, a theme that has defined clinical immunosuppression almost since its inception: drugs with differing mechanisms of action are administered to inhibit immune responses at multiple steps in the rejection cascade. This approach is thought to enable use of lower doses of each individual agent to minimize toxicity, while also most effectively preventing or treating allograft rejection. Induction is now a widely accepted concept, referring to immunosuppression administered in the initial peri-transplant period, usually antibody-based, to prevent early rejection and set the stage for long-term therapy. The primary purpose of induction therapy is immediate establishment of effective immunosuppression, with secondary goals of delaying administration of potentially nephrotoxic agents (calcineurin inhibitors, CNI) and modifying immune responses to enhance long-term engraftment. Maintenance immunosuppression is the long-term therapy required to ensure allograft survival, administered with the dual intentions of avoiding both immunological injury and drug-related toxicity.

Induction

Induction agents can be sub-classified as depletional or non-depletional. Depletional agents including polyclonal (ATG) and monoclonal (alemtuzumab) preparations reduce lymphocyte populations in both central and peripheral lymphoid tissue, with a long-lasting impact on absolute lymphocyte counts. Non-depletional agents modulate immune responses without altering lymphocyte counts and include basiliximab and OKT3.

Polyclonal ATG (or ALG) is manufactured by immunizing animals with crude preparations of human thymocytes (or cultured lymphoblasts). Serum from the animals (horses or rabbits) is then recovered and purified to its immunoglobulin G (IgG) component. Not only is there activity against lymphocytes, but these preparations also contain non-specific IgG reactivity against platelets and other leukocyte receptors. Administration in humans is thought to induce both complement-dependent cytolysis and apoptosis, resulting in lymphodepletion that may require 6–9 months to return to baseline. A depletional effect on other lymphoid cells (including B lymphocytes and natural killer [NK] cells) may also contribute to ATG efficacy.

Rabbit ATG (rATG), which received FDA approval for treatment of acute rejection after kidney transplantation, is now more commonly used as an induction agent. Dosage and timing of administration are widely variable, but a usual dose of rATG is 0.5–1.5 mg/kg/day for a total of 3–5 doses. The maximal total per treatment course is generally limited to 10 mg/kg, with larger doses thought to be associated with increased risk of complications, notably post-transplant lymphoproliferative disease (PTLD). Infusion-related side effects are seen with the first or second dose, generally within the first few hours of infusion, and are typically related to cytokine release syndrome or potentially anaphylaxis. Thus rATG is most commonly administered after pretreatment with corticosteroids, acetaminophen, and anti-histamine. Serum sickness is infrequent with this preparation, but can occur in some cases. Common early adverse effects include leukopenia and thrombocytopenia, with the latter considered an indication for dose reduction. Long-term side effects generally reflect burden of overall immunosuppression. Despite its cost (as much as USD 1000 per dose), rATG is the most commonly used induction agent in the United States.

Alemtuzumab is available in the United States after FDA approval as therapy for chronic lymphocytic leukemia; its use in transplantation has grown in part due to its low cost relative to other depletional agents. The potent and long-lasting effects of alemtuzumab have been viewed as enabling minimization protocols in which one or more maintenance agents (usually corticosteroids or CNIs) are avoided. Several single and multi-center studies support its utility in this regard. Various dosing regimens have been used, including repetitive dosing of alemtuzumab as monotherapy after kidney or pancreas transplantation. Most commonly, alemtuzumab is administered at the time of transplantation as a single 30-mg intravenous dose. There appear to be few adverse effects associated with infusion; most long-term side effects are a consequence of its potent, long-lasting lymphodepletion.

The only current agent actually approved for induction usage is basiliximab, available since 1997. Compared with placebo, and combined with CyA-based regimens that did not include MMF or SRL, this agent, when administered at the time of transplantation, reduced the incidence of acute rejection by half, with few, if any, significant adverse effects. Although shown unequivocally to reduce incidence of acute rejection compared with placebo, efficacy of basiliximab has been thought by some to be limited to relatively low-risk patients. In a subsequent randomized trial, with a study population enriched for high-risk patients (African Americans, highly sensitized), basiliximab was shown to be less effective than rATG in preventing rejection, although graft survival was identical among treatment groups. A more recent trial found more effective prevention of acute rejection with alemtuzumab compared with basiliximab in a corticosteroid-free protocol. Thus use of basiliximab tends to be limited to relatively low-risk patients. As the only antibody preparation FDA-approved

Table 3.1 Calcineurin inhibitors (CNI) and drug interactions

Effect	Drugs
Drugs that increase CNI levels	**Calcium Channel Blockers**: diltiazem, nicardipine, verapamil **Antifungals**: fluconazole, itraconazole, ketoconazole, voriconazole **Macrolides**: erythromycin, azithromycin, clarithromycin **Gastric acid suppressants**: lansoprazole, rabeprazole, cimetidine **Others**: methylprednisolone, allopurinol, colchicine, bromocriptine, metoclopramide, amiodarone, grapefruit juice, INH, protease inhibitors, statins
Drugs that reduce CNI levels	**Anti-tubercular drugs**: rifabutin, rifampin **Anti-convulsants**: carbamazepine, phenobarbital, phenytoin **Others:** octreotide, ticlopidine, St. Johns wort, orlistat, bosentan, nafcillin,
Drugs levels increased by CNI	Statins, methotrexate
Drugs levels decreased by CNI	Digoxin

for induction therapy, however, basiliximab is also commonly used in registration trials of novel immunosuppressants. Basiliximab is administered intravenously as a fixed-dose 20-mg infusion on days 0 and 4 after transplantation. It has not been shown to be effective in reversing established rejection.

Maintenance immunosuppression

Despite the potency of induction therapy, it is generally accepted that without long-term immunosuppression, allografts would fail. Although TAC and MMF, among others, have been shown to reverse established rejection at times, they are, in general, considered to be less potent than induction agents (or high-dose corticosteroids), and their primary purpose is to prevent acute rejection with a tolerable profile regarding adverse effects.

CNI (TAC and CyA)

TAC has been viewed by many, but not all, as an improvement over CyA. These agents are not used together, but one or the other forms the basis of most immunosuppressive protocols. CyA is usually initiated at a dose of 4–8 mg/kg/day, with target trough levels (depending on the assay used) of 100–300 ng/ml. Current practices with TAC typically involve a starting dose of 0.05–0.15 mg/kg/day and a maintenance dose of 0.05–0.1 mg/kg/day (6–36 months after transplantation), especially when used in conjunction with MMF. There is a wide range of acceptable TAC levels for solid organ transplant recipients; however, when used in combination with MMF, data indicate therapeutic efficacy at a trough level between 5 ng/ml and 10 ng/ml. Significant drug–drug interactions impact serum levels of both TAC and CyA (Table 3.1).

Studies comparing efficacy between TAC and CyA have consistently shown little difference in patient and allograft survival, with most, however, indicating less acute rejection, and although both drugs are nephrotoxic, higher glomerular filtration rate (GFR) is demonstrated (at least in the short term) with TAC usage. In general, TAC demonstrates a more favorable cardiovascular disease risk profile (in terms of less hyperlipidemia and less hypertension) than CyA. Alternatively, although both agents are associated with glucose intolerance and new-onset diabetes after transplantation (NODAT), incidence is generally greater with TAC than CsA. Cosmetically, more hirsutism and gingival hyperplasia occur with CsA, whereas a small percentage of TAC-treated patients experience alopecia.

MMF and MPS

MMF dosing was derived from the phase 3 trials noted earlier. From this experience, recommended oral or intravenous dosage for MMF is 1000 mg administered twice daily, with doses not to exceed 3000 mg/day. It is recommended that MMF be administered on an empty stomach due to clinical evidence that food decreases MPA maximum concentration (C_{max}) by 40%. Extensive safety data are available from the clinical trials of MMF, with the most common adverse events related to the gastrointestinal tract: diarrhea, nausea, bloating, dyspepsia, and rarely gastrointestinal bleeds. Enteric-coated mycophenolate sodium (EC-MPS) is thought to be therapeutically equivalent to MMF at comparable doses. Claims of fewer gastrointestinal side effects with EC-MPS compared with MMF have not been substantiated by randomized trials, although some patients clearly benefit. Other adverse effects of both MMF and AZA include hepatotoxicity, bone marrow suppression (anemia, thrombocytopenia, and leukopenia), and macrocytosis. The manufacturers of MMF do not recommend use during pregnancy, although some centers report successful outcomes of pregnancy on MMF. Switching immunosuppression in preparation for pregnancy has inherent risks, in particular, rejection.

As noted above, MMF and EC-MPS dosing were developed empirically in combination with CyA. It is now apparent that pharmacokinetic (PK) profiles vary considerably when both preparations are used in combination with other agents, including TAC and SRL. It is now known that CyA inhibits enterohepatic recirculation of MPA, lowering plasma levels and overall exposure by as much as 50%, and that bioavailability increases dramatically in most patients over the first 4–6 weeks after transplantation. The effect can be highly variable, although a recent study documented intra-patient pharmacokinetic variability as very low. Some have advocated monitoring of MPA drug levels as a guide to proper dosing, with AUC measurements more predictive of outcomes than trough levels. A recent consensus panel recommended that for standard-risk patients, MPA monitoring may not be necessary. Empiric doses of 3000 mg/day during the peri-transplant period, with subsequent reduction to 2000 mg/day, provided adequate MPA exposure for most CyA-treated patients. For TAC-treated recipients, an initial dose of 2000 mg/day, with subsequent reduction to 1500 mg/day, was adequate for most. In patient sub-groups deemed at higher risk for rejection (e.g., diabetics or others with altered gut absorption; elevated immunological risk; or undergoing CNI or corticosteroid withdrawal), MPA monitoring may be beneficial in establishing the correct dose. Because of the altered PK profile associated with its enteric coating, the relationship of trough levels to overall MPA exposure with EC-MPS is not reliable.

SRL

Although approved as a fixed-dose adjunct to CyA, SRL is seldom used in this fashion in the present day. Trough level monitoring, with appropriate dose adjustment, is now recommended. A loading dose of 4–6 mg/day followed by a maintenance dose of 2 mg/day is recommended with a targeted trough level between 5 and 15 ng/ml. When used in non-CNI combinations, some recommended higher trough levels (10–25 ng/ml), although side ffects are more common with higher levels. SRL, administered concomitantly with CyA, seems to exacerbate the nephrotoxicity and increases the risk of acute rejection compared with combinations. Apart from this nephrotoxic effect, common reasons for discontinuation of SRL include hyperlipidemia, proteinuria, mouth ulcers, peripheral edema, pneumonitis, impaired wound healing, lymphocele, and anemia/thrombocytopenia. Everolimus, also known as RAD during development, is another mammalian target of rapamycin (mTOR) inhibitor with a shorter half-life. Its more benign side effect profile may represent usage in phase 3 trials at a relatively lower dose and target levels than SRL.

SRL, when administered concomitantly with TAC, shows less potential to exacerbate CNI-related adverse effects. In several randomized trials, outcomes with the TAC/SRL combination appear comparable to those of TAC/MMF and superior to those of CyA/SRL. SRL or everolimus used in a non-CNI combination has been used de novo following transplantation (although with greater risk of acute rejection) but may be useful late after transplantation when there is significant nephrotoxicity and may allow some recovery or delay progression to ESRD. There is also the suggestion that the anti-proliferative effects may be useful in patients with evidence of vasculopathy or after treatment for malignancy.

Prophylaxis of acute rejection

The primary goal of current immunosuppressive protocols is to prevent acute rejection, a goal achievable with numerous combinations. Most common approaches begin with an induction agent in the peri-operative period, accompanied by high-dose corticosteroids. Appropriate doses of maintenance agents are instituted during this period; once desirable therapeutic levels of maintenance agents are achieved, induction is discontinued. Given the multitude of agents available, there is wide center-to-center and geographic variation, driven by drug availability, cost, and physician preference.

Standard of care in kidney transplantation in the United States is use of antibody induction (78% of recipients) with either rATG or basiliximab (given

Table 3.2 Immunosuppression use for induction and maintenance in the United States

	2007	1998
Functioning graft at initial discharge	16 252	12 002
With immunosuppression information	15 884	11 933
Induction (%)		
rATG (Thymoglobulin)	43	0.2
Basiliximab/daclizumab	26	17
Alemtuzumab	9	0
ATGAM/OKT3	2	22
Information not recorded	20	61
Maintenance regimen (%)		
TAC + MMF/MPA + steroids	51	20
TAC + MMF/MPA	28	0.6
CsA+ MMF/MPA + steroids	5.4	48
CsA + Ever/sirolimus + steroids	1	3
CsA + Anti-metabolite + steroids	0.1	9

Source: Organ Procurement and Transplantation Network/SRTR Data as of May 1, 2008.

limited availability of daclizumab), TAC, MMF, and corticosteroids (prednisone, tapered to 5–10 mg/day by 4–6 weeks after transplant). Induction is less common in lung (62%), heart (54%), small bowel (49%), and liver (25%) according to 2007 data from the US Scientific Registry of Transplant Recipients (SRTR). Overall, use of antibody induction is less common in Europe. Although TAC is the preferred CNI in 80% of patients, CyA is still widely used at some centers in the US and Europe. Likewise, although MMF is used in 87% of kidney recipients, some choose SRL or AZA instead. Triple therapy remains the standard in thoracic transplantation, with TAC/steroids (and no induction) the most common approach in hepatic transplantation (Table 3.2).

Numerous studies support current therapies in kidney transplantation. Mourad and colleagues studied rATG induction in an open-label multi-center study using a TAC-based regimen in kidney transplant recipients. Compared with a non-induction protocol, there was comparable graft survival between the two approaches but less rejection in the rATG group. Recently, the Efficacy Limiting Toxicity Elimination (ELITE)–Symphony study, a global project that involved 1600 subjects in 83 centers randomized to four different protocols, was completed. All groups received standard dosing of MMF and corticosteroids. The control group was standard dosing of CyA without antibody induction. The other groups all received daclizumab induction with low-dose CyA, TAC, or SRL. Patients in the TAC group had the fewest episodes of acute rejection after 1 and 3 years, with better allograft survival and better preservation of renal function than the other groups. Serious adverse events were most common among patients in the SRL group, which also had the most rejection and, despite the avoidance of CNI, inferior renal allograft function. NODAT and diarrhea were more common in patients treated with tacrolimus.

Beyond current standards, trends in maintenance immunosuppression are to minimize or avoid those agents most associated with long-term toxicity, notably corticosteroids and CNIs. In renal transplantation, minimization is perceived to be more dependent on depletional induction than standard therapy, with rATG and alemtuzumab as the agents of choice. A recent randomized multicenter study indicated that early corticosteroid withdrawal can best be accomplished with the least risk of acute rejection in the intermediate term (3 years) with either rATG or alemtuzumab as compared with basiliximab. Alemtuzumab was associated with fewer infectious complications than rATG and was administered at a lower cost. It is in this context that alemtuzumab use is increasing rapidly in the United States.

A 5-year, randomized, double-blind study comparing early corticosteroid withdrawal to maintenance steroid therapy (5–10 mg/day) after antibody induction with concomitant TAC/MMF was recently completed. Overall, there was no difference in graft or patient survival after 5 years. However, there was significantly more acute rejection (27% versus 17%) in the steroid-free group, with more interstitial fibrosis and tubular atrophy (IF/TA) in for-cause biopsies taken from the same group. However, some metabolic benefits did accrue to the steroid-free group, with less NODAT and better preservation of bone histology. Overall, about 25% of US kidney recipients are now on steroid-free protocols.

As documented in the ELITE-Symphony trial, CNI minimization or avoidance has, to the present time, been perceived as relatively ineffective because of the inability of alternative agents to prevent rejection. With risk of acute rejection highest in the first 90 days after transplantation, and risk of SRL adverse effects most daunting during the same period, several studies of planned conversion from CNI to SRL have been conducted. Although one study in liver and one in kidney documented little associated rejection and improved renal function with conversion to SRL, others have indicated excessive rejection complicated by proteinuria, anemia, and graft failure. It would appear that widespread adoption of CNI minimization or avoidance will not occur until late after transplant, when the risk of rejection is lower or more effective alternative agents become available.

Treatment of acute rejection

The traditional approach for treatment of acute rejection in organ transplantation is high-dose corticosteroid followed by anti-lymphocyte therapy for "steroid-resistant" rejection. In renal transplantation this approach is falling rapidly out of favor following the introduction of the Banff schema using histologic findings to define therapeutic approaches to rejection. Acute cellular rejection of the milder variety (Banff 1A or B) is generally treated with intravenous methylprednisolone (10 mg/kg/day for 3 days) up to a total of 1–3 g. More severe acute cellular rejection or refractory acute cellular rejection (incomplete clinical response to IV corticosteroids) generally becomes an indication for use of antibody therapy, with rATG (dosed similarly to induction protocols) as the most commonly used agent. Strategies for treating recurrent or persistent rejection include drug changes (converting AZA to MMF and CyA to TAC; increasing baseline steroid dose), photopheresis, and total lymphoid irradiation.

The relatively recent appreciation of a different phenotype of acute rejection (antibody-mediated rejection, AMR) has resulted in a different approach to therapy for patients with this diagnosis. Until AMR is fully characterized and understood, the protocols for treatment remain variable and not evidenced-based. Treatment is targeted at removing antibodies (usually anti-HLA) from circulation, inhibiting antibody binding to cells, and/or manipulating antibody production. Early AMR within the first 3–6 months after transplantation is usually treated with a combination of plasmapheresis (with therapeutic plasma exchange, TPEX) followed by low-dose intravenous immunoglobulin (IVIg) at 100 mg/kg for a total of 3–5 cycles. Some centers use a single dose of rituximab at 1000 mg or 375 mg/m^2 at the end of treatment cycles to reduce further B-cell maturation. Others utilize very high-dose IVIg (2 g/kg, with a second dose 1 month later). As time elapses following transplantation, the phenotype of AMR is often less simple and may be co-existent with cell-mediated and chronic injury. The benefit of the protocols outlined above (IVIg, TPEX, with or without rituximab) become less well defined, though still often implemented. Several novel therapies (see next section) are currently undergoing investigation.

Generic drugs

Generic substitution of immunosuppressants remains a topic of considerable debate within the transplant community. Clearly, the costs associated with life-long maintenance therapy can be daunting for patients and payers alike, with some grafts clearly lost as a consequence of financial challenges. AZA and prednisone were the first agents to transition to generic status, with little or no apparent negative impact. The emergence of generic CyA preparations in the late 1990s was complicated by confusion, uncertainty regarding financial impact, and an extremely slow transition away from branded preparations despite several studies indicating no adverse impact of the switch. In the past 2–3 years, generic formulations of MMF and TAC have been introduced with bioequivalence data but no published experience in transplant recipients. Criteria for approval of generics in the United States are single-dose trials in fed and fasted control subjects demonstrating bioequivalence in terms of absorption of active ingredient with major PK measures, with a 90% confidence interval within 0.8 and 1.25 ratio with reference product. Despite aggressive introduction of these agents into the community and some confusion on the part of patients, there appears to be little negative impact on patient outcomes to this point.

In 2001, The American Society of Transplantation invited experts to review generic immunosuppressants. Alloway and colleagues published a summary statement (*American Journal of Transplantation*, 2003) that underscored the welfare of the individual patient as the preeminent concern and supported the availability of efficacious less expensive immunosuppressive medications as helping improve patient adherence. They further endorsed the FDA process as appropriately rigorous, with FDA-approved generic narrow therapeutic index immunosuppressive agents appearing to provide adequate immunosuppression to low-risk transplant patients. However, they cautioned that the standards may not be adequate for higher risk patients, and approval of new generic preparations should include studies in at-risk patient populations. The International Society for Heart and Lung Transplantation released a Consensus Statement on generic immunosuppression in 2009. The recommendations cautioned against use of generics in patients with critical drug dosing requirements and that regulating agencies should approve only those generics studied with concomitant interacting medications or in transplant recipients. In addition, the transplant recipient and center should have greater vigilance to adverse sequelae and closer therapeutic drug monitoring following conversion.

Immunosuppression: future

As implied in the previous section, despite the remarkable advances of the last half-century, current immunosuppression remains a less than ideal approach to support solid organ transplantation. Each agent is associated with its own set of toxicities in addition to the shared adverse consequences of long-term immunosuppression: infection and malignancy. As also noted above, drug minimization to avoid these adverse effects now appears directly associated with immunological graft failure as we increase our understanding of previously unrecognized immune responses. It seems unlikely that additional permutations of currently available therapies will be able to alter this dynamic. Although the promise of manipulating immune response at the time of transplantation to induce long-term graft acceptance (tolerance induction) remains an ultimate goal, techniques to apply these approaches on a widespread basis still seem far in the future.

In the near future, therefore, further improvement in outcomes for transplant recipients is likely to reflect progress along two fronts. First is the increasing ability of new approaches to define subgroups of transplant recipients at different immunological risk using novel biomarkers and microarrays. Although such immunological monitoring has been attempted throughout the history of the field, these new technologies seem on the verge of moving from the laboratory to the clinic and providing a mechanism to define who does and does not need potent immunosuppression. The second approach likely to contribute to better outcomes is development of novel immunosuppressant pharmacotherapies. Discovery of new agents is informed by our evolving understanding of how immunological processes injure allografts, with substantial attention now being devoted to antibody-mediated injury and lymphoid tissue of B-cell lineage (Figures 3.1 and 3.2).

Small molecules

Agents now under development in this category follow in the tradition of most current maintenance immunosuppression: oral agents that will be ingested on a daily basis in combination with other agents. They differ from current therapeutic approaches by targeting different pathways, with hopes of better efficacy and fewer side effects.

Tafocitinib (CP-690550)

With the discovery of the importance of Janus kinases (Jak) in mediating cytokine-driven lymphocyte activation, and that congenital deficiency of Jak3 results in severe combined immunodeficiency in children, partial inhibition of this pathway became an attractive target for immunosuppression. Given widespread expression of Janus kinases in other tissues, especially hematopoietic, specificity for Jak3 was essential, as well as the ability to inhibit lymphocyte activation in a dose-dependent fashion. Both of these prerequisites have been met by the Pfizer compound tafocitinib. In rheumatoid arthritis, doses ranging from 5–30 mg twice daily are effective in improving symptomatology, with relatively few adverse effects. A pilot study in renal transplant recipients comparing two dosage regimens of tafocitinib in a CNI-free protocol that included basiliximab, MMF, and steroids documented comparable rates of acute rejection after 6 months to a TAC-based control group. However, the higher-dose tafocitinib patients (30 mg twice daily) appeared over-immunosuppressed, with complications including BK nephropathy and cytomegalovirus disease. There also appeared to be additive hematopoietic toxicity in combination with MMF and a trend to higher plasma lipid levels. Additional studies are underway to better define proper dosing and the most beneficial drug combinations for use with this novel agent, with an initial phase 3 trial being organized at the time of writing.

Sotrastaurin (AEB071)

Protein kinase C (PKC) occupies a central point in mechanisms of T-cell activation via both the T-cell receptor and costimulation pathways; PKC activity is crucial for production of inflammatory cytokines, including interleukin-2 (IL-2) and interferon γ. Sotrastaurin, by inhibiting PKC, blocks T-cell

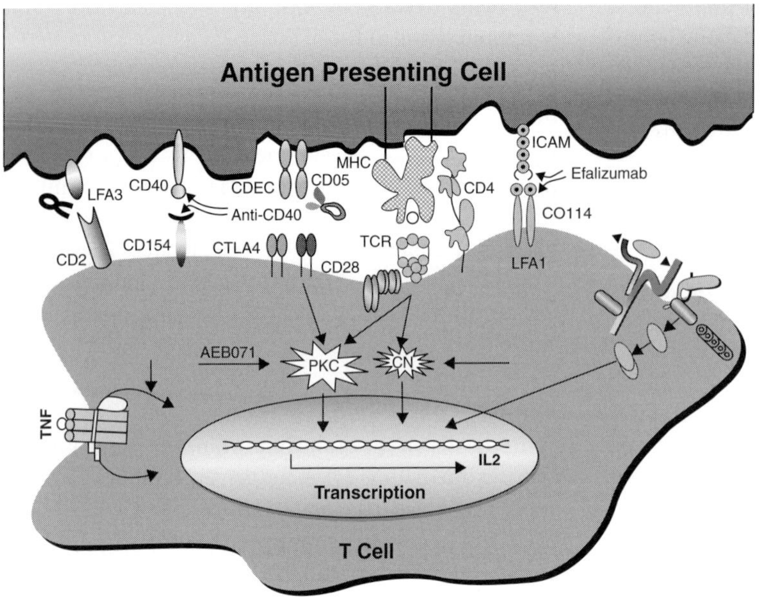

Figure 3.1 Novel biologics and small molecules targeting cell surface receptors and intracellular pathways of the T cell. PKC: protein kinase C; CN: calcineurin. Reproduced from Vincenti F and Krik AD, What's next in the pipeline, *American Journal of Transplantation*, 2008, with permission from John Wiley & Sons Inc.

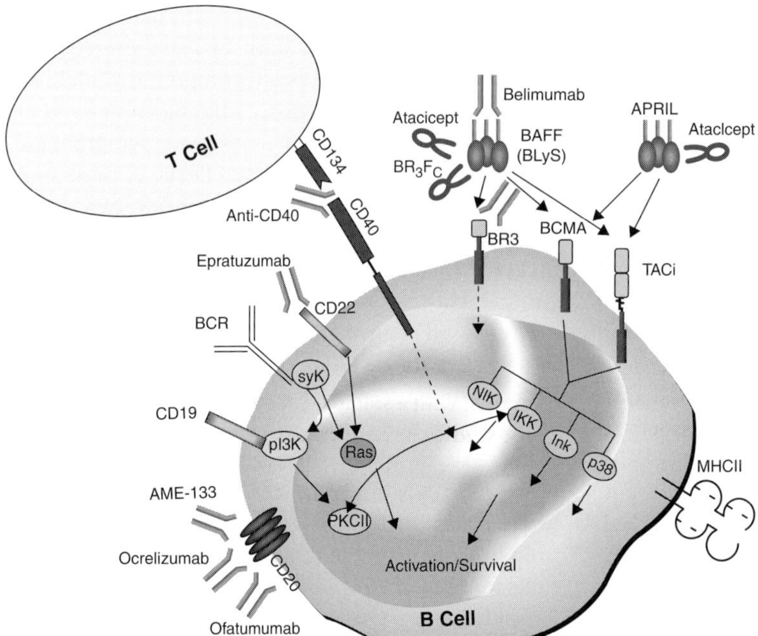

Figure 3.2 Novel monoclonal antibodies and fusion receptor proteins that deplete and/or block activation of B cells. Reproduced from Vincenti F and Krik AD, What's next in the pipeline, *American Journal of Transplantation*, 2008, with permission from John Wiley & Sons Inc.

activation in a CNI-independent fashion and in primate models has been shown to prolong kidney and heart allograft survival. Results from two large phase 2 trials in de novo kidney allograft recipients using sotrastaurin with MPS and corticosteroids as an alternative to TAC-based therapy were disappointing due to excess acute rejection. However, patients receiving a TAC/sotrastaurin-based regimen for 90 days prior to substitution of MPS for TAC experienced little acute rejection and a relative dearth of adverse events. A third phase 2 trial with sotrastaurin in combination with everolimus is underway, with more trials planned using sotrastaurin with a variety of agents in kidney and liver transplantation.

Bortezomib

Bortezomib is a reversible inhibitor of the 26S proteasome in mammalian cells. This proteasome degrades ubiquitinated proteins, thus playing an essential role in maintaining cell homeostasis. Inhibition of this proteasome prevents targeted proteolysis, leading to cell death, especially in rapidly dividing cells. It is administered intravenously and is approved by the FDA for treatment of multiple myeloma, shown to be effective in decreasing plasma cell burden in some refractory cases. Its use in kidney transplant recipients has been anecdotal, primarily as therapy for refractory antibody-mediated rejection.

Biologics

It is now common to use biologics, such as polyclonal or monoclonal antibodies, for a short time as induction or treatment of acute rejection. Under development are several monoclonal antibodies, usually humanized, that target specific cell surface proteins to alter immunological responses for long-term administration. This is analogous to increasing use of agents such as etanercept and adalimumab in autoimmune diseases; in fact, some of the agents studied in transplantation are already marketed for these indications. Efalizumab is a humanized monoclonal antibody directed against lymphocyte-function associated antigen-1 (LFA-1), an adhesion molecule expressed on multiple cell populations including T cells, B cells, and NK cells. LFA-1 is important in facilitating cell migration and homing. It had been used for psoriasis and showed promise in clinical trials for solid organ transplant recipients but was withdrawn from the market when a small number of psoriasis patients developed progressive multifocal leukoencephalopathy (PML), a fatal central nervous system infection caused by JC polyomavirus, after 3 years on the drug. There are no current trials using efalizumab, and existing patients have been transitioned to other immunosuppression.

Belatacept

Belatacept is a novel biologic fusion protein composed of the non-binding portion of IgG fused to the extracellular domain of cytotoxic T-lymphocyte antigen 4 (CTLA-4). As mentioned earlier, CTLA-4 has a high affinity for CD80/86 and therefore prevents the CD80/86-CD28 interaction required for costimulation, raising the threshold for activation of T cells, effectively downregulating the immune response. The agent is administered intravenously at intervals ranging from 1–4 weeks in clinical trials. Two large phase 3 trials of belatacept-based maintenance therapy have recently been completed. In both studies conducted in differing patient populations all thought to be at relatively low immunological risk, maintenance therapy with two different regimens of belatacept dosing was compared with CyA in regimens that also included basiliximab induction, along with MMF and corticosteroids. Despite a higher incidence of acute rejection with belatacept, the newer agent seemed associated with equivalent graft and patient survival at 1 and 2 years and better allograft function. However, although the overall rates of infection and malignancy were similar among treatment groups, PTLD occurred more frequently among belatacept-treated subjects, primarily those who were naive for Epstein-Barr virus before transplantation. Data after 1 year indicate a possible beneficial impact of belatacept on anti-donor antibody formation.

Patients in the phase 2 belatacept trial were offered enrollment in an extension, allowing follow-up in a small cohort of patients beyond 5 years after transplant. There did not appear to be an increasing incidence of rejection, graft failure, or malignancy in these patients, with a stable GFR over time. Additional small pilot studies have been performed using belatacept in combination with either TAC or SRL, with favorable short-term outcomes. FDA approval of belatacept for routine usage in the United States is anticipated in 2010.

Alefacept

Alefacept is a dimeric, humanized fusion protein that targets the extracellular CD2 receptors expressed on T lymphocytes and inhibits the CD2/LFA-3 interaction, thereby inhibiting lymphocyte activation. T cells of the memory effector phenotype may be more sensitive to the effect than other T-lymphocyte populations.

Treatment with alefacept reduces the circulating total CD4 and CD8 counts. As CD2 is also expressed on the surface of other lymphoid tissue (such as NK cells and some B cells), there may be additional effects as well. Alefacept, available for subcutaneous injection, is already FDA-approved as treatment for chronic plaque psoriasis, with a known safety profile as monotherapy. A global phase 2 trial to define the proper dosing and explore combination therapy in kidney transplantation has recently completed enrollment.

Eculizumab

Eculizumab is a recombinant humanized monoclonal IgG that specifically binds, with high affinity, to the complement component, C5, and prevents development of the terminal complement complex, C5b-9. It thus blocks complement-mediated cell lysis and is FDA approved for treatment of paroxysmal nocturnal hemoglobinuria (intravascular hemolysis). It is also an intravenous preparation, administered at intervals of 1–4 weeks. Anecdotal use in transplantation is to prevent (in patients at high risk) or treat antibody-mediated rejection. By blocking the terminal effector component of the injury response, preliminary data indicate that eculizumab is highly effective in preserving allograft function in highly sensitized kidney allograft recipients, at least for intermediate-term periods.

Further reading

Brennan DC, Daller JA, Lake KD, Cibrisk D, Del Castillo D. Rabbit antithymocyte globulin versus basiliximab in renal transplantation. *N Engl J Med* 2006; **355**: 1967–77.

Ekberg H, Tedesco-Silva H, Demirbas A, *et al.* Reduced exposure to calcineurin inhibitors in renal transplantation. *N Engl J Med* 2007; **357**: 2562–75.

Kirk AD. Induction immunosuppression. *Transplantation* 2006; **82**: 593–602.

Kuypers DR, Le Meur Y, Cantarovich M, *et al.* Consensus report on therapeutic drug monitoring of mycophenolic acid in solid organ transplantation. *Clin J Am Soc Nephrol* 2010; **5**: 341–58.

Scientific Registry of Transplant Recipients. 2008 Annual Data Report. Available at: www.ustransplant.org (accessed on January 14, 2011).

Vincenti F, Kirk AD. What's next in the pipeline. *Am J Transplant* 2008; **8**: 1972–81.

Chapter 4A

Major complications – cancer

Bimalangshu R. Dey and Thomas R. Spitzer

Key points

- Malignancy may occur due to transplantation in patients with pre-existing malignancy, transmission from donor to recipient, and de novo in the recipient following transplantation. Transplant outcomes are adversely affected by recipient malignancy.
- Incidence of de novo malignancy increases cumulatively following transplantation, with 20% after 10 years and nearly 30% after 20 years, and is three to four times more common in transplant recipients compared with age-matched controls.
- Cutaneous and lip malignancies are the most common malignancies, comprising approximately 36% of all post-transplant neoplasms.
- Post-transplant lymphoproliferative disorder is Epstein-Barr virus driven, with an incidence of 1–5% after renal transplant and 5–15% after lung, small bowel, and multi-organ transplants.
- Careful surveillance for occurrence of malignancy, investigation of symptoms, and early treatment are important in post-transplant care.

Malignancy in recipients of solid organ transplants (SOT) occurs due to transplantation in patients with pre-existing malignancies, transmission from donor to recipient, and de novo following transplantation. The outcomes for recipients who develop malignancy following transplantation are significantly worse, and therefore close consideration must be given to donor and recipient selection.

Recurrence of pre-existing malignancy is an important consideration when selecting transplant recipients. Studies in renal and cardiothoracic organ transplant patients with pre-existing malignancies suggests a recurrence rate of approximately 20%, with the majority occurring in patients who remain disease free for more than 5 years. Tumor recurrence is more common following previous cancer of lung, skin, bladder, pancreas, and lymphoma. The length of the surveillance period until true remission is achieved has to be balanced against the known outcomes for individual cancers, their grade, and the degree of organ failure.

Transmission of donor malignancy to a recipient has been described in the Cincinnati Transplant Tumor Registry (CTTR) and United Network for Organ Sharing (UNOS) Registries, often with subsequent poor outcome. Close consideration should be given to unexpected donor malignancy during work-up from a detailed history and during organ procurement. Non-melanoma skin cancers, primary cerebral malignancies (except astrocytomas, glioblastomas, and medulloblastomas) and those who remain cancer-free more than 5 years following treatment are generally considered to have an acceptable risk.

Recipients are at high risk of developing de novo cancers, both epithelial and lymphohematopoietic malignancies, due to complex interactions of several factors, among which oncogenic viruses and impaired immunity as a result of chronic immunosuppression are the major causes. The prevalence of post-transplant malignancies (PTM) ranges from 4–18%. The incidence of malignancy increases with the length of follow-up after transplantation, with a cumulative cancer incidence of 20% after 10 years and nearly 30% after 20 years. Overall, the incidence of cancer is increased three- to four-fold in transplant recipients compared

Organ Transplantation: A Clinical Guide, ed. A.A. Klein, C.J. Lewis, and J.C. Madsen. Published by Cambridge University Press.

Table 4A.1 Incidence of neoplasms in general population versus Cincinnati Transplant Tumor Registry patients

Neoplasm	General population	Transplant recipients
Lymphoma	5%	24%
Carcinoma of the lip	0.2%	6.7%
Kaposi's sarcoma	0.02%	5.6%
Carcinoma of vulva/perineum	0.5%	3.5%
Carcinoma of the kidney	2.3%	4.8%
Hepatobiliary carcinoma	1.5%	2.4%

Reproduced from Ginns LC, Cosimi AB, and Morris PJ, *Immunosuppression in Transplantation*, 1999, p. 771, with permission from John Wiley & Sons Inc.

with age-matched controls in the general population. Cancer has become the second cause of late mortality following transplantation after late graft failure. Fast progression, unfavorable prognosis, and poor response to treatment are the general characteristics of post-transplant tumors. Once a diagnosis of PTM is made, staging evaluation should be done specific to the diagnosis.

This chapter is based on the study of data collected by CTTR and the available literature published by both North American and European organ transplant centers. We have attempted to review the characteristics of the most important de novo malignancies in organ allograft recipients, although it is outside the scope of this chapter to discuss diagnosis and treatment of less common malignancies.

Types of de novo malignancies

The most frequent cancers in transplant recipients are skin and lip cancer, solid organ malignancies, and post-transplant lymphoproliferative disorder (PTLD). Table 4A.1 illustrates the incidence of certain cancers in SOT recipients in contrast to that in the general population (Table 4A.1).

Skin and lip cancers

Cutaneous and lip malignancies are the most common neoplasms, comprising approximately 36% of all PTMs, appearing on sun-exposed areas, particularly of the head and neck and upper limbs, especially in light-skinned individuals with blue eyes and blonde or red hair. The incidence of non-melanoma skin cancers in renal recipients, according to a Dutch study, was 10% at 10 years, rising to 40% after 20 years. Similarly, an Australian study showed a linear increase in skin cancers with the length of time after transplantation, approaching 70% at 20 years. The increase is mostly seen with squamous cell carcinoma (SCC). The incidence of SCC in transplant recipients is 40 to 250 times higher than in the general population, basal cell cancer (BCC) 10 times higher, and malignant melanoma 5 times higher. Precancerous keratoses, Bowen's disease, and keratoacanthomas are also seen and can be treated with topical 5-fluorouracil or tretinoin. Melanomas comprised 5.4% of skin cancers in the CTTR in contrast to the incidence of 2.7% in general population. BCC outnumbers SCC in the general population by 5 to 1, but in transplant recipients SCC outnumbers BCC by 1.8 to 1.0. The characteristics of SCC differ in many ways from those seen in the general population. In the general population, skin cancers cause only 1–2% of all cancer deaths, the great majority from melanoma. SCC in transplant recipients is much more aggressive, accounting for the majority of lymph node metastases, and approximately 5% of patients die from their SCC. Allograft recipients with skin cancers are more likely to have other, more aggressive types of neoplasia than transplant recipients without skin cancer. Specialist dermatology input is required, but treatment options include reduction in immunosuppression (especially stopping anti-metabolites), cryotherapy, and surgical excision.

Kaposi's sarcoma

The incidence of Kaposi's sarcoma (KS), which is a human herpes virus type 8 (HHV-8)–related cancer, in allograft recipients is markedly increased, comprising approximately 5.6% of all neoplasms, in contrast to its incidence of 0.02–0.07% of all cancers in the general population. The risk of developing KS in transplant recipients is more than 100-fold compared with age-matched controls in the general population, with the risk being much higher in allograft recipients who are Arab, Italian, Jewish, black, or Greek, likely reflecting the greater prevalence of HHV-8 infection. Reddish-blue macules or plaques in the skin or oropharyngeal mucosa in allograft recipients, particularly in those at risk, must be investigated for KS. One study showed that KS was the most common cancer in renal recipients in Saudi Arabia, comprising up to 76% of all cancers. In the CTTR, a little over 50% had non-visceral disease confined to the skin, conjunctiva, or oropharynx. The rest had visceral KS mainly involving the gastrointestinal tract, lungs, or lymph nodes, but other organs may also be affected as well. The relatively short period of latency between transplantation and the diagnosis of KS suggest that KS development in transplant recipients is associated with rapid reactivation of latent HHV-8 infection.

According to the CTTR, 54% of patients with non-visceral KS achieved complete remission (CR) following treatment, including 32% of these CRs occurring following reduction in immunosuppressive therapy. Patients with visceral KS fared worse, with only 27% achieving CR following therapy. Surprisingly, 63% of CRs in visceral KS resulted from a decrease or discontinuation of immunosuppressive therapy only. Fifty-six percent of patients with visceral KS died. Interestingly, 16 of 39 renal allograft recipients in whom immunosuppression was reduced or stopped had long-term stable renal function, 21 lost their allografts to rejection, and 2 had impaired renal function.

Lymphoproliferative disorders

PTLD, mostly driven by Epstein-Barr virus (EBV), is a potentially fatal complication of transplantation and spans the spectrum from early lesions, including infectious mononucleosis-like PTLD, to frank monoclonal malignant lymphoma. In the CTTR, of a total of 1560 lymphomas, only 42 (2.7%) were Hodgkin's lymphoma, compared with a 10% incidence of lymphomas in the general population; multiple myeloma and plasmacytoma constituted only 58 cases (3.7%) in contrast to a 19% incidence of all lymphomas in the general population. The great majority of post-transplant lymphomas were non-Hodgkin's lymphoma (NHL), making up 93.6% of the cases, as compared with 71% in the general population.

In transplant recipients, PTLD is predominantly of recipient origin. Multiple single-center reviews suggest two important risk factors for the development of PTLD: the degree of immunosuppression and negative EBV recipient serology, i.e., development of primary infection after transplantation. A recent study from Ann Arbor, Michigan, showed that transplant recipients with lymphoma, compared with all other patients who received allografts, were more likely to have negative pretransplant EBV serology (48% versus 7%) and to have received an organ from an EBV-positive donor. The incidence of PTLD is lowest after renal transplantation (1–5%) and highest after lung, small bowel, and multi-organ transplants (5–15%). Overall, more than one third of PTLD cases develop within 2 years after transplantation, and approximately 20% develop 10 or more years following transplantation. Available histologic analysis of tumor tissue in the Ann Arbor study showed that 62% of PTLD cases were EBV positive, and EBV-positive tumors occurred sooner after transplantation than EBV-negative tumors (mean, 29 months versus 66 months).

EBV is a human herpes virus that infects more than 90% of adults. EBV is highly immunogenic, and during primary infection, a vigorous cellular and humoral immune response occurs, with the cellular component consisting of both CD4 and CD8 T cells, which control both primary infection and the periodic reactivation that occurs in all EBV-seropositive individuals. After clearance of primary infection, EBV persists in B cells, establishing latent infection. Immunosuppressive agents in allograft recipients disrupt the balance between latently infected B-cell proliferation and the EBV-specific T-cell response, allowing the increased population of latently infected B cells to develop into PTLD. Several lines of evidence support a causative role of EBV in the pathogenesis of PTLD. First, EBV-naive patients who experience primary infection after transplantation are at the highest risk for PTLD. Second, both EBV genomes and gene products are found frequently in the tumor cells of PTLD. Third, EBV can express type III latency in B cells, which is the most promiscuous, antigenic, and growth-promoting stimulator of B cells. Based on the data on histological detection of EBV in tumor cells in the Ann Arbor study, 66% of patients with diffuse large B-cell lymphoma and 60% of patients with polymorphic PTLD were EBV positive. EBV positivity was detected in 100% of patients with Hodgkin's lymphoma and 75% of patients with multiple myeloma/plasmacytoma, whereas 75% of patients with Burkitt's lymphoma were EBV negative.

In transplant recipients, PTLD is predominantly of recipient origin. In the CTTR, 86.3% of PTLD arose from B lymphocytes and 13.3% were of T-cell origin. Histologically, PTLD includes a heterogeneous group of disorders ranging from reactive, polyclonal hyperplasia to aggressive NHL. The World Health Organization classifies PTLD into four categories: (1) early lesions such as plasmacytic hyperplasia and infectious mononucleosis-like lesion; (2) polymorphic PTLD, which is composed of a mixture of small- and medium-sized lymphocytes, immunoblasts, and plasma cells; (3) monomorphic PTLD, which has sufficient architectural and cytopathic atypia to be diagnosed as frank lymphoma; and (4) classic Hodgkin's lymphoma-like PTLD. A great majority of all types are associated with EBV. Despite this and previous efforts to standardize the pathological classification of PTLD, neither histology nor clonality consistently predicts outcome. PTLD may occasionally present as more diffuse disease that is more difficult to diagnose and may be mistaken for a fulminant sepsis syndrome.

Although extralymphatic disease occurs in 24–48% of NHL patients in the general population, extranodal disease is present in 69–79% of NHLs in allograft recipients. Central nervous system (CNS) is one of the most common extranodal sites, being involved in 21% of lymphoma patients in the CTTR. Of these cases, 9% were patients with systemic disease involving both CNS and other organs, whereas 12% were confined to the CNS only. This 12% CNS-only PTLD contrasts markedly with the general population, in which there is only a 1–2% incidence of primary CNS involvement. Macroscopic or microscopic allograft involvement can occur in 23% of NHLs in SOT recipients. According to the Ann Arbor study, frequent involvement of extranodal sites (79%), poor performance status (68%), elevated lactate dehydrogenase (LDH; 71%), and advanced-stage disease (68%) are all common at the time of diagnosis of PTLD.

Diagnosis of PTLD

Patients with PTLD may often be asymptomatic, whereas others may present with fever, night sweats, weight loss, lymphadenopathy, and so forth. Occasionally, PTLD may present as a diffuse disease involving multiple organs and running a fulminant clinical course. As the gastrointestinal tract is often involved by PTLD, any signs suggesting perforation, peritonitis, or intestinal obstruction should be pursued seriously for a conclusive diagnosis. The possibility of CNS lymphoma must be suspected when a transplant recipient develops neurological symptoms, including a change in mental status.

As PTLD may evolve progressively from a polyclonal entity to a more aggressive monoclonal variant, early diagnosis is important. Therefore, there has been interest in designing predictive assays to identify patients who are at high risk for developing PTLD. Initial studies in recipients of T-cell–depleted (TCD) hematopoietic stem cell transplantation (HSCT) indicated that an elevated serum EBV-DNA measured by quantitative polymerase chain reaction amplification assays was highly predictive of EBV-PTLD. Subsequent studies showed that only 50% of patients with elevated EBV-DNA developed PTLD. Up to 50% of transplant patients may have an elevated EBV-DNA after transplantation, but only a small subset will develop PTLD. Serial monitoring of EBV-DNA is important to distinguish patients with stable-elevated EBV-DNA from the patients with increasing EBV-DNA. A rising EBV-DNA load is more predictive of PTLD than stable-elevated EBV-DNA load. Combined monitoring of EBV-DNA and EBV-specific CTL responses has been found to be more predictive of subsequent development of PTLD.

Treatment of PTLD

Reduction of immunosuppression

There is increasing evidence that reducing immunosuppression may decrease the development of PTLD in high-risk patients, i.e., patients with a rising EBV-DNA load. With overt PTLD, reducing immunosuppression has yielded variable results. Single-center studies report overall response rates of up to 75% in patients treated with this modality alone or in combination with surgery, and one study showed complete remissions in 20% of patients. If EBV is actively promoting B-cell proliferation at the time of PTLD diagnosis, as is believed to be the case in PTLD that occurs early after transplantation, reducing immunosuppression appears to have a better therapeutic influence than in late PTLD.

EBV-specific cytotoxic T cells

Donor-derived EBV-specific cytotoxic T cells (CTLs) given to the high-risk patients after HSCT have been found to be highly effective as prophylaxis, and they have also proved to be effective as treatment for PTLD in more than 80% of patients. In solid allograft recipients, there are additional challenges because patients remain on long-term immunosuppression. However, studies have demonstrated that it is possible to generate autologous EBV-specific CTLs from transplant recipients, which restores EBV-specific immunity, albeit short-term, that controls disease progression. Long-term persistence of EBV-specific immunity has not been feasible in patients who remain on immunosuppression.

CD20 monoclonal antibody (rituximab)

Because EBV-driven neoplastic B cells routinely express CD20 antigen, rituximab, a humanized

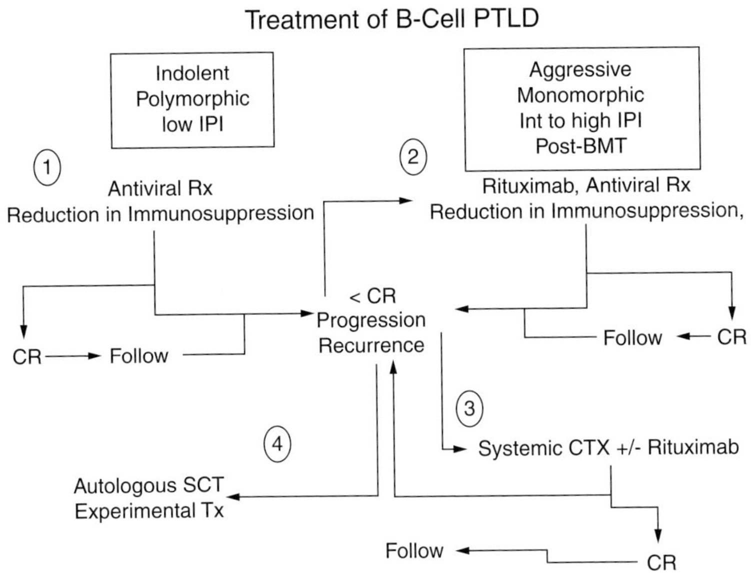

Figure 4A.1 An algorithm for the treatment of B-cell post-transplant lymphoproliferative disorder (PTLD). BMT: bone marrow transplantation; CR: complete remission; CTX: chemotherapy; Int: Intermediate; IPI: International Prognostic Index; SCT: stem cell transplantation; Tx: treatment.

anti-CD20 monoclonal antibody, has become an attractive approach to eliminate EBV-transformed malignant cells. Rituximab has significant activity against PTLD in transplant recipients, with response rates of 44–100% in several small series. A recent phase 2 clinical trial that included patients who had reduction of immunosuppression as their only previous therapy, but excluded patients with CNS PTLD, reported a response rate of 44% at day 80. However, a long-term follow-up study of transplant recipients treated with rituximab demonstrated that 57% had progressive disease at 12 months, and another study showed recurrence of PTLD in 50% of patients.

Surgery and radiotherapy

If the staging evaluation confirms localized disease confined to one site, then radiation and/or surgery can be an effective approach. In one study on the outcome of PTLD occurring late after transplantation, patients with localized disease achieved sustained remissions following surgery or radiotherapy and reduction of immunosuppression.

Chemotherapy

PTLD is generally chemotherapy-sensitive after progression or failure to respond to rituximab and reduction of immunosuppression, and cyclophosphamide, doxorubicin, vincristine, and prednisone (CHOP) salvage therapy has been associated with an overall response rate of up to 75% in patients with NHL-type PTLD. Similarly, patients with Hodgkin's lymphoma-like PTLD can be treated with doxorubicin, bleomycin, vinblastine, and dacarbazine (ABVD) chemotherapy. Some centers are reporting high response rates using chemotherapy as first-line treatment in addition to reduction in immunosuppression.

Hepatocellular carcinoma

In the CTTR, hepatocellular carcinoma (HCC), which represents the great majority of hepatobiliary tumors in transplant recipients, constitutes 2.4% of all PTMs, compared with an incidence of 1.5% in the general population. Two epidemiological studies have shown a 20- to 40-fold increased incidence of HCC in transplant recipients compared with age-matched controls. Hoffmann *et al.* from the Johns Hopkins University School of Medicine demonstrated an incidence of HCC of 6.5 per 100 000 person-years among kidney, heart, and lung (non-liver) recipients and 25 per 100 000 person-years among liver recipients. HCC incidence among non-liver recipients was independently associated with hepatitis B virus (HBV) surface antigenemia, hepatitis C virus (HCV) infection, and diabetes mellitus. Among liver recipients, HCC incidence was associated with advancing age, male sex, HCV infection, and diabetes mellitus. In the

Johns Hopkins study, although HCC incidence in liver transplant recipients was overall elevated, the overall incidence of HCC among non-liver recipients was similar to that of the general population, but increased among those with HCV and HBV antigenemia.

Renal cell carcinoma

Carcinoma of the kidney in the CTTR comprised 4.8% of all PTMs in comparison with a 2.3% incidence in the general population. Renal cell carcinoma (RCC) represents approximately 80% of all renal tumors, whereas 12% are represented by transitional cell carcinoma. The incidence of RCC in transplant recipients is increased by 30- to 40-fold over its incidence in the general population. Most malignancies in kidney transplant recipients arose in their own diseased kidneys, whereas 9% were found in the kidney allografts; 24% of RCCs were discovered at the time of native nephrectomy for hypertension or other reasons. One predisposing cause of cancers in renal allograft recipients is acquired cystic disease (ACD) of the native kidneys, which occurs in 30–95% of patients receiving hemodialysis and which is known to be complicated by RCC.

Tobacco- and alcohol-related cancers

Several series have not shown an appreciably higher incidence of lung and head and neck malignancies in allograft recipients as compared with the general population. However, recently, Medina *et al.* from Spain examined PTMs in liver allograft recipients and demonstrated an increased prevalence of lung, oropharyngeal, laryngeal, and esophageal cancers. This may be explained by the fact that a good proportion of their patients underwent liver transplants due to alcoholic liver disease and they also had significant exposure to tobacco. Lung cancer is the most common non-cutaneous malignancy after heart transplantation and often occurs in patients with a significant tobacco history. Although the success of surgical treatment for early-stage lung cancer is good, most present with metastatic disease, despite frequent surveillance post-transplant, with poor survival despite treatment. There have also been reports of tobacco-related lung cancers following transplantation of lungs from known smokers.

Carcinoma of the vulva and perineum

The incidence of carcinomas of vulva/perineum in allograft recipients is 3.5% in the CTTR compared with its 0.5% incidence in the general population. In general, males outnumber females by more than 2:1 in regard to the distribution of all PTM. In contrast, with carcinomas of the vulva, perineum, or anus, females outnumber males by 2.5:1. Approximately 50% of patients have a history of preceding condyloma acuminatum, which should be regarded as a premalignant lesion. Many patients can be successfully treated with local or extensive surgery, but 12% of patients in the CTTR died from their malignancy.

Other PTMs

The Australia and New Zealand Dialysis and Transplant Registry noted a 289-fold increased incidence of endocrine cancers, a 5.6-fold increase in leukemia, a 2.5-fold increase in cancers of the digestive tracts, and a 2-fold increase in pulmonary tumors. Recently, a study from Spain showed an increased risk of acute myeloid leukemia in liver allograft recipients. Malignancies have been reported from most organ systems in addition to those discussed already. Sarcomas, breast carcinoma, bladder, and bowel cancers are particularly seen after transplantation.

PTMs in children

Post-transplant malignancies in children are different from those in the general childhood population and from those observed in adult transplant recipients. In a recent study from France in which 1326 children underwent SOT, 80 patients (6%) were diagnosed with PTMs; EBV-related PTLD was the most common, comprising 80% of all tumors, with 52% of cases occurring within the first 6 months after transplant. PTLD was associated with primary EBV infection in 81% of cases and EBV reactivation in the remaining 19% of patients. The prevalence of PTLD in SOT children in this study was 5%, but it was disproportionately higher (18%) among combined liver and small bowel recipients. EBV-negative lymphomas were rare and occurred more evenly throughout the 10-year period after transplantation. Skin cancer is the second most common malignancy after PTLD, and melanomas comprised 16% of all skin cancers in children compared with 5% among adults.

Management of PTM

Prevention and surveillance

In principle, the level of immunosuppression should be kept as low as possible in order to maintain good allograft function. Whenever possible, viral infection should be prevented in immunocompromised patients. Because the incidence of HCC is increased in transplant recipients, mainly in non-liver recipients, and as this is frequently associated with HBV infection, vaccination of potential organ allograft recipients with the HBV vaccine may prevent HCC. Because human papillomavirus (HPV) infections, suspected of having a pathogenetic role in carcinomas of the vulva, perineum, and cervix, are transmitted sexually, patients should use barrier methods of contraception and undergo HPV vaccination where available. Premalignant lesions such as condyloma acuminatum or cervical dysplasia should be treated adequately to prevent progression to invasive cancers. Light-skinned patients should avoid excessive sunlight exposure. In many institutions, antiviral drugs such as acyclovir or ganciclovir are used prophylactically to prevent viral infections including EBV infection, but whether or not this prophylactic strategy will reduce the incidence of EBV-related malignancies, including PTLD, remains debatable. Reduction in immunosuppression in response to a rising EBV viral load, which indicates a high risk of developing PTLD, has reduced the incidence of PTLD in pediatric liver transplant patients.

Understanding the increased risk of malignancy of transplant recipients, careful surveillance and screening for selected malignancy should be undertaken. Careful examination is required at follow-up, including examination of skin, mucosa, and lymph nodes. In some centers periodic screening investigations include fecal occult blood, flexible sigmoidoscopy, colonoscopy, prostate-specific antigen, mammography, chest X-ray, and cervical smear. Regular dermatology review with biopsy of suspicious skin or lip lesions should also be undertaken. Symptoms or suspicious findings on routine examination and testing require further investigation, imaging, biopsy, or specialist referral as necessary.

Treatment

PTM has a poor prognosis in general, and cancers in allograft recipients frequently demonstrate a more aggressive behavior than do similar cancers in the general population. In principle, reduction or cessation of immunosuppressive therapy, as clinically feasible, must be considered a central component of the therapeutic strategy for PTM. Cessation or reduction of immunosuppression may lead to significant antitumor responses, including sustained remissions of PTLD and KS, but such treatment by itself rarely causes regression of epithelial tumors.

Conclusion

Malignancies of both epithelial and lymphohematopoietic cell origin are common, often life-threatening complications of transplantation and underscore the delicate balance between providing adequate immunosuppression to prevent allograft rejection and allowing sufficient restoration of immune surveillance to prevent causative mechanisms of these PTM (such as oncogenic viruses). More targeted immunosuppressive strategies in the future will hopefully lessen the global immunosuppression that complicates conventional anti-rejection approaches and diminish the risk of these malignancies. In the meantime, diligent preventive strategies, early diagnosis (with, e.g., monitoring of EBV-DNA) leading to successful preemptive treatment, and aggressive treatment of established PTM will remain the cornerstones of management of this serious complication of transplantation.

Further reading

Heslop H. How do I treat EBV lymphoproliferation. *Blood* 1009; **114**: 4002–8.

Hoffmann CJ, Subramanian AK, Cameron AM, *et al.* Incidence and risk factors for hepatocellular carcinoma after solid organ transplantation. *Transplantation* 2008; **86**: 784–90.

Medina EM, Romero CJ, Camara AG, *et al.* Malignancy after liver transplantation: cumulative risk for development. *Transplant Proc* 2009; **41**: 2447–9.

Navaro MD, Lopez-Andreu M, Rodriguez-Benot A, *et al.* Cancer incidence and survival in kidney transplant patients. *Transplant Proc* 2008; **40**: 2936–40.

Penn I. Neoplastic complications of organ transplantation. In: Ginns LC, Cosimi AB, Morris PJ (eds). *Transplantation*. Blackwell Science, Oxford, 1999, pp. 770–86.

Chapter 4B

Major complications – pathology of chronic rejection

Yael B. Kushner and Robert B. Colvin

Key points

- Chronic rejection is a major cause of late allograft loss in solid organ transplants and is due to repeated or sustained alloimmune graft injury.
- T-cell mediated and antibody-mediated rejection as well as innate immunity can all lead to chronic rejection as a common outcome.
- The final pathway leading to late graft loss likely includes non-immune vascular pathology such as atherosclerosis, hypertension, and chronic drug toxicities.
- Treatment for chronic rejection is limited by a lack of agents that affect antibody production, tissue repair, and fibrosis.
- Originally thought to be irreversible and untreatable, the lesions of chronic rejection can be responsive to certain regimens and possibly show resolution over time if the offending insult is removed.
- New techniques are needed to assess the activity of chronic rejection and the molecular pathways involved and to direct targeted therapy.

Chronic rejection is a major problem and the most common cause of late graft injury in solid organ transplantation. It causes late graft loss in approximately 25% of recipients of kidney, heart, and lung allografts and is a significant factor in liver allografts. Chronic rejection is widely regarded as difficult to diagnose, of obscure etiology, untreatable, and irreversible. We attempt herein to convince the reader that none of these attributes are necessarily true.

Definition

Chronic rejection is defined as the slowly evolving injury and response of a solid organ graft to persistent or recurrent alloimmune attack. Progression of chronic rejection occurs over weeks to months to years and depends on two main factors. The first is the intensity of the alloimmune response and the second is the resistance of the organ to the assault. All tissue structures within organs are potential targets; however, most commonly affected are the arteries (transplant arteriopathy or vasculopathy), capillaries (chronic humoral rejection), and the epithelium. Organ-specific targets include the glomeruli (transplant glomerulopathy), biliary tree (vanishing bile duct syndrome), and bronchioles (bronchiolitis obliterans). Chronic rejection is a major cause of late graft injury and mortality. Other causes of late graft injury, such as infection and recurrent disease, can generally be distinguished histologically.

Transplant arteriopathy

Definition

Transplant arteriopathy (TA) is the main lesion of chronic rejection. TA describes the effects of the immune system on arteries in solid organ transplants. It is variously termed *chronic allograft vasculopathy*, *sclerosing transplant vasculopathy*, *accelerated atherosclerosis*, *chronic allograft arteriopathy*, and *transplant arteriopathy*. Transplant arteriopathy (TA) is our preferred designation, because the disease is

Organ Transplantation: A Clinical Guide, ed. A.A. Klein, C.J. Lewis, and J.C. Madsen. Published by Cambridge University Press.

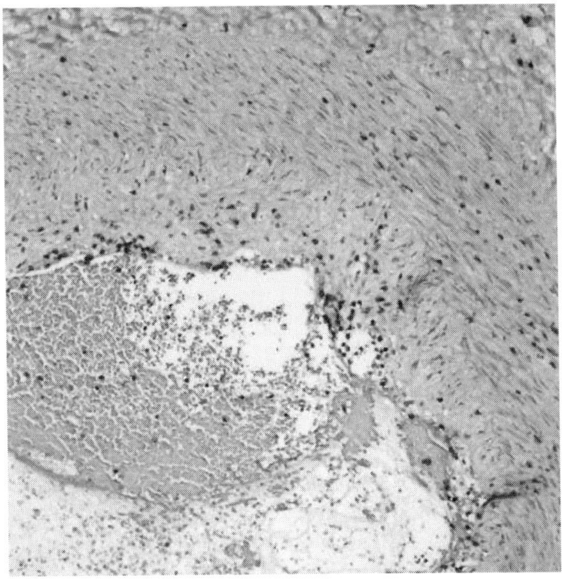

Figure 4B.1 Chronic, active TA can be identified by the inflammatory infiltrate that is typically under the endothelium and accompanied by intimal fibrosis. This artery from a renal allograft shows T cells within an arterial wall and focally lifting the endothelium of an affected vessel stained for CD3 by immunohistochemistry. Antibody also may play a role in the pathogenesis of TA, as shown in experimental studies. See color section.

restricted to arteries, and this nomenclature does not implicate a specific mechanism.

Pathological diagnosis

The stages of TA have been well documented histologically. Typically, the first stage detectable is endarteritis, with inflammatory cells (primarily T cells) infiltrating and lifting off vascular endothelium (Figure 4B.1). Endarteritis in a previous biopsy is a strong risk factor for later TA.

Following endarteritis, concentric intimal fibrosis ensues, with eventual vascular luminal narrowing leading to graft ischemia and failure. The lesions of TA are most prominent in larger caliber arteries but extend to peripheral arterial branches, sparing only arterioles. Activity of the lesion is suggested by loose stroma, density of the lymphocytic infiltrate, stromal proliferation, and the occasional presence of fibrin.

Diagnostic difficulty is encountered when attempting to distinguish chronic TA from atherosclerotic lesions that develop in patients with organ transplants due to hypertension or other risk factors. Certain features are thought to be helpful in this regard. In TA, there is intimal fibrosis but a relative paucity of elastic fibers in the neointima, with occasional infiltrating mononuclear cells. In contrast, in native organs with atherosclerotic vascular disease, there is duplication of the internal elastica and few inflammatory cells (Figures 4B.2A and 4B.2B). In TA, lipid deposition is usually modest and consists of foamy macrophages abutting the internal elastic, whereas it is more substantial and diffuse in atherosclerosis. In addition, atherosclerosis typically affects vessels in an eccentric distribution and tends to spare the small arteries, in contrast to TA, which is concentric and frequently affects small vessels. Although many authors have noted these differing features, it has been shown that there is great synergy between immune and non-immune vascular injury. For example, conditions such as hypercholesterolemia are also risk factors for TA, and protocol biopsies have shown evolution from lesions that resemble TA to those resembling atherosclerosis over time. Certain authors feel that transplant patients are simply at risk for accelerated arteriosclerosis for various reasons and that these lesions would all fall under the guise of immune and non-immune mediated TA.

Pathogenesis and experimental models

Intimal proliferation is thought to be due to increased numbers of myofibroblasts or smooth muscle cells as well as increased deposition of extracellular matrix. These proliferating myofibroblasts stain with alpha-smooth muscle actin. The myofibroblasts/smooth muscle cells express endothelin-1, iNOS, β-actin (a marker of synthetic myocytes), and the anti-apoptotic molecule Bcl-xL. The extracellular matrix material is composed of collagen, fibronectin, tenascin, biglycan, decorin, and acid mucopolysaccharides and is believed to be in part produced by the myofibroblasts themselves. Collagen IV and later I and III are deposited first against the internal elastica and then progressively toward the vessel lumen. Both the inflammatory cells and about half of the spindle-shaped myofibroblasts are of recipient origin.

The immunological basis of TA is under active investigation. The belief that the process is immunologically mediated is based on the observations that TA rarely arises in autografts. Three separate and possibly synergistic pathways have been identified: T cells, antibody-mediated injury, and natural killer (NK) cells. Macrophages, although unlikely primary responders to donor antigen, are thought to be important

(A)

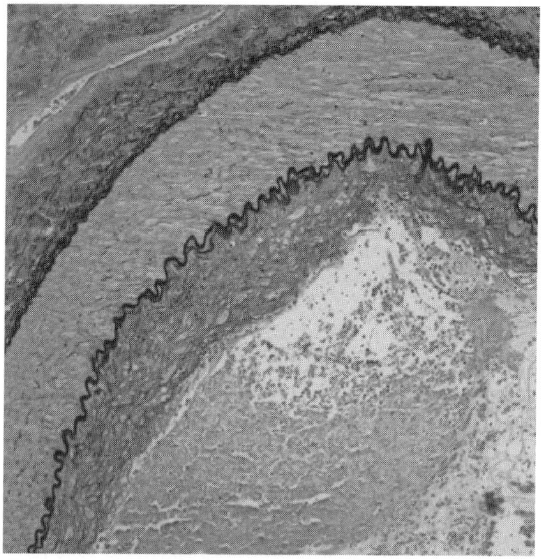

(B)

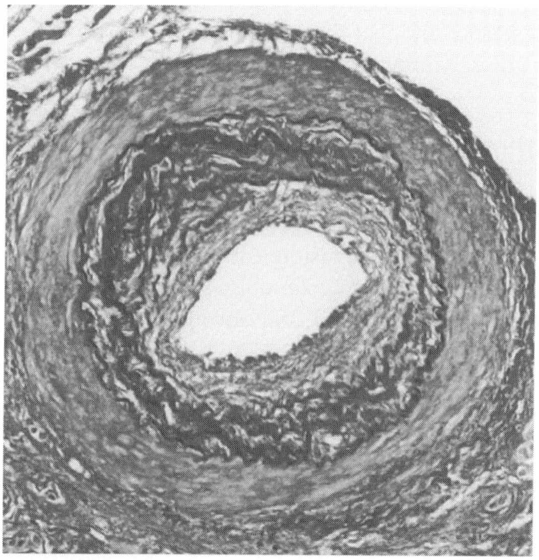

Figure 4B.2 Contrasting appearances of TA and non-immunologic arteriosclerosis can be appreciated in sections stained for elastic fibers. (A) An artery from a renal allograft with TA shows intimal fibrosis without an increase in elastic fibers and with infiltrating inflammatory cells. (B) An artery from a native kidney with arteriosclerosis shows duplication of the elastic lamina, termed *fibroelastosis*, and few inflammatory cells. A and B, Weigert elastic stain. See color section.

secondary participants in all three pathways. The target antigens are mainly major or minor histocompatibility antigens. The possibility of other autoantigens such as vimentin and collagen V has been raised, but the evidence is not yet convincing to these authors. The primary target cell in TA is probably the endothelium, although the medial smooth muscle cells may also be affected.

T cells are sufficient immunological instigators of TA, as judged by animal studies, and provide the first etiologic pathway of TA. TA lesions readily arise in settings without antibody production or NK cell activity. This has been shown in B-cell deficient allograft recipients, murine male-to-female heart grafts, and other minor histoincompatible grafts. In vitro, T-cell supernatants from patients with chronic rejection enhance the proliferative effects of cultured smooth muscle cells via platelet-derived growth factor (PDGF). T cells in the lesions of human TA express a cytotoxic phenotype (perforin, GMP-17). In murine models lacking cytotoxic molecules perforin or granzyme B, the lesions of TA are inhibited. Blocking the alternative cytotoxic pathway with soluble Fas also inhibits TA in rats. Thus repeated or sustained T-cell mediated rejection, as evidenced in the kidney by inflammatory cells infiltrating renal compartments (interstitial inflammation, tubulitis, endarteritis), is sufficient to cause chronic rejection.

Antibodies, the second pathway of TA, are also sufficient to produce TA. Acute humoral or antibody-mediated rejection (AHR) is typically diagnosed in the presence of serum donor-specific antibodies (DSA), complement split-product complement component 4d (C4d) deposition in capillary walls as seen on immunofluorescence or immunohistochemistry, and histological signs of humoral rejection, such as inflammatory cells in peritubular capillaries or fibrinoid necrosis of vessel walls. It is thought that repeated or sustained episodes of AHR can lead to chronic rejection. Antibody-mediated rejection is independently linked to chronic rejection as well: DSA to major histocompatibility complex (MHC) antigens (class I and II) are associated with transplant glomerulopathy (TG) in the kidney and accelerated progression of TA. In non-human primates, TA in renal allografts is strongly associated with prior DSA and C4d deposition in the graft. In vitro antibody to MHC class I promotes endothelial proliferation via upregulation of FGF-1 receptors and RhoA and phosphorylation of Src. Endothelial proliferation is inhibited by simvastatin or complement component 3 (C3) exoenzyme, which also inhibit RhoA. In Rag-1 knockout mice that lack T and B cells, adoptive transfer of DSA causes TA over 3–4 weeks in heart allografts. In humans, TA is often associated with C4d deposition in

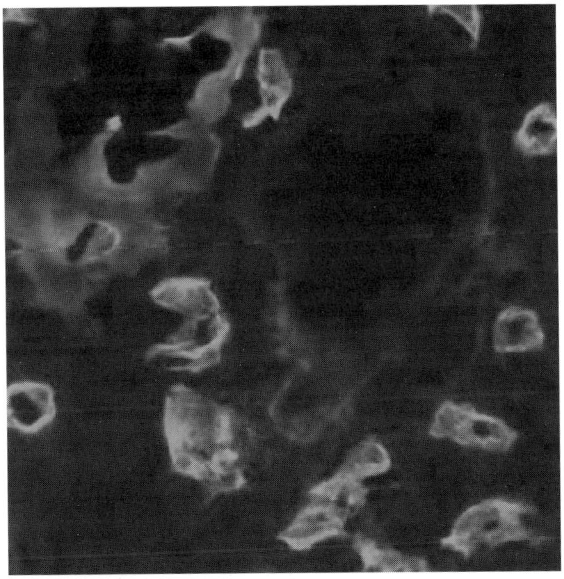

Figure 4B.3 In chronic antibody-mediated rejection CHR, C4d is deposited in peritubular capillary walls, as shown in this immunofluorescence micrograph of an allograft kidney cryostat section stained with anti-C4d monoclonal antibody. CHR is well documented in the kidney but not yet in other organs, although it probably exists. See color section.

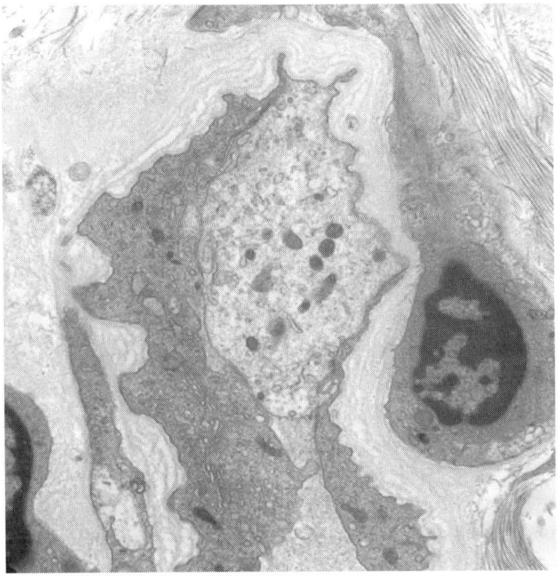

Figure 4B.4 In CHR, multi-lamination of peritubular capillary walls occurs in renal allografts, best shown by electron microscopy. This is a manifestation of repeated episodes of endothelial injury and repair mediated by antibodies. Similar changes occur in glomerular capillaries, where it is termed *transplant glomerulopathy*. See color section.

myocardial capillaries. However, animal studies indicate that complement fixation is not necessary for antibody-mediated TA. This may explain the variable association of C4d deposition and TA in humans.

The third pathway of chronic rejection involves the innate immune system and NK cells. This has been most clearly demonstrated in animal studies in which MHC compatibility and immune reactivity can be better controlled. The first evidence came from murine models that had become tolerant of donor skin tissue by neonatal exposure to donor cells or later by induction of mixed chimerism. Curiously, these recipients showed no acute rejection of donor strain hearts, but later developed TA. In parent to F1 heart grafts, in which T or B cells are tolerant to the graft (self) and only NK cells are expected to respond to the lack of self on the graft, TA also developed. In these same models, TA could be inhibited by blocking NK cells. In Rag-1 knockout mice (who lack T or B cells), when parent to F1 grafts are performed, viral infection promotes the ability of NK cells to produce TA. These results are particularly interesting in conjunction with the clinical evidence that viral infection (cytomegalovirus, CMV) is a risk factor for TA in the kidney and in the heart.

Chronic humoral rejection in the kidney

The concept of chronic humoral rejection (CHR) was introduced with diagnostic criteria by Mauiyyedi and colleagues in studies of kidney allografts and was soon confirmed and expanded by Regele. In the kidney, the hallmarks of chronic antibody-mediated injury include C4d deposition in peritubular and glomerular capillary walls, multi-lamination of the basement membrane of peritubular and glomerular capillaries, and the presence of circulating DSAs. The combination of these features define CHR in the Banff schema.

C4d deposition in capillary walls, as seen by immunofluorescence or immunohistochemistry, is pathognomonic for humoral rejection, both acute and chronic (Figure 4B.3). Because C4d is cleared by allografts in 1–2 weeks, visualization of C4d deposition serves as a marker of current immunological activity. Multi-lamination of peritubular capillary walls is thought to arise from repeated endothelial injury and healing deposition of new basement membrane material (Figure 4B.4). This multi-lamination is best appreciated on electron microscopic studies, but can also be highlighted by special stains that have an

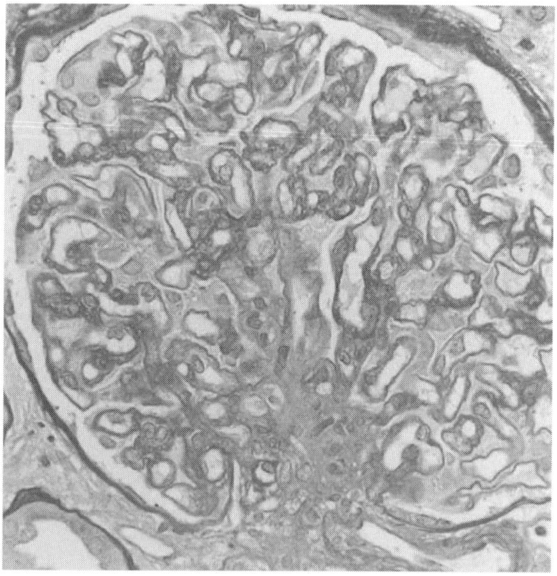

Figure 4B.5 Transplant glomerulopathy (TG) is defined by duplication of the glomerular basement membrane, easily appreciated when severe by light microscopy in sections stained with PAS. This is highly associated with circulating anti-donor antibodies and deposition of C4d. However, the pattern of injury can be due to other causes, such as thrombotic microangiopathy. See color section.

affinity for the basement membrane, such as Periodic Acid-Schiff (PAS) or silver stains. A similar etiology is thought to underlie duplication of the glomerular basement membrane (GBM), which, when found in allografts, is termed *transplant glomerulopathy* (TG) (Figure 4B.5). Repeated or sustained endothelial injury leads to deposition of new basement membrane material within the capillary loops and eventual duplication of the GBM. This can be easily observed by light microscopy as well as electron microscopy. The finding of GBM duplication/TG is not pathognomonic for CHR. Other causes of chronic endothelial injury, such as thrombotic microangiopathy (TMA), also lead to GBM duplication in allografts and native kidneys. Because transplant recipients can often develop TMA due to drug toxicities as well as recurrent disease (membranoproliferative glomerulonephritis [MPGN] pattern) in addition to CHR, TG has an etiologic differential diagnosis when seen on a biopsy. Other findings, such as intraluminal thrombi (TMA), immune-complex deposits (recurrent or de novo glomerulonephritis), and C4d (CHR), can be helpful when assessing TG in renal allografts. Repeated antibody-mediated capillary injury in CHR causes eventual loss of capillary density, and this contributes to secondary ischemic injury. The loss of capillaries may make it more difficult to interpret C4d stains because fewer target vessels are present.

Other, less specific histological features of CHR may be present in the kidney, such as interstitial fibrosis, tubular atrophy, and TA. Interstitial fibrosis and tubular atrophy, a manifestation of any chronic injury to these renal compartments, can frequently be accompanied by lymphoid aggregates. Although TA is thought to be a major factor in chronic rejection, it is not considered in the definitive histological diagnosis of chronic rejection because chronic vascular injury due to ischemia, hypertension, atherosclerosis, drug toxicities, and more can all have a similar histological end point.

The majority (57%) of late kidney graft losses are associated with DSA and/or C4d deposition, and the risk of subsequent graft failure is significantly worse after a C4d+ biopsy. Increased transcription of endothelial-specific genes has been detected in patients who have DSA and is correlated with an adverse outcome, even in the absence of detectable C4d. Thus antibody-mediated rejection is a significant clinical barrier to long-term success of kidney allografts. It is likely that CHR also occurs in other organs and will be one day be identified by appropriate clinicopathological studies.

Chronic rejection in the liver

Although liver allografts are relatively resistant to rejection, features of chronic rejection have been described, primarily consisting of TA (difficult to detect in needle biopsies) and immune destruction of the biliary tree, termed *vanishing bile duct syndrome* (VBDS). VBDS is manifested in biopsies or liver resections by loss of bile ducts within portal tracts and eventual signs of biliary obstruction such as cholestasis, but without ductular proliferation (Figure 4B.6A). VBDS also occurs in native livers under certain conditions (lymphoma, drug toxicity, and viral infection); therefore, it may or may not be a direct effect of immunological rejection. Bile duct epithelium manifests molecular markers of senescence (p21) in early chronic rejection, a process that can be reversed by conversion from cyclosporine to tacrolimus. Transient lobular hepatitis may also be a feature of chronic rejection and is potentially reversible, although VBDS and TA (Figure 4B.6B) are resistant to current therapy.

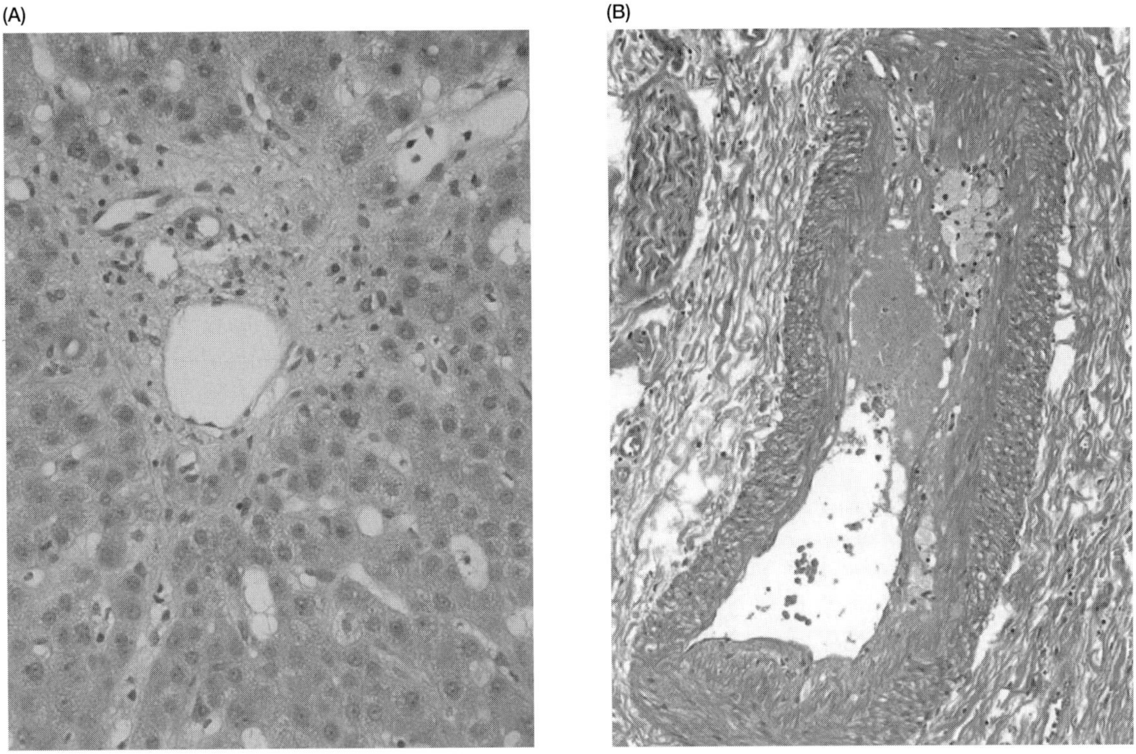

Figure 4B.6 Chronic rejection in the liver affects bile ducts and vessels. (A) In vanishing bile duct syndrome, a manifestation of chronic rejection in the liver, there is loss of bile ducts in portal tracts with associated cholestasis. (B) Chronic allograft vasculopathy in an hepatic artery shows prominent foam cells in the intima. Foam cells, which are macrophages filled with lipid, are characteristic of chronic rejection and are probably related to hyperlipidemia. Photomicrographs courtesy of Dr. V.A. Marcus, McGill University (A) and A.J. Demetris, University of Pittsburgh (B). See color section.

Features predicting irreversibility included bile duct loss of greater than 50%, bridging perivenular fibrosis, and the presence of foam cell clusters within portal tracts. The role of antibodies in hepatic chronic rejection is not clear, although DSA is associated with late graft loss, and several studies have detected endothelial C4d in liver grafts with ductopenic chronic rejection and TA.

Chronic rejection in the heart

The study of rejection in cardiac allografts has been greatly limited by the difficulty in obtaining real-time histological material for examination. TA is the main lesion in heart transplants that leads to late graft loss, ischemia, and death; in the heart, by convention it is termed *cardiac allograft vasculopathy* (CAV). TA in the heart has a similar appearance as in other organs, with concentric intimal fibrosis leading to luminal occlusion (Figure 4B.7). However, for practical reasons, TA and luminal occlusion can only be assessed by imaging or catheterization, or histologically at the time of explant or autopsy. In addition, because the cardiac vasculature is a terminal circulation, patients with severe CAV are in immediate danger, as opposed to renal transplant patients who could feasibly return to dialysis. In the heart, TA is felt to be multi-factorial and attributable to both cell-mediated and humoral factors, as well as non-immune injury due to hypertension, metabolic derangements, perioperative ischemia, and infection. Interferon γ (IFNγ) is thought to be a critical mediator of CAV, originating from lymphocytes, macrophages, and even medial smooth muscle cells.

Chronic rejection in the lung

The lesions of chronic rejection in the lung consist of TA and a lesion occluding airways that is termed *obliterative bronchiolitis* (OB). OB describes edematous myofibroblastic obliteration of membranous and respiratory bronchioles, leading to partial or complete

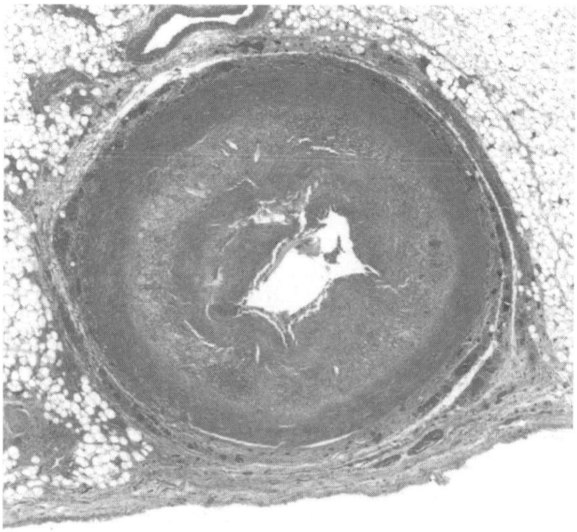

Figure 4B.7 Chronic rejection in heart allografts is generally best appreciated in angiographic studies, such as intravascular ultrasound, because the diagnostic lesion is in the small-to-large arteries not typically sampled in endomyocardial biopsies. TA is manifested in the heart by the same features as in other organs, namely, concentric intimal fibrosis leading to luminal stenosis and eventual occlusion with intramural chronic inflammation, as shown in this explant sample (Courtesy of Dr. J.R. Stone, Massachusetts General Hospital). See color section.

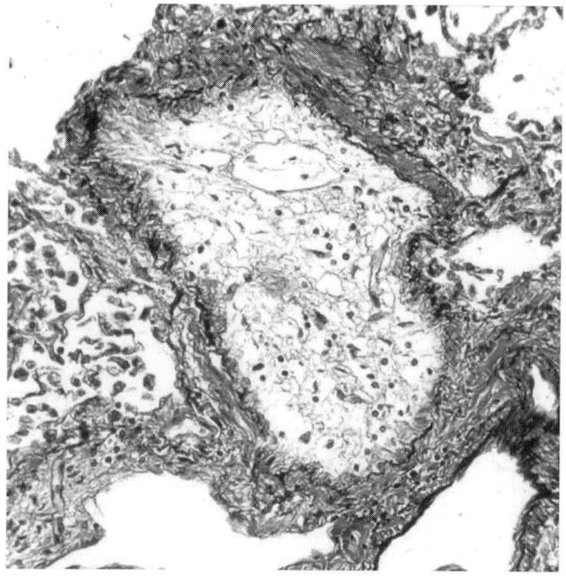

Figure 4B.8 In addition to TA, chronic rejection in the lung results in edematous myofibroblastic obliteration of a bronchiolar lumen, termed *obliterative bronchiolitis*, which can be identified in biopsies and has characteristic effects on pulmonary function (Courtesy of Dr. E.J. Mark, Massachusetts General Hospital). See color section.

luminal occlusion (Figure 4B.8). The fibrosis can also be more hyalinized, with an eccentric or concentric distribution, and is often associated with fragmentation and destruction of the smooth muscle and elastica of the airway wall. Mononuclear inflammation is frequently detected within the obliterative fibrosis. At times, the only clue to the previous presence of an airway is a focus of dense laminated fibrosis adjacent to a pulmonary artery. The pathogenesis of OB is probably a mixture of immune and non-immune mechanisms. In miniature pigs with MHC identical, minor-mismatched lung allografts, classic OB lesions develop. Although certain studies have shown evidence of acute antibody-mediated lung rejection, pulmonary CHR per se has not yet been specifically defined. However, DSA and autoantibodies have been associated with OB. OB was more frequent in patients with anti-HLA antibody and was preceded by circulating antibody. Pulmonary alveolar septal C4d and C3d deposition predicted graft failure and was correlated with bronchial wall fibrosis. In murine models, when anti-class I antibodies were introduced into native lungs via tracheal lavage, lesions resembling OB were induced. Experimental studies therefore support a possible role for antibodies in chronic rejection in the lung. TA in the lung is similar to that found in other solid organ transplants, with intimal fibrosis and a possible link to CHR.

Comments on treatment and reversibility

Several issues impede the treatment of chronic rejection: diagnostic accuracy, detection of activity, and availability of appropriate therapy. The availability of C4d staining and solid-phase antibody testing has improved the sensitivity and specificity of diagnosis of CHR. Standard histopathology, sometimes coupled with immunophenotyping of inflammatory cells, is helpful in the diagnosis of T-cell–mediated lesions. However, there is no test analogous to C4d to show the T cells' direct effect on graft tissue. When contemplating treatment of CHR, presence or absence of lesional activity (i.e., C4d deposition) is of great importance. For T-cell–mediated rejection, perhaps the best measure of activity would be detection of cytokines and cytotoxic molecules in tissue (e.g., granzyme B, IFNγ, and T-bet); however, this is not yet routinely available. Immunohistochemistry or immunofluorescence may prove useful, especially when multiple markers can be combined. Although staining for cytokines themselves is difficult, other possibilities include cytokine target detection (e.g., IDO for IFNγ, and Smad3 for transforming growth factor β) and cell proliferation markers (Ki67).

A major limitation is the current lack of effective treatment for chronic rejection. Agents in current use are primarily directed against acute rejection and thereby reduce recurrent or sustained episodes of acute rejection as a cause of eventual chronic rejection. They therefore indirectly have beneficial effects on the prevention of chronic rejection. Cellular pathways involved in chronic rejection need to be defined at the molecular level. Missing from our current repertoire are drugs that will halt antibody production at the level of the plasma cell, inhibit myofibroblast-related fibrosis, and restore cell longevity and tissue repair. Further exploration of additional and largely unknown pathways of chronic rejection is needed. Only when we have investigated these pathways and developed appropriate targeted agents will we be in a position to determine whether or not lesions of chronic rejection are indeed treatable and potentially reversible.

Further reading

Colvin RB. Pathology of chronic humoral rejection. *Contrib Nephrol* 2009; **162**: 75–86.

Gaston RS, Cecka JM, Kasiske BL, *et al.* Evidence for antibody-mediated injury as a major determinant of late kidney allograft failure. *Transplantation* 2010; **90**: 68–74.

Hill GS, Nochy D, Loupy A. Accelerated atherosclerosis: a form of transplant arteriopathy. *Curr Opin Organ Transplant* 2010; **15**: 11–15.

Mitchell RN. Graft vascular disease: immune response meets the vessel wall. *Ann Rev Pathol Mech Dis* 2009; **4**: 19–47.

Sis B, Halloran PF. Endothelial transcripts uncover a previously unknown phenotype: C4d-negative antibody-mediated rejection. *Curr Opin Organ Transplant* 2010; **15**: 42–8.

Weigt SS, Wallace WD, Derhovanessian A, *et al.* Chronic allograft rejection: epidemiology, diagnosis, pathogenesis, and treatment. *Semin Respir Crit Care Med* 2010; **31**: 189–207.

Zhang X, Reed EF. Effect of antibodies on endothelium. *Am J Transplant* 2009; **9**: 2459–65.

Chapter 4C

Major complications – infection

Camille Nelson Kotton

Key points

- Infections are among the most common complications after transplantation and greatly increase the morbidity and mortality of transplantation and decrease graft survival.
- Improved understanding of various infections, diagnostics, therapeutics, and prevention has allowed for improvement of outcomes after infection in transplant recipients.
- Prophylactic measures and medications can significantly decrease the risk of infection after transplantation.
- Pretransplant evaluation for latent infections and optimization of vaccination can help mitigate the risk of infection after transplant.

Infections are among the most common complications after transplantation and greatly increase the morbidity and mortality of transplantation while decreasing graft survival. New infections occur from acquisition of infections in the hospital, from the organ transplant or blood product donor, or in the community. Reactivation of latent infections encompasses another significant number of infections. In general, the intensity of immunosuppression is considered highest for a year after solid organ transplant and for 2 years after hematopoietic stem cell transplant. Clinically focused guidelines on diagnosis, treatment, and prevention of many infections after solid organ transplant have recently been published by the Infectious Disease Community of Practice of the American Society of Transplantation (2009).

A timeline of infection after transplantation has been described (Figure 4C.1). In the first month after organ transplant, infections tend to be related to the surgical procedure and hospital stay and include wound infection, anastomotic leaks and ischemia, aspiration pneumonia, catheter infection, and *Clostridium difficile* colitis. They are more likely to be due to resistant pathogens in this population with frequent health care exposure, including methicillin-resistant *Staphylococcus aureus* (MRSA), vancomycin-resistant *Enterococcus faecalis* (VRE), and non-*albicans Candida*. Donor-derived infections and recipient-derived infection due to prior colonization with agents such as *Aspergillus* or *Pseudomonas* may present in this phase.

The next 5 months are often the period when the classic opportunistic infections occur; their risk can be mitigated or delayed by prophylaxis and increased by intensified immunosuppression, leukopenia, or immunomodulatory (and usually endogenous) viral infections. Although relatively standard prophylaxis (e.g., trimethoprim-sulfamethoxazole and an antiviral [acyclovir or ganciclovir or related products]) mitigates the risk of many infections, certain infections are still seen, including BK reactivation, hepatitis C infection (HCV), adenovirus and influenza infections (especially seasonally), and *Cryptococcus neoformans* infection. Without prophylaxis, numerous additional infections are seen (especially those in the herpes virus family and hepatitis B [HBV]), as well as *Pneumocystis jiroveci* pneumonia and infections with *Listeria*, *Nocardia*, *Mycobacterium tuberculosis* (TB), *Toxoplasma*, *Strongyloides*, *Leishmania*, and *Trypanosoma cruzi* (*T. cruzi;* the etiologic agent of Chagas disease).

The stable and relatively healthy organ transplant recipient who is more than 6 months out

Organ Transplantation: A Clinical Guide, ed. A.A. Klein, C.J. Lewis, and J.C. Madsen. Published by Cambridge University Press.

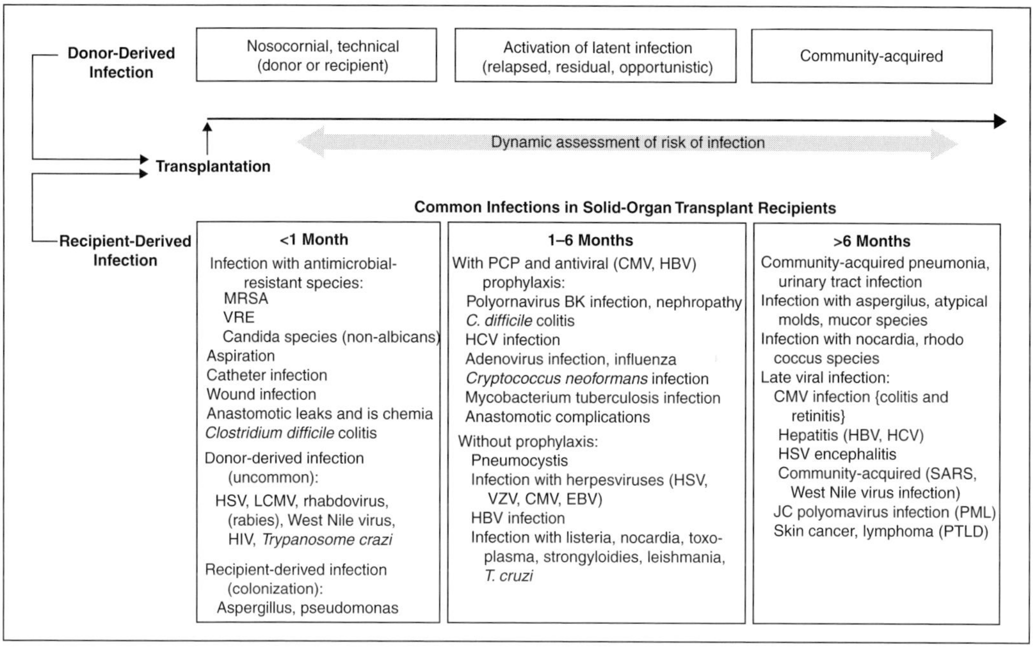

Figure 4C.1 Trends in the timings of infection after organ transplantation. Reproduced with permission from Fishman JA, Infection in solid-organ transplant recipients, *N Engl J Med* 2007; **357**: 2601–14. © Massachusetts Medical Society. All rights reserved.

from transplant tends to develop community-acquired or routine infections, including urinary tract infections, upper respiratory infections and pneumonia, gastroenteritis, and varicella zoster virus (VZV). Infections with unusual and opportunistic pathogens such as *Aspergillus*, unusual fungi, *Nocardia*, and *Rhodococcus* are still seen. In the era of effective prophylaxis with valganciclovir, an increased risk of late cytomegalovirus (CMV; occurring more than 6 months after organ transplant) has been noted, primarily in the few months after prophylaxis has been stopped. Other late viral infections include polyomavirus infections (from BK, causing nephropathy primarily in renal transplant recipients, or JC, causing progressive multifocal leukoencephalopathy) and Epstein-Barr virus (EBV)–related post-transplant lymphoproliferative infections.

Pretransplant evaluation can help mitigate the risk of some infections, especially latent ones. Knowledge of serostatus for CMV, EBV, HBV, and HCV can help optimize post-transplant management. Potential transplant recipients should be screened for latent TB, either by skin testing or use of the QuantiFERON-TB Gold (in vitro test for TB and latency). Recipients from or in endemic regions should be screened for latent infections such as *T. cruzi*, *Coccidioides*, and *Strongyloides*. Those seronegative for measles, mumps, rubella, hepatitis A and B, and varicella should undergo important pretransplant vaccination, as some are with live viral vaccines that can not be given after transplant when a recipient is significantly immunosuppressed, leaving them possibly permanently vulnerable to potentially life-threatening infection(s).

Atypical presentation of infection is more common in immunosuppressed hosts. Clinical presentations may be subtler, yet the patients more ill compared with normal hosts. For example, transplant recipients with West Nile virus infection are much more likely to have clinical illness and succumb to infection. Clinicians need to expand their differential diagnoses when caring for transplant recipients. Diagnosis of emerging, novel, and atypical pathogens is especially challenging in this vulnerable population, as has been seen with cases of lymphocytic choriomeningitis virus, tuberculosis, Chagas disease, strongyloidiasis, and numerous others.

The importance of donor-derived infections has been increasingly recognized in recent times. Such infection occurs in at least 1% of deceased donor organ transplants and are significantly higher in some organs, e.g., lung transplants. Although some transmission of some infections is expected, such as CMV and EBV, others have been a surprise to clinicians caring for patients. Such unanticipated donor-derived infections range from viruses such as rabies, lymphocytic choriomeningitis, and West Nile virus, to bacteria including bacteremias and tuberculosis, fungi including cryptococcosis and histoplasmosis, and parasites including *T. cruzi* (causing Chagas disease) and *Strongyloides*. Enhanced appreciation of donor-derived infections has resulted in better screening and use of diagnostics.

Post-transplant infections can be mitigated by preventative methods as described next in individual sections, as well as routine vaccinations, intake of clean food and water, preventative measures during times of outbreaks (as with severe acute respiratory syndrome [SARS] and H1N1 influenza), visits with travel medicine specialists prior to visiting high risk regions, safer sexual practices for non-monogamous recipients, and guidance on better tattoo acquisition.

Viruses

Viral infections are the most common type of infection after transplantation. They encompass a broad array of viruses, ranging from herpes to respiratory to hepatitis and other viruses. In addition to the direct effects (i.e., clinical syndromes) caused by viruses, they can be quite immunomodulatory, especially CMV, HCV, or EBV, resulting in both inflammation (perhaps mitigating graft tolerance) as well as increased immunosuppression (increasing the risk of infection from other opportunistic pathogens). Because many of the important viruses after transplantation remain latent, their ongoing management is a fine balance between optimal levels of immunosuppression and reactivation of infection.

The human herpes viruses (HHV) are the most common etiologic agents of infection after transplantation. The family includes eight viruses: herpes simplex type 1 and type 2 (HSV-1, -2), VZV, EBV, CMV, the roseola-like human herpes virus 6 and 7 (HHV-6, -7), and human herpes virus 8 (HHV-8, the etiologic agent of Kaposi's sarcoma). The alpha herpes virus family (HSV-1, -2, VZV) establishes latent infections primarily in sensory ganglia, whereas the beta herpes viruses (CMV, HHV-6, -7) maintain latency in leukocytes, endothelium, and other tissues, and the gamma herpes viruses (EBV and HHV-8) are latent in lymphoid tissue. Disseminated infection from any of the human herpes viruses can be life-threatening.

Numerous other types of viruses cause disease in transplant recipients. Respiratory viruses such as influenza, respiratory syncytial virus (RSV), adenovirus, parainfluenza, and human metapneumovirus are common and may present more subtly or with fulminate disease. Hepatitis viruses (primarily B and C) are common causes for liver transplantation and also common complications after transplant, predominantly as reactivation of latent infections. In addition, the primarily zoonotic hepatitis E has been reported as an emerging pathogen in transplant recipients. Most adults have latent infection with the polyoma viruses BK and JC. Although BK is predominantly a pathogen in kidney transplant recipients, it can cause disease in other transplant recipients. Risk of BK reactivation relates directly to the intensity of the immunosuppression, and early diagnosis of BK replication and subsequent reduction in the immunosuppressive regimen largely abrogates the risk of BK nephropathy, which generally has poor outcomes in kidney transplant recipients, with high rates of graft loss. JC virus causes progressive multifocal leukoencephalopathy, which is often mortal but fortunately is also fairly rare. Numerous other viruses have been shown to cause disease in transplant recipients, including parvovirus B19, West Nile virus, lymphocytic choriomeningitis virus, and others.

Viral diagnostics have improved exponentially with the onset of molecular techniques. Viral culture is progressively being replaced by more rapid and specific molecular assays. Within a matter of hours, various amplification methods can document active replicating viral infections. In the era of quantitative assays, trends in infection can be followed over time, as is seen with serial assays for response to CMV treatment or for BK viremia/viruria or EBV viremia. Molecular diagnostics have given us powerful assays for infections that were previously very challenging (or even impossible) to diagnose in this population, such as parvovirus B19, HHV-6 and -7, and others. Knowledge of serostatus for some viruses, such as CMV, EBV, and the hepatitis viruses, can be helpful in management. Immunohistochemistry can be very helpful for various herpes infections, including HSV, VZV, EBV, CMV, and HHV-8.

Effective treatment of viral infections may involve a multi-pronged approach: use of antiviral agents, reduction of immunosuppression when possible, and augmentation of immunity through the use of immunoglobulins and sometimes adoptive infusions of CMV-specific T cells. Common antiviral treatments include the acyclovir family (including famciclovir and valacyclovir, primarily for HSV and VZV infections), ganciclovir (with the oral prodrug valganciclovir for CMV and other infections), foscarnet (predominantly for resistant CMV), cidofovir (for resistant CMV, BK virus, and others), and ribavirin (for RSV and other less common infections). Hepatitis B has numerous antiviral agents for treatment, and hepatitis C is primarily treated with ribavirin and interferon. Reducing the intensity of immunosuppression (even transiently) may allow for more rapid clearance of a viral infection. Although not always well evidence-based, repleting recipients who have hypogammaglobulinemia with intravenous immunoglobulin may help clear infection. Some centers use CMV immunoglobulin in seronegative recipients with active disease. The novel use of adoptive infusions of CMV- or EBV-specific T cells has been shown to be effective especially in hematopoietic stem cell recipients and increasingly in organ transplant recipients.

Prevention of viral infections can be achieved by the use of antiviral medications, judicious use of immunosuppression, occasional use of immunoglobulins, careful monitoring, and vaccination. The most common antiviral medications used for prevention include the acyclovir family, primarily for HSV and VZV prophylaxis, and (val)/ganciclovir, which is targeted at CMV prevention but also successfully decreases the rates of other herpes virus infection to varying extents, as well as anti-hepatitis B agents. The duration of prevention varies considerably among institutions, but many programs use antivirals for 3–6 months after organ transplant (especially with high-risk situations where the donor is CMV seropositive and the recipient seronegative, or with lung transplant), often with either a ganciclovir family agent to prevent CMV or an acyclovir-type drug to prevent disseminated VZV infection. Although some organ transplant centers use antiviral agents in certain cohorts of patients at risk for CMV (termed *universal prophylaxis*), other use *preemptive therapy*, where treatment is begun only when routine monitoring tests show evidence of active infection. Guidelines for optimal management of CMV after solid organ transplant have been published. Because the severity of many viral infections relates to the intensity of immunosuppression, careful management of the regimen can result in a decreased risk of viral infections, especially with latent viruses. CMV immunoglobulin and HBV and VZV hyperimmune globulins have been shown to be effective in preventing infection in certain settings; repleting recipients with hypogammaglobulinemia with intravenous immunoglobulin can reduce their net risk of infection. In addition, periodic monitoring has been shown to be helpful, as with CMV, EBV, and BK viruses. Vaccination against influenza, hepatitis A and B, human papillomavirus, and other viral pathogens can provide additional protection.

Bacteria

Bacterial infections occur at increased frequency in the vulnerable transplant recipient. They range from routine infections such as urinary tract infections, pneumonias, and bacteremias to more exotic infections with *Nocardia*, *Rhodococcus*, *Listeria*, and other pathogens. Frequent exposure to health care settings increases the risk of resistant pathogens, including MRSA, VRE, *Pseudomonas*, *Stenotrophomonas*, and others. TB reactivates at much higher rates in those with renal and hepatic failure, as well as in the post-transplant period.

Diagnosis of bacterial infections still relies heavily on culture techniques. In order to optimize the diagnostic yield of cultures, clinicians should notify the laboratory when usual organisms are suspected, such as *Listeria*, *Rhodococcus*, TB, and *Nocardia*. Expanding the standard panel of antibiotic sensitivity at the time of initial diagnosis may help with subsequent therapy, especially given the increased risk of drug interactions and side effects, partly due to concomitant use of multiple medications (i.e., increased risks of leukopenia, nephrotoxicity, etc.). Molecular diagnostics are emerging as a diagnostic methodology for bacterial infections. Serologic techniques tend to yield diagnoses less frequently in this population due to a more muted immunological response. Histopathology, especially with special stains for microorganisms, can sometimes be helpful in achieving a diagnosis.

Treatment often begins in febrile or ill-appearing transplant recipients with empiric antibacterial therapy, which should be chosen based on local epidemiology. This approach appears to be justified by the significant incidence of bacteremia in the post-transplant period and by the concomitant high mortality rate when appropriate treatment is delayed, especially in infections caused by certain pathogens. Transplant patients are at higher risk for resistant pathogens, and the empiric antibiotic choice should reflect this. Once a culture diagnosis has been made and antibiotic susceptibilities are available, the antibiotic regimen may be tailored. Because of the increased rates of resistance, intravenous (IV) therapy is more common in this population, which requires the use of prolonged IV access. In general, arm veins should be avoided and preserved for future hemodialysis access in this population at higher risk for chronic kidney disease. Optimizing the drainage of collections via the use of radiographically or surgically placed drains may help clear infection and prevent recurrent infection. Preventative measures include eliminating any nidi of infection (such as IV catheters, skin defects that encourage abscess formation, etc.) and optimizing foci of recurrent infections (i.e., urinary tract infections). The use of trimethoprim-sulfamethoxazole after transplant to prevent *Pneumocystis* has the additional advantage of preventing other bacterial infections, ranging from *Streptococcus* to *Listeria* to *Nocardia* and many others. Vaccination against *Streptococcus pneumoniae, Clostridium tetani, Corynebacterium diphtheriae*, and other bacterial pathogens may provide additional protection.

Fungi

Invasive fungal disease, particularly aspergillosis, are significant causes of morbidity and mortality in transplant recipients and are among the most dreaded of the infectious complications. Although infections from *Candida* tend to be more manageable, infections such as zygomycosis have very high mortality rates. Iron overload in liver transplant recipients may explain their propensity to develop more fulminant disease presentation and a higher risk of disseminated disease due to a number of opportunistic infections, including invasive aspergillosis, cryptococcosis, and zygomycosis. Although these have a predilection to occur in the early post-transplant period, they may also occur years later, for example, *Pneumocystis jiroveci* and *Cryptococcus neoformans*, which may cause late meningitis.

Fungal diagnostics utilize dedicated fungal stains and culture as well as detection of fungal antigens in blood, urine, and other fluids. Fungi may be harder to grow in culture and harder to diagnose than other pathogens. A high level of suspicion, as well as multiple diagnostic approaches, is imperative in the diagnosis of these potential more elusive pathogens. Some pathogens such as *Candida* will usually grow on routine culture, whereas others require fungal culture media to promote growth. Fungal antigens, including the 1,3-β–D-glucan, galactomannan, and cryptococcal assays, have increased diagnostic capacity in recent times. The 1,3-β–D-glucan assay can be positive with a variety of fungal pathogens ranging from *Candida* to *Aspergillus* and numerous others including *Fusarium* spp., *Trichosporon* spp., *Saccharomyces cerevisiae, Acremonium, Coccidioides immitis, Histoplasma capsulatum, Sporothrix schenckii, Blastomyces dermatitidis*, and *Pneumocystis carinii*. The galactomannan antigen has been used on a variety of specimens and is relatively specific for *Aspergillus*. Serology may sometimes be helpful (i.e., *Coccidioides*). Histopathology can also provide diagnostic input, especially with special stains.

Treatment of fungal infections may involve use of one or more antifungal agents, as well as surgical debulking (especially with zygomycosis and sometimes aspergillosis). *Candida* infection may be treated with an azole (primarily fluconazole) or with an echinocandin (i.e., micafungin, caspofungin, anidulafungin). Depending on the individual pathogen, the filamentous fungal infections are treated with an amphotericin B product, often a lipid-based one for better tolerability, or with a higher level azole, such as voriconazole or posaconazole. The echinocandins are sometimes used in salvage regimens or as part of a multi-drug regimen, albeit with very little available data for multi-drug regimens in this setting. Antifungal susceptibilities are increasingly being used to guide optimal treatment, as is therapeutic drug monitoring for the higher level azoles. There are important drug interactions between the immunosuppressive agents (especially tacrolimus, cyclosporine [CyA], and sirolimus) and the azoles (especially the higher level ones), necessitating reductions in doses of the immunosuppressive agents. *P. jiroveci* is treated with agents such as trimethoprim-sulfamethoxazole, clindamycin, primaquine, atovaquone, and others.

Preventing fungal infections involves a combination of avoidance measures, filtered air systems in hospitals, recognition of existing infection or colonization, and evidence-based targeted antifungal prophylaxis. Fungal spores are ubiquitous in the environment. It is very rarely possible to reliably distinguish community-acquired from nosocomial aspergillosis. Transplant recipients should wear gloves while gardening or touching plants or soil, and they should avoid inhaling or creating soil or dust aerosols that may contain fungal spores. They may wish to wear well-fitting face masks (FFP2/N95 masks) in some unavoidable situations and should always wash their hands after such contact and care for skin abrasions or cuts sustained during soil or plant contact. Invasive fungal infections in the explanted lungs, more common in those with cystic fibrosis, are often not recognized before lung transplantation and have been associated with poor outcomes; similarly, airway colonization with fungus in other organ recipients may blossom into a full infection after transplant; thus knowledge of culture data at or before the time of transplant may help target therapy and mitigate infection. Antifungal prophylaxis varies broadly among transplant centers; in general, most centers would only give prophylaxis against *Aspergillosis* and other fungi for a relatively brief period, if at all. Many centers recommend prophylaxis against *P. jiroveci*, often with trimethoprim-sulfamethoxazole, atovaquone, or dapsone. Adherence to avoidance measures, acknowledging their limitations, combined with antifungal prophylaxis, is likely to be the most effective approach to prevent invasive fungal disease.

Parasites

Parasitic infections tend to be less common than the previously mentioned pathogens. The more clinically significant parasites include *Toxoplasma gondii, Strongyloides stercoralis, T. cruzi, Leishmania*, and intestinal parasites. The incidence of parasitic infection is anticipated to increase in transplant recipients due to multiple factors, including increases in active organ transplant programs in geographic areas where parasitic infections are highly prevalent; increases in travel and migration of donors and recipients from endemic areas, with latent or asymptomatic infections, as well as patients from developed countries undergoing transplantation in endemic areas (transplant tourism); increases in leisure tourism to endemic regions by transplant recipients; and decreases in CyA-based immunosuppressive regimens and the increased use of newer drugs that lack the anti-parasitic effects of CyA metabolites.

Diagnosis of parasitic infections in solid organ transplant recipients can be complex. Depending on the parasite, a variety of techniques may be used, ranging from rapid diagnostics on stool, peripheral blood smears (*Babesia*, malaria, *T. cruzi*), special stains and microscopic exam of various specimens or tissues (blood, stool, biopsy), culture, serology (which may be less helpful in this population), and histopathology. Molecular diagnostics, when available, can be quite helpful. Use of clinical measures such as eosinophilia may be muted in this population, in whom the immunosuppressive regimen (especially steroids) may cause false-negative results.

Treatment of individual parasitic infections can involve medications that may interact with transplant medications, or have significant side effects, and should be used carefully. Immunocompromised hosts are more likely to have relapses of certain parasitic infections (i.e., *Babesia, T. cruzi, Strongyloides*) and should be monitored after treatment.

Parasitic infections can be prevented by avoiding ingestion of contaminated food and water (predominantly for intestinal pathogens), by screening recipients for latent infection prior to transplant as well as organ and blood product donors in endemic regions (i.e., toxoplasmosis, Chagas disease, malaria, babesiosis), and by use of preventative medications such as trimethoprim-sulfamethoxazole (used chronically to prevent *T. gondii* infection) or ivermectin (to treat active or latent *Strongyloides*). Once a more common infection after solid organ transplant, toxoplasmosis has become a largely preventable disease in the era of trimethoprim-sulfamethoxazole or atovaquone prophylaxis. Use of anti-malarial prophylaxis in endemic regions is recommended for all transplant recipients. Avoidance of tick and other insect bites will also decrease risk of transmission.

Infections tend to occur in fairly predictable phases after solid organ transplant. Although many of the classic opportunistic infections occur in the first 6 months, during what is usually the period of most intense immunosuppression, the risk of such infection remains for the duration of time that the recipient is on immunosuppressive medications. The risk of infection is decreased by the use of prophylaxis and augmented by the use of more potent immunosuppression (both in the induction and maintenance phases, as well as during treatment of rejection), allograft rejection, concomitant infections, leucopenia, and technical surgical issues.

Further reading

American Society of Transplantation Infectious Diseases Guidelines 2nd Edition. *Am J Transplant* 2009; **9**: S1–S281.

Fishman JA. Infection in solid-organ transplant recipients. *N Engl J Med* 2007; **357**: 2601–14.

Ison MG, Hager J, Blumberg E, *et al.* Donor-derived disease transmission events in the United States: data reviewed by the OPTN/UNOS Disease Transmission Advisory Committee. *Am J Transplant* 2009; **9**: 1929–35.

Jong EC, Freedman DO. Chapter 8: Advising Travelers with Specific Needs: The Immunocompromised Traveler. *2010 Health Information for International Travel.* 2010 ed, Atlanta, GA: Centers for Disease Control and Prevention. Available at: http://wwwnc.cdc.gov/travel/yellowbook/2010/chapter-8/immunocompromised-traveler.aspx (accessed January 14, 2011).

Kotton CN, Kumar D, Caliendo AM, *et al.* International Consensus Guidelines on the Management of Cytomegalovirus in Solid Organ Transplantation. *Transplantation* 2010; **89**: 779.

Chapter 5

Organ donor management and procurement

Edward Cantu III and David W. Zaas

Key points

- Traumatic brain injury accounts for one third of all trauma-related deaths; however, only 20% of these potential donors become actual donors.
- Somatic organ donor identification, management, and procurement requires intensive coordinated effort in order to abrogate the negative consequences of brainstem death and avoid donor loss.
- Physiological derangements during the process of brain death are induced via diffuse vascular regulatory perturbation and metabolic cellular injury.
- Care of potential donors is goal-directed, with emphasis on minimizing further brain injury by maximizing cerebral perfusion and preventing or treating systemic morbidity.
- Interest in non–heart-beating donors and ex vivo perfusion systems continues to grow and may make significantly more organs available.

In many patients with end-stage organ dysfunction, solid organ transplantation has emerged as the treatment of choice; however, the paucity of suitable organ donors has placed severe limits on the number of transplants being performed. Given the limitation of available organ donors and number of deaths on the waiting list, many transplant programs have expanded selection criteria to include older, higher risk donors in order to offer transplants to more patients. Despite the increased use of higher risk donors, outcomes have continued to improve as experience has accrued. Unfortunately, the number of patients awaiting transplantation continues to grow at a faster rate than the number of available donors.

The number of potential donors in the United States is believed to be between 10 000 and 14 000 per year, with actual donation rates at about 26 donors per million population. The United Kingdom remains relatively low at 15 donors per million population, although steps are in place to try to increase rates of donation. Spain has the highest rate of cadaveric organ donation of any country, with an annual donor rate of 30–35 donors per million population. This is due to a unique organizational model that has been implemented in other countries, with similar though somewhat less success (see Chapters 40 and 41). The percentage of donors utilized for lung transplant in the United States is only 19%, significantly lower than most other countries. Concerns about the risk for poor outcomes create conservative practice styles, but also increase the number of deaths on the waiting list.

Reasons for limited recovery of organs include (1) failure to identify potential donors, (2) inability to obtain consent for donation, (3) donor loss due to cardiovascular collapse, and (4) unsuitability of organ(s) for transplantation. This chapter discusses the physiological changes of brain death, the management of these complex patients, the organization of the recovery, and new technologies that may allow increased number of organs available for transplantation.

Physiology of brain and brainstem death

Brain death has been defined as the complete and irreversible cessation of all brain and brainstem function. Diagnosis is usually made by clinical examination documenting no brainstem reflexes and a lack of spontaneous respiratory effort. Several confounders

Organ Transplantation: A Clinical Guide, ed. A.A. Klein, C.J. Lewis, and J.C. Madsen. Published by Cambridge University Press.

must also be ruled out, including hypothermia (<32°C) and drug or metabolic intoxication. However, the legal definition does vary from state to state and country to country.

As the brain is dying, physiological derangements are induced via two major mechanisms, the first being through a diffuse vascular regulatory perturbation and the second through a diffuse metabolic cellular injury. Severe alterations in endocrine function, immunology, and coagulopathy also commonly manifest. These diffuse physiological insults contribute to numerous complications that compromise end-organ function and result in significant donor loss; therefore, a thorough understanding of the events leading to and following brain death must be clearly understood.

Most lethal brain injuries follow a common pathway whereby a patient suffers brainstem death secondary to sudden or gradual increases in intracranial pressure (ICP). The mass effect from the initial injury self-potentiates, with further progression of ischemia, venous congestion, and edema subsequently leading to more mass effect. The brainstem is compromised by arterial compression when it herniates through the foramen magnum, further promoting ischemia and edema, resulting in continued increases in ICP until cessation of cerebral blood flow occurs.

A characteristic sequence of physiological changes occurs as ischemia propagates caudally from the cerebrum to the spinal cord. Pontine ischemia leads to a mixed sympathetic and vagal stimulation resulting in hypertension and bradycardia, commonly referred to as the "Cushing reflex." This, in turn, is followed by an unopposed sympathetic stimulation as ischemia progresses more caudally to the distal medulla oblongata, involving the vagal nuclei. This period is characterized by severe hypertension and tachycardia, often referred to as "sympathetic storm." Finally, as herniation is completed and ischemia of the spinal cord occurs, there is a progressive loss of spinal sympathetic stimulation, leading to a loss of all vascular tone, hypotension, and cardiovascular collapse. Homeostatic control pathways mediated by the hypothalamus and pituitary axis are also lost, resulting in endocrine and cellular metabolic dysfunction. Although many lethal brain injuries follow these typical changes, there is some variability with respect to time course, speed of deterioration, and time spent at each stage. This is likely due to etiology of brain injury, clinical treatments, and biological variability.

Cardiovascular changes

Cardiac function is reduced after brain death, which has been attributed to catecholamine cardiotoxicity. The myocardial damage and morphological changes seen after brain death (myocytolysis, contraction band necrosis, subendocardial hemorrhage, edema, and interstitial mononuclear cell infiltration) are similar to those described after high-dose catecholamine infusion. Further, these changes could be abrogated by total cardiac sympathectomy before cerebral insult. The extreme sympathetic surge seen after vagal nuclear death leads to profound increases in circulating catecholamines and have been shown to correlate with the speed of ICP elevation. In animal models evaluating rate of increase in ICP, it has been demonstrated that slow gradual increases in ICP resulted in 175-fold increase in epinephrine and a 40-fold increase in norepinephrine plasma levels, with only mild ischemic injury to the myocardium, whereas rapid increases in ICP resulted in 750-fold and 400-fold increase in epinephrine and norepinephrine plasma levels accompanied by extensive ischemic injury to the myocardium. This sympathetic surge increases myocardial oxygen demand and results in large increases in intracellular calcium, leading to impaired high-energy phosphate production and increased free-radical generation, leading to further cellular damage.

Morphometric analysis has demonstrated contraction band necrosis in 89% of inpatients without previous heart disease who have succumbed to brain death. Furthermore, myocardial gene expression in animal models has also demonstrated significant perturbation after brain death. The sympathetic storm seen initially followed by massive loss of vasomotor tone are related by time course and severity. Experiments evaluating velocity of ICP and time to cardiovascular collapse noted that in the rapid elevation group, death occurred within 1 hour, whereas in the gradual elevation group, animals survived until the experiments were terminated at 3 hours. Further studies by other groups discovered that rapid induction of brain death resulted in more precipitous decrease in systemic vascular tone, which could be mitigated by volume infusion.

Hemodynamic instability seen after brain death is also consequent to loading conditions imposed on the heart. Additional evidence from animal studies has shown that profound vasodilation and afterload reduction results in reduced coronary perfusion pressure, relative intravascular hypovolemia, and decreased preload. In canine cross-circulation studies, if loading conditions and coronary perfusion pressure were kept constant, no cardiac dysfunction was seen. Coronary blood flow is reduced secondary to dysfunction of endothelial-dependent vasodilatory mechanisms after brain death, but the significance of this finding is not settled. It is likely that because of alterations in loading conditions, profound vasodilatation, and loss of autoregulatory control in coronary arteries, deterioration of cardiac function is even seen in donors without pre-existing cardiovascular disease.

Pulmonary changes

The physiological changes of brain death have direct and indirect effects on lung function. The direct effects are related to neurogenic pulmonary edema and inflammatory acute lung injury. The indirect effects are secondary to respiratory complications of severe brain injury (pneumonia, aspiration, pulmonary contusion, and barotraumas). Neurogenic pulmonary edema was initially recognized at autopsy in combat casualties who had traumatic brain injuries. This constellation of pulmonary microvascular hemorrhage and pulmonary edema has also been documented in patients who experience sudden death after intracranial hemorrhage. The pathological mechanism results from the sympathetic storm seen in brain death. Unopposed catecholamine excess results in systemic vasoconstriction, which in turn increases left ventricular afterload and end-diastolic pressure. Accordingly, the left atrial pressure rises, resulting in shunting of blood to the central compartment. Together with increased pulmonary vasoconstriction, pulmonary capillary pressures experience dramatic increases, resulting in pulmonary edema and hemorrhage due to the significantly elevated hydrostatic pressure and mechanical disruption of the endothelium.

There is also some evidence that α-adrenergic receptor stimulation may cause an increase in pulmonary capillary permeability independent of its hemodynamic effects. Several studies have demonstrated that α-adrenergic receptor blockade reduced systemic inflammation and preserved capillary-alveolar membrane integrity.

Acute inflammatory lung injury has been experimentally induced after cerebral hemorrhage in animal models. Circulating levels of tissue factor and increased intracellular adhesion molecule expression have been documented, resulting in progressive neutrophil recruitment and alveolar disruption seen in the lung. In rats, traumatic brain injury has demonstrated increased lipid peroxidation and intracellular membrane damage in type II pneumocytes. Additionally, structural damage to tracheal-bronchial epithelium (and possibly airway defense mechanisms) has been seen and may help explain why there is such a high airway complication rate after severe head injury.

Endocrine changes

Many hormonal changes have been noted after brain death and are consequent to the loss of the hypothalamic–hypophyseal axis. The most common and immediate manifestation is the early depletion of anti-diuretic hormone (ADH) and development of diabetes insipidus. Greater than 75% of brain death donors have undetectable levels of ADH. This leads to inappropriate diuresis of dilute urine, resulting in severe hypovolemia, hyperosmolarity, and hypernatremia.

The anterior pituitary receives some of its blood supply from the inferior hypophyseal artery, a branch off the extradural internal carotid artery. In animal models, brain death results in rapid decrease in free triiodothyronine (T3) from diminished peripheral conversion of tetraiodothyronine (T4) and impaired thyroid-stimulating hormone (TSH) secretion. Decreased circulating T3 is thought to play a role in the deterioration of cardiac function after brain death. Furthermore, studies in pigs and baboons demonstrated that decreased T3 levels are associated with changes in cellular energy utilization due to the conversion from aerobic to anaerobic metabolism. Administration of T3 in animal studies has been shown to enhance cardiovascular function with abrogation of hemodynamic collapse and improvement in myocardial contractile function. However, in human studies there have been conflicting results, and a recent clinical trial demonstrated no efficacy with respect to cardiac performance or heart retrieval rate with infusion of intravenous T3.

Plasma cortisol levels are relatively preserved in most brain dead donors; however, the capacity to increase secretion with adrenocorticotropic hormone stimulation appears attenuated. The clinical significance of this is not entirely known.

Immediately after brain death, plasma insulin levels begin to decrease, leading to increased extracellular glucose concentration, shift toward anaerobic metabolism, and acidosis. Coupled with the ongoing resuscitation with free water to combat hypernatremia that typically occurs, this insulin deficiency can quickly lead to profound increases in osmolarity, excessive diuresis, and hypovolemia.

Inflammatory and immunological changes

A generalized inflammatory state has been documented after severe brain injury and brain death, with increased serum levels of several cytokines such as interleukin (IL)-6, IL-8, IL-1β, IL-2R and tumor necrosis factor alpha (TNF-α). Increased expression of IL-6 and TNF-α in donor hearts has been correlated with donor heart dysfunction. Furthermore, increased cytokine levels in blood and kidneys of brain death donors are predictive of worse short- and long-term outcomes as compared with living unrelated donors. Diffuse cytokine-stimulated inflammatory responses have been documented in all organ systems evaluated. Upregulated adhesion molecule expression and leukocyte adhesion and activation has been demonstrated. This increased cytokine release results in further inflammation and increase major histocompatibility complex (MHC) expression on donor cells, which increases its immunogenicity. This has been confirmed by more frequent higher grade rejection occurrence rates in organs from donors after brain death than those of living donors.

Although increased cytokine levels have been documented, there remains uncertainty regarding the cell of origin of these cytokines. It is likely that contributions from multiple sources (endothelial cells, platelets, circulating leucocytes, and brain) result in the pro-inflammatory states seen. It is also likely that the hemodynamic perturbations seen with severe brain injury and brain death lead to ischemic changes within end organs, which also contribute to the inflammatory state.

Other systemic perturbations

Temperature regulation is significantly altered, with loss of hypothalamic control. Hypothermia is not uncommon in brain death donors consequent to peripheral dilatation and decreased metabolic rate. Severe brain injury results in blood–brain barrier compromise and release of large amounts of tissue factor. Circulating tissue factor coupled with systemic inflammation and endothelial activation results in consumptive coagulopathy in up to 28% of brain death donors.

Optimization of donor organ function for donation after brain death (DBD)

Initial resuscitative measures

Traumatic brain injury occurs every 7 seconds and results in death every 5 minutes, making it the largest cause of brain death in the United States. Traumatic brain injury accounts for one third of all trauma-related deaths. Unfortunately, only 20% of these potential donors become actual donors. This is in part the result of marked pathophysiological changes experienced by the brain-injured patient and the extremely labor-intensive management required to support these patients prior to organ recovery. These patients are typically treated in the intensive care unit, according to evidence-based guidelines advocated by the Brain Trauma Foundation in the United States. Care is goal-directed, with emphasis on minimizing further brain injury by maximizing cerebral perfusion and preventing or treating systemic morbidity. This may include but may not be limited to supporting blood pressure, reducing ICP, maintaining euthermia and euglycemia, maintaining adequate intravascular volume, and correcting anemia and coagulopathy. The goal during this phase of care is brain protection.

Once brain death has been diagnosed, the emphasis of patient care changes based on patient and family preference. The challenge is to recognize lethal or irreversible brain injury prior to other end-organ damage. During the 1990s, potential donor identification rates improved significantly. This improvement was likely the result of implementation of the Medicare Conditions of Participation requirements of hospitals, which required deaths to be reported to organ-procurement organizations for evaluation and that request for organ donation be made by specially trained personnel. This also, in part, has contributed to the improvement in conversion rate (ratio of actual donors/potential donors) seen from 33% in 1990 to 66% in 2008. Increasing conversion rate is one way to address the current organ shortage.

Post-consent donor management

Consent to organ donation realigns care to that of end-organ preservation and prevention of somatic donor loss. Prior to consent, treatment may require many strategies that result in end-organ damage and

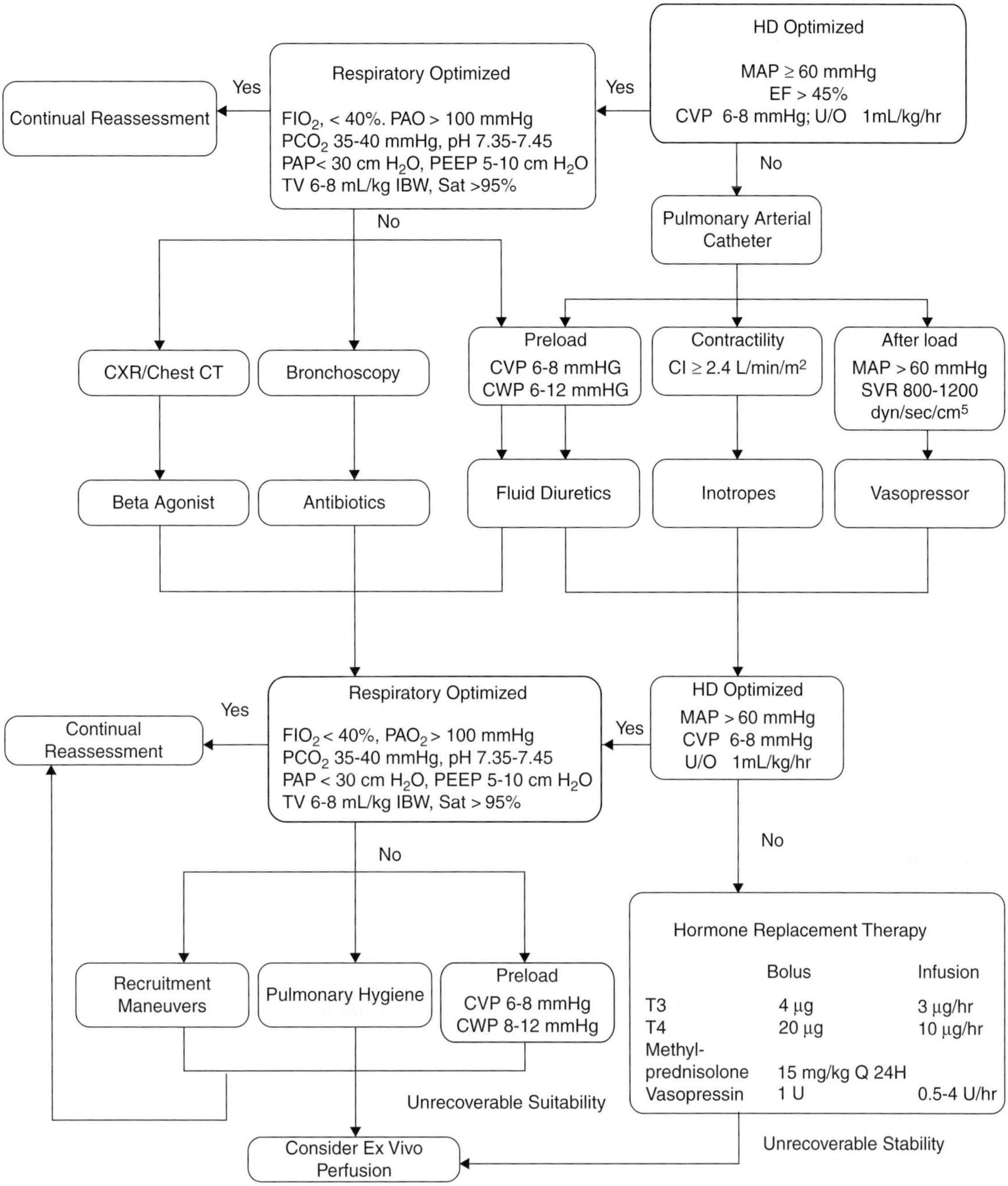

Figure 5.1 Donor management algorithm (modified from Wood *et al*., 2004).

increase the risk of organ dysfunction after transplant (Figure 5.1). The period between consent for donation and organ procurement can be tumultuous, and it requires intense medical management to avoid somatic donor loss. Up to 20% of potential donors are lost during this timeframe, and risk of loss increases with time from brain death. Therefore, care must be delivered in a timely, efficient, and standardized manner. The following sections will specifically address donor management concepts in sequence, which ordinarily are addressed at the same time.

Cardiovascular management

As previously discussed, brain death may result in severe cardiovascular perturbations as a consequence of cardiac dysfunction and loss of vasomotor tone. Therefore, the central goal in donor management is to maintain hemodynamic stability with good end-organ perfusion while maintaining euvolemia with minimal to no inotropic or pressor support. Generally, care occurs within the intensive care unit, where arterial and central venous pressure monitoring is available. Continual reassessment is the rule, with targeted mean arterial pressure ≥60 mmHg, central venous pressure (CVP) 6–8 mmHg, and urine output ≥1 ml/kg/hr.

Echocardiographic assessment should be obtained in all potential heart donors. This provides valuable information regarding heart function and structural abnormalities that may complicate donor management and/or preclude heart donation. It is important to recognize that early poor cardiac function may improve with time and should not in and of itself preclude heart donation. Many centers, but particularly in patients with depressed cardiac function (ejection fraction <45%) or hemodynamic instability, use pulmonary artery catheterization to assess ventricular loading conditions (ideally capillary wedge pressure 8–12 mmHg, CVP 6–8 mmHg), cardiac contractile function (cardiac index ≥ 2.4 l/min/m^2), and vasomotor tone (systemic vascular resistance 800–1200 dyne/s/cm^5); see Figure 5.1. This aggressive approach has resulted in significant improvements in hemodynamics, somatic donor salvage, and organ recovery rates.

Hypotension is the most common clinical scenario encountered, with incidence of up to 80% and the most common precipitator of cardiac arrest and somatic loss. Twenty percent of donors may remain hypotensive despite vasoactive drug support, with this being more common in donors who are hypovolemic or who have diabetes insipidus and who are not on vasopressin. Therefore, it is imperative to continuously reevaluate volume status, contractile function, and vasomotor tone.

With low CVP and hypotension, volume should be administered. Colloid or crystalloid should be used based on clinical scenario. For example, if the hematocrit is less than 30%, then packed red blood cells should be transfused. If the donor is hypernatremic and acidotic, bicarbonate buffered (50 mmol/l) half-normal saline should be administered. Care should be taken when administering large amounts of glucose-containing free water when treating hypernatremia, because this may precipitate hyperglycemia, resulting in osmotic diuresis, further hypovolemia, and electrolyte disorders. In these situations, insulin infusion should be maintained to achieve target glucose levels between 80 and 150 mg/dl. Also, care must be taken when administering hydroxyethyl starch, which has been implicated in injury to renal tubular cells and early renal graft dysfunction. Given the high incidence of temperature dysregulation seen in donors, all fluids should be warmed to 37°C.

Euvolemic donors with hypotension require vasoactive drug support. The choice between inotrope and pressor is dependent on cardiac function. If cardiac function is preserved and the donor is experiencing loss of vasomotor tone, then dopamine, vasopressin, or phenylephrine can be used based on the specific clinical scenario. The use of any one particular agent is not based on randomized clinical trials, but rather on individual opinion, which varies widely. However, norepinephrine has traditionally been avoided, and vasopressin has traditionally been the first choice in this clinical scenario. That being said, in most donors, homodynamic stability can be maintained with volume replacement and moderate doses of dopamine (0–5 μg/kg/min). Requirements higher than 10 μg/kg/min may require the addition of additional vasoactive support and suggest serious cardiac dysfunction.

There are no guidelines for specific combinations of vasoactive drugs. Clearly, combinations of drugs that work synergistically and decrease dosages of each agent (thereby reducing the α-adrenergic effects) are beneficial. With respect to kidney transplantation, this strategy has resulted in decreased rates of acute rejection and improved graft survival. Catecholamine excess, as seen during sympathetic storm or when administered to experimental animals in very high concentrations, results in damage to the myocardium, as previously described. For this reason, many donors who are on high doses of catecholamines are not used by cardiac surgeons. There is some evidence, however, that the combination of dopamine and norepinephrine, even at high doses, has resulted in excellent outcomes in heart recipients. Unfortunately, there are also data that demonstrate increased incidence of primary graft dysfunction, reduced right ventricular contractility, and reduced 1-year survival with use of norepinephrine. Currently, there are no data conclusively demonstrating superiority of one vasopressor over another. However, the dominant opinion is the norepinephrine should be studiously avoided due to its β-adrenergic effects.

In the event that hemodynamic stability cannot be achieved with volume optimization and combination vasopressor therapy, hormone replacement therapy should be initiated early. As previously discussed, the hypothalamic–pituitary axis becomes dysfunctional, resulting in depletion of ADH and insulin and decreases in thyroid hormone and relative cortisol levels. Early practice utilized a combination of vasopressin, insulin, thyroid hormone, and steroids. Today, insulin is begun prior to brain death and vasopressin is begun once diabetes insipidus is recognized or as a pressor agent for hypotension. Although use of thyroid hormone is controversial, in the scenario in which donor loss is inevitable, if hemodynamic stability is not achieved, thyroid hormone is reasonable. Dramatic improvement in hemodynamics and acid–base status and improvement in the rate of organ recovery have been demonstrated with T3 infusion (4-μg bolus followed by 3 μg/hr). Similarly, steroid administration (methylprednisolone 15 mg/kg bolus repeated every 24 hours) may enhance vascular reactivity and is associated with improved short- and long-term outcome for most transplanted organs.

Arrhythmias are common and difficult to treat. They can be a result of catecholamine surge during herniation or initiation of pharmacological drug support or as a terminal event after brain death 48–72 hours later. Atrial and ventricular tachyarrhythmias can be treated with amiodarone. Bradyarrhythmias do not respond to atropine and must be treated with epinephrine or isoproterenol. Cardiac arrest is treated as in non–brain-dead individuals with advanced cardiac life support protocols because recovery of cardiac function will allow for organ donation.

Respiratory management

The medical optimization of respiratory function in brain death donors has not been rigorously evaluated by clinical trials. The medical suitability of lungs for procurement lags significantly behind that of all other solid organs. Published results from one institution comparing lung procurement with that of all other solid organs using the same potential donor population demonstrated a conversion rate of 17% and 70%, respectively. This huge disparity is mainly the result of the myriad of pulmonary complications that occur in this patient population, which include aspiration pneumonia, trauma, inflammatory mediated acute lung injury, and neurogenic pulmonary edema. However, standardized goal-directed therapy has improved conversion rates without jeopardizing other organs for recovery.

Most guidelines advocate a lung-protective strategy with judicious use of fluid for resuscitation and aggressive pulmonary toilet in order to optimize gas exchange and maintenance of adequate hemodynamics. Low-pressure ventilation with end-inspiratory pressures <30 cm of water, tidal volumes of 6–8 ml/kg, moderate amounts of positive end-expiratory pressure (5–10 cm of water), and the lowest fraction of inspired oxygen possible that achieves PaO2 > 100 mmHg are recommended. Bronchoscopy, frequent suctioning, and recruitment maneuvers counteract mechanical reasons for poor gas exchange and have also been demonstrated to improve lung recovery.

Early management of the somatic donor often requires adjustments to minute ventilation in order to normalize carbon dioxide levels (often resulting in a rise in carbon dioxide), reduce barotrauma, and improve oxygen extraction (allow oxyhemoglobin curve to shift to the right). Furthermore, judicious use of diuretics may be necessary to decrease CVP to 6–8 mmHg and/or pulmonary capillary wedge pressure to 8–12 mmHg, as the lungs will be exquisitely sensitive to small hydrostatic pressure changes given the inflammatory and neurogenic lung injury so common in brain death donors. Additionally, evidence from animal and ex vivo studies suggests that inhalation of a beta agonist may accelerate the rate of alveolar fluid clearance. Steroids abrogate the inflammatory effects of brain death and have been demonstrated to reduce fluid accumulation in the lung and be the most significant predictor of successful lung donation in multivariate analysis of lung procurement. All somatic donors should receive steroids as soon as possible after brain death.

Organization of procurement

After brain death has been certified and consent has been obtained, the recovery time is determined and procurement teams are notified. Aggressive donor care continues in the operating room. The donor is placed supine on the operating table with arms tucked and is prepped from chin to knees. A midline incision from sternal notch to pubis is made. What follows next is a description of the thoracic recovery.

The sternum is divided, the pericardium opened, and a pericardial cradle created. The heart and lungs are inspected and assessment of organ suitability is communicated to the implanting surgeon. Mobilization of the superior vena cava (SVC), inferior vena cava (IVC), intra-atrial groove, aorta, and pulmonary artery is performed. Once the abdominal procurement teams have completed their dissection, 30 000 U of heparin is administered intravenously. Purse-string sutures are placed in the ascending aorta and pulmonary artery and perfusion cannulas are placed. The azygous vein is ligated and divided. Five hundred micrograms of prostaglandin E1 is injected into the pulmonary artery. The SVC is ligated or clamped distal to the azygous vein. The left heart is vented through the left inferior pulmonary vein (or the left atrial appendage if the lungs are being procured) and the IVC is vented at the pericardial reflection. The aortic cross clamp is applied and the heart and lungs are perfused with 4°C preservation solutions. Crushed ice is placed over both the heart and lungs. Care is taken to ensure no dilatation of the heart occurs and the lungs blanche. After arrest has occurred, completion of the cardiectomy takes place. The SVC is divided distal to the azygous, taking care not to injure the right pulmonary artery. Next, the IVC is divided at the pericardial reflection. The aorta and pulmonary arteries are then divided, with sufficient length for subsequent transplantation of both the heart and lungs. The apex of the heart is then elevated, and midway between the coronary sinus and the pulmonary veins, the left atrium is divided. This division is carried around the left atrium, maintaining adequate cuff for both heart and lung teams. The heart is then removed and inspected and preservation solution infused into the coronary arteries prior to placement in two cold saline–filled bags and then a hard container of ice for transport.

Ventilation continues with room air. The lung team then retrograde flushes the pulmonary vein with the cold preservation fluid to remove any pulmonary emboli. Next the trachea is identified and divided and stapled with the lungs at almost maximal inflation, 2–3 rings above the carina. Lastly, heavy scissors are used to quickly divide all posterior mediastinal tissue just anterior to the esophagus. The lungs are then removed, inspected, and bagged for transport. The implanting surgeon is notified of cross-clamp time and expected time of arrival.

Abdominal organs

Maintenance of cardiac output following confirmation of death allows a significant proportion of dissection to be performed prior to cold perfusion with preservation solution ("warm dissection"). This has the distinct advantage that important structures are much easier to identify and can be prepared with greater precision, minimizing organ damage and shortening dissection following perfusion ("cold dissection"), during which suboptimal cooling of the organs may occur. A midline laparotomy and sternotomy is performed and can be extended using transverse abdominal incisions to maximize surgical access. A full exploratory laparotomy is undertaken to exclude intra-abdominal sepsis or malignancy, and any suspicious lesions are biopsied and sent for urgent histological analysis. Early assessment of renal and liver quality is performed, in particular the degree of steatosis and, in cases of donor death secondary to trauma, exclusion of liver injury. The procurement of the liver is discussed in detail in Chapter 22. Both kidneys are inspected for transplant suitability; however, if only one kidney is required, the left is preferred because the renal vein is longer, making recipient transplantation easier to perform. Multiple renal arteries exist in approximately 20% of potential donors, and removal of the kidney with a single renal artery is preferred (cadaveric donor nephrectomy is discussed further in Chapter 29).

Non–heart-beating donors

Despite efforts to expand the donor pool, there still remains a significant shortage of donor organs. In an effort to make more organs available for transplantation, the transplantation community, government regulators, and United Network for Organ Sharing have reintroduced policies for the donation of organs after cardiac death. Historically, organs were recovered from non–heart-beating donors, also termed *donation after cardiac death* (DCD); however, the introduction of the concept of brain death decreased enthusiasm for this population of donors, given the numerous uncertainties involved. Recently, mounting pressure to make more organs available has renewed interest in DCD (see Chapter 41).

Ex vivo perfusion

In our current era, more organs are procured from older, marginal, and non–heart-beating donors than ever before. From 1988–2009, there has been a 630% increase in donors greater than 50 years of age and an 800% increase in donors who experienced a cardiovascular cause of death. Given the increased use of higher risk donors and DCD, improvements in organ preservation techniques are required to help expand the number of suitable donors.

Today, most centers use static cold storage as the preferred organ preservation method. Static cold storage begins after cold perfusion of a preservative solution (varies by center and organ) to displace blood components within the vasculature and to achieve a hypothermic equilibrium within the organ. In the early 1960s, cooling alone was demonstrated to be an effective preservation strategy. Metabolic rate is halved by each 10°C drop in temperature, reaching its nadir at about 10% of normal at 4°C. Unfortunately, impaired activity of the Na^+/K^+ ATPase results in passive sodium entry to the cell and consequent cell swelling. Cell swelling, acidosis secondary to metabolic shifts, and generation of reactive oxygen species have led to many developments in organ preservation solutions. The preservation solutions currently available for use vary with respect to impermeants, buffers, electrolyte compositions, reactive oxygen species scavengers, and additives. Each solution has been optimized for specific organ use. The perfect universal preservation solution remains to be discovered and has therefore led many groups to investigate ex vivo perfusion.

Much of the conceptual basis for current practice originated from the Medical College of Georgia's pioneering work on hypothermic ex vivo renal perfusion systems. In 2006, 20% of all kidneys were preserved using a hypothermic ex vivo perfusion system. In extended criteria kidney donors, static cold storage has been demonstrated to increase the risk of graft dysfunction and loss. Given these limitations, a prospective randomized controlled study was performed in 336 consecutive donors in which one kidney was preserved using the static cold storage techniques and the other kidney was preserved using a hypothermic ex vivo perfusion system. At 1-year follow-up, the ex vivo perfusion grafts experienced less delayed graft function and improved graft survival. Further, the upfront cost of the perfusion system was more than offset by the additional costs incurred in the static cold storage group for graft-related complications.

As a result of the impressive results in kidney preservation, interest has also increased in liver, pancreas, heart, and lung ex vivo preservation systems. Studies with warm blood perfusion of beating donor hearts have shown promising early results, allowing longer distance procurement and potentially further assessment of marginal hearts. Given the increasing pressure for more transplantable organs and the extremely low conversion rates seen in lung transplantation, considerable research has been directed in evaluating and optimizing donors prior to DBD and DCD. Early experiments in dogs demonstrated that lungs transplanted with 1 hour of non-ventilated warm ischemic time could function well with good gas exchange. Additional studies by the same group demonstrated that up to 4 hours of ventilated warm ischemic time was tolerable. Encouraged by these results, since 1995, several clinical groups have transplanted DCD lungs from Maastricht category III donors using ex vivo lung perfusion (EVLP) rigs to first assess the organ. Total published experience of category III somatic donors to date is about 100 patients worldwide.

Interest in EVLP assessment and optimization has continued to increase. Described systems allow for visual evaluation, hemodynamic and ventilatory mechanics, and gas exchange to be followed over time. The circuit consists of a blood reservoir, a pump, a leukocyte filter, a gas exchanger, an in-line blood gas monitoring system, and a heat exchanger. Perfusion cannulas are connected to the main pulmonary artery and the left atrium, the trachea is intubated using a standard endotracheal tube, and the lungs are placed in a sterile box. Perfusion is maintained at pressures no greater than 20 mmHg at 37°C with varying perfusion solutions and additives. Successful normothermic perfusion has been described up to 12 hours without inducing edema and preserving stable pulmonary vascular resistance, gas exchange, and mechanics.

The University of Toronto has recently presented their outcomes in more than 20 patients who underwent lung transplant with donor lungs treated with EVLP for 12 hours. Initial results showed that graft function and short-term survival were not significantly different from those of DBD. These early reports have increased enthusiasm for the introduction of EVLP in an increasing number of centers to improve utilization of marginal lung donors.

These reports open the possibility of extended evaluation and repair of marginal donors and potentially further expanding the donor pool. Treatment of lungs during EVLP has great potential to significantly improve graft function. It has been shown that treatment of ex vivo human lungs with an adenoviral vector encoding for IL-10 decreased inflammatory cytokine expression and led to significant improvements in graft function. Clearly more research is needed, but there remains conservative optimism that many more organs will be rehabilitated and transplanted.

Further reading

Bugge JF. Brain death and its implications for management of the potential organ donor. *Acta Anaesthesiol Scan* 2009; **53**: 1239–50.

Jenkins DH, Reilly PM, Schwab C W. Improving the approach to organ donation: a review. *World J Sur* 1999; **23**: 644–9.

Smith M. Physiologic changes during brain stem death–lessons for management of the organ donor. *J Heart Lung Transplant* 2004; **23**: S217–22.

Wood KE, Becker BN, McCartney JG, D'Alessandro AM, Coursin DB. Care of the potential organ donor. *N Engl J Med* 2004; **351**: 2730–9.

Yeung JC, Cypel M, Waddell TK, Van Raemdonck D, Keshavjee S. Update on donor assessment, resuscitation, and acceptance criteria, including novel techniques–non-heart-beating donor lung retrieval and ex vivo donor lung perfusion. *Thorac Surg Clin* 2009; **19**: 261–74.

Chapter 6

Recipient selection

R.V. Venkateswaran and Jayan Parameshwar

Key points

- Advances in the management of heart failure have significantly improved the outcome of patients with this condition.
- Heart transplantation remains the best treatment for selected patients with advanced heart failure.
- The number of donor hearts available for transplantation continues to fall; careful assessment of potential candidates for transplantation is therefore crucial to ensure optimal use of this scarce resource.
- Pulmonary vascular resistance is a continuous variable for risk of an adverse outcome after transplantation.
- Cardiopulmonary exercise testing with measurement of gas exchange is generally thought to be the best method of assessing functional capacity in the ambulant heart failure patient.

Heart transplantation (HT) is the treatment of choice for selected patients with advanced heart failure (HF). Despite the success of the procedure and improvements in long-term recipient outcome, only a small fraction of advanced HF patients can be treated by this modality. Unfortunately, the number of heart transplants performed worldwide every year is declining. This trend is seen in Europe, particularly in the United Kingdom, whereas the number of hearts transplanted in the United States remains fairly static (Figure 6.1). The increasing numbers of patients referred for transplantation has lead to a major imbalance between supply and demand. Mortality on the HT waiting list is also increasing. Allocation of a scarce resource (the donor heart) requires two different perspectives. From the recipient's point of view, it could be argued that the organ should be allocated to the most ill patient. From the point of view of the wider community of HF patients, society in general, and the donor family, it might be argued that the organ is given to the recipient predicted to have the best long-term outcome after a transplant. In practice, a compromise between these two positions is required.

Recipient selection

Patients with New York Heart Association (NYHA) class IIIB and class IV HF are best discussed with the local heart failure/transplant center to optimize medical management and to consider high-risk non-transplant surgery where appropriate. Examples include valvular heart disease and reversible ischemia that could be managed by conventional surgery. It is imperative that every effort is made to optimize medical therapy. Particular attention must be paid to fluid restriction and elimination of potential contributors such as excessive alcohol intake. Every attempt must be made to maximize the dose of prognostically beneficial agents such as angiotensin-converting enzyme (ACE) inhibitors and beta-blockers. Patients who may benefit from cardiac resynchronization therapy (CRT) should be identified and referred for bi-ventricular pacing. Patients with chronic HF should be referred before they develop significant renal and hepatic dysfunction and irreversible pulmonary hypertension. Finally, it is important to continually reassess the response to changes in therapy.

Indications for heart transplantation

Patients with NYHA class IV heart failure despite best medical therapy will generally derive prognostic benefit from heart transplantation. Patients with

Organ Transplantation: A Clinical Guide, ed. A.A. Klein, C.J. Lewis, and J.C. Madsen. Published by Cambridge University Press.

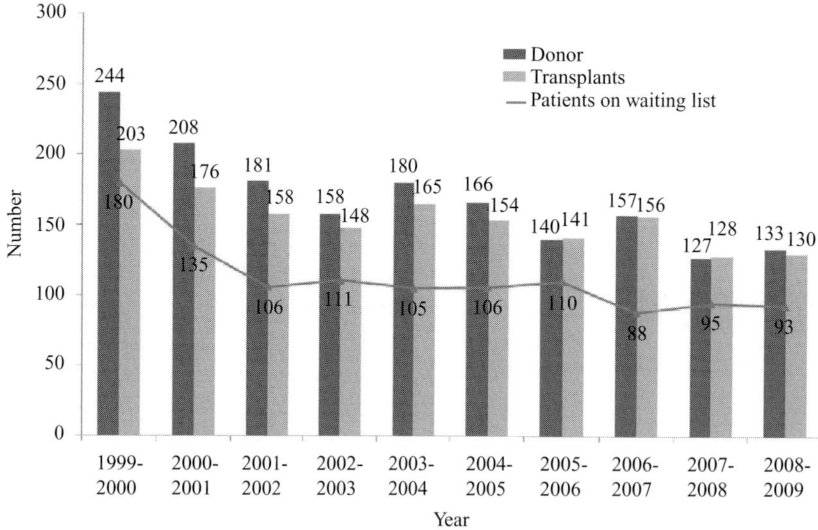

Figure 6.1 Deceased donor heart program in the United Kingdom, April 1, 1999–March 31, 2009. Number of donors, transplants, and patients on the active transplant list at March 31, 2009.

Table 6.1 Indications for heart transplantation

Heart failure	Ongoing symptoms of HF at rest or minimal exertion despite optimal medical therapy. Functional capacity measured by peak oxygen uptake on exercise less than 14 ml/kg/min (or 50% predicted peak VO_2 normalized for age and sex). For patients receiving beta-blockers, a value of 12 ml/kg/min has been recommended.
Recurrent admission	History of recurrent admission to hospital with worsening HF despite compliance with optimal medical therapy.
Ischemia	Refractory ischemia not amenable to revascularization associated with severe impairment of left ventricular function.
Arrhythmia	Recurrent symptomatic ventricular arrhythmia associated with severe impairment of ventricular function.

NYHA class III heart failure need careful assessment of prognosis. Table 6.1 shows the usual indications for heart transplantation; Table 6.2 outlines the usual contraindications. Most of these are relative rather than absolute contraindications.

Table 6.2 Absolute and relative contraindications to heart transplantation

Active infection (including chronic active viral infections, e.g., HIV, HBV)
Symptomatic peripheral or cerebrovascular disease
Diabetes mellitus with end-organ damage (nephropathy, neuropathy, proliferative retinopathy)
Coexistent or recent neoplasm (within 5 years)
Severe lung disease (FEV_1 and FVC <50% predicted)
Renal dysfunction: estimated glomerular filtration rate <40 ml/min/1.73 m^2 (consider combined heart and kidney transplantation)
Recent pulmonary thromboembolism
Pulmonary hypertension: pulmonary artery systolic pressure >60 mmHg, transpulmonary gradient ≥15 mmHg, and/or pulmonary vascular resistance >5 Wood units.
Psychosocial factors including history of non-compliance with medication, inadequate social support, drug or alcohol abuse
Obesity: body mass index >34 or weight >140% of ideal body weight
Age: usually >70 years

FEV_1: forced expiratory volume in 1 second; FVC: forced vital capacity.

Ventricular dysfunction

Patients who require heart transplantation invariably have severe ventricular dysfunction, but the converse is not true; many patients with severe ventricular dysfunction have well-controlled heart failure and do not require listing for a transplant. Although the severity of ventricular dysfunction and increasing ventricular volume is a predictor of adverse outcome in HF, there is no cut-off level of ejection fraction (EF) or left ventricular dimension that mandates listing for transplantation.

Cardiopulmonary exercise testing

Exercise capacity is known to correlate with prognosis in advanced HF. Assessment of this variable by history is usually expressed in terms of NYHA class. An objective measure of functional capacity is essential to compare patients and to assess response to treatment. The 6-minute walk test is a simple tool to assess exercise capacity in advanced HF, but cardiopulmonary exercise testing (CPEX) with measurement of gas exchange is generally thought to be the best method of assessing functional capacity in the ambulant HF patient. This tool was introduced into the HF clinic in the 1980s by Weber and Janicki and was rapidly adopted by transplant centers to guide listing for heart transplantation following a publication by Mancini and colleagues in 1991. Patients with advanced HF were stratified based on peak VO_2 levels: (1) peak VO_2 < 14 ml/kg/min and suitable for HT; (2) peak VO2 < 14 ml/kg/min but with contraindications to HT; (3) peak $VO_2 > 14$ ml/kg/min. One-year survival was 94% for patients with peak $VO_2 \geq 14$ ml/kg/min compared with 74% for patients with peak VO_2 < 14 ml/kg/min who were suitable for HT. In patients who were unfit for HT, the 1-year survival rate on medical treatment was only 47%. To use the measured peak VO_2 for prognostic purposes, it is important to establish that the patient has achieved the anaerobic threshold. In practice, a respiratory exchange ratio (RER) of >1.05 is used to define a maximal CPEX.

The widespread introduction of beta-blockade and implantable cardioverter-defibrillators (ICDs), which improve survival but have little effect on exercise capacity, has prompted revision of the level of peak VO_2 that is used to guide listing for transplant. There have also been advances in the interpretation of CPEX. In the presence of a beta-blocker, it has been suggested that a level of 12 ml/kg/min is used. Normalizing peak VO_2 for age and gender is particularly useful for young patients and women. It may also be preferable to use a level of 50% predicted rather than an absolute value of peak VO_2 to guide listing. When a patient is unable to perform a maximal CPEX, the ventilatory efficiency or minute ventilation to carbon dioxide production relationship (VE/VCO_2 slope) may be used. A slope >35 is used as a determinant for listing. Finally, it has been suggested that in obese patients, a lean body mass adjusted peak VO_2 of <19 ml/kg/min is used to guide listing.

Right heart catheterization

Invasive right heart pressure measurement gives important information regarding the filling pressures and cardiac output in patients with HF. It is also essential to measure the transpulmonary pressure gradient (TPG) and pulmonary vascular resistance (PVR). Chronic HF is associated with a high left ventricular end-diastolic pressure (LVEDP), which in turn leads to pulmonary venous and pulmonary arterial hypertension. This is usually reversible following transplantation. However, acute right ventricular (RV) failure is an important cause of peri-operative mortality following heart transplantation (up to 20% of early deaths), and it was recognized early in the 1970s that a high PVR was a predictor of this complication. The donor RV is particularly susceptible to injury following brainstem death and organ retrieval, and there is a complex interaction between PVR and RV dysfunction.

There is evidence that when HF therapy achieves low filling (near normal) pressures with a cardiac index $>2\ l/min/m^2$, medium-term prognosis is good enough to defer listing for transplantation. PVR is a continuous variable for risk of an adverse outcome after transplantation, as discussed later. The exact levels of pulmonary artery (PA) pressure, TPG, and PVR that preclude transplantation are uncertain. A reasonable guide would be a combination of PA systolic pressure >60 mmHg, TPG > 15 mmHg, and fixed PVR above 5 Wood units (WU). Reversibility, as defined by the acute response to a pulmonary vasodilator, may be used to refine selection of patients, but there is no consensus on the best agent or the fall in PVR that predicts a satisfactory outcome. Longer term reversibility studies, e.g. with intra-aortic balloon pumping and a phosphodiesterase inhibitor (e.g., enoximone or milrinone), may be more useful in practice. It is important to repeat right heart catheterization while patients wait for a suitable donor heart; this helps to identify those in whom the PVR is rising, but also those patients who improve on continued medical therapy and may therefore no longer require transplantation.

Role of HF prognostic scores

Several survival scores have been developed to help define prognosis in HF. The best studied scoring system in the context of predicting the need for HT is the Heart Failure Survival Score (HFSS). HFSS includes CPEX in addition to serum sodium, resting heart rate, ischemic etiology, QRS duration, EF, and mean arterial blood pressure. The score is calculated as the absolute value of the sum of products of the prognostic variables and their computed coefficients. Based on final HFSS, the patients are graded as low risk (≥8.10), medium risk (7.20–8.09), and high-risk (<7.20). This score was developed and validated in patients undergoing transplant evaluation and has been extensively re-validated. On continued medical therapy, patients in the three risk strata had a 1-year survival of 88%, 60%, and 35%, respectively. However, the HFSS was developed before widespread use of CRT, ICDs, and beta-blockers. Introduction of these treatments has altered the prognostic variables used in computing the score. Nevertheless, a number of studies have evaluated the role of HFSS in the current therapeutic era and confirmed the validity of the score in assessing prognosis.

The Seattle HF Score may be easier to use in the heart failure clinic and can guide the physician in referring a patient to a transplant center at the appropriate time. It is a 21-variable model derived from data collected during the PRAISE (Prospective Randomized Amlodipine Survival Evaluation) study and validated on subsequent clinical trial data. Five of the seven variables of the HFSS are included in this model (heart rate and peak VO_2 are not). There is relatively good concordance between the two models.

Comorbidity (relative contraindications)

Age

The long-term outcome following HT has been shown to be worse with increased recipient age (discussed further in Chapter 12). However, chronological age alone should not be considered an absolute contraindication to transplant evaluation. Patients greater than 70 years of age have generally been reported to have a worse survival following transplantation. Older patients run a higher risk of post-transplant malignancy and renal dysfunction as compared with younger recipients. In contrast, the incidence of rejection is lower in older recipients. This is perhaps due to reduced immunological activity that occurs with aging. This immune senescence has also been linked with increased risk of development of opportunistic infections and post-transplant malignancies. In patients who are older than 65 years, the decision regarding listing should be individualized; careful attention to comorbidity, including renal function, pulmonary function, and general fitness, helps to define a group with acceptable outcome.

Malignancy

Patients with a recent history of malignancy (<5 years) are generally not considered suitable for HT. Potential recipients with some hematological malignancies in remission with very low rate of recurrence may be considered for HT within shorter time periods. However, each patient should be assessed carefully, and discussions should involve oncologists to establish the long-term prognosis. If the expected survival for patients with the malignancy in question exceeds the median survival following heart transplantation, it may not be considered a contraindication. The possible effect of immunosuppression on the malignancy also needs to be taken into account. Low-grade tumors such as prostate carcinoma may not be a contraindication to HT.

Renal dysfunction

Renal dysfunction is common in patients with advanced HF. It is a marker of adverse outcome in patients on optimal medical therapy; severe renal dysfunction also affects outcome after HT. Serum creatinine will often rise in the immediate post-transplant period, in part due to the effects of cardiopulmonary bypass. Hemodynamic instability and the introduction of a calcineurin inhibitor compound this problem. If renal size is normal and there is no proteinuria, an estimated glomerular filtration rate of above 40 ml/min/1.73m^2 is considered adequate to list patients for HT. Occasionally a trial of IV inotropic therapy to increase cardiac output is warranted; if there is a substantial fall in the serum creatinine, the patient can be listed for HT. The duration of abnormal renal function may also be an important variable. There may be an indication in individually assessed cases for combined heart and kidney transplantation.

Obesity

Patients with obesity (>140% of ideal body weight or body mass index >3.5) have increased morbidity and mortality in the medium term. The Cardiac Transplant Research Database identified this variable as a risk factor for infection and death. Ideally, such patients should be strongly advised and helped to lose weight before listing for transplantation.

Chronic viral infection

Infection with human immunodeficiency virus (HIV), hepatitis B virus (HBV), and hepatitis C virus (HCV) has generally been considered a contraindication to heart transplantation. The reasons include viral multiplication in the face of immunosuppression, the potential for dysfunction of other affected organs (liver and kidney), toxicity of antiviral drugs, and the possible association of viruses (including cytomegalovirus and hepatitis viruses) in the acceleration of coronary artery disease. The advent of effective therapy for HBV and HIV has led to this position being challenged by several groups who hold that the outcome in selected patients is no worse than that of the general population of HF patients. Data on long-term outcome in any of these groups are lacking (particularly in the context of HT), but there are several reports of acceptable short- and medium-term outcome in small numbers of patients. Although there is no consensus on the best approach, HIV patients who have normal CD4 counts and no evidence of the acquired immune deficiency syndrome (AIDS)–related complex may be considered for transplantation. Similarly, patients who are HBV surface antigen–positive but have no detectable viral load by polymerase chain reaction may have an acceptable outcome after transplantation. In addition, some centers advocate the use of hearts from HCV-positive donors for transplantation into HCV-positive recipients.

Congenital heart disease

Growing populations of young adults who have survived palliative surgery for congenital heart disease are likely to be referred for transplant evaluation in the next 10 to 20 years. The operative mortality and 1-year survival for these patients is inferior to that of other recipients. This is due to the operative difficulties caused by adhesions, increased risk of bleeding, and complex anatomy. Despite these difficulties, long-term outcome for patients who survive the HT operation is excellent. Although these patients should not be denied transplant evaluation, their risk should be carefully assessed and consideration given to concentrating expertise in a few centers.

Smoking and alcohol abuse

Smokers have a decreased survival following HT, which in one study was apparent at 4 years. They have a higher incidence of cardiac allograft vasculopathy (CAV) and malignancy than non-smokers. Smoking cessation, ideally for 6 months, before transplantation is required by many programs. A recent history of alcoholism or drug abuse is usually considered an absolute contraindication to transplantation because of the association with non-compliance in such patients.

HLA tissue typing and sensitization

The most important alloantibodies are directed against human leukocyte antigen (HLA) and are formed in response to foreign HLA molecules, often at the time of blood product transfusion, previous transplantation, or pregnancy. All potential recipients require tissue typing to identify any preformed HLA antibodies, which would result in hyperacute rejection at the time of transplant and should therefore be avoided. Potential recipients with very high levels of antibody will inevitably wait longer for a compatible donor heart and may therefore never undergo transplantation, even in the context of a separate national "sensitized patient" list. Recipients for heart transplants are not prospectively HLA matched with donors as would be performed for renal transplantation. This is due to concerns about smaller numbers of donor hearts, ischemic time, and clinical urgency of recipients. Outcomes transplanting across HLA-A, -B, or -DR appear to improve with increasing matching (risk reduction of 1 or 2 matches, 0.8 and for 4–6 matches, 0.6), although the DR mismatch appears to have the greatest short- and long-term impact on outcome. In the presence of HLA antibodies, traditionally, prospective complement-dependant cross-match and flow cytometry cross-match would be performed by the tissue-typing laboratory prior to proceeding with a heart transplant. In many centers, this has been replaced by virtual cross-match, which allows prediction of a significant antibody-mediated immune event between donor heart and recipient and can thus be used in pretransplant risk assessment and organ allocation. Desensitization of presensitized patients with donor-reactive HLA to reduce antibody levels to levels that make transplantation safe have been reported prior to heart transplantation (discussed in Chapter 33). Evidenced-based protocols and outcome data remain to be defined.

Re-transplantation

Early re-transplantation in patients with multiple episodes of acute rejection has been associated with a poor outcome. In selected patients with CAV and HF, late post-transplant acceptable outcomes have been achieved. However, in general, survival is worse than in patients receiving their first transplant. Allosensitization complicates donor organ allocation in many of these patients. In an era of decreasing donor organs, there is also the ethical issue of whether re-transplantation is justified. In carefully selected patients, we feel it is reasonable to consider re-transplantation, but patients must be made aware at initial evaluation that, for most, this will not be an option.

Bridging to transplant with mechanical circulatory support

The percentage of donor hearts implanted in patients who are classed as in "urgent" need of a transplant (usually patients who are inotrope dependent in critical care units) is rising as the overall number of donor organs has declined. These patients are at risk of sudden deterioration and have a high short-term mortality rate. Mechanical circulatory support may be needed in many of these patients to bridge them to a heart transplant. Assessment of the appropriateness of such therapy should ideally be carried out at the same time as transplant evaluation (Discussed further in Chapter 8).

Estimated waiting time for a transplant

The estimated waiting time for patients after listing depends on blood group, allosensitization, and patient height and weight. In general, patients who carry blood group O and who are of large build have a longer wait. Patients who are sensitized to a significant proportion of donors will also have a long wait and, in some cases, are unlikely to receive a donor heart. These factors must be taken into account when the decision to list for transplant is considered. They may also drive earlier use of mechanical circulatory support at a time when end-organ function is preserved and the risk of surgery is lower.

Combined heart–kidney and heart–liver transplantation

Combined heart–kidney transplantation with allografts from the same donor is regularly but rarely performed (1.4% of the total heart and kidney transplantation experiences). Since the initial report of simultaneous heart–kidney transplantation with allografts from the same donor in 1978, multiple solid organ transplantation has evolved into an acceptable approach, with satisfactory short and intermediate results. In carefully selected patients, long-term survival is similar to that of separate heart and kidney transplantation, although rejection can occur in both allografts individually. No HLA matching is performed in heart or combined heart–kidney transplantation.

Combined heart–liver transplantation has been increasingly performed, but data on patient and graft outcomes remain limited. A recent study described 47 cases of combined heart–liver (n = 41) and heart–liver–kidney transplantation (n = 6) reported to the United Network for Organ Sharing registry over an 18-year period. Indications include cardiac disease with cardiac cirrhosis, amyloidosis, and hemochromatosis. One-year patient, heart, and liver graft survival rates were 84.8%, 84.8%, and 82.4% at 1 year and 75.6%, 75.6%, and 73.5% at 5 years, respectively. Combined heart–liver transplantation is a viable option, with outcomes comparable to those of single-organ recipients.

Further reading

Anyanwu AC, Rogers CA, Murday AJ. Intrathoracic organ transplantation in the United Kingdom 1995–99: results from the UK cardiothoracic transplant audit. *Heart* 2002; **87**: 449–54.

Kirklin J, Banner NR, Jessup M (eds). *Advanced Heart Failure. ISHLT monograph series*, Vol. 3, Part 1 & 2. Addison, TX: International Society for Heart and Lung Transplantation, 2009.

Mancini D, Lietz K. Selection of cardiac transplantation candidates in 2010. *Circulation* 2010; **122**: 173–83.

Mehra MR, Kobashigawa J, Starling R, *et al.* Listing criteria for heart transplantation: International Society for Heart and Lung Transplantation guidelines for the care of cardiac transplant candidate. *J Heart Lung Transplant* 2006; **25**: 1024–42.

Taylor DO, Stehlik J, Edwards LB, *et al.* Registry of the international society for heart and lung transplantation: twenty-sixth official adult heart transplant report. *J Heart Lung Transplant* 2009; **28**: 1007–22.

Section 2 Heart

Chapter 7

Donor heart selection

Kiran K. Khush and Jonathan G. Zaroff

Key points

- Availability of donor organs limits heart transplantation rates today.
- Judicious liberalization of graft acceptance criteria would increase transplant rates.
- The risks of transplantation with a marginal graft must be weighed against the risk of remaining on the transplant waiting list.
- Many criteria previously thought to be "absolute" contraindications to transplantation are now considered "relative" contraindications.
- Marginal donor hearts may be safely utilized for high-risk transplant recipients who would not otherwise be suitable candidates for heart transplantation.

Advances in surgical techniques, postoperative care, and immunosuppression have led to greatly improved survival following cardiac transplantation in the past two decades. The success of heart transplantation, however, has led to a large disparity between the number of available donor organs and the number of patients on the waiting list. Thus wait-list mortality remains unacceptably high, at up to 30 deaths per 100 patient-years for critically ill (status 1A) recipients. Numerous proposals have therefore been put forward to liberalize donor organ acceptance criteria. Although use of "extended-criteria donors" presents some risk to the recipient, this risk must be balanced against the risk of remaining on the waiting list. Efforts to increase donor heart utilization are therefore needed, but caution must be exercised, as early allograft failure accounts for up to 25% of deaths in heart transplant recipients.

Donor selection

Absolute contraindications

Donor sepsis and severe infections

Patients expiring from overwhelming infection have traditionally been excluded from donor evaluation due to potential transmission of pathogens (discussed further in Chapter 4C). A retrospective study of 599 donors whose organs were used for transplantation identified 46 donors (7.5%) with positive blood cultures and 25 donors (4.5%) with positive urine cultures. A total of 179 patients received organs from these contaminated donors, including 11 heart transplant recipients. Three of the heart recipients grew organisms in the postoperative period that were similar to those found in the corresponding donors; however, no patient suffered significant morbidity and mortality from these infections. These data suggest that in the era of rapid and accurate identification of pathogens in the transplant donor and effective antibiotic therapy, contamination of organs should not be an absolute contraindication to graft utilization.

Donor hepatitis B and C virus infection

Hearts from donors infected with hepatitis C virus (HCV) carry a substantial risk of transmission to the recipient, as evidenced by a report of five HCV-naive recipients who were transplanted with hearts from HCV-positive donors, of whom four developed evidence of infection. A subsequent study examined outcomes of 261 heart transplants involving an HCV-positive donor. This analysis revealed higher 1-, 5-, and 10-year mortality in recipients of HCV-positive donor hearts. These transplant recipients were more likely to die of liver disease and cardiac allograft

Organ Transplantation: A Clinical Guide, ed. A.A. Klein, C.J. Lewis, and J.C. Madsen. Published by Cambridge University Press.

vasculopathy (CAV), suggesting a viral trigger for this common post-transplant complication.

This discovery led to interest in other viral infections, including hepatitis B virus (HBV). An analysis of coronary angiograms from 13 patients in whom the heart transplant (HT) donor or recipient was positive for HBV also revealed a significant increase in CAV at 1 year post transplant (31% versus 5% in control patients), suggesting that HBV may be a trigger for the development of CAV. Despite the possible association with CAV, there is currently no evidence that recipients of cardiac allografts from HBV-positive donors have reduced survival. Currently, grafts from HBV core antibody–positive donors may be safely accepted for heart transplantation into HBV-negative recipients, followed by post-transplant prophylactic lamivudine to prevent viral transmission.

Donor human immunodeficiency virus (HIV) infection

There is a paucity of data regarding transmission of the HIV virus in the setting of heart transplantation. A 1991 multi-center review of 88 HIV-infected recipients of solid organ transplants in whom HIV was presumably transmitted via organs or peri-operative blood transfusions showed that 28% of the recipients developed acquired immune deficiency syndrome (AIDS), and 80% of these patients died of AIDS-related complications. Another 10% of recipients developed HIV-related diseases. In the majority of cases, transplantation occurred before routine donor screening for HIV antibody began. With current screening practices, HIV transmission by transplantation is rare, and donor HIV seropositivity is an absolute contraindication to graft utilization.

Donors with extracranial malignancies

Studies of donor-related tumor transmission to transplant recipients usually distinguish between central nervous system (CNS) and non-CNS donor malignancies. The risk of cancer transmission in HT from donors with a CNS malignancy appears to be very low, provided that there are no detectable metastases. Non-CNS malignancies, however, do have a significant risk of transmission from donor to recipient in HT as in other organs, with multiple reports of transmission of melanoma, choriocarcinoma, and cancers of the lung, kidney, and breast. Currently, most surgeons will accept grafts from non-skin and non-CNS cancer donors with a 5–10-year "disease free" interval, using this time period as evidence for "cure." There are also data suggesting that donors with subcapsular renal cell carcinomas may be considered. Given these precautions, the current risk of donor-related tumor transmission appears to be extremely low. These data support a careful risk/benefit assessment by the transplant team, reviewing donor cancer history and the recipient's urgency of need for transplantation in order to safely expand the donor pool.

Donors exposed to myocardial toxins

Carbon monoxide (CO) poisoning causes pathological myocardial changes from tissue hypoxia. Use of cardiac allografts from CO-poisoned donors can result in early recipient deaths due to graft failure. Since adoption of standardized donor management protocols, longer donor management periods have allowed adequate time to evaluate and reject irreversibly damaged organs. Several centers have since published results of small case series ($n = 5$–7) of heart transplantation with organs from CO-poisoned donors, demonstrating acceptable recipient outcomes. Given the limited data available, caution is warranted when evaluating potential grafts from CO-poisoned donors. Ideally, the donor should be hemodynamically stable for at least 36 hours from the time of poisoning in order to select organs with a low risk of graft failure.

Case reports have described the transplantation of hearts from donors poisoned with tricyclic antidepressants with satisfactory graft function. Successful heart transplantation has also been reported after donor death from poisoning with barbiturates, cyanide, methanol, serotonin antagonists, and 3,4-methylenedioxymethamphetamine ("Ecstasy"). Given the relatively small number of cases, consensus guidelines are unlikely to be proposed for evaluation of donors exposed to myocardial toxins. Nevertheless, it is reasonable to conclude that hearts from these donors should not be summarily rejected (Figure 7.1).

Relative contraindications

Advanced donor age

The acceptance cut-off for donor age has increased significantly in the setting of the donor organ shortage. In the early days of HT, the upper limit for donor age was 35 years. However, older donors are now used frequently, with hearts from donors aged 50–55 years being accepted at many centers, especially for older recipients. Donors $\geq$ 50 years of age now account for approximately 12% of all cardiac donors. The effect

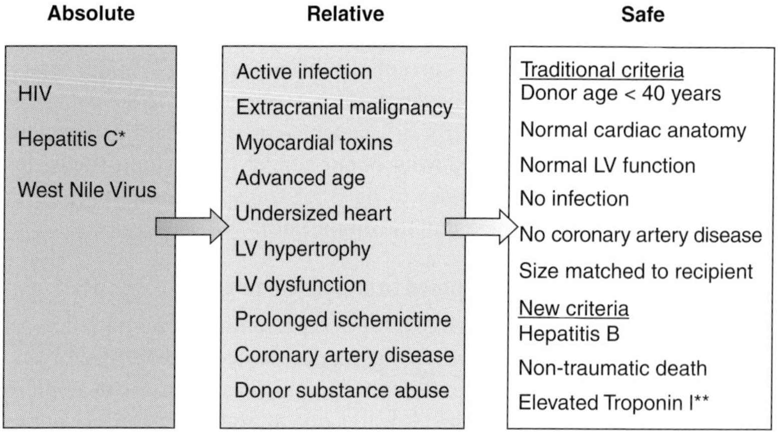

Figure 7.1 Donor contraindications to graft utilization: a changing paradigm. *Consider for HCV-positive recipients. **Assuming other cardiovascular factors are favorable. HIV: human immunodeficiency virus; LV: left ventricular.

of donor age liberalization on post-transplant outcomes has been debated, and the International Society for Heart and Lung Transplantation Registry has reported increased recipient mortality (discussed further in Chapter 12). An analysis of recipient survival at the Columbia University transplant program showed a 30-day mortality rate of 5% in recipients of hearts from donors less than 40 years of age, 13% in recipients of hearts from donors 40–50 years of age, and 22% in recipients of hearts from donors more than 50 years of age. After the first 30 days, however, they did not find any association between advanced donor age and recipient mortality. These early mortality data must be interpreted in light of the significant risk of death while awaiting heart transplantation. A risk/benefit analysis performed by the same authors concluded that expansion of the donor age to greater than 40 years is more beneficial than indefinitely remaining on the waiting list, especially for critically ill patients.

Undersized donor hearts

Traditional rules dictate that cardiac allografts should only be accepted from donors within 20–30% of the recipient's weight. However, undersized donor hearts have been used successfully with excellent long-term outcomes. In a prospective study of 14 undersized donor hearts, investigators demonstrated an increase in left ventricular mass and internal dimensions post transplant, suggesting that the donor left ventricle adapts to the larger recipient circulation.

One area of concern lies in transplanting undersized hearts into recipients with preoperative pulmonary hypertension, due to the risk of acute right ventricle (RV) failure. Several case series demonstrate that undersized donor hearts can be safely utilized for heart transplantation, even in recipients with high pulmonary vascular resistance, provided that postoperative care is tailored to maximize cardiac output and reduce the risk of acute RV failure. As is often the case, the decision regarding whether to accept an undersized donor heart must be informed by individual donor and recipient characteristics.

Donor left ventricular hypertrophy

Recent case series report a 15–30% prevalence of left ventricular hypertrophy (LVH) in donor hearts accepted for transplantation, suggesting that this is a fairly common finding. It is unclear, however, whether increased left ventricular (LV) wall thickness detected during the donor evaluation period represents transient myocardial edema in the setting of brain death, or actual myocyte hypertrophy. Furthermore, the impact of donor LVH on graft and recipient outcomes remains in question. Initial reports suggesting that donor LVH portends reduced recipient survival included very few donor hearts with LVH (n = 6–9), and LVH was frequently diagnosed by electrocardiography or qualitative interpretation of echocardiograms. Later series studied larger numbers of donors (n = 47–62) and used echocardiographic measurements, but definitions of LVH varied (e.g., LV septal wall thickness > 1.1–1.4 cm). Thus it is not surprising that results vary widely between studies. In donors with a history of hypertension, LVH had an unfavorable impact on late survival, suggesting that those patients had more advanced changes in myocardial structure and diastolic function. Finally, several studies have reported an interaction between donor LVH and prolonged ischemic time, which in combination portend poor recipient outcomes.

Donor left ventricular dysfunction

LV dysfunction is the most frequently cited reason for non-utilization of potential cardiac allografts. A review of non-transplanted donor hearts managed by the California Transplant Donor Network demonstrated that LV dysfunction was the cause for graft refusal in 26% of cases.

The pathogenesis of brain death–induced LV dysfunction is complex, but acute catecholamine toxicity likely plays a central role. Regardless of the underlying mechanism, there is evidence that brain death–induced cardiac dysfunction is highly reversible. Serial echocardiograms performed on 13 brain dead organ donors with an initial LV ejection fraction of less than 50% demonstrated an improvement in LV function in 12 of the 13 donors after extended donor management. Hearts from these donors were subsequently accepted for transplantation, with a recipient survival rate of 92% at 16 months.

Encouragingly, single-center studies have reported good results after transplantation of donor hearts with LV dysfunction. Although an analysis of risk factors affecting recipient survival in a multi-institutional study found that diffuse echocardiographic wall motion abnormalities are an independent risk factor, with 22% recipient mortality in the early post-transplant period, this study was performed before the era of extended donor management and tailored hemodynamic protocols. More recent evidence has demonstrated the reversibility of brain death–induced LV dysfunction, suggesting that these hearts may be acceptable for transplantation.

The debate regarding whether to accept a graft with LV dysfunction for heart transplantation is likely to continue. Evaluation of donor hearts with depressed function is difficult, because none of the commonly used tests, such as electrocardiography, echocardiography, and coronary angiography, distinguish between reversible ischemic injury and irreversibly damaged tissue. Such cases are best evaluated in the context of donor management guidelines discussed in Chapter 5. Furthermore, extended donor management times enable organ procurement organizations to assess for reversibility of graft dysfunction, such as with serial echocardiograms, and may therefore improve graft utilization rates and recipient outcomes.

Prolonged ischemic time

Our need to transfer organs between centers has spurred innovations that allow for longer cold ischemic time (CIT). Current practice generally uses a CIT threshold of 4 hours for cardiac allografts. Data from the Collaborative Transplant Study, which included 104 centers in 24 countries, demonstrated a significant survival difference at 3 years between hearts preserved for $\leq$ 4 hours (73%, $n = 7589$) compared with those preserved for more than 4 hours (65%, $n = 630$) ($p < 0.001$). In an analysis of the United Network for Organ Sharing (UNOS) database, the authors found a significant interaction, with a greater tolerance for prolonged ischemic times among grafts from younger donors, especially those less than 19 years of age. In aggregate, these data support an extension of the CIT to more than 4 hours for young donors with excellent graft function. In older donors, efforts should be made to minimize the CIT, especially given the concern that endothelial injury during the ischemic period could predispose grafts to the development of CAV. Newer, improved preservation solutions and continuous organ perfusion may allow further extension of ischemic times.

Donor coronary artery disease

With the increasing acceptance of older donor hearts for transplantation comes the likelihood that a significant number of these hearts will have coronary atherosclerosis. Several case series have been published describing coronary artery bypass grafting performed at the time of the transplant surgery, demonstrating that the surgery is technically feasible. However, there appears to be a high risk of early graft failure. The University of California, Los Angeles (UCLA) heart transplant group demonstrated that the prevalence of CAV at 3 years post transplant appears to be higher in recipients of hearts with donor coronary artery disease than in recipients without donor atherosclerosis (25% versus 4%; $p < 0.001$). CAV did not appear to preferentially develop at sites of pre-existing donor lesions, but rather in a diffuse distribution, perhaps secondary to coronary endothelial dysfunction in older donor hearts. This observation has been reported by other centers, suggesting that the use of donor hearts with coronary atherosclerosis is associated with development of CAV in the transplant recipient; however, it is unclear whether this translates to significant differences in quality of life, graft function, or survival.

Elevated donor troponin (Tn) levels

The lack of echocardiography and angiography at many hospitals where donors are evaluated underscores the need for simpler methods for expedited and accurate evaluation. The use of serum markers that reliably predict graft function and survival is therefore attractive as a simple, non-invasive screening tool. Circulating cardiac Tn levels are highly sensitive and specific markers of myocardial cell injury and are therefore often measured during organ donor assessment; however, their utility in donor selection remains controversial. Riou and colleagues initially observed that an elevated cardiac troponin T level was associated with a severe decrease in LV function in brain-dead patients and expressed concern that this finding could represent irreversible myocardial cell damage. Small-scale retrospective and prospective studies in heart transplantation have yielded conflicting results; although most confirm that elevated Tn levels are associated with graft LV dysfunction, some show an association with early graft failure, whereas others failed to find an association between elevated donor Tn levels and recipient mortality. All studies had major limitations, and well-designed prospective studies with serial, standardized Tn assays are needed to determine whether there is a Tn threshold level above which grafts may be unsuitable for transplantation.

Donor cause of death

Experimental studies in animals have shown that acute increases in intracranial pressure as a result of traumatic brain injury or atraumatic intracranial bleeds (aICB) cause a dramatic upregulation of pro-inflammatory cascades and an exaggerated catecholamine response compared with other modes of brain death. The combination of this catecholamine "storm" and upregulation of pro-inflammatory mediators is associated with hemodynamic impairment and persistent myocardial dysfunction. Several studies have suggested that donor brain death caused by aICB is a potential risk factor for early recipient mortality. A recent analysis of the UNOS database reported that recipients of donors who died from cerebrovascular accidents have mildly worse survival when compared with recipients whose donors died from head trauma (relative risk = 1.1; 95% confidence interval, 1.01–1.12). Given the current donor organ shortage, mode of death should not preclude grafts from acceptance; rather, careful evaluation of graft function should be performed in donors who die from aICB or traumatic brain injury. Innovative cardioprotective strategies aimed at preventing graft dysfunction in this setting, such as the use of short-acting anti-hypertensive medications and CO-releasing preservation solutions, are needed.

Donor substance abuse

There is widespread use of substances such as cigarettes and alcohol in the donor pool. Several retrospective studies have attempted to determine whether donor substance abuse is associated with adverse recipient outcomes.

Significant alcohol consumption (>equivalent of 60 ml 100% alcohol daily for $\geq$3 months) is present in 15–25% of the donor pool, and concern exists due to the association between heavy alcohol consumption and cardiomyopathy. However, in a relatively large study of 437 heart transplants, De La Zerda noted the opposite effect: chronic alcoholism in donors appeared to be protective, with higher recipient survival. The data regarding cocaine use is similarly contradictory. High catecholamine levels in the setting of cocaine use may cause coronary and systemic vasoconstriction, myocardial microinfarction, increases in heart rate, systemic arterial pressure, and myocardial demand. Great concern therefore exists regarding the use of cardiac grafts from cocaine-abusing donors. A recently published analysis of the UNOS Registry, however, is reassuring: In 9217 adult heart transplant recipients, the incidence of donor cocaine use was 10%, with no difference in mortality or development of angiographic CAV at 1 and 5 years.

Donor cigarette smoking is a cause for concern given the link between smoking and endothelial dysfunction, atherosclerosis, and other pathological processes. This is especially concerning given the high prevalence of smoking in the donor pool, with estimates of up to 76%. Of interest is a prospective study by Rickenbacher in which coronary angiography with intravascular ultrasound was performed to identify donor factors that predispose recipients to CAV. These investigators found a significant association ($p < 0.02$) between donor smoking history and coronary artery intimal thickening within the first year after transplantation, suggesting that early intimal thickening reflects a predisposition to myointimal proliferation mediated by smoking, which is then accelerated following the initiation of the alloimmune response.

Non-standard donors and the alternate list

Due to the severe donor organ shortage, with long recipient waiting times, "non-standard" or "marginal" donor hearts are increasingly being used for higher risk recipients and critically ill patients, leading to an expansion of both the donor and recipient pools. The UCLA group first reported experience with such a listing policy. In their scheme, recipients who otherwise would have been excluded for transplantation (due to advanced age, renal insufficiency, re-transplantation, or peripheral vascular disease) were matched with non-standard donor hearts that otherwise would not have been used for transplantation (due to donor coronary artery disease, illicit drug use, HBV, HCV, LV dysfunction, high inotropic requirement, LVH, age >55 years, small size, or a reused transplanted heart). Although early recipient mortality was higher in this alternate group than among patients on the standard transplant list, conditional mid-term outcomes were comparable. Recently, a review of all heart transplants reported to UNOS from 1999–2005 (n = 13 024, including 347 alternate list transplants) revealed higher morbidity and mortality in the alternate-list group, with a 5-year survival rate of 51.4% compared with 75.1% in the standard transplant group. Even with worse outcomes, however, this strategy offers a median survival of 5.2 years to patients with end-stage heart disease who otherwise would be expected to live for less than 1 year.

Conclusion

Liberalizing donor criteria has already saved or at least extended the lives of many individuals who would otherwise have died while awaiting organs. It is difficult to quantify the impact of a single donor risk factor on recipient survival, because few randomized trials with higher-risk donor organs have been conducted, due to ethical and practical considerations. Similarly, the combination of donor and recipient features may also play an important role. Moreover, the decision about whether or not to proceed with transplantation must be weighed against the risk of remaining on the transplant waiting list. Given these considerations, it is encouraging that use of non-standard donors appears to be safe and provides acceptable long-term results.

Further reading

Ardehali A, Bresson J, Fonarow GC, *et al.* Use of two recipient lists for adults requiring heart transplantation. *J Thorac Cardiovasc Surg* 2003; **125**: 49–59.

Armstrong WF, Babcock WD, D'Alessandro A, *et al.* Consensus conference report: maximizing the use of organs recovered from the cadaver donor: cardiac recommendations, March 28–29, 2001, Crystal City, Va. *Circulation* 2002; **106**: 836–41.

Aurora P, Christie JD, Dobbels F, *et al.* Registry of the International Society for Heart and Lung Transplantation: Twenty-sixth Official Adult Heart Transplant Report – 2009. *J Heart Lung Transplant* 2009; **28**: 1007–22.

Edwards NM, John R, Lietz K, *et al.* Outcomes in cardiac transplant recipients using allografts from older donors versus mortality on the transplant waiting list: Implications for donor selection criteria. *J Am Coll Cardiol* 2004; **9**: 1553–61.

Fishman JA, Grossi PA. Donor-derived infections in solid organ transplant recipients. *Am J Transplant* 2009; **9**: S19–26.

Large SR, Oduro A, Potter CD, *et al.* Transforming the "unacceptable" donor: outcomes from the adoption of a standardized donor management technique. *J Heart Lung Transplant* 1995; **14**: 734–42.

Chapter 8 Ventricular assist devices

David G. Healy and Steven S.L. Tsui

Key points

- Ventricular assist devices (VAD) are increasingly used in the management of acute cardiogenic shock to support the circulation until either myocardial recovery (bridge to recovery) or a more definitive treatment is decided upon (bridge to decision).
- The type of device used is influenced by the acuteness of the patient and the projected duration of support required.
- Preoperative preparation should focus on optimizing end-organ function and right ventricular function.
- Overall survival with left ventricular assist device placement (not device-specific) is 74% at 1 year. This compares with 50% 1-year survival for bi-ventricular assist device support.
- The most common causes of death following VAD insertion are cardiac failure, infection, and neurological events.

Chronic heart failure (HF) remains a persistent global problem despite advances in preventive and therapeutic developments. Considering that the primary function of the heart is to act as a blood pump, it might be expected that such a role could easily be replaced with contemporary technology. Numerous attempts to create artificial blood pumps have been made since the early 1960s. The initial hope of developing a pump that would completely replace the function of the heart has proven to be challenging. However, significant progress has been made, particularly in recent years, and there are now a number of reliable mechanical replacements for the failed heart.

Mechanical circulatory support devices (MCSD) include the use of extra corporeal circulatory support, implantable ventricular assist devices, and total artificial hearts. These devices are increasingly used in the management of acute cardiogenic shock to support the circulation until either myocardial recovery (bridge to recovery) or a more definitive treatment is decided upon (bridge to decision). In patients who are decompensating from chronic heart failure, MCSD is used as a bridge to transplantation or as a permanent form of therapy in those with contraindications for heart transplantation (HT). For the purposes of this chapter, we confine our focus on the role of ventricular assist devices (VAD) in HT.

History

Attempts to develop VADs was spearheaded by Michael DeBakey, who performed the first clinical VAD implant in 1963 (Table 8.1). By 1966, he achieved the first successful bridge to recovery in a post-cardiotomy HF patient who was weaned from a para-corporeal device after 10 days of support. The first total artificial heart (TAH) was used by Denton Cooley in 1969. This is noteworthy not only as a historical medical event, but also as a legal milestone, as the patient's wife filed an action claiming failure of consent in relation to an experimental procedure. It remains a reference case in issues of consent. The early enthusiasm for MCSD was fueled by optimism, rather than by clinical outcomes. There were expectations that once minor technical challenges were overcome, success would inevitably follow. An Artificial Heart Program was formed in the United States with the aim of developing an artificial heart by 1970. The contemporary thinking included an implantable nuclear energy source to power the device long term. This

Organ Transplantation: A Clinical Guide, ed. A.A. Klein, C.J. Lewis, and J.C. Madsen. Published by Cambridge University Press.

Table 8.1 Milestones in the evolution of mechanical circulatory support

Date	Event
1953	Gibbon performs first ASD closure with aid of cardiopulmonary bypass circuit
1963	DeBakey (Texas) – first ventricular assist device case
1967	Bernard (Cape Town) performs the first successful heart transplantation
1969	Cooley (Texas) implants first total artificial heart
1971	First patient discharged home with MCS
1982	De Vries (Utah) implants a total artificial heart as destination therapy
1984	First successful bridge to transplantation with a Novacor LVAD
1985	First survivor for 1 year on MCS
1995	First (Berlin) successful VAD bridge to recovery
1996	First survivor for 2 years with MCS
1999	First rotary pump implantation
2001	REMATCH trial: Randomized trial comparing optimal medical therapy against pulsative VAD as destination therapy
2009	HeartMate II Study: Randomized trial of pulsatile versus continuous flow VAD as destination therapy

developmental phase spawned a number of commercially available devices such as the Thoratec paracorporeal VAD, the Novacor left ventricular assist device (LVAD), the HeartMate, and Abiomed devices. However, although the initial goal was long-term replacement of the heart with a mechanical pump, problems with device durability and device-related morbidity resulted in a switch in focus from developing a device as an end point or destination therapy to a device to support an HF patient to an allograft HT (bridging to transplant, BTT). The first BTT was performed in 1978, but it wasn't until 1984 that the first survivor was seen. These first-generation devices were large and generally could only be sited in recipients above a certain size. The recipient was also trapped in the hospital due to the large and unwieldy drive consoles. The need for smaller implantable devices, with control systems that facilitated return to community living, motivated the next generation of devices. In addition, improving device reliability and reducing morbidity were important priorities. To achieve these aims, the focus shifted away from total heart replacement to ventricular assistance, and from pulsatile to continuous-flow devices, e.g., Thoratec HeartMate II, HeartWare HVAD. With improving clinical

Table 8.2 INTERMACS classification system

INTERMACS Level	Patient status	NYHA
1	Critical cardiogenic shock	IV
2	Progressive decline	IV
3	Stable but inotrope dependent	IV
4	Recurrent advanced HF	Ambulatory IV
5	Exertion intolerant	Ambulatory IV
6	Exertion limited	IIIB
7	Advanced NYHA III	III

outcomes, confidence has grown, and these devices are increasingly used in the clinical management of advanced HF.

Indications

The predominant indication for mechanical circulatory support is to augment the systemic circulation in the presence of a failing native heart. The median survival after diagnosis of heart failure is 3 years in medically managed patients. A decision regarding elective placement of a VAD in the chronic HF setting must balance the predicted survival without VAD, the likelihood of a timely heart transplant, and their survival on the VAD. The International Registry for Mechanically Assisted Circulatory Support (INTERMACS) has developed a classification system of HF that best identifies their urgency and status and is tailored to the indications of MCS (Table 8.2).

In this system, MCSD is considered for INTERMACS level 1–4 patients. To date, there is no evidence supporting the use of MCSD in INTERMACS level 5 patients. The choice of device used is influenced by the acuteness of the patient and the projected duration of support required. When the etiology suggests rapid recovery is possible (e.g., fulminant myocarditis) or when the patient's systemic suitability for a permanent device is doubtful (e.g., possible neurological dysfunction), support with a temporary device is warranted. This allows bridge to recovery or bridge to decision regarding the placement of a longer-term VAD, listing for transplantation, or withdrawal of support. In less urgent situations and when the patient has been fully assessed, a long-term implantation device can be sited from the outset.

Patient selection

Careful selection of patients is a cornerstone in a successful VAD program. Worldwide, 78% of VAD recipients are male; 51% of patients are aged between 40 and 59 years and 18% between 19 and 39 years. The majority are sited in an acute phase, with 30% placed in the presence of critical cardiogenic shock and 40% in the case of progressive decline. BTT candidates must be suitable for transplantation or likely to be transplant candidates after a period of VAD support, e.g., patient with raised pulmonary vascular resistance (PVR) or borderline renal function. Patient selection for transplantation is discussed in Chapter 6. Among those being considered for destination therapy, an approach similar to that of heart transplant assessment is required. Ideally the patient should demonstrate single organ failure, with minimal or reversible hepatic or renal impairment. A number of scoring systems are available to predict survival following VAD placement.

Ventricular assist devices

VADs provide either left-, right-, or bi-ventricular support. A left-sided VAD (LVAD) withdraws oxygenated blood from the left atrium or LV and returns it to the aorta; a right-sided VAD (RVAD) draws venous blood from the right atrium or right ventricle (RV), and returns it to the pulmonary artery. In general, it is preferable to cannulate the ventricle for VAD inflow, as this provides superior ventricular decompression, avoids ventricular stasis, and affords higher VAD flow rates.

Bi-ventricular versus uni-ventricular support

The output of an LVAD is dependent on adequate RV function to propel sufficient blood across the lungs into the left heart chambers for the LVAD to pump. Likewise, an RVAD can only provide benefit if the native left ventricle can match the output of the RVAD. If both native ventricles are failing, two VADs are required in order to provide bi-ventricular assistance to support the circulation.

Pre-implantation factors can often predict the success of uni-ventricular support with LVAD alone. Poor RV stroke work index, older age, and non-ischemic cardiomyopathy predict poor RV function in the post-implantation period and a high requirement for inotropic support. High pulmonary pressures are also associated with RV impairment. RVAD use is associated with higher rate of bleeding and thromboembolic complications. In a HeartMate II series, 6% of LVAD patients required additional RVAD support. In cases in which the initial strategy was to site an LVAD but RV dysfunction becomes an impediment, late conversion from a uni-ventricular LVAD to bi-ventricular support is associated with poorer outcomes. Bi-ventricular support as an initial therapy is indicated for patients with arrhythmia likely to threaten the function of the remaining ventricle if a uni-ventricular approach is used, or those with multi-organ failure associated with right heart dysfunction. The final decision to use bi-ventricular support should be made intraoperatively, with direct inspection of the right ventricle and the aid of transesophageal echocardiography (TEE).

Classification

MCSD are classified according to the duration of support, flow characteristics, and/or pump mechanism. Classification based on support duration reflects the durability of the pump and ease of placement. Generally, short-term devices can be inserted quickly and are usually paracorporeal or extra-corporeal. They are only designed for days or weeks of support but cost a fraction of the price of longer term devices. Longer term devices are usually implanted inside the chest or the anterior abdominal wall. They have portable controllers that are designed to allow patient discharge from hospital.

The flow generated by these blood pumps may be pulsatile or non-pulsatile. The first-generation devices produce flow by volume displacement, and therefore, they generate pulsatile flows (e.g., Thoratec PVAD and IVAD, Novacor, HeartMate XVE). These devices are relatively bulky and noisy in operation due to the multiple moving parts. The latter predisposes to wear and tear and therefore finite durability. Second- and third-generation devices are rotary blood pumps that produce continuous flows with reduced pulsability. These devices are smaller, quiet in operation, and do not require valves or compliance chambers. Instead, without a valve, there is the potential for regurgitant flow if the device is stopped. Second-generation devices have mechanical bearings (e.g., Jarvik 2000, HeartMate II). Third-generation devices, however, do not require mechanical bearings. Instead, the impeller is either suspended by magnetic levitation (e.g., Berlin Incor, Terumo DuraHeart) or hydrodynamic suspension (e.g., HeartWare HVAD).

Peri-operative considerations

Preoperative preparation

Preoperative preparation should focus on optimizing end-organ function and RV function. Ideally, all sources of sepsis are eradicated. Optimization of renal function may require administration of inotropes and/or intra-aortic balloon pump to augment cardiac output and renal perfusion. RV function can also be improved by normalizing fluid status to achieve right atrial pressures <12 cmH_2O with diuretics or veno-venous hemofiltration. In the emergency situation, the use of a short term MCSD might enable recovery of end-organ function prior to committing to a longer-term device (bridge). Nutritional status should also be optimized.

Implantation

The implant procedure should be covered with broad-spectrum prophylactic antibiotics. Anti-fibrinolytic agents may reduce the risk of postoperative blood loss (e.g., tranexamic acid 2 g IV followed by an infusion of 1 g/hr). TEE is used to confirm aortic valve competence and to exclude the presence of a septal defect. Normothermic cardiopulmonary bypass is used, but the lungs are kept ventilated throughout the bypass period, often with the addition of nitric oxide (NO) at 5–20 parts per million to minimize atelectasis and pulmonary vasoconstriction respectively. The use of NO has been shown to reduce the need for RV support. The patient is filtered on bypass to maintain hemoglobin concentration greater than 10 g/dL and base excess within ± 2 mEq. The VAD cannulae are implanted on a beating heart, thus avoiding aortic cross-clamping and cardiac ischemia. The pericardial space is flooded with carbon dioxide so that gas entrained into cardiac chambers can dissolve more readily. The RV is supported by inotropes as appropriate. Heart rate is optimized with temporary pacing at 90–100 bpm. SVR is maintained between 800 and 1000 dyne.sec.cm^{-5} using an infusion of vasopressin or with an alpha agonist. Thorough de-airing is confirmed prior to wean from bypass. At the end of the procedure, careful hemostasis is crucial to minimize hemorrhage. The percutaneous cannula or driveline must be secured externally to minimize movement and trauma to the exit sites.

Table 8.3 Potential complications of LVAD use

Air embolism
Bleeding
Thromboembolism
Neurological injury
Right ventricular failure in the setting of LVAD placement
Hemolysis
Infection
Device failure

Once returned to the intensive care unit, patients must be closely monitored for early complications. Coagulation defects should be corrected without waiting for signs of significant bleeding. RV failure can be precipitated by excessive LVAD flow or elevated PVR. Therefore, it is advisable to limit the LVAD flow rate in the first few days to avoid overwhelming the RV. It is essential to avoid factors that may predispose to increases in PVR, such as hypoxia and acidosis. Anticoagulation is usually omitted in the first 48 hours and is only started when the patient has stopped bleeding (test tube drainage <30 ml/hr for 3 consecutive hours). Rising right atrial pressures associated with a fall in pump flow are signs of impending RV failure or tamponade. RV failure could be confirmed with TEE, which would demonstrate full right-sided chambers and empty left chambers. Under these circumstances, it is important not to increase the pre-load further with more fluid infusions. Immediate treatment consists of a combination of inotropes and pulmonary vasodilators. If the situation does not respond readily, early consideration should be given to re-exploring the patient and addition of right ventricular assist device.

Operative outcomes

Data from the 2010 INTERMACS Register showed an overall 1-year survival of 74% after LVAD placement (not device specific). This compares with 50% 1-year survival for Bi-VAD support. In selected series using only rotary LVAD, 1-year survival rates of 74% and 85% have been achieved for DT and BTT, respectively. Bleeding and infection are the most common early complications (Table 8.3). Neurological events are most likely to occur in the first 1–2 months after implant. The most common causes of death are cardiac failure, including right ventricular failure and ventricular arrhythmias, infections, and neurological events. At 1 year after implant for bridge to transplant, 52% have undergone heart transplant, 35% remain alive on LVAD support, and 12% have died on support.

Physiological response to VAD – remodeling of heart failure

Cardiac response

The benefits of angiotensin-converting enzyme (ACE) inhibitors in HF through afterload reduction leading to ventricular remodeling are well established. A more direct unloading of the LV with a VAD offers similar remodeling potential. An effective LVAD will unload the LV, which results in restoration of pressure-volume relationships, reduction in end-diastolic ventricular dimensions, reduction in cardiac mass, and improved contractility and cardiac index. Normalization of β-adrenergic receptor function is also seen. Histology samples taken at the time of LVAD placement compared with those taken at the time of subsequent transplantation have shown reversal of myocardial hypertrophy, attenuation of the myocardial apoptotic profile seen in HF, and improved myocardial mitochondrial function. There is reduced ventricular expression of atrial natriuretic peptide and reduced tumor necrosis factor alpha production. Cases of complete myocardial recovery have also been reported, allowing LVAD explant.

Pulmonary response

Improved LV unloading has sequential effects on the pulmonary circulation. VADs have been shown to reduce pulmonary hypertension, with both systolic and diastolic pressures falling significantly. The pulmonary capillary wedge pressure is reduced, as are the PVR and transpulmonary pressure gradient. This may render a patient with prohibitive pulmonary hypertension secondary to LV failure to HT candidacy.

Systemic responses

The improved cardiac output has beneficial effects on end organs and on systemic neurohormonal and cytokine signaling. Improved hemodynamics lead to improvements in renal and hepatic function and facilitate physical exercise and rehabilitation. There is a fall in plasma renin, angiotensin II, plasma epinephrine, and norepinephrine levels and reductions in cytokine and neuroendocrine responses. There is much interest in the systemic effects of reduced pulsativity with continuous flow devices. So far, there does not appear to be any detriment to renal and hepatic functions even after years of support with such devices. However, reduced systemic pulsatility appears to be associated with a higher incidence of gastrointestinal bleeding.

Outpatient management

Hospital discharge

Early mobilization is essential to successful outcomes. Many candidates have been in the intensive care unit for prolonged periods prior to device implant, with significant physical deconditioning. Physiotherapy involvement and patient motivation will be required at an early stage. Although full fitness may take some time to restore, there must be a program to optimize independence and to provide education for the patients and their caregivers to facilitate hospital discharge. This can be a staged process, with intermediate discharge to a nearby hostel prior to discharge home.

Outpatient management represents more efficient use of health care resources and is of high importance for patient quality of life. Prior to discharge, patients need to be mobilizing independently, feeding adequately, have good pain control, and be able to manage the device in conjunction with their home support. Arrangements must be in place to provide VAD patients in the community access to advice and assistance round-the-clock. Regular outpatient follow-ups are arranged at intervals.

Patient education

The patient and their family must be trained in managing the device (including emergencies) and prescription medications. This requires a period of familiarization prior to discharge, during which the patient should manage the device, power supply, and all their own medications. The patient and their caregivers should be comfortable with battery and controller changes prior to discharge.

Monitoring

Monitoring of patients implanted with a continuous flow device can be challenging for the unfamiliar. With a weak or absent pulse, blood pressure can often only be measured with a blood pressure cuff and a hand-held Doppler. Interpretation of the device control display and alarm record is likely only possible by those familiar with the device. Monitoring for hemolysis with bilirubin, hemoglobin, and plasma free hemoglobin should be performed at intervals. Anticoagulation will require careful monitoring with INR measurements.

Quality of life

Most patients report significant improvement in symptoms to New York Heart Association (NYHA) class I or II. Patient satisfaction and improved objective measures are noted in small studies. Patients can travel freely by road or by plane. Some countries still impose restrictions on driving for patients implanted with a VAD. Contact with water will damage the device, and so VAD patients are not allowed to swim or bathe. Showering is performed ideally with a hand-held shower head to avoid wetting the power supply. Some VAD manufacturers provide special equipment to protect the driveline and controller during showering. Sporting activities are limited to land-based sports that are non-contact. As a result, some VAD recipients remain dissatisfied with living with a VAD implant. Psychological support is often helpful and necessary, as there are reports of self-harm among VAD patients.

Transplantation after VAD therapy

The first successful bridge to a heart transplant with a VAD was performed in a patient at Stanford University. Although technically challenging, the 1-year post-transplant survival for patients bridged to transplant with an LVAD is similar to that of those without an LVAD (discussed further in Chapter 12). During the procedure, the re-opening and dissection phase is the most challenging. It is helpful if the implanting surgeon used a membrane under the sternum overlying any cannula and device. A good operative note or diagram is useful, but a preoperative chest computed tomography is helpful to identify VAD and conduit positioning. Some operators prefer initiating cardiopulmonary bypass by femoral or axillary cannulation prior to sternotomy.

Myocardial recovery and VAD removal

LVAD support can result in significant ventricular remodeling, as previously discussed. In 1995, a patient with an LVAD for 160 days at the Berlin Heart Institute demonstrated such an improvement in cardiac function that it became possible to remove the LVAD. This started the bridge to recovery program, with good success reported both in Berlin and in London using the Harefield Protocol. Successful weaning from the LVAD is predicted by LV size (<50 mm LV end-diastolic diameter) and ejection fraction.

Destination therapy

Long-term permanent MCS for patients not suitable for transplantation is sometimes called *destination therapy*. This is perhaps the ultimate goal of MCS development. It may be appropriate in selected patients with INTERMACS 1–4 (NYHA IV) heart failure status on optimum medical therapy. The first piece of good evidence for destination therapy came from the REMATCH trial with the Thoratec Heartmate VE. This demonstrated a 1-year and 2-year survival rate of 52% and 23%, respectively, in the VAD group compared with 25% and 8%, respectively, in the medical therapy group. Subsequent comparison of the pulsatile HeartMate XVE with a continuous-flow device (Heartmate II) showed 2-year survival rates for the Heartmate XVE of 24% and the Heartmate II of 58%. However, there is currently no trial data to support the use of LVADs in NYHA class III patients.

The future

Science fiction has often used the theme of the bionic man of the future. MCS is certainly in that realm but is now of our time. The latest generation of devices offer clinical reliability, and the limitation of their widespread application is largely due to cost and a limited pool of expertise in their use. The use of VAD in transplantation will always be limited by the number of available hearts. Unless the number of donor hearts increases, using VADs to bridge patients to transplant will only serve to select which patient receives a heart. The more likely scenario is that VADs will see greater application outside of transplantation as destination therapy. However, as the duration of support for bridge to transplant increases, these two indications are becoming increasingly blurred. Using VAD as bridge to recovery is a very exciting prospect and deserves further study. However, the proportion of VAD patients successfully recovered and explanted remains small at present. Adjuncts in regenerative medicine, including gene therapy and cell transplantation, may enhance and realize the full potential of this approach.

With regard to device technology, further improvements are desirable. A modular component system would enable surgical replacement of failing parts rather than replacement of the entire VAD system if a problem develops. The size of the VADs has reduced considerably, but further size reduction may confer additional benefit. Some of these are now small enough to be used as a pair of devices for Bi-VAD support. The Achilles heel of all currently available LVAD systems is the need for a percutaneous driveline. Eliminating such a requirement is likely to minimize infection risks, remove the onerous burden of driveline management, and improve body image and the psychological impact of the device and, therefore, quality of life of VAD recipients. The development of fully implantable VADs hinges on a better power delivery system and control mechanism. Improvements in battery technology will also enable a patient to charge overnight while sleeping and mobilize for the full day on a small and light battery pack. The main challenge, however, remains affordability. These devices are most likely to be used in an older patient population, possibly retired and not contributing to the state economy and without independent income to cover the cost of their treatment. The potential number of people who might benefit from such devices is unknown. Can we afford to offer this to the entire HF population, and what is the opportunity cost of resources directed into this area in the Western world? Perhaps a bigger challenge is the ethical and moral dilemma of the appropriate healthcare resource allocation in the world.

Further reading

Feller E, Sorensen E, Haddad M, *et al.* Clinical outcomes are similar in pulsatile and nonpulsatile left ventricular assist device recipients. *Ann Thorac Surg* 2007; **83**: 1082–8.

Kirklin J, Naftel D, Kormos R, *et al.* Second INTERMACS annual report: More than 1,000 primary left ventricular assist device implants. *J Heart Lung Transplant* 2010; **29**: 1–10.

Liang H, Lin H, Weng Y, Dandel M, Hetzer R. Prediction of cardiac function after weaning from ventricular assist devices. *J Thorac Cardiovasc Surg* 2005; **130**: 1555–60.

Lietz K, Long J, Kfoury K, *et al.* Outcomes of left ventricular assist device implantation as destination therapy in the post-REMATCH era: Implications for patient selection. *Circulation* 2007; **116**; 497–505.

McMurray J. Systolic heart failure. *N Engl J Med* 2010; **362**: 228–38.

Ochiai Y, McCarthy P, Smedira N, *et al.* Predictors of severe right ventricular failure after implantable left ventricular assist device insertion: analysis of 245 patients. *Circulation* 2002; **106**: I198–202.

Slaughter M, Rogers J, Milano C, *et al.* Advanced heart failure treated with continuous-flow left ventricular assist device. *N Engl J Med* 2009; **361**: 2241–51.

Tsui S, Parameshwar J. Shock due to catastrophic loss of myocardium. In Banner N, Jessup M (eds). *ISHLT Monograph Series: Advanced Heart Failure*. Philadelphia: Elsevier, 2009, pp. 509–23.

Chapter 9

Surgical procedure

R.V. Venkateswaran and David P. Jenkins

Key points

- Median sternotomy is the standard approach for heart transplantation.
- The bicaval technique of implantation is most commonly employed.
- Previous sternotomy makes the procedure considerably more complicated and may lead to increased postoperative bleeding.
- Ventricular assist devices and implantable defibrillator devices should be removed concurrently.

Heart transplantation, like any other procedure, requires careful selection of the recipient and donor graft. It is medically and ethically vital to select recipients who need the most and have the best chance of good outcome. It also requires an excellent coordination and communication between the donor and recipient teams. The surgical procedure and immediate postoperative care are discussed in this section.

Preoperative preparation

Donor to recipient matching is based primarily on ABO blood group compatibility. Other variables that may play a role in optimally matching donor and recipients are age, height, weight, and gender. In general, the height disparity between the donor and recipient should be restricted to within 10%. Recipients' invasive hemodynamic parameters such as transpulmonary gradient (TPG) and pulmonary vascular resistance (PVR) must be taken into account when accepting a marginal heart donor. Recipients with more than 10% of panel reactive antibodies in serum suggesting presensitization to alloantigen usually require cytotoxic or virtual cross-matching prior to transplantation. Assessment and management of potential donor hearts is discussed in Chapter 5.

Technique of orthotopic heart transplantation

Preparation

The patient is painted with standard antiseptic solutions and draped. Both groins should be prepared and draped for access to the femoral vessels either for cannulation or for insertion of intra-aortic balloon pump. In the current era, many recipients have cardiac resynchronization therapy (CRT) devices with or without implantable cardioverter-defibrillators (ICDs). These should also be included in draping so that after heart implantation, these leads and the generator can be removed at the end of the procedure.

Incision and cardiopulmonary bypass

Median sternotomy is the standard approach for heart transplantation. The pericardium is opened and the edges sutured to the skin edges. The plane between aorta and pulmonary artery is separated using diathermy. In difficult circumstances, the aorta may be encircled with a nylon tape to get easy access to ascending aorta for cannulation. Following systemic heparinization, the ascending aorta is cannulated as high as possible just below the origin of innominate artery. The superior and inferior vena cavae (SVC and IVC) are cannulated separately for venous drainage. A size 24 or 28 right-angled cannula is preferred for the SVC and a size 30 or 32 malleable straight cannula for the IVC. Care must be taken during cannulation, especially if the CVP is very high. Following cannulation,

Organ Transplantation: A Clinical Guide, ed. A.A. Klein, C.J. Lewis, and J.C. Madsen. Published by Cambridge University Press.

cardiopulmonary bypass is initiated, and the patient is cooled to 30°C. Both cavae should be encircled using nylon tapes and snared to avoid draining air into the bypass circuit.

Recipient cardiectomy

Explantation of the heart is commenced after making sure that the donor heart is within 20 minutes from the recipient hospital. The aorta is clamped and the cavae snared, but cardioplegic arrest is unnecessary. However, sometimes with a large heart, venting is useful to aid cardiectomy, either via the left ventricular (LV) apex or right superior pulmonary vein to keep the field clear. An alternating current fibrillator is used by some to induce ventricular fibrillation.

The right atrium is opened along the atrioventricular groove, leaving an adequate cuff along the lateral wall toward the appendage. The interatrial septum is opened along the fossa ovalis and blood drained from the left atrium. The incision is extended cranially around the roof of the left atrium. Then the aorta and pulmonary arteries are divided immediately distal to their valves. The interatrial septum is further divided caudally into coronary sinus, and the incision follows the course of the sinus around the heart. The heart is explanted, leaving a large cuff of left atrium by dividing left atrium close to the posterior annulus of the mitral valve. Both atrial appendages are excised to reduce the risk of postoperative thrombus formation. This should leave a cuff of right and left atrium and the two major arteries. The left and right atrial cuffs can be further fashioned to match the size of the donor heart.

Implantation of donor heart

Biatrial technique

Lower and Shumway initially described the technique of biatrial anastomosis, which has been widely used in cardiac transplantation. The heart is removed from the ice box and prepared on a table in a cold saline container. It is examined for any damage during retrieval, and the interatrial septum is examined for any septal defect or persistent foramen ovale, which may then be closed. The aorta and pulmonary artery are separated. The left atrium is fashioned for anastomosis by incisions between the origins of the pulmonary veins to create a circular cuff of atrium to match that of the recipient. The left atrial appendage is inspected, and any venting incisions made at retrieval are oversewn. A curvilinear incision is made on the lateral wall of right atrium from the IVC opening toward the right atrial appendage. This reduces the risk of injuring thesinoatrial node. The SVC is oversewn.

Using a long length of double-ended 3–0 Prolene, the anastomosis is started at the left atrial appendage of the donor heart to the recipient's left atrial cuff at the level of the left superior pulmonary vein. After two or three stitches, the heart is lowered into the pericardial cavity over a cold swab, and further cold swabs are placed anteriorly. A Prolene stay suture at the level of the left inferior pulmonary vein on both donor and recipient left atrium can aid accurate approximation and reduce the risk of torsion. The posterior lateral left atrial cuff is sutured, and then the second arm of the 3–0 Prolene is used to complete the anterior medial left atrial cuff. If a right superior pulmonary vein vent was used prior to explantation, the same could be used to vent the left ventricle of the donor heart to avoid any distension during the implantation. A cold saline irrigation or a cold jacket may be used to keep the heart cold during the rest of the implantation.

Next the pulmonary artery anastomosis is commenced, using a continuous 4–0 Prolene suture. Care is taken to avoid any twist, and the length should be kept short to avoid any kinking. To reduce the ischemic time, the anterior wall of pulmonary artery anastomosis can be completed after reperfusion of the heart. The aortic anastomosis is next completed using a continuous 4–0 Prolene suture. Any discrepancy in size should be adjusted on the anterior wall so that any suture line bleeding can be controlled easily. A 4–0 Prolene purse string suture is placed on the ascending aorta, and an aortic root vent cannula is inserted. The cold saline or the jacket is removed, and the patient is placed in the Trendelenburg position. The heart is filled with blood, and thorough deairing is done through both aortic root and pulmonary vein vent if present. Carbon-dioxide insufflation of the surgical wound may be used to aid deairing. The cross-clamp is then removed, and the perfusionist is advised to open the arterial circuit with a leucocyte filter.

During reperfusion, the anterior wall of the pulmonary artery anastomosis is performed, if not completed earlier. The right atrial anastomosis is completed using continuous 3–0 Prolene with the heart perfused and beating to reduce "warm" ischemic time. The patient is re-warmed, and the caval snares are removed.

Following the completion of all anastomoses, the heart is reperfused and the patient is rewarmed. During this time, ventilation of the lungs may be recommenced. Both atrial and ventricular temporary pacing wires are inserted and connected to a dual-chamber pacing device. Temporary pacing and isoprenaline infusion are useful to keep a higher heart rate in the denervated heart. The patient is weaned off from cardiopulmonary bypass, and the heart is decannulated and hemostasis is achieved. The right pleural cavity is opened widely to create a large window to avoid postoperative pericardial effusion.

Bicaval technique

In the early 1990s, the bicaval technique of heart transplantation was first introduced, and currently, it is most widely used technique. The recognition of complications related to atrial enlargement in the biatrial anastomosis led to the development of the bicaval and total heart transplant techniques to preserve atrial size. The donor retrieval team should dissect the entire length of the SVC and ligate the azygos vein in order to get adequate length of SVC. After confirming the adequacy of the length of donor SVC, the recipient right atrial cuff is excised, leaving separate SVC and IVC cuff for bicaval anastomosis. The caval anastomosis can be constructed after reperfusing the heart during systemic rewarming. A sump sucker inserted through the SVC orifice into the right atrium would aid in dry field during IVC anastomosis, which is performed using 3–0 Prolene suture. The SVC anastomosis is finally completed using 4–0 or 5–0 Prolene sutures. Care is taken to avoid any twisting and narrowing by purse-string effect on the SVC anastomosis. Total heart transplantation involves excision of the recipient heart, including the left atrium, leaving two separate pulmonary venous cuffs for each side and anastomosis of the pulmonary venous cuffs and separate caval anastomosis.

These techniques are more technically demanding and may lead to increased implantation and warm ischemic time. However, several series of retrospective studies have shown that the bicaval technique has been associated with reduced hospital stay; lower incidence of atrial arrhythmia, pacemaker requirement, and diuretic dependence; early return to sinus rhythm; and reduced incidence of postoperative tricuspid regurgitation and RV dysfunction. However, the long-term outcome of heart transplantation does not differ between both techniques. Prospective randomized trials are unlikely to be done to evaluate the outcome between both techniques due to a major shift to the bicaval technique of implantation.

Special considerations

Although the surgical technique of heart transplantation is simple, there are certain specific circumstances in which the operation can be technically demanding and require careful planning to get the best outcome.

Redo-sternotomy

Patients who have had previous cardiac surgery either for ischemic or valvular heart disease are increasingly referred or listed for heart transplantation. In these patients, the recipient dissection and cardiectomy will take longer, and adjustment of timings is necessary. The retrieval of the donor heart may have to be delayed until the recipient team has completed the dissection and are ready to institute cardiopulmonary bypass. Some units advocate exposure of the femoral vessels in particularly complex cases in the event that cannulation for bypass is necessary. Following sternotomy, the aim is directed toward dissecting the aorta and right atrium and both cavae to establish cardiopulmonary bypass. The rest of the dissection can be performed after establishing bypass. It is preferable to use diathermy dissection to have a dry field. Once the dissection is complete, the remaining operation is carried out as a standard procedure.

Explantation of ventricular assist devices

Ventricular assist devices (VADs) are more commonly used as a bridge to transplantation, and many patients wait for heart transplantation with a functioning VAD or are listed for urgent procedure due to VAD-related complications. The procedure is technically more challenging in these circumstances, and we recommend 2 to 3 hours dissection time to explant the recipient heart. During the initial VAD procedure, it is advisable to avoid dissection around the aorta and pulmonary artery and both cavae to minimize pericardial adhesions. Use of silastic membrane around the VAD inflow cannula and partial closure of the pericardium at the time of initial surgery may help reduce adhesions. Good communication is even more essential between the donor and recipient team to avoid a long ischemic time. A preoperative computed tomography scan of the chest may aid in clear demarcation of the VAD outflow graft and its relationship to the posterior sternal table.

At redo sternotomy, care is taken to avoid injury to the drive line, which normally crosses the midline at the lower end of sternum, and the VAD outflow graft, which may lie anteriorly beneath the sternum. If there is difficulty in identifying the aorta, the VAD outflow graft can be used for arterial cannulation. Once the cavae and aorta are dissected, cardiopulmonary bypass is established in the usual manner and the VAD is turned off and the outflow graft isolated and clamped. The VAD itself can be removed with the heart, but if time is short, it can be removed following implantation of the donor heart. If there is any infection around the driveline, it is dealt with at the end of the procedure after closure of the sternotomy wound to avoid any contamination.

Heart transplantation for congenital heart disease

Due to advances in the management of congenital heart disease, many patients present in early or later adult life with end-stage heart failure and are listed for heart transplantation. These patients may have had multiple operations in the past, and dissection and explantation of their heart can be a challenge. Surgical planning due to the variability of anatomical findings is essential with the aid of appropriate radiological imaging. There are a number of particular problems encountered with heart transplantation in this group of patients. Recipients with atrial switch palliation (Mustard/Senning procedure) for transposition of great arteries in the earlier era pose particular difficulty for venous cannulation. In these patients, the atrial baffle prevents the insertion of venous cannula through the right atrium. The SVC is preferably cannulated high up near the junction with innominate vein. After establishing cardiopulmonary bypass using single venous cannula, the atrium can be opened and the baffle incised to allow the insertion of IVC cannula. An alternative is cannulation of the femoral vein. In some patients, the pulmonary artery lies posterior to the aorta, and it is preferable to have an adequate length of pulmonary artery to allow tension-free anastomosis. In addition, bleeding from the anastomosis will be difficult to control due to the poor access. In patients with single ventricular palliation (Fontan type procedure), heart transplantation is specifically complicated, in particular by the short length of the recipient SVC. The donor retrieval team should dissect the SVC, including the innominate vein, for tension-free SVC anastomosis. In patients following previous systemic to pulmonary artery shunts or bidirectional Glenn procedure, the pulmonary arteries may be narrowed and require surgical correction of stenosis at the time of heart transplantation.

Left-sided SVC

Patients with left-sided SVC pose difficulty in establishing adequate venous drainage and cardiopulmonary bypass. It may only be detected at the time of surgery due to the absence or smaller size of the recipient SVC. It may be associated with a small or absent innominate vein. If detected, the left SVC should be cannulated to avoid venous congestion of the brain and left side of the upper torso. After explantation of the heart, the transplant operation is performed as usual. The donor SVC is anastomosed to the innominate vein high up. If the innominate vein is absent, then the donor team should retrieve the heart, including the innominate vein, and this can be used to create a new SVC innominate vein junction. At the end of procedure, the left SVC cannula is removed and it is oversewn.

Domino heart transplantation

In patients undergoing heart–lung transplantation, especially small cystic fibrotic recipients, their explanted heart can be used for transplantation. This procedure is called domino heart transplantation. Technically, the surgical procedure is not different from that of standard heart transplantation. However, the SVC may not be long enough in the explanted heart and may require biatrial anastomosis in the domino recipient. The outcome following domino heart transplantation has been shown to be comparable to that of cadaveric donor transplantation. Heart–lung transplantation and domino heart transplantation have largely been superseded by bilateral sequential lung transplantation.

Heterotopic transplantation

This procedure was rarely performed in the recent era but may have a place in the modern era to make use of small hearts that might otherwise not be used to maximize organ utilization. Heterotopic HT may be performed as either a bi-ventricular or left ventricular assist configuration. The donor heart is placed usually in the right side of the chest and anastomosed to the recipient's heart, which remains in situ. For bi-ventricular support, after institution of cardiopulmonary bypass, the posterior pericardium is divided to create space for the donor heart. The left atrial anastomosis is first performed by placing the donor heart in the chest with the right ventricle facing posteriorly. After completing left and right atrial anastomosis, the donor aorta is connected to the recipient's aorta using side-biting clamp. The pulmonary artery anastomosis is performed last, and both this and the aortic anastomosis may require vascular grafts due to length limitations. Heterotopic transplantation allows much more leniency on the donor and recipient mismatching. As the recipient heart is not excised, this could be particularly useful in patients with elevated TPG and PVR. However, patients may continue to suffer from symptoms of angina or thromboembolism from the diseased heart.

Immediate postoperative management

Postoperative management will be discussed in more detail in the following chapter. Post-transplant recipients are preferably managed in an isolated intensive care unit bed to avoid cross-infection. Careful consideration should be given to the adequacy of cardiac output in maintaining oxygen delivery to the tissues, bleeding, collections, pneumothorax, and position of the monitoring lines. The patient is slowly warmed using warming blankets and inotropes are continued to maintain stability. After achieving stability for a few hours, the patient may be woken up from the anesthesia for planned extubation.

Further reading

Christie JD, Edwards LB, Aurora P, *et al.* The Registry of the International Society for Heart and Lung Transplantation: Twenty-sixth Official Adult Lung and Heart-Lung Transplantation Report – 2009. *J Heart Lung Transplant* 2009; **28**:1031–49.

Jacob S, Sellke F. Is bicaval orthotopic heart transplantation superior to the biatrial technique? *Interact Cardiovasc Thorac Surg* 2009; **9**: 333–42.

Luckraz H, Charman SC, Parameshwar J, *et al.* Are non-brain stem-dead cardiac donors acceptable donors? *J Heart Lung Transplant* 2004; **23**: 330–3.

Potter CD, Wheeldon DR, Wallwork J. Functional assessment and management of heart donors: a rationale for characterization and a guide to therapy. *J Heart Lung Transplant* 1995; **14**: 59–65.

Chapter 10

Management during surgery

Kate Drummond and Andrew A. Klein

Key points

- Commencing an infusion of an inotropic agent before induction of anesthesia may improve hemodynamic stability.
- Donor heart failure is not uncommon, and mechanical support may be required in order to separate successfully from CPB.
- Management of right ventricular dysfunction includes optimization of fluid status, judicious lung ventilation strategies, and use of pulmonary vasodilators.
- Transesophageal echocardiography may aid diagnosis and guide management of hypotension after heart transplantation.

Heart transplant surgery is almost inevitably emergency in nature, happening often with minimal notice and out of hours. It requires a rapid response to minimize ischemic time for the transplanted organ, and good communication between the retrieval and the operating team is essential. Optimal timing of anesthesia and surgery will ensure that the recipient is prepared and ready for cardiopulmonary bypass as the donor organ arrives. From the time the anesthetic team is alerted to the possibility of organ transplantation and the arrival of the organ, the patient must be assessed and prepared and anesthesia induced and maintained. Following transplantation itself, the perioperative team must be prepared to deal with a number of potential complications that may arise in this complex surgical group after weaning from cardiopulmonary bypass (CPB). This chapter covers the preoperative considerations and reviews the intraoperative management of heart transplant patients.

Preoperative considerations

Heart transplantation is considered emergency surgery, and there is often little time for extensive evaluation in the immediate preoperative period. In order to determine their need for transplantation, all patients will have had an extensive multidisciplinary assessment prior to being listed for transplantation. In order to identify and plan for all potential anesthetic complications, some centers review potential heart transplant recipients in preanesthetic assessment clinics. Regardless of this, there will be some degree of assessment required prior to induction of anesthesia. A quick medical history, examination, and review of recent investigations may be all there is time for prior to induction.

Patients presenting for heart transplantation by their nature have severe cardiac disease. Many have subsequent end-organ dysfunction due to chronic low perfusion. Serum chemistry, electrolytes, and liver and renal function should be checked, along with hematological and clotting studies. Blood should also be taken for blood typing and antibody screening. Cross-matching of blood can be difficult in these patients due to the presence of antibodies, so the anesthetist should liaise with the laboratory ensure there is enough compatible blood products on site. In addition, consideration should be given to the cytomegalovirus status of donor and recipient when ordering blood for transfusion.

It is not uncommon for patients to be on long-term therapeutic anti-coagulation due to the high incidence of atrial fibrillation and risk of atrial thrombus. Liver dysfunction due to hepatic congestion may also complicate this. Surgery should of course proceed without delay, but correction in the immediate post-CPB period may be required with fresh-frozen plasma or prothrombin complex concentrate.

Organ Transplantation: A Clinical Guide, ed. A.A. Klein, C.J. Lewis, and J.C. Madsen. Published by Cambridge University Press.

Patients with severe heart failure are often on many drugs, including diuretics, angiotensin-converting enzyme (ACE) inhibitors and calcium antagonists. Many of these drugs interact with anesthesia and should be taken into account.

Preoperative pulmonary hypertension is a significant risk factor for postoperative right heart failure. Elevated preoperative pulmonary artery pressure (PAP) is associated with increased postoperative complications, including death. Although this relationship is not linear, the information obtained from routine preoperative right heart catheterization can assist the anesthetist in predicting and preparing for problems with right heart dysfunction after bypass.

Any history of previous surgery should be clarified, as at least 30% of patients will have had a previous sternotomy incision. Usual precautions for resternotomy should be taken, including obtaining large-bore venous access, placing external defibrillator pads, and having cross-matched blood checked and available in the operating theatre prior to commencing surgery. In some cases the femoral vessels may be prepared for cannulation before commencing resternotomy.

Preoperative left ventricular assist device (LVAD) use presents a number of unique problems for the anesthetist, but most importantly preload must be maintained as hypovolemia can result in inadequate ventricular assist device (VAD) output and hypotension. Patients with VADs are usually on some form of anti-coagulation that will need to be managed.

Implanted defibrillators and pacemakers are common in this patient group due to the high incidence of malignant supraventricular and ventricular arrhythmias. Implantable defibrillators should be turned off immediately prior to induction of anaesthesia to prevent inadvertent discharge during surgery. External defibrillator pads should be applied. Pacemakers should be reprogrammed to asynchronous (fixed rate) mode.

Intraoperative considerations

Induction and maintenance

Following pre-anaesthetic assessment, induction of anesthesia should be performed after placement of essential monitoring. Large-bore intravenous access should be inserted, and pulse oximetry and ECG monitoring applied. Commonly placed in radial or femoral arteries, arterial lines should be inserted prior to induction for both invasive blood pressure monitoring and access to arterial blood sampling.

Central venous access and introducers for pulmonary artery catheters are often placed after induction of anesthesia for patient comfort, but may be placed in advance of this if clinically indicated. The internal jugular approach allows easier access during surgery but, although uncommon, may interfere with future endomyocardial biopsies due to vascular thrombosis. The pulmonary artery catheter should be placed so that it lies within the superior vena cava (SVC) so that it does not interfere with surgical bicaval anastomosis. Patients with severe heart failure may be transferred to the operating theatre straight from the intensive care unit and already have these lines and monitors in situ. The anesthetist should check their position and patency prior to surgery, as access will be limited once the patient is positioned and draped and surgery has commenced. All lines should be placed with strict aseptic technique due to the risk of infection from immunosuppression.

Cerebral oximetry by using near-infrared spectroscopy is increasing in use in cardiac anesthesia. It has the advantage of being non-invasive compared with other methods such as jugular venous bulb saturation monitoring. Prolonged cerebral oxygen desaturation (SrO2) is associated with a higher risk of postoperative cognitive dysfunction and longer hospital stay in general cardiac surgery populations. Despite this, the ideal treatment strategy for when confronted with low SrO2 is still unknown. The use of depth of anesthesia monitors, such as the bispectral monitor, although not in routine use, can be a useful additional tool for the titration of anesthetic agents and has also been shown to correlate with cerebral oxygenation.

There is often inadequate time to observe conventional fasting periods in transplant surgery. If this is the case, a modified rapid sequence induction should be performed. Preoperative use of prokinetics such as metoclopramide or drugs to lower gastric pH such as sodium citrate or proton pump inhibitors are useful. Cricoid pressure may be indicated if gastric emptying is considered likely to be incomplete, in which case either suxamethonium or a longer acting muscle relaxant such as rocuronium may be administered. Both have been used successfully in heart transplant surgery.

Patients with severe heart failure are dependent on preload for ventricular filling and elevated sympathetic tone to ensure cardiac output and tissue perfusion. Acutely unwell patients may already be on significant doses of inotropic agents preoperatively. In other patients, commencement of an infusion of inotrope such as dopamine or epinephrine prior to induction is prudent and may minimize hypotension and hemodynamic instability prior to commencement of CPB.

Although most anesthetic agents have been successfully used in cardiac transplantation, all will unfavorably alter hemodynamics. Traditionally, opioid- or benzodiazepine-based induction is used, with fentanyl 5–10 μg/kg and midazolam 0.1–0.2 mg/kg commonly used. Ketamine has also been used at a low dose of 1–2 mg/kg. Anesthesia can then be maintained with total intravenous anesthesia (TIVA), volatile agents, or a combination of both. Institutional or individual anesthetist preference will ultimately decide which drug combination is used. Regardless of the agents used, dosing should be judicious and titrated carefully, as overdose is easy in patients with low cardiac output state. Changes in preload, systemic vascular resistance (SVR), and heart rate must be aggressively managed with fluids, inotropes, and/or vasopressors. The use of intraoperative transesophageal echocardiography (TEE) can be a useful guide to hemodynamic management as well as diagnosing intracardiac thrombi, which are common in this population.

Infection control and maintenance of aseptic technique is essential due to infection risk. Most transplant centers have protocols including prophylactic antibiotics and pre- or intraoperative administration of immunosuppression including induction.

Since the voluntary withdrawal of aprotinin in 2007, there has been much discussion in the literature about the use of anti-fibrinolytic agents in cardiac surgery. Currently, two lysine analogues are available and commonly used (epsilon amino-caproic acid and tranexamic acid). The Society of Thoracic Surgeons Blood Conservation Guideline Task Force recommends the use of these anti-fibrinolytic agents as part of a comprehensive strategy to reduce blood loss and transfusion requirements in routine and high-risk cardiac surgery. Many centers have also incorporated their use into cardiac transplant surgery. There is a paucity of evidence regarding potential complications of the lysine analogues currently in use; however, the risk of thrombotic complications appears to be low.

Preparation to come off bypass

Preparation to discontinue CPB should be undertaken as per any other cardiac case. The anesthetist should ensure that the patient's electrolytes, pH status, and oxygenation are adequate. Ventilation should be commenced gently to reinflate the lungs and aid in the deairing process. TEE examination looking for residual air should be performed. The transplanted heart is denervated, so reflex-mediated heart rate responses will be absent. Baseline heart rate is usually around 100 beats per minute in a denervated heart. Any ischemia or damage to the sinoatrial (SA) or atrioventricular (AV) nodes may result in severe bradycardia. Indirectly acting chronotropic agents will be ineffective, so direct-acting agents such as isoproterenol at 0.005 to 0.05 μg/kg/min are recommended for chronotropic support. In addition, temporary epicardial pacing wires may be used with AV sequential pacing at approximately 90–100 beats per minute, as it may take several minutes for spontaneous rhythm to resume after release of the aortic cross-clamp. Failure of the return of SA node activity or adequate AV conduction requires permanent pacemaker implantation early after transplant in 5–10% of patients after HT following biatrial anastomosis, with a lower rate in bicaval transplants.

Pharmacological support

Initial pharmacological support is required during the period of weaning from CPB, and this initial management is described here, with ongoing support and choice of agent discussed in the following chapter. Mean arterial pressure should be kept above 60 mmHg with vasopressor or inotropic agents as clinically indicated. Ideally, short-acting, titratable agents should be used. A mean arterial pressure greater than 80 mmHg is undesirable, and a short-acting vasodilator should be available for use if the need arises. Following separation from bypass, taking care not to disrupt suture lines, a pulmonary artery catheter can be passed into the pulmonary artery. The inotrope of choice will depend on patient variables derived from this, TEE evaluation, and institutional and the individual anesthetist's practice.

Care must be taken with the use of systemic vasopressors, because although they increase MAP and coronary perfusion pressure, they may also increase pulmonary vascular resistance and worsen right heart function. Noradrenaline, adrenaline, dopamine, and phenylephrine have all been used successfully in cardiac transplantation surgery. Phenylephrine is most likely to worsen right ventricular (RV) function in patients with chronic pulmonary hypertension. Vasopressin has been used to elevate SVR and has minimal effects on PVR.

Isoproterenol is a non-selective beta-agonist. Along with its chronotropic properties, it has inotropic activity and produces systemic and pulmonary vasodilatation and has been advocated as the inotrope of choice after cardiac transplantation. If used, it should not be discontinued abruptly, as PVR will rapidly rise to baseline levels. Dobutamine, a synthetic catecholamine with predominantly beta-agonist effects and minimal alpha-agonist activity, is also a useful agent when aiming to avoid vasoconstriction. Phosphodiesterase III inhibitors such as milrinone and enoximone have been used successfully due to their positive inotropic action coupled with vascular smooth-muscle relaxing activity. These drugs are particularly useful, as this group of patients often have beta-adrenergic receptor downregulation. Enoximone is incompatible with many other commonly used cardiac drugs and should be infused via a dedicated line. It is not uncommon for a combination of agents to be required in order to achieve optimal cardiac and vascular conditions.

Mechanical support

If cardiac function following bypass remains inadequate after implementation of all other strategies, the use of mechanical support should be considered. An intra-aortic balloon pump will assist in supporting the left ventricle predominately but will also aid the right ventricle by ensuring adequate perfusion pressure for the coronary vessels and limiting ischemia. Temporary left, right, or bi-ventricular mechanical assist devices, together with extracorporeal membrane oxygenation (ECMO), have been used successfully in cases of extremely poor ventricular function after transplantation. The particular device used will depend on which ventricle is failing. Their use should be considered earlier rather than later to avoid prolonged periods of organ hypoperfusion and ischemia. The heart usually recovers quickly, and nearly half of these devices may be weaned within 4 days.

Right heart dysfunction

Acute RV dysfunction is the most common cause of difficulty weaning from CPB, and this initial management to aide weaning is described here. The etiology is multifactorial: pulmonary hypertension is common in this population, and elevated PVR will be worsened temporarily by the release of vasoactive substances associated with cardiopulmonary bypass. The donor heart, although able to increase contractility, may be unable to cope with such a high afterload. Surgical manipulation, tricuspid or pulmonary insufficiency, denervation, and ischemia may all contribute to right heart dysfunction. Additionally, although temporary, the RV is more commonly affected by intracoronary air, as the right coronary artery is most anterior. This can cause acute and catastrophic right heart ischemia and failure until the air is expelled from the coronary vessel.

Right heart failure results in a reduction in pulmonary blood flow and left ventricular (LV) preload. In addition, dilation of the failing RV causes the interventricular septum to bulge leftward, impinging on LV filling. The overall result is a reduction in cardiac output and aortic root pressure. Reduction in coronary blood flow ensues and further ischemia occurs, leading to a downward spiral of RV function.

Right heart failure can be identified using TEE, which will show a dilated, poorly contracting right ventricle. The left ventricle will be underfilled, with a septum bulging leftward in systole. There may be severe tricuspid regurgitation secondary to a dilated tricuspid annulus. Mean PAP will be elevated, typically above 25–30 mmHg.

Treatment of RV failure involves temporary supportive measures until the ventricle recovers. In order to maximize RV function, a number of strategies are useful:

1. Optimizing ventilation to minimize PVR
2. Optimizing fluid status and RV preload
3. Managing PVR to minimize RV afterload
4. Pharmacological and mechanically supporting RV function
5. Preservation of coronary blood flow by maintaining aortic root pressure

Ventilation strategies for RV dysfunction

Although there is little evidence for any specific ventilation strategies in preventing RV decompensation, it would seem reasonable to avoid factors that increase pulmonary artery pressure (PAP) and employ strategies known to reduce PAP. Avoiding hypoventilation by providing adequate minute ventilation and inspired oxygen is essential. Hypercarbia increases systolic PAP predominantly by increasing PVR. High inspired oxygen concentrations should be used to avoid hypoxic pulmonary vasoconstriction in the presence of low alveolar oxygen concentrations. Although this reduces hypoxemia from shunting, it results in elevated PVR. It is also stimulated by acidosis and inhibited by alkalosis. The use of positive end expiratory pressure (PEEP) in cardiac transplantation remains controversial. PVR is minimal at functional residual capacity (FRC). The judicious application of PEEP reduces atelectasis and aids in maintaining FRC. Excessive PEEP or high inflation pressures, however, will cause a rise in PVR and RV dilation.

Fluid management in RV dysfunction

Fluid management in patients with a failing RV is critical, as the heart will be preload-dependent. Hypovolemia will result in reduced preload and RV output, whereas any large increase in fluid volume may result in RV distension at the expense of LV preload and output. Observation of the heart directly through the sternotomy, TEE, and CVP or pulmonary artery catheter monitoring are all useful measures to employ when determining the volume of fluid to be administered.

Selective pulmonary vasodilators for RV dysfunction

The use of pulmonary vasodilators in cardiac transplantation has been well studied. A number are available in current practice. Intravenous prostaglandin E2 (PGE2) is a potent pulmonary vasodilator that undergoes extensive metabolism in pulmonary vessels. It is widely used to facilitate weaning from CPB, as it reduces PVR and improves RV function. Vasodilatation and hypotension due to its effects on SVR can limit its use. Inotrope or vasopressors are often required to counteract this.

Another commonly used selective pulmonary vasodilator, inhaled nitric oxide, produces vasodilation of smooth muscle in pulmonary vessels by increasing production of cyclic GMP. Systemic absorption is minimal, resulting in fewer systemic side effects. Rebound pulmonary hypertension may occur when it is withdrawn. Nitric oxide has been show to reduce PVR immediately after heart transplantation by 50%, whereas PGE1 decreased resistance only 10%.

Transesophageal echocardiography

Recent updated guidelines from the American Society of Anesthesiologists and the Society of Cardiovascular Anesthesiologists on TEE recommend its use in all open heart procedures. A complete examination of the heart should be performed prior to bypass in order to assess the likelihood of potential complications following transplantation of the donor heart and to look for intracardiac thrombi. If any thrombi are identified, the surgeon should be alerted in order to avoid manipulation that may cause embolization.

After CPB, the TEE should focus on the ventricular function, particularly that of the RV, as described earlier. It is often more practical to determine preload status with TEE rather that intermittent pulmonary artery catheter measurements. Filling can be undertaken with TEE guidance in order to avoid ventricular over distension. The surgical anastomoses of the main pulmonary arteries should be evaluated with Doppler pressure gradients. Mild mitral, tricuspid, and pulmonary regurgitation is not uncommon after transplantation, but aortic regurgitation should be cause for concern. Distortion of the atria, depending on surgical technique used, may cause significant mitral regurgitation. A higher incidence of systolic anterior motion of the anterior mitral leaflet has also been described after heart transplantation.

Management of coagulopathy

Significant coagulopathy is not uncommon following CPB in heart transplantation procedures. This may be due to residual preoperative anticoagulation, CPB-induced platelet dysfunction, dilution of clotting factors, and hypothermia.

Heparin should be reversed with protamine once the patient is stable and off bypass. It should be administered slowly due to the risk of pulmonary vasoconstriction and its effect measured using activated clotting time (ACT). Thromboelastography (TEG) can be used to determine clotting status and has the advantage that it can be performed while still on bypass (by using a cup with heparinase added to negate the effect of heparin) in order to allow time for thawing of fresh-frozen plasma and cryoprecipitate if necessary. Formal clotting studies should also be performed once CPB has been discontinued.

Clotting factor concentrates, fibrinogen concentrates, and recombinant single factors (e.g., factor VIIa) can be considered in patients with clotting deficiencies who cannot tolerate administration of large fluid volumes. Platelet count and hemoglobin should be maintained as per institutional transfusion guidelines. Input from an experienced hematologist can help guide management of any coagulopathy. Meticulous surgical technique will aid in reducing blood loss. The surgical field should be thoroughly checked for bleeding points before the chest is closed and the patient leaves the operating theatre.

Hand-over

Finally, there should be a careful and thorough hand-over to the team taking over the patient's care following transfer to the intensive care unit. All observations and interventions should be documented for later review if necessary.

Further reading

Shanewise J. Cardiac transplantation. *Anesthesiol Clin North Am* 2004; **22**: 753–65.

Thys DM, Abel MD, Brooker ER, *et al.* Practice guidelines for perioperative transesophageal echocardiography: an updated report by the American Society of Anesthesiologists and the Society of Cardiovascular Anesthesiologists Task Force on Transesophageal Echocardiography. *Anesthesiology* 2010; **112**: 1084–96.

Chapter 11

Postoperative care and early complications

Mandeep R. Mehra

Key points

- In the immediate postoperative period, close attention must be paid to hemodynamic stability by focusing on preventing right ventricular failure and maintaining chronotropic competence.
- Infection prophylaxis is essential and structured protocols must be devised, targeted against superficial candida infection, cytomegalovirus, toxoplasmosis, and anti-protozoal infections.
- Induction immunosuppression may be helpful when primary graft failure ensues, renal dysfunction forces a delay in calcineurin inhibitor initiation, or a high risk for rejection is evident, as with a positive cross-match.
- Statins should be used early and universally in the post-transplantation phase to improve outcomes from rejection and cardiac allograft vasculopathy.
- Two distinct types of rejection exist, with distinct allograft outcomes and responses to therapy.

During procurement and implantation, the cardiac allograft suffers a series of insults, ranging from the effects of donor brain death and cold ischemic injury during transport and then subsequent ischemia-reperfusion injury as engraftment ensues. Immediately, the denervated cardiac allograft encounters a hostile circulation in the recipient, with aberrant neurohormonal reflexes and an inability to match its function to the hostile vasculature. As such, the principle focus of early postoperative management is on achieving hemodynamic stability in the setting of renal dysfunction, pulmonary hypertension, fluid overload, unexpected bleeding, and immunological interactions.

Early allograft-related hemodynamic events

Normal systolic function of the left ventricle (LV) coupled with restrictive physiology is typical; however, the function of the right ventricle (RV) can often be variable. This is highly dependent on donor and recipient size match, the pulmonary vascular resistance (PVR) of the recipient, cold ischemic time, and aggressiveness of fluid loading. Furthermore, damage to the susceptible RV can also ensue from air embolism or technical difficulties such as pulmonary artery torsion.

Importantly, cardiac allografts that display excellent early function can suffer a functional decline over the first 6–24 postoperative hours. This may be due to development of RV failure or development of myocardial edema that leads to restrictive physiology by diminishing diastolic filling and subsequent poor stroke volume. In this setting, the denervated cardiac allograft often is required to maintain overall cardiac output by a reliance on increased heart rate, and thus bradycardia is very poorly tolerated.

Bradycardia can occur from the effects of preexisting medications (particularly amiodarone), prolonged cold ischemia, and even direct injury to the sinoatrial (SA) node. The rhythm in these circumstances is most likely an accelerated junctional rhythm, and such SA node dysfunction is usually transient, with full recovery occurring in 2–6 weeks. However, a permanent pacemaker may be required in rare instances (<5%). The incidence of SA node

Organ Transplantation: A Clinical Guide, ed. A.A. Klein, C.J. Lewis, and J.C. Madsen. Published by Cambridge University Press.

dysfunction is low when a cavo-caval technique as opposed to a bi-atrial technique for transplantation is used. Temporary atrioventricular (AV) pacing (using surgically implanted temporary wires), isoproterenol, and even oral beta-2 receptor agonists can be used to maintain cardiac output by increasing the heart rate in this situation. The general clinical recommendation is to maintain the heart rate between 90 and 110 bpm; however, a higher rate is recommended if significant donor under-sizing with respect to the recipient (donor weight >30% below recipient weight) occurred.

The cardiac allograft may require inotropic support for the first 24–72 hours as it begins to replenish itself and adapt to the new circulation. Early on, myocardial contractility may be decreased due to edema. In addition, myofibril necrosis can also occur, an event that can be picked up by serum biomarker assessment.

Primary graft failure in the absence of hyperacute rejection after cardiac transplantation is said to occur if more than two inotropes, or the need for mechanical circulatory support, is required early (24 hours) after engraftment. Isolated RV failure is more common than bi-ventricular failure. This is typically exhibited by elevated right atrial pressure ≥20 mmHg with a left atrial pressure ≤12 mmHg, elevated PVR, and resultant decreasing cardiac output. Typically, these are accompanied by instability of the peripheral circulation and hypotension.

Primary cardiac allograft failure accounts for 40% of mortality within 30 days of heart transplantation (HT) and 18% of mortality for the second through the 12th months. General risk markers include preoperative use of a mechanical circulatory support device, female donors, and "marginal" donor hearts (e.g., positive viral serology, older donor, diabetic donor, reduced cardiac function, coronary artery disease, moderate to severe left ventricular hypertrophy, and high preoperative catecholamine requirements).

Preoperative support of the recipient circulation by mechanical assist devices appears to significantly increase the risk of post-transplantation primary graft failure. The reasons underlying this observation are unclear but may have to do with the general inflammatory response provoked by the prolonged operation that is required to separate the recipient from the mechanical device. Whether other articulated associations with primary cardiac failure truly influence survival is uncertain.

Maintenance of hemodynamic stability

1. ***Choice of inotropic therapy:*** Isoproterenol has been the time-honored agent used to provide hemodynamic support. This is because of its chronotropic and pulmonary vasodilating properties in addition to inotropism. However, in the setting of a cavo-caval transplant, the chronotropic property may cause excess tachycardia because the incidence of SA node dysfunction is reduced by that technique. The combination of dobutamine with temporary pacing may allow for similar outcomes without the excess tachycardia, but effects on pulmonary vasodilation are less forthcoming. Dopamine alone may not be effective as it requires an intact nerve supply to the cardiac allograft.
2. ***Unique vasodilators:*** Prostacyclins, such as PGE1 or PGEI2, are used to maintain low pulmonary pressures and may improve renal perfusion. However, when systemic hypotension is a concern, inhaled nitric oxide may be used.
3. ***Systemic hypotension:*** More often than not, systemic blood pressure is reduced after cardiac transplantation. This is due to the presence of acidosis and cytokine-related vasodilatation. Continuous infusion of vasoconstrictor such as phenylephrine, norepinephrine, or vasopressin may be required. The guanylate cyclase inhibitor methylene blue has been successfully used for the treatment of catecholamine-refractory vasoplegia.
4. ***Mitral and tricuspid valve regurgitation:*** Early after transplantation, it is not uncommon to discover mild grades of mitral insufficiency. This is due to poor coaptation of the mitral leaflets as a result of loss of diastolic function of the left atrium and development of mechanical dyssynchrony. Active management is usually not necessary. On the other hand, the occurrence of tricuspid valve disease is vastly more common, a result of the effects of damage to the right ventricle and in the setting of pulmonary hypertension. In situations of persistent hemodynamic compromise and severe dilation of the tricuspid annulus, valve repair can be considered. In small series, this has been shown to improve cardiac allograft outcomes. Typically, the RV remodels favorably and the tricuspid regurgitation either reduces or is eliminated by 1 year.

5. *Pericardial effusion:* Although commonly encountered in one fifth of transplanted hearts, this not usually hemodynamically significant and resolves within 4–6 weeks after transplantation. Vigilance for a pericardial hematoma and compressive physiology must be maintained and resternotomy may be required.

Atrioventricular arrhythmias

Despite the physiological insults and pathological injury accorded to the donor allograft, the frequency of AV arrhythmias is relatively low. Atrial fibrillation is more common than atrial flutter and occurs with a frequency of 7–25%. It should be noted that this frequency is lower than the anticipated frequency in comparison with traditional cardiac surgery, and although the reasons are not clear, the use of steroids has recently been shown to lower the risk of atrial fibrillation in general cardiac surgery. Because these patients are ubiquitously given steroid therapy, one can speculate that this may be an operative factor in determining a lower than expected occurrence of atrial arrhythmias. Ventricular arrhythmias are even uncommon and typically seen in <2% of cases. When they occur, the etiology can usually be traced to excessive pathological ischemic injury in the allograft or to a causative drug exposure. Although infrequent, some principles of therapy must be kept in mind. Digitalis and its analogues do not work effectively due to vagal denervation. Beta-blockers can slow the rate of atrial arrhythmias, but in the early postoperative period, their use can worsen RV failure and hemodynamics. Some intensify anti-rejection therapy when atrial arrhythmias are encountered. However, it is rare for rejection to be a culprit in those arrhythmias occurring within the first 2 weeks of engraftment. Typically, a rapid reduction in catecholamine exposure coupled with anti-arrhythmic therapy is usually effective. Amiodarone can be used in these patients, but drugs like calcium channel blockers (negative inotropism), sotalol (beta blockade and renal dysfunction), and dofetilide (multiple drug interactions) should be avoided.

Special early perioperative circumstances

1. *Diabetes mellitus:* Postoperative hyperglycemia is an important occurrence and may be due to worsening of pre-existing diabetes, stress-induced uncovering of hyperglycemia, or corticosteroid-induced hyperglycemia. Because advanced diabetes can cause worsening of acidosis and increased propensity for infection, it is important to control blood sugars within a range of <200 mg/dl blood glucose. Importantly, metformin should be withheld because it can precipitate lactic acidosis. The development of hypoglycemia must be avoided because in non-transplant settings, hypoglycemic episodes are associated with worse cardiac outcomes.
2. *Renal failure:* Many patients have pre-existing renal failure. Additionally, the exposure to hemodynamic instability and fluid shifts in addition to the pro-inflammatory effects of cardiopulmonary bypass worsen kidney function. Strategies include optimizing RV function and reducing exposure to nephrotoxic drugs and immunosuppressant. If renal replacement therapy is required (1–15% of patients) early after transplantation, outcome is quite poor (mortality up to 50%). Despite this tendency to worse outcome, consideration should be given to early renal replacement therapy if there is renal failure in the context of RV dysfunction and rising right atrial pressures.
3. *Infection prophylaxis:* Early after transplantation, bacterial infections predominate, and therefore, institution-specific flora and sensitivity-based regimens must be used. Prophylaxis is similar to that of other transplants, as described in Chapter 4C. Importantly, cytomegalovirus (CMV) infection is a critical target for prophylaxis, and the appropriate regimen is based on the donor and recipient serological status. Those at high risk of primary infection (donor positive/recipient negative) or reactivation (recipient positive) should receive targeted prophylaxis with either oral valganciclovir (900 mg daily) or initial 4–6 weeks of intravenous ganciclovir (5–10 mg/kg/day). Some centers use CMV-specific immunoglobulin initially, and this has support from observational trials in reducing infection-related complications and also the occurrence of cardiac allograft vasculopathy. Oral therapy is usually continued for 3 months. Similarly, therapy to prevent toxoplasmosis and pneumocystis jiroveci infection using

trimethoprim-sulfamethoxazole–based therapy, or, if allergic, dapsone or pyrimethamine is also advocated. At the time of hospital discharge, anti-fungal prophylaxis to prevent mucocutaneous candidiasis should be initiated with nystatin (4–6 mL [400 000–600 000 units] 4 times daily, swish and swallow) or clotrimazole lozenges (10 mg).

Clinical principles of immunosuppression

Development of a rational immunosuppressant regime requires assessment of the donor and recipient immunological match as well as comorbidities likely to interact with the immunosuppressants within the host environment (see Chapter 3). Following HT, the use of intraoperative and peri-operative corticosteroids remains the mainstay of early therapy. Typically, high-dose corticosteroids are administered before induction of anesthesia and during reperfusion after implantation. Thereafter, induction therapy may or may not be used, followed by the establishment of a calcineurin-based regimen (cyclosporine or tacrolimus) with an adjunctive agent (mycophenolate mofetil, mammalian target of rapamycin [mTOR] inhibitors, or azathioprine). In all cases, steroids are prescribed with intent to rapidly wean off by 6 months. Up to 44% of all cardiac transplant recipients are able to wean off steroids completely by 1 year.

Induction therapy

The concept of induction therapy applies to the use of very intensive immunosuppression designed to deplete entire cell lines in an effort to abrogate the immune response. Unlike in other organ transplants, the use of polyclonal or monoclonal antibodies in HT is unproven. Muromonab-CD3 (OKT3), the old monoclonal antibody of choice, has now been replaced by anti–interleukin-2 (IL-2) receptor blockers (used in approximately 30% of induction cases). More commonly, the new polyclonal preparations (Thymoglobulin, antithymocyte globulin [ATG]) have replaced the antibodies used in the past (ATGAM). Two CD25 (IL-2 receptor blockers) specific chimerical monoclonal antibodies, daclizumab and basiliximab, have been designed to reduce the limitations of non-human antibodies. The inclusion of human proteins prevents the destruction of the therapeutic antibodies by the recipient's anti-mouse antibodies (daclizumab: 10% murine, 90% human protein; basiliximab: 30% murine, 70% human protein) and the development of serum sickness associated with mouse-, rabbit-, or horse-derived proteins. Alemtuzumab has been associated with prolonged leukopenia in renal and lung transplant recipients, and few multi-center data exist in cardiac transplantation. Of the polyclonal antibodies, ATG has the most support. In recent years, investigators have evaluated a shorter ATG course (5 versus 7 days) or adjustment of ATG dose to achieve a lymphocyte count below $<100/\mu l$. Shorter duration of ATG therapy was associated with higher rejection rates. In contrast, adjustment of ATG doses according to T-cell counts was associated with lower rejection rates as well as lower or fewer ATG doses. Although there is little universal support for using induction therapy, it should be considered in special circumstances in which a calcineurin inhibitor (CNI) delay is desired due to renal insufficiency. However, at this time, CNI-free protocols cannot be considered a standard of care in de novo HT. In situations in which the risk of early rejection is high (sensitized patients with a positive cross-match) or when primary graft failure has ensued, the use of induction agents may be particularly useful.

Calcineurin inhibitors and adjunctive therapy

The major randomized clinical trials of immunosuppression in heart transplantation have allowed us to alter our clinical management options, but a close examination of these data suggest that one can interpret the findings broadly. On an intent-to-treat basis, these trials have not shown differential effects on survival with various immunosuppressive regimens. Although the 1998 mycophenolate mofetil (MMF) trial resulted in a large shift in replacing azathioprine with this agent, the data show that MMF did not improve 1-year survival compared with azathioprine (AZA). However, in this study, randomization occurred preoperatively, and 11% of recipients never received the study drug. When the analysis was restricted to patients who received at least one dose of MMF (treated-patient analysis), 1-year survival was greater in the MMF than in the AZA group (6.2% versus 11.4%; $p = 0.031$). Two trials of CNIs within Europe and the United States comparing tacrolimus (TAC) and cyclosporine (CyA)-based immunosuppression found similar rejection rates. More recently, a three-arm trial comparing regimens of TAC/MMF, TAC/sirolimus (SRL) and CyA/MMF showed that both TAC-based regimens were associated with significantly lower 6-month rates of any treated rejection than the CyA/MMF regimen. Furthermore, TAC/MMF-treated patients had lower rates of cellular rejection (International Society for Heart and Lung Transplantation [ISHLT] grade >3A) and of any treated rejection than the CyA/MMF-treated subjects. Another trial suggested that the combination of TAC/MMF is ideal across ethnic populations, with evidence of enhanced survival in African-American heart transplant recipients. Thus the combination of TAC/MMF appears to possess the most optimum risk-benefit ratio in treating cardiac transplant recipients and may therefore represent the drug strategy of choice.

Therapeutic drug monitoring

Monitoring of therapeutic drug levels is important but there is some controversy in how best to monitor the target levels of CNIs. At present, 2-hour post-dose (C2) levels should not replace 12-hour trough (C0) concentrations for routine monitoring of CyA exposure in most patients, but may be useful in selected patients in whom a better characterization of the pharmacokinetic profile of CyA is desired. Measurement of 12-hour trough CyA concentration is the recommended form of therapeutic drug monitoring for routine clinical use. In general, when used in conjunction with azathioprine, or MMF preparations, the average CyA trough concentration target using the Abbot TDX assay (or equivalent) is 325 ng/ml (range 275–375 ng/ml) for the first 6 postoperative weeks, 275 ng/ml (range 200–350 ng/ml) for weeks 6–12, 225 ng/ml (range 150–300 ng/mL) for months 3–6, and 200 ng/ml (range 150–250 ng/mL) from month 6 onward, although this needs to be balanced against renal function.

Measurement of 12-hour trough concentration for twice-daily TAC and a 24-hour trough concentration for once-daily TAC is the recommended drug monitoring method for routine clinical use. The therapeutic range of TAC levels varies depending on concomitant drugs, toxicity concerns, and time after HT. In general, when used in conjunction with AZA or an MMF, TAC trough concentration targets range between 10 and 15 ng/ml during the early postoperative period (days 0–60), between 8 and 12 ng/ml for the next 3–6 months, and between 5 and 10 ng/ml in stable patients 6 months after HT.

Therapeutic drug monitoring for mTOR inhibitors, SRL, or everolimus (EVL) using trough concentration levels is recommended. Levels should be measured at least 5 days after adjustment of the dose, when a new steady state is achieved. When used in combination with CyA, the optimal trough target levels range for EVL is between 3 and 8 ng/ml. The corresponding optimal trough level range for SRL is 4 to 12 ng/ml. The optimal levels for these agents with TAC remain uncertain, and the safety of this combination remains in doubt. Routine therapeutic drug monitoring of mycophenolic acid levels to adjust MMF doses is not recommended.

Statins

Three-hydroxy-3-methylglutaryl coenzyme A (HMG-CoA) reductase inhibitors, or statins, function as both lipid-lowering and immunomodulating agents. Statins are used early post-transplant irrespective of lipid levels in an effort to employ their immune-modifying properties. Evidence with pravastatin and then subsequently with simvastatin has suggested that this may represent a class effect of immunomodulation and anti-inflammatory effects. In aggregate, the evidence supports a reduction in mortality, decrease in hemodynamically compromising rejection, and amelioration of cardiac allograft vasculopathy. One must remain vigilant for the development of sympathy or rhabdomyolysis with statins in this vulnerable population, particularly with simvastatin, due to interaction with CNIs.

Clinical principles in rejection surveillance, detection, and management

Types of rejection

Hyperacute rejection, which occurs within hours of engraftment, is uniformly fatal but very rare, due to immunological matching and monitoring. On the other hand, *acute cellular rejection* (ACR) is most common in the first 6 months after heart transplantation and is a predominantly T-cell–mediated phenomenon. It occurs in 20% of recipients in the first

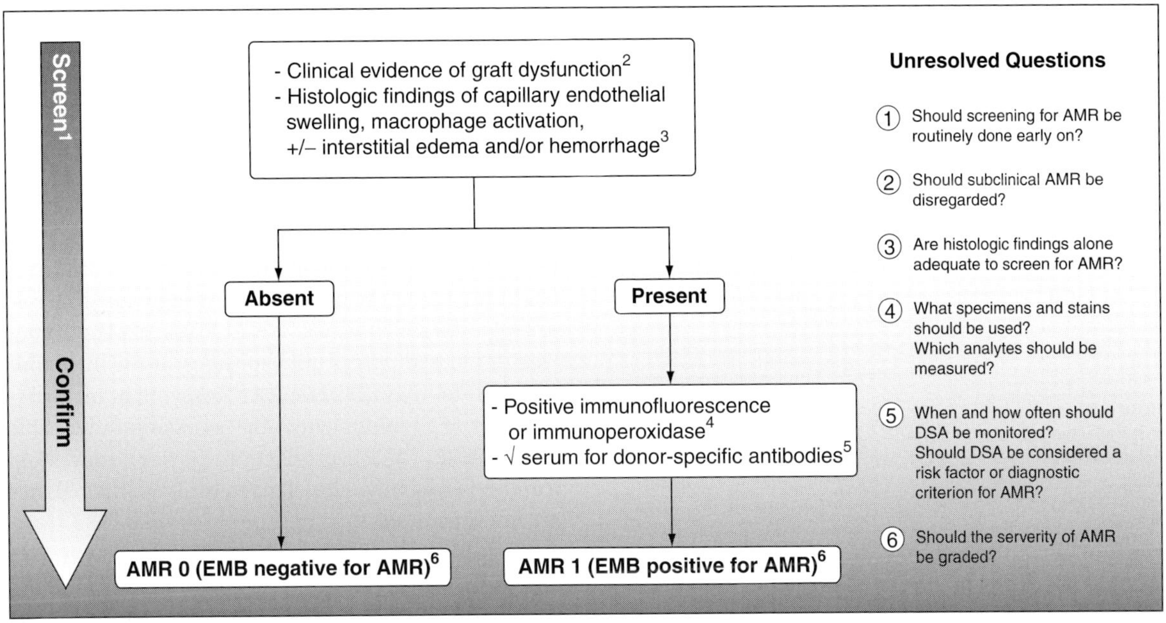

Figure 11.1 Understanding antibody-mediated rejection (AMR) in cardiac transplantation. DSA, donor-specific antibodies; EMB, endomyocardial biopsy. Reprinted with permission from Kfoury AG, Hammond ME, Controversies in defining cardiac antibody-mediated rejection: need for updated criteria, *J Heart Lung Transplant* 2010; **29**: 389–94.

year, and this frequency is declining as a result of improvements in the intensity of immunosuppressants. More recently acknowledged as a clinically valid entity, acute *antibody-mediated rejection* (AMR) is less common than ACR, occurring in approximately 10% of patients, but is more dreaded because it is accompanied by hemodynamic compromise, is difficult to treat, and leads to late sequelae, particularly cardiac allograft vasculopathy. Acute AMR consists of antibodies directed against donor vascular endothelial antigens. It is not uncommon for both ACR and AMR to coexist. The allograft demonstrates recruitment of neutrophils, interstitial edema, and intravascular thrombus and subsequent myocyte necrosis. The presence of immunoglobulin (IgG, IgM, or IgA), complement fragments (C3d, C4d, C1q), or CD68-positive cells (macrophages), as well as the appearance of circulating de novo anti-donor human leukocyte antigen (HLA) antibodies, are sentinel peripheral and allograft events that form the signature for AMR (Figure 11.1).

Monitoring for rejection

Because the signs and symptoms of rejection are few, surveillance with invasive endomyocardial biopsy is advised. In advanced cases, the patient may present with symptoms of allograft failure, and echocardiography will signal the presence of myocardial thickening (due to edema) or restrictive physiology. In overt rejection, systolic dysfunction ensues, signaling the immense gravity of this rejection episode.

Early after transplantation, particularly in the first 3 months when the risk of rejection is highest, invasive biopsies are recommended at decreasing intervals. Thus weekly biopsies are advised in the first month, fortnightly in the next month, and then monthly thereafter until 6 months. After that a lower frequency is undertaken, usually at 3 monthly intervals until the end of the first year. There is much controversy regarding the value of performing routine biopsy beyond the first year of transplantation (Figure 11.2). An invasive biopsy is reassuring but is not without risk. Complications may occur in 2–3% of procedures, including access-related vascular or bleeding problems, pneumothorax, arrhythmias, heart block, or even tricuspid valve injury. Pericardial tamponade can occur due to right ventricular perforation.

Classification of rejection

The histology of the allograft is evaluated pathologically based on a uniform ISHLT grading scale,

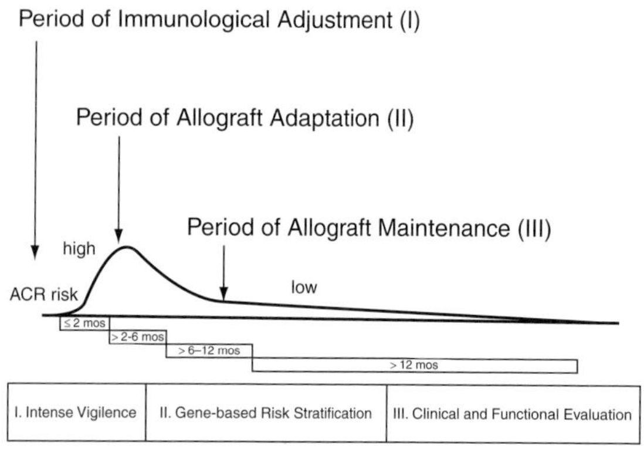

Figure 11.2 Phases of cardiac adaptation and time-dependency of cardiac rejection. Reprinted with permission from Kfoury AG, Hammond ME, Controversies in defining cardiac antibody-mediated rejection: need for updated criteria, *J Heart Lung Transplant* 2010; **29**:599–602.

initially described in 1990 and subsequently updated in 2005 to include a definition for AMR. Due to intra- and inter-observer variability in the determination of the different grades of mild or moderate rejection and the observation that grades 1 and 2 were mostly self-limiting, the revised heart allograft rejection grading system in 2005 divided the various grades; grade 0 (no cellular rejection) was now named grade 0R ("R" added to reflect the revised 2005 scale). The intermediate grades of 1A, 1B, and 2 were re-classified as grade 1R, or mild acute cellular rejection. Grade 3A was re-classified as grade 2R, moderate acute cellular rejection, and grades 3B and 4 were re-classified as grade 3R, severe acute cellular rejection. In addition, AMR was recognized as a clinical entity, and recommendation was issued for determination of its presence (AMR1) or absence (AMR0). Non-invasive monitoring for rejection has been attempted, and more recently a gene based biosignature has shown promise. However, this particular signature should not yet be applied in the early post-transplant period, within the first 6 months.

Management of rejection

Early after transplantation, even asymptomatic allograft histology restricted ACR is treated with augmentation using corticosteroids. Although most use a high-dose intravenous pulse of steroids daily for 3 days, in the absence of allograft failure, oral steroids at a dose of 1 mg/kg of prednisone for 3 days followed by immediate return to the baseline dose is quite adequate in treating the episode to histological resolution. Background immunosuppression must be adjusted by evaluating trough levels, and attempts to wean corticosteroids must be slowed down. Most episodes of ACR resolve within 3 weeks. Interestingly, two thirds of ACR episodes that are untreated tend to resolve spontaneously as well. This data accrues from later phases of transplantation, and most clinicians would rather err on treating during the early phase of transplantation. However, it is perhaps prudent to not over-immunosuppress mild episodes, as the incidence of infection may increase. An assay that measures activated T lymphocytes by assessing adenosine triphosphate (ATP) production (Cylex) may hold promise in allowing clinicians to evaluate the balance of immunosuppression and infection risk. The treatment of AMR is quite distinct from that of ACR, and although the scope of this chapter is to not detail these issues, it is important to provide some clinical implications of available therapy. There are three distinct goals of AMR therapy, which include protection of the allograft from further injury, reduction of circulating donor-specific antibodies, and suppression of production of these deleterious antibodies. The allograft is typically protected by the administration of high-dose steroids and therapy targeted to prevent thrombosis. Circulating antibodies are decreased by the use of plasmapheresis, typically used 3–5 consecutive times followed by intravenous IgG; cytolytic induction antibodies such as ATG and rituximab are then used to diminish T- and B-cell responses. In the late phase, suppressive therapy with cyclophosphamide or, in recalcitrant cases, photopheresis or total lymphoid irradiation may be used. Close vigilance for re-emergence of circulating antibodies is needed, and newer approaches using complement inhibitors or intensive B-cell modulating drugs such as bortezomib are being studied. The long-term outcomes for these patients deserves further study because it is uncertain whether these anecdotally derived treatments influence late outcomes from AMR.

Further reading

Costanzo MR, Dipchand A, Starling R, *et al.* The International Society of Heart and Lung Transplantation Guidelines for the care of heart transplant recipients. *J Heart Lung Transplant* 2010; **29**: 914–56.

Kfoury AG, Hammond ME. Controversies in defining cardiac antibody-mediated rejection: need for updated criteria. *J Heart Lung Transplant* 2010; **29**: 389–94.

Kobashigawa J, Mehra M, West L, *et al.* Report from a consensus conference on the sensitized patient awaiting heart transplantation. *J Heart Lung Transplant* 2009; **28**: 213–25.

Uber PA, Mehra MR. Induction therapy in heart transplantation: is there a role? *J Heart Lung Transplant* 2007; **26**: 205–9.

Chapter 12

Long-term management and outcomes

Hari K. Parthasarathy and Clive J. Lewis

Key points

- Heart transplantation has excellent long-term survival, with 50% of patients living 10 years, and significant improvement in quality of life.
- Early graft failure, rejection, and infection contribute most to mortality in the first year. Cardiac allograft vasculopathy and malignancy contribute most to late mortality.
- Complications continue to limit long-term survival following heart transplantation.
- The incidence of vasculopathy at 10 years after heart transplant is 50% and causes late graft dysfunction, myocardial infarction, arrhythmia, and sudden cardiac death.
- Malignancy, severe renal dysfunction, and metabolic syndrome (hyperlipidemia, hypertension, diabetes and obesity) are common comorbidities both early and late after heart transplantation.

Since Christiaan Barnard performed the first human heart transplantation over 40 years ago, more than 85 000 heart transplants have been performed worldwide. On average, more than 5000 heart transplants are undertaken every year in more than 225 centers. Understanding the short- and long-term survival is important to determine the place of transplantation within the success of other medical and surgical therapies. In the early years, survival after heart transplantation was limited to the medium term, with mortality due to rejection and severe infection (1-year survival 30% in 1967–1973, 60% in 1974–1980). Subsequently, survival has increased with each decade, although the major improvement has been during the first year after transplant due to advances in donor management, cardioplegia, and intensive care, but particularly immunosuppression with the introduction of cyclosporine. The International Society for Heart and Lung Transplantation (ISHLT) Registry is the largest dataset for heart transplantation worldwide and shows the half-life to be 10 years following transplant, with a half-life conditional on surviving the first year of 13 years (Figure 12.1). Importantly, there is also significant improvement in functional status and quality of life, with more than 90% of recipients having no functional limitations during the first 7 years, more than 50% working or retired at 1, 3, and 5 years, and rehospitalization in fewer than 25% of patients 1 year after heart transplant.

Between 1982–1991 and 2002–2007, survival increased by 4% at 1 month and 6% at 6 months in spite of higher risk donor and recipient profiles. The improvement in early mortality following heart transplantation has led to a longer half-life, from 8.8 to 10.5 years, in the two decades above. Short and long-term survival is also determined by the underlying diagnosis: cardiomyopathy (84% 1-year survival), coronary artery disease (82%), valvular heart disease (78%), congenital heart disease (76%), and re-transplantation (68%), and this effect persists in subsequent years. Survival has greatly improved in recent patient cohorts undergoing re-transplantation, mainly attributed to careful patient selection and improvement in post-transplant management.

Disappointingly, however, long-term complications continue to limit survival, with an attrition rate of 3–4% annually in all decades, including the most recent. Cumulative causes of death from the ISHLT Registry following transplantation are shown in Figure 12.2. Understanding causes of death after transplant continues to have a significant impact on directing preventative, surveillance, and treatment strategies to reduce the incidence of long-term complications.

Organ Transplantation: A Clinical Guide, ed. A.A. Klein, C.J. Lewis, and J.C. Madsen. Published by Cambridge University Press.

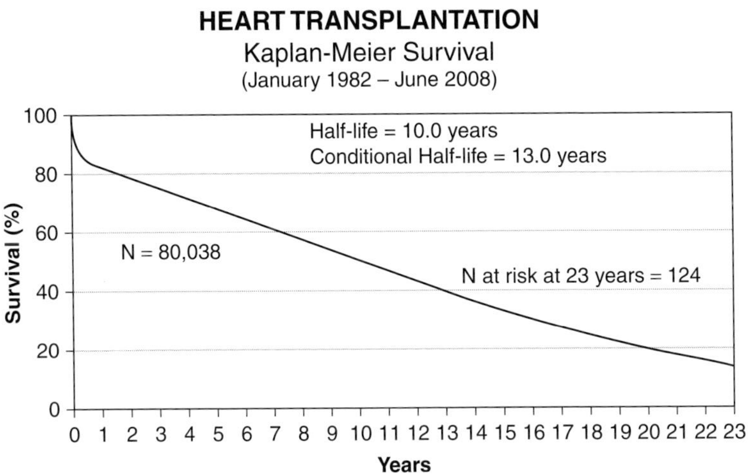

Figure 12.1 Survival following heart transplantation in adult transplant recipients from ISHLT Registry, 1982–2008. From *J Heart Lung Transplant*, 2010; **29**(10): 1083–141. Reproduced with permission from the International Society for Heart and Lung Transplantation.

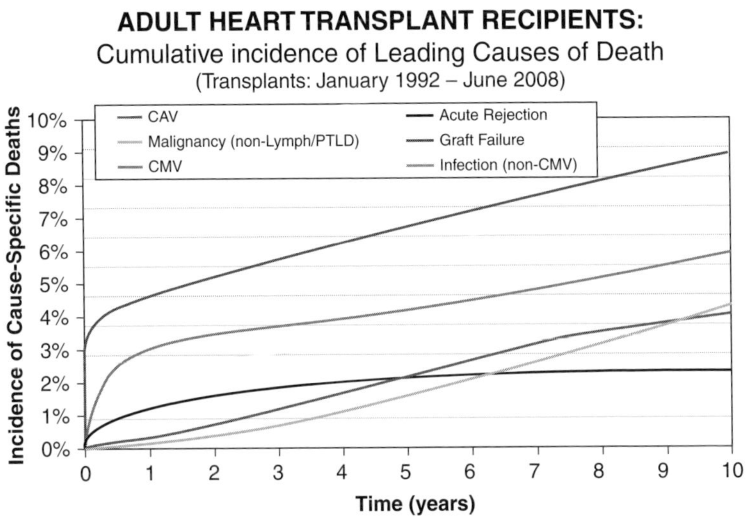

Figure 12.2 Cumulative incidence of leading causes of death in adult transplant recipients from ISHLT Registry, 1992–2008. From *J Heart Lung Transplant*, 2010; **29**(10): 1083–141. Reproduced with permission from the International Society for Heart and Lung Transplantation.

Mortality following heart transplantation

The outcome following transplantation can be usefully divided into short (30 day and 1 year) and long-term mortality (>1 year). The major causes of death alter with the length of survival after transplant (Figure 12.3). Within the first 30 days post-transplant, graft failure is the leading cause of death (41%), followed by multi-organ failure (13%) and non-cytomegalovirus (CMV) infection (13%). Between 31 and 365 days, non-CMV infection is the leading cause and accounts for 30% of the deaths, followed by graft failure (18%) and acute rejection (12%). Long-term mortality is due to coronary artery vasculopathy (CAV) and late graft failure (likely due to CAV), which together account for 32% of deaths 5 years following transplantation, followed by malignancy (23%) and non-CMV infections (10%).

Mortality during the first year

Various factors contribute to increased early graft failure and morality, including changing donor and recipient profiles in recent years (Table 12.1). Continuous risk factors for worse outcome include increasing recipient age and body mass index (BMI), increasing donor age and BMI, smaller transplant center volume, longer ischemic time, borderline pulmonary wedge pressure, and rising bilirubin, creatinine, and pulmonary vascular resistance (PVR).

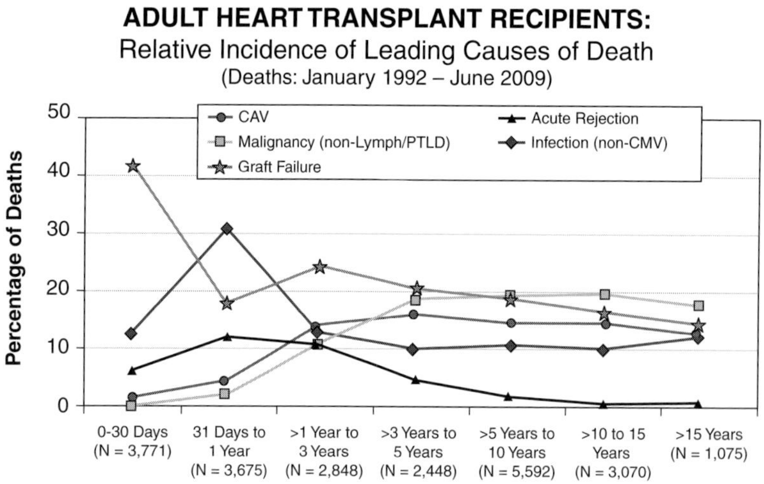

Figure 12.3 The relative incidence of causes of death in adult transplant recipients over time from transplant, ISHLT Registry, 1992–2008. From *J Heart Lung Transplant*, 2010; **29**(10): 1083–141. Reproduced with permission from the International Society for Heart and Lung Transplantation.

Donor selection

Patient selection for transplant remains the most important predictor of outcome, with the adage "poor donor and poor recipient leads to poor outcomes." Optimization and careful selection of the donor (Chapter 7) prior to harvesting the organ will improve outcomes. Careful selection and optimization of sick heart failure patients is critically important to reduce the chance of early and late mortality. A range of treatments from conventional heart failure drugs to cardiac resynchronization therapy (CRT) and implantable cardioverter-defibrillator (ICD) mean that patients are often referred with very poor cardiac reserve and are too sick to remain ambulant while awaiting transplantation. Patients may be optimized in high-dependency wards with inotrope, intra-aortic balloon pump, ultra/hemofiltration, and mechanical support to improve otherwise adverse prognostic indicators for mortality after transplant.

Rejection

Hyperacute rejection is rarely seen after heart transplantation and is usually due to a rapid overwhelming immune attack on the graft due to preformed antibodies directed against human leukocyte antigen (HLA) or ABO blood group systems but may also occur with non-HLA antibodies. Avoiding transplant against known recipient HLA antibodies and ABO-incompatible transplants should avoid hyperacute rejection.

Acute cellular rejection contributes to up to 40% of early death following transplant and is especially common in the first month and months 2–6 and is unusual after the first year, but the risk of fatal rejection never disappears completely. Some centers continue to biopsy annually in subsequent years, but studies have shown no difference in outcome without annual surveillance. Histological rejection grade 2R requires treatment, especially when associated with allograft dysfunction (ISHLT Consensus on Diagnosis of Heart Rejection, 2005). Treatment of lower grades of rejection (1R) is controversial but is warranted if recurrent within the first 6 months. Acute cell-medicated rejection may be treated conventionally as for other organs with high-dose steroid, augmenting or switching oral immunosuppression, intravenous (IV) antithymocyte globulin (ATG)/muromonab-CD3 (OKT3), plasmapheresis, and total lymphoid irradiation, as discussed in Chapter 11.

Antibody or humoral rejection is increasingly recognized as an important form of rejection even without evidence of acute cellular rejection and leads to reduced graft survival and increased incidence of early vasculopathy. Strategies for treatment include rituximab, plasmapheresis, and immunoglobulin. Risk factors for rejection are shown in Table 12.2.

Infection

Infection is the cause of death in 10–15% of patients during month 1 and the leading cause of death in the first year. Decreased resistance to infection arises

Table 12.1 Donor and recipient risk factors associated with increased early graft failure and mortality 1 year following heart transplantation

Donor factors
Increasing age (25% of recipients in current era, RR = 1.5 age 40 years, 2.4 age 50 years)
Decreasing BMI
Increasing allograft ischemic time (RR = 1.4 after 5 hours)
High-dose inotropic support
Reduced systolic function
"Marginal" or extended criteria donors (especially in higher risk recipients)
Recipient factors
Significant donor/recipient size mismatch (especially female donor to male recipient)
Younger and older age (RR = 1.33 for 18-year-old; survival 77% over 70 years vs. 84% 30–39 years)
Increasing BMI (RR = 1.3 over BMI of 34)
Decreasing transplant center volume (RR = 0.9 for > 55 transplants/year)
Increasing pretransplant serum bilirubin (RR = 1.3 > 3.5 mg/dl) and creatinine (RR = 2.1 > 2.5 mg/dl or dialysis requirement)
Pulmonary vascular resistance > 3–5 Wood Units (PVR > 5 increases mortality by 3% and 5% at 1 and 5 years; survival improved by donor over-sizing)
Trans pulmonary gradient > 15
High right atrial pressure
Higher rates of diabetes mellitus
Higher rates of nicotine use
Recipient panel-reactive antibody (PRA) > 10%
Congenital heart disease (RR = 2.3) or coronary artery disease (RR = 1.2)
Ventilated patients (RR = 1.6)
Dialysis at transplant (RR = 1.6)
Recent infection
Higher incidence of temporary (RR = 3) or long-term left ventricular assist device (LVAD, RR = 1.25)
Compatible but non-identical ABO matching (RR = 1.2)

LVAD: left ventricular assist device; RR: relative risk.

from recipient older age, high or low BMI, lung disease, pretransplant ventilation, smoking history, diabetes, previous intervention (sternotomy, mechanical support), and critically illness. As in other organ recipients, following heart transplantation, bacterial and viral infections are common, but consideration should be given to protozoal and fungal infection, which carry the highest mortality. CMV infection may occur in up to 20% of recipients but does not predict worse outcome, although there may be a higher incidence of early vasculopathy. Antibiotic prophylaxis should routinely be given in the postoperative period. Longer term prophylaxis is given for pneumocystis and toxoplasmosis with cotrimoxazole (may be stopped when levels of immunosuppression are lower); CMV (unless donor and recipient CMV negative) with IV ganciclovir then oral valganciclovir for 3–12 months; and herpes viruses with acyclovir if not on valganciclovir. Physicians need a systematic approach to diagnosing infection, with consideration given to time since transplant, donor infection, recipient serology, degree of immunosuppression (recent treatment for rejection), and recent exposure. Ongoing post-transplant surveillance by specialists is important to detect unusual infection. Up-to-date immunization should be checked pretransplant and continue (except live vaccine) as usual post-transplant, including annual influenza, pandemic influenza, and pneumococcal vaccination.

Table 12.2 Risk factors for acute cellular rejection

Younger recipient age
Black or Hispanic recipient
CMV mismatch
HLA mismatch
Older donor age
High TPG (may represent poor cardiac reserve to hemodynamic stress of rejection)

TPG: transpulmonary gradient.

Survival after the first post-transplant year

Coronary vasculopathy and malignancy account for more than 50% of the mortality at 5 years. The risk factors for 1-year mortality remain powerful predictors for 5-year outcomes (Table 12.3). The factors affecting 5-year survival also affect the longer term survival to 10 and 20 years or longer. It is important to note that the data collected for these analyses are not as comprehensive as that of the modern era, and the number of patients reaching more than 20 years is small (144 at 22 years in the ISHLT dataset). Changes in recent years that have improved very long-term survival include modern immunosuppression, statin use,

Table 12.3 Risk factors affecting 5-year survival conditional on surviving the first year post-transplant

Donor factors
Older age (RR = 1.35 age 55 years)
Recipient factors
Allograft vasculopathy within first year
Rejection episodes in first year (especially if graft dysfunction)
Ventilator at the time of transplant
Diabetes
Coronary artery disease
Age (U-shaped: RR = 1.5 age 20, RR = 1.4 age 65 years)
High BMI
Decreasing transplant center volume (RR = 0.8 > 55 transplants/year)
Re-transplantation
Ischemic time (RR = 1.36 > 5 years)

BMI: body mass index; RR = relative risk.

systematic post-transplant care/surveillance, and better management of renal dysfunction.

Long-term complications after heart transplant

The long-term complications following heart transplantation are similar to those of other organ transplants and include vasculopathy and complications of immunosuppressants. Consideration is given here to complications and management that are specific to the cardiac allograft; other principles of pathophysiology and management are discussed elsewhere. Table 12.4 illustrates the incidence of complications 10 years after heart transplant (ISHLT 2009 Registry data).

Cardiac allograft vasculopathy

CAV or chronic rejection is a leading cause of graft failure and mortality following heart transplantation, with the incidence approaching 8% at 1 year, 31% at 5 years, and 52% at 10 years after heart transplantation. There is a small reduction in CAV incidence in the most recent era, possibly due to improved patient selection, post-transplant management, and in particular the widespread use of statins. CAV has a complex pathophysiology, and the detailed mechanisms are largely unknown but involve both immune-mediated endothelial damage and conventional atherosclerosis

Table 12.4 Comorbidities 10 years following heart transplantation

Angiographic CAV, 52%
Severe renal insufficiency, 14%
Dialysis, 4.7%
Renal transplant, 1.5%
Hypertension, 97%
Hyperlipidemia, 93%
Diabetes, 39%
Malignancy, 30%

Table 12.5 Risk factors for development of cardiac allograft vasculopathy

Donor factors
Hypertension
Active infection
Increasing donor age
Recipient factors
Pretransplant coronary artery disease
Mismatches at DR locus/class 1 mismatch
Decreasing recipient age
Antibody-mediated rejection
Recurrent cell-mediated rejection
CMV infection
Smoking history (particularly post-transplant)

(see Chapter 4B). It may be regarded as an accelerated form of atherosclerosis, but is usually a diffuse process affecting the entire coronary artery tree, including epicardial, intra-myocardial branches, and veins. This process is distinct from that of the usual coronary atherosclerosis in which the lesions are often eccentric and more focal, the elastic lamina is extensively involved, and calcification is common. Donor-related coronary atherosclerosis may be recognized early following transplantation but tends to have a differing pathophysiology, slower progression, and better prognosis than CAV. The risk factors for developing CAV in addition to those involved in traditional atherosclerosis (hypertension, diabetes, dyslipidemia) are shown in Table 12.5.

Pathophysiology

The process of CAV involves coronary endothelial cell damage since this is the barrier between recipient blood carrying immune cells and donor tissue in addition to being a site of donor antigen presentation (see Chapter 4B). Endothelial injury may be immune (HLA mismatch, antibody- and cell-mediated rejection) or non-immune mediated (e.g., due to ischemia/reperfusion injury, atherosclerotic risk factors, CMV infection).

Clinical presentation and diagnosis

The clinical presentation of CAV is often atypical, and diagnosis may be challenging due to denervation of the transplanted heart. Patients often lack chest pain and suffer from silent myocardial ischemia, although re-innervation may occur to a variable degree a few years after transplant. Presentation may therefore be asymptomatic (surveillance angiography) or present with new-onset heart failure, arrhythmia, myocardial infarction, syncope, or sudden cardiac death. Following exclusion of acute cellular rejection, the diagnosis of CAV must be considered in the presence of signs/symptoms of heart failure, ECG changes, changes in systolic or diastolic function on echo, arrhythmia (especially ventricular), bradycardia, and heart block. Regular surveillance for CAV is performed, often annually and using a variety of different investigations. Coronary angiography has remained the "gold standard" for diagnosis of CAV since the early days of heart transplantation.

Angiography has the advantage of being widely available but may under-diagnose CAV because of the diffuse and concentric nature of vessel involvement. Careful comparison of previous angiograms may help to identify the progressive loss of the lumen calibre and smaller branches. In 2010, the ISHLT published a standardized nomenclature for CAV (Table 12.6). Lesions may be classified as type A (discrete, tubular, or multiple stenoses), type B1 (abrupt ending with distal diffuse narrowing and obliterated vessels), type B2 (gradual tapering with remnant distal lumen), and type C (narrowed irregular and blunt ending distal vessels).

Intravascular ultrasound (IVUS) of at least one epicardial vessel over 40–50 mm appears very sensitive to identify early CAV with very good negative predictive value. IVUS can be used to assess various parameters, including intimal thickness and luminal and external elastic membrane cross-sectional areas. IVUS may provide evidence of subclinical CAV but probably does not add incremental information when the angiogram appears normal. Increasing intimal thickness predicts development of angiographic CAV, guides treatment, and is associated with adverse outcomes: intimal thickening of $\geq$0.5 mm in the first year after transplant appears to be a reliable surrogate marker for subsequent development of CAV and mortality up to 5 years after heart transplantation.

Table 12.6 ISHLT nomenclature for cardiac allograft vasculopathy

ISHLT CAV0 (Not significant)	No detectable angiographic lesion
ISHLT CAV1 (Mild)	Angiographic left main (LM) 50%, or primary vessel with maximum lesion of 70%, or any branch stenosis 70% (including diffuse narrowing) without allograft dysfunction.
ISHLT CAV2 (Moderate)	Angiographic LM 50%; a single primary vessel 70%, or isolated branch stenosis 70% in branches of two systems, without allograft dysfunction.
ISHLT CAV3 (Severe)	Angiographic LM 50%, or two or more primary vessels 70% stenosis, or isolated branch stenosis 70% in all three systems; or ISHLT CAV1 or CAV2 with allograft dysfunction (defined as LVEF 45% usually in the presence of regional wall motion abnormalities) or evidence of significant restrictive physiology.

LVEF: left ventricular ejection fraction.

Other diagnostic investigations include non-invasive computed tomography–based angiography (sensitivity and specificity remain low, and distal branch vessel anatomical definition is poor); coronary flow reserve quantification (abnormal endothelial responses associated with vasculopathy); non-invasive imaging and perfusion studies (nuclear, magnetic resonance imaging [MRI], and echo stress testing); Myocardial biopsy, immune-based markers, gene and protein biomarkers (B-type natriuretic peptide [BNP], troponin, high-sensitivity C-reactive protein [CRP]). None of these investigations are recommended for CAV surveillance due to lack of sufficient sensitivity or specificity for diagnosis and issues of reproducibility or standardization of performance.

Outcomes in CAV

CAV reduces short-term survival and remains the main cause of death in long-term survivors after cardiac transplantation. A cohort of patients has a

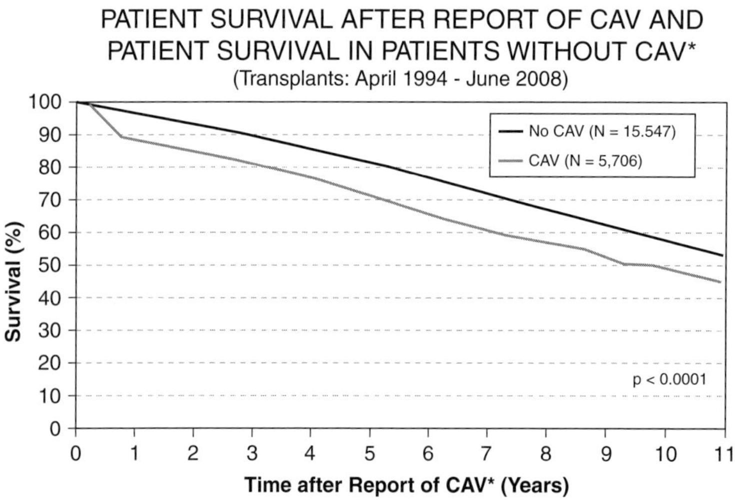

Figure 12.4 Survival following diagnosis of CAV from ISHLT Registry, 1994–2008. From *J Heart Lung Transplant*, 2010; **29**(10): 1083–141. Reproduced with permission from the International Society for Heart and Lung Transplantation.

more rapidly progressive CAV, with overall survival reduced by approximately 7% 1 year after diagnosis and increasing to 11% 5 and 10 years after diagnosis (Figure 12.4). A worse prognosis appears to be related to early development of CAV, rapid progression, and more severe disease (widespread, multi-vessel, and lesions >70% luminal diameter).

Treatment

Because the development of CAV is generally slow, early recognition of the presence of disease may allow early intervention and prevent graft dysfunction. Rapid progression of CAV may also be recognized, allowing consideration of re-transplantation. Prevention of CAV by modification of conventional atherosclerotic risk factors is the current therapeutic strategy, specifically control of hypertension, hyperlipidemia, obesity, and diabetes mellitus; abstinence from smoking; and exercise. Potential therapeutic strategies to treat CAV are listed in Table 12.7, although few have clinical evidence in human heart transplantation. Among other therapeutic agents, newer immunosuppression regimens may reduce the immunological risk for CAV and have anti-proliferative effects. In symptomatic CAV, medical treatment is similar to that of traditional coronary artery disease. Revascularization has no proven prognostic value but may provide symptomatic relief in selected cases. In any case, percutaneous coronary interventional and surgical treatments are often not possible in view of the diffuse nature and small caliber of vessels and carry a higher risk of re-stenosis. Conventional cardiac surgery on a transplanted heart carries higher risk due to associated comorbidities, including previous sternotomies, renal dysfunction, hypertension, immunosuppression, and poor wound healing. However, the only definitive treatment for established CAV is re-transplantation.

Metabolic syndrome

The incidences of various metabolic syndrome risk factors including hypertension, obesity, diabetes mellitus, and hyperlipidemia are increasingly seen after heart transplantation. The following sections give consideration to aspects of these complications, which are specific to patients after heart transplantation.

Systemic hypertension

Systemic hypertension is seen in the majority of patients after transplantation and often develops early (73% in year 1, 93% by year 5). The risk factors for hypertension in the general population apply post-transplant but are more likely to be pre-existing in heart transplant recipients, leading to increased incidence. The use of CNIs as described earlier is directly linked to the development of post-transplant hypertension.

Mechanisms include both neurohormonal and sympathetic nervous activation and direct cyclosporine (CyA)-induced renal vasoconstriction. CyA stimulates the release of endothelin and thromboxane

Table 12.7 Potential therapeutic strategies of treatment of cardiac allograft vasculopathy

Antihypertensives
Calcium antagonists
ACE inhibitors
Alpha and beta-blockers
Antioxidants
Omega-3
Fish oils
Vitamins E, B6
Folic acid
Antiplatelet
Aspirin
Clopidogrel
Antiproliferative
Low-molecular-weight heparin
mTOR inhibitors
Antivirals
Ganciclovir/valganciclovir
Endothelial protection
Better myocardial preservation
Strategies to reduce ischemia/reperfusion
Strategies to reduce effects of brainstem death
Immunosuppression
MMF
mTOR inhibitors
Anti-cytokines/adhesion molecules
Lipid modification
Statins
Apheresis
Re-transplantation
Revascularization
Percutaneous coronary intervention
Coronary bypass surgery
Transmyocardial laser revascularization

A_2. The end point is renal vascular bed vasoconstriction and salt and fluid retention. Other causes include corticosteroids (salt and fluid retention), loss of autonomic regulation due to cardiac denervation, and lack of nocturnal dip of blood pressure. Abnormal responsiveness of the renin–angiotensin–aldosterone system to salt and fluid retention is seen in post-transplant patients. Hypertension leads to allograft dysfunction through left ventricular hypertrophy and both systolic and diastolic dysfunction. Treatment follows usual guidelines for management of hypertension; however, patients are often resistant to treatment, and multiple drug combinations are needed. Calcium antagonists have the advantage of also reducing CAV and are not nephrotoxic. Diuretics may also be useful due to the increasing circulating volume after heart transplant, especially in the context of right heart dysfunction early after transplant, or in the presence of tricuspid regurgitation. Beta-blockers exacerbate autonomic dysfunction and prevent chronotropic response to exercise and have traditionally been avoided, although they may be used safely in selected patients.

Hyperlipidemia

Heart transplant patients require tight control of hyperlipidemia due to the impact on CAV. There is a high incidence of hyperlipidemia, with 58% of patients affected 1 year and 88% 5 years after heart transplantation. Causes include immunosuppressants, high-cholesterol diet, excessive weight gain (possibly related to reversal of ghrelin resistance), and genetic factors (familial hypercholesterolemia), which may be present pretransplant, particularly in patients with an ischemic etiology. Pravastatin has been shown to reduce cholesterol after heart transplant but also to reduce the incidence of CAV and should be used first line. Other statins and lipid-lowering therapies (fibrates, nicotinic acid) may be useful but should be used with caution to avoid rhabdomyolysis. Because CAV predicts long-term survival after heart transplant, consideration should be given to alteration in immunosuppression if lipid reduction is suboptimal.

Hyperglycemia

Diabetes mellitus and glucose intolerance are common after transplantation due to steroid and CNI use. The incidence of diabetes after heart transplantation is 28% at 1 year and 36% at 5 years, although the incidence remains higher in those with an ischemic cardiomyopathy pretransplant. Usual treatment and surveillance for diabetes should be instigated, but metformin should be avoided in patients with renal dysfunction.

Chronic renal dysfunction

Acute and chronic renal failure are common after heart transplantation. Due to the 50% increase in relative risk of 1-year mortality for creatinine >2.5 mg/dl, consideration should be given to combined heart–kidney transplant in carefully selected patients with moderate to severe renal dysfunction. The incidence of severe renal dysfunction (creatinine >2.5 mg/dl, dialysis, or renal transplant) is 7–12% at 1 year and 40% at 10 years after transplant. Over the last decade, the rate of development of severe renal dysfunction seemed to have lessened significantly. This could be attributed to better patient selection, improved management, and modern immunosuppression regimens. Risk factors include pre-existing renal dysfunction from chronic heart failure, diabetes, hypertension, and atherosclerosis, but CNI usage is undoubtedly the major factor for chronic renal dysfunction. CNI nephrotoxicity is discussed elsewhere but results in glomerulosclerosis, tubulo-interstitial fibrosis, and obliterative afferent arteriolopathy.

Prevention by minimizing CNI levels may be helpful balanced against the risk of rejection, although higher levels of immunosuppression are often required after heart transplantation compared with other transplanted organs. Other strategies include minimizing exposure to any additive medication with nephrotoxic potential, using CNI-sparing immunosuppression (mycophenolate mofetil [MMF]- and mammalian target of rapamycin [mTOR]-based regimens), secondary prevention (tight control of blood pressure, diabetes, and cholesterol), and use of calcium channel blockers where appropriate (afferent arteriolar vasodilatation). Care should be taken to minimize use of contrast agents for various investigations, especially for coronary angiography. Progression to dialysis predicts poor outcome after heart transplant, and if allograft function remains well preserved and other factors would predict reasonable medium-term prognosis (e.g., absence of CAV), then renal transplantation should be considered.

Malignancy after heart transplant

Malignancy is a major cause of late morbidity and mortality after heart transplantation, with mortality increasing cumulatively over time and accounting for approximately 10% of deaths at 5 years and 20% at 10 years. Cumulative prevalence is approximately 3% at 1 year, 15% at 5 years, and 30% at 10 years after heart transplant. In common with other transplants, the major malignancies are skin cancers and post-transplant lymphoproliferative disorder (PTLD), which together form about 80% of malignancies in 10-year survivors and may present early after transplant (Table 12.8).

Table 12.8 Proportion of malignancies after heart transplant in 10-year survivors (ISHLT 1994–2008)

Malignancy	%
Skin cancer	72
Lymphoma	8
Prostate	2
Adenocarcinoma	1
Lung	1
Bladder	4
Kaposi's sarcoma	1
Breast	2
Cervical	2
Colon	1
Renal	1
Indeterminate	5

A reduction in late malignancy can only be achieved by lower levels of induction and maintenance immunosuppression, induction of tolerance, and earlier detection through close surveillance. Improved immunosuppressive regimes in the modern era may explain the lower incidence of malignancies seen over the last decade. Recurrence of pre-existing treated malignancy in heart transplant recipients, following careful selection, is similar to that of other organ transplants at 20%. The pathogenesis, risk factors, and treatments are similar to those of other transplanted organs and are discussed elsewhere, but it is worth noting that the incidence of malignancy, particularly PTLD, is somewhat higher in cardiac transplantation due to the generally higher levels of immunosuppression required to prevent rejection. Urological and lung cancers are also common after heart transplant, in part due to the high incidence of smoking prior to transplant.

Late cardiac allograft dysfunction

Arrhythmia

Atrial arrhythmia late after heart transplant is common due to atrial enlargement (in biatrial anastomosis), allograft dysfunction, and late tricuspid regurgitation. Consideration should always be given to the possibility of acute rejection in the presence of arrhythmia. The loss of atrial contribution to ventricular contraction is particularly important in transplant patients. Management algorithms follow usual treatment for atrial arrhythmia, although beta-blockers may be less well tolerated and electrophysiological procedures are more anatomically challenging. Ventricular arrhythmia is usually pathological and suggests the presence of CAV and allograft dysfunction. Late bradyarrhythmia due to sinus or AV node dysfunction is unusual (1–2% of patients) and may also be related to acute rejection or CAV. Permanent pacing to preserve atrial contraction is preferred.

Tricuspid regurgitation

Mild and moderate late tricuspid regurgitation (TR) is common after heart transplant and is usually slowly progressive. Severe TR requiring treatment or surgical intervention is more unusual, seen in 1–5% of patients 5 years after transplant. Causes include multiple endomyocardial biopsies, tricuspid annular distortion in the biatrial anastomosis, right heart dilatation (in pulmonary hypertension), and torsion of atria during cardiac contraction. Diuresis is sufficient therapy in most patients, but surgical repair may be of benefit in patients with severe right heart failure symptoms.

Cardiac allograft failure

Systolic and diastolic heart failure are seen late after transplant, most commonly due to CAV, hypertension, and left ventricular hypertrophy, although acute rejection should always be considered because impaired function may improve with treatment. Treatment with conventional heart failure medication is instigated, although there is no evidence base after heart transplant. No place has been established for cardiac resynchronization or implantable defibrillator therapy. More important perhaps is the recognition of end of life, counseling the patient, and access to palliative care.

Quality of life after heart transplant

There is excellent improvement in quality of life in addition to the improved mortality following heart transplantation. In common with other transplants, there remain problems with the demands of a complex medical regimen, altered body image due to immunosuppression, stress about uncertainty of complications, unfulfilled expectations about exercise capacity, anxiety/depression, and other psychosocial difficulties. Involvement of psychological and psychiatric support is especially important following heart transplantation.

Further reading

Costanzo MR, Dipchand A, Starling R, *et al.* The International Society of Heart and Lung Transplantation Guidelines for the care of heart transplant recipients. *J Heart Lung Transplant* 2010; **29**: 914–56.

Kirklin JK, Young JB, McGiffin DC. *Heart Transplantation.* Philadelphia: Churchill Livingstone, 2002.

Mehra MR, Crespo-Leiro MG, Dipchand A, *et al.* International Society for Heart and Lung Transplantation working formulation of a standardized nomenclature for cardiac allograft vasculopathy. *J Heart Lung Transplant* 2010; **29**: 717–27.

Stehlik J, Edwards LB, Kucheryavaya AY, *et al.* The Registry of the International Society for Heart and Lung Transplantation: Twenty-seventh official adult heart transplant report – 2010. *J Heart Lung Transplant* 2010; **29**: 1089–103.

Section 2 Heart

Chapter 13

Pediatric heart transplantation

Jacob Simmonds and Michael Burch

Key points

- ABO-incompatible transplantation is possible in infants and young children. The precise level of isohemagglutinins at which it is safe to perform ABO mismatch transplant remains unclear; however, a dilution of 1:16 may be used.
- In ambulatory children with chronic heart failure a VO2 max of <50% of predicted, blunted blood pressure and heart rate responses, and a B-type natriuretic peptide level of >300 pg/ml are all associated with a poor outcome and can be considered in the transplant listing process.
- Transplant for congenital heart disease has a varied peri-operative risk. Previous Senning and Mustard patients have a relatively low risk, but Fontan patients have a relative risk of death of 8.6 compared with other congenital patients.
- The risk for Fontan patients appears greater if the circulation is failing because of pulmonary resistance rather than ventricular failure.
- Post-transplant lymphoproliferative disease is the predominant malignancy in pediatric transplantation. Epstein-Barr viral load on polymerase chain reaction may be helpful in diagnosing incipient lymphoma or guiding treatment, although this remains unproven.
- Cardiac allograft vasculopathy is the main cause of late graft loss and the major reason for re-transplantation in children, as in adults. Inflammatory factors such as cytomegalovirus and recurrent rejection appear to be important in progression, although the exact cause is unknown.

Heart transplantation remains the only realistic therapeutic option for children with end-stage heart disease. Although the first pediatric heart transplant was performed by Kantrowitz in New York in 1967 only 3 days after Barnard's celebrated first adult transplant, it was soon understood that the discipline was not a mere extension of transplantation in adults, but rather a distinct clinical entity with its own set of principles, techniques, and goals. Of course, there is much overlap with adult transplantation, and much of what we know and practice is a direct extrapolation of that much larger experience. However, although broad surgical techniques, postoperative intensive care, and ongoing pharmacological management share much in common between the age groups, there are vital differences that must be taken into account if a center is going to produce a successful pediatric transplant program.

It is also important to state that pediatric heart transplantation is itself a very heterogeneous subspecialty. Whereas approximately 90% of adult transplants are performed for cardiomyopathy (either ischemic or non-ischemic), up to one in three pediatric recipients has a diagnosis of congenital heart disease. The use of the word "diagnosis" in the singular form is somewhat of a misnomer, however, since this subgroup of patients is further subdivided into a wide variation of congenital heart defects, with the possibility of multiple previous surgical interventions and wide diversity in clinical status. This variability in anatomic substrate must be thought about carefully and on an individual by individual basis by the surgical team prior to heart transplant listing; it is also accompanied by

Organ Transplantation: A Clinical Guide, ed. A.A. Klein, C.J. Lewis, and J.C. Madsen. Published by Cambridge University Press.

variability in physiological status that requires skilful management by the anesthetic and intensive care specialists. Further complexity arises from the significant differences between neonates, young children, and adolescents, again with regard to anatomy and physiology, but also in regard to psychology and social background. In addition, patients requiring heart transplantation in childhood often have coexisting conditions or syndromes that must be considered throughout the transplant process.

With this heterogeneity in mind, pediatric transplant teams have been set up in many centers worldwide as distinct entities to their adult counterparts, with obvious benefits from the subspecialization. However, the experience of these teams is generally much less than that of their adult counterparts. The latest data from the International Society for Heart and Lung Transplantation (ISHLT) reveal that only 11% of pediatric transplant centers performed more than 10 per year since 2001, compared with 58% of adult centers. Low volume of cases is known to be a risk factor for mortality post-transplantation, and it is easy to understand how increased experience and familiarity of every aspect of transplantation would lead to a more successful program. The small numbers of procedures per center also greatly limit both quantity and quality of research possibilities, yet this is counterbalanced by effective multi-center clinical audit and research, such as with the Pediatric Heart Transplant Study Group. However, even with these caveats, complications, and complexities, pediatric heart transplantation has survival rates slightly better than that of adults.

One further important difference between pediatric and adult heart transplantation is how to define success for the pediatric transplant program and for the individual patient. If a 55-year-old man with coronary artery disease survived 15 years after transplantation, it would be considered by many patients and health care providers alike as a successful and worthwhile intervention with obvious benefit to the patient and society as a whole. Although the success and worth of 15-year survival following infant transplantation could never be questioned, the prospect of re-transplantation or death in adolescence or early adulthood invites further philosophical, ethical, and economic questions. Although difficult, these issues must be discussed with any prospective patient and family to allow careful consideration before agreeing to be transplant listed.

Indications

Improvements to every stage of transplantation have greatly increased the success of the procedure, both in terms of longevity and quality of life of the childhood recipients. Simultaneously, there have been great strides made in the treatment of heart failure (HF) and the surgical treatment of congenital heart disease, allowing transplantation to be postponed or completely avoided in some patients. With this in mind, in 2007 the American Heart Association Council on Cardiovascular Disease in the Young developed a document describing the current indications for pediatric heart transplantation.

Predictably, the guidelines are largely based on non-randomized studies or on consensus clinical expert opinion, rather than large, multi-center randomized controlled trials. In evidence-based medicine terms, these are level of evidence B and C. The main indication for transplantation in children that is widely agreed (class I indication) is severe HF associated with impaired function of the systemic ventricle (usually of left ventricular [LV] morphology but sometimes right ventricular [RV] morphology in some types of congenital heart disease). However, it is also considered reasonable to list children with moderate HF if they have severe limitation of activity/exercise or significant growth failure as a result of the chronic HF. Exercise testing can aid listing such patients, although it is difficult in children (as discussed in the next section, Timing of listing). Intractable arrhythmias are considered an indication for listing, provided all treatment options including an implantable defibrillator have been considered. Heart transplantation for restrictive cardiomyopathy is considered appropriate if there is evidence of reactive pulmonary hypertension within safe limits. That is, when the pulmonary vascular resistance (PVR) can be reduced using pulmonary vasodilators to a transpulmonary gradient (TPG) of under 15mmHg and a PVR of $\leq$6 Wood units·m^2. The latter PVR rule applies to the other main indications for transplant previously mentioned.

Less strong indications without universal agreement but for which the weight of evidence is broadly in favor (class II) include children whose heart disease is inoperable and may lead to development of irreversible pulmonary vascular disease; e.g., restrictive cardiomyopathy with mildly elevated pulmonary pressures. There are also some other congenital problems for which the prognosis for conventional surgery is so bad that transplantation listing can be considered, such as coronary atresia/stenoses or severe valve regurgitation or impaired ventricular function.

Cardiac re-transplantation in children is mainly indicated when there is poor ventricular function and significant coronary artery vasculopathy (class I indication). It is more controversial when ventricular function is preserved (class II indication). There is general agreement that re-transplantation should not be performed during an episode of acute rejection. Early re-transplantation has a poor outcome, and there is consensus that this should not be performed within 6 months of transplant.

It is important to stress that HT should not be used as the primary therapy for any infant with congenital heart disease without the presence of concomitant coronary, valvular, or ventricular impairment. It is, however, reasonable to consider transplantation in the setting of previously repaired congenital heart disease without ventricular dysfunction if there is risk of developing fixed raised PVR that could preclude future transplantation, severe aortic or systemic valve insufficiency, severe cyanosis, persistent arrhythmia, or persistent protein-losing enteropathy.

Timing of listing for transplant of ambulatory patients

Although increasing proportions of HT are performed in very ill patients on high-dose inotropes or mechanical support, some patients undergo transplantation while still ambulatory and at home. Many pediatric cardiologists base timing on evidence of LV systolic dysfunction and symptoms of HF. Severity of ventricular dysfunction has been found to be predictive of outcome in some studies but not in others. Symptoms appear to provide poor prognostic capability too, because even asymptomatic children with incidental discovery of cardiomyopathy can have a poor prognosis. Finding ways to identify those patients with the highest risk of clinical deterioration and/or death would greatly assist in clinical decision making, including the indication and prioritization for transplant.

Extensive evidence supports the use of cardiopulmonary exercise testing as a tool to select patients with increased short-term mortality who should be offered transplantation. Besides peak oxygen uptake, several additional variables, such as ventilatory efficiency, have been shown to have high prognostic value in adults with HF. However, despite widespread use in the adult population, information regarding the practical clinical value of exercise testing as a prognostic tool in pediatrics is very limited. Our own experience is that exercise testing is possible in children over 10 years of age and sometimes younger. Our data are broadly supportive of a peak oxygen consumption of less than 50% of predicted for age, although we have also found peak blood pressure response to exercise to be an important prognostic test.

Exercise testing is complicated in congenital heart disease. Peak heart rate appears to be a useful prognostic marker. Oxygen consumption and ventilatory efficiency are also useful. However, the values at which transplantation should be considered vary with the type of congenital heart disease. Patients with a Fontan circulation have much lower baseline levels of oxygen consumption and ventilatory efficiency. A simple 6-minute flat walking test is still valuable in congenital heart disease.

For younger children, pre-school age and infants, exercise testing is impossible. It is in this age group that biomarkers of HF are particularly useful. In patients with chronic HF, B-type natriuretic peptide level of over 300 pg/ml may be predictive of poor outcome in pediatric cardiomyopathy. Other biomarkers are currently being assessed.

Transplantation for congenital heart disease

Transplantation for congenital heart disease illustrates best many of the peculiarities of heart transplant in the pediatric age group. As experience with pediatric transplant has grown, the boundaries of what anatomy is considered transplantable have extended to the point now that the only contraindications from a purely anatomical point of view are severe pulmonary artery hypoplasia and pulmonary vein stenosis. However, these may be correctable by combined heart–lung transplantation or using extended donor pulmonary arteries for pulmonary hypoplasia.

Concurrently, improved conventional surgical techniques have led to the treatment of more and more congenital heart disease without the need for early transplantation. However, these, along with the success of non-curative surgical procedures such as the Fontan pathway, have only postponed the need for transplant in many patients, reducing strain on the youngest, most scarce donors, but in many cases adding to the waiting list in later childhood. In reality, these improvements may have even increased the overall numbers of potential recipients, as many infants would previously have died during neonatal operations or on neonatal transplant waiting lists. Many of these children are now surviving infancy, but with circulatory systems that are destined to fail at some point, and by the time a heart transplant is required, some families are finding transplantation a more attractive option, and palliative care strategies less so.

In most registries, congenital heart disease remains a risk factor for transplantation. Attrition is early and related to the complexity of the reconstruction. Yet it would be wrong to be uniformly negative about transplantation for congenital heart disease. Registry data have shown that transplantation for previous Senning or Mustard procedures can be achieved with a low mortality rate. Previously palliated infants and young children with a Glenn circulation also appear to have relatively low risk. However, it is the Fontan patients who represent the highest risk, with a recent paper showing a relative risk of death of 8.6 compared with that of other congenital operations. The Fontan patients often have liver or renal problems and may suffer more infections by virtue of protein-losing enteropathy and lymphopenia. Protein-losing enteropathy increases the risk of transplant, perhaps because it may be a marker of increased pulmonary vascular resistance. Resistance is hard to calculate in the Fontan patient with multiple sources of pulmonary blood supply, pulmonary arteriovenous malformations, collaterals, and fenestrations.

For all congenital patients, it is obvious that risk can be reduced by having an experienced congenital surgeon perform the operation with appropriate anesthetic and intensive care teams. This is particularly important in adult congenital heart disease, where few adult transplant teams have extensive congenital experience.

Because the lifespan of a transplanted organ is limited, no potential recipient should be transplanted too early. The aim of pediatric programs is often to delay transplantation for as long as possible by optimizing medical management. However, this delay must not be at the expense of other organ damage (most notably renal failure or cirrhosis in Fontan patients), increasing pulmonary resistance, or inducing human leukocyte antigen (HLA) sensitization by virtue of blood transfusions. Any of these complications of delaying transplant may reduce the success of future transplantation and have the effect of an overall decrease in life expectancy.

Prior to listing for transplantation, detailed scanning of the heart and pulmonary vasculature with an appropriate combination of echocardiography, angiography, computed tomography (CT), or magnetic resonance imaging (MRI) must be undertaken to ensure that the anatomy is favorable. These scans must be available to the surgeon before accepting an offer of a potential organ so he can request extended portions of the great vessels, which may be required to facilitate non-standard anastomoses. Because it is likely that other organs may be being harvested from the same donor, it is important for the cardiac surgeon to speak to other transplant teams to enable the most judicious use of donor vessels, or perhaps arrange for alternative tissue to be collected. For instance, if the heart transplant surgeon feels he is unable to harvest enough of the pulmonary arteries for a particular recipient, he may be able to use donor pericardium or descending aorta.

Pulmonary vascular resistance

The assessment of PVR is particularly crucial in order to reduce the rate of right HF post-transplant, but it can be technically difficult, particularly in congenital heart disease. In general the guidelines document referred to previously advises that transplantation is possible if PVR can be reduced using pulmonary vasodilators to a TPG under 15 mmHg and a PVR of $\leq$6 Wood units·m^2. There is a tendency for pediatric centers to push the boundaries of transplantable PVR, and some units will take on children with resistance higher than this, but it is clear that risk is increased. A long period of inotrope or vasodilator therapy may reduce PVR, as may a period of mechanical support by reducing LV end-diastolic pressure.

Mechanical support

Traditionally pediatric units offered extracorporeal membrane oxygenation (ECMO) support as a bridge to transplant, as most ventricular assist devices (VADs) were not suitable for small children. This strategy allowed only a short time for support before serious complications ensued. The development of the pneumatic assist device suitable for children, the Berlin Heart, has allowed long-term bridge to transplant in young children. Successful support is possible for many months, although few children are discharged from hospital. Most experience has been obtained in children with dilated cardiomyopathy who are older than 1 month of age. Usually the device is implanted in children with progressive cardiac failure and inotrope dependency. Few data exist on support for very young children who weigh less than 4 kg. It seems likely that the neonatal group will be more difficult to manage, with the small 10-ml pumps and anticoagulation complexities increasing their risk of thromboembolic complications. Typically the device is used as a bridge to transplant, although there are reports of use as bridge to recovery, and it has been used in myocarditis. In general, fulminant myocarditis is still treated with ECMO in most centers, although this may change as experience with the Berlin Heart increases. However, ECMO does avoid an LV scar. Conversion from ECMO to Berlin Heart is often performed, although primary implantation of Berlin Heart is preferred in most units. The use in single-ventricle circulations and particularly the Fontan circulation also appears more complex. The limited data available do suggest a higher mortality in the single-ventricle group. However, the recent huge increase in Berlin Heart insertion in the United States illustrates the success of this device.

Surgical modifications

The particular anatomy in each case of congenital heart disease will require adaptation by the surgeon. Previous sternotomy may have produced significant mediastinal adhesions, which can cause heavy intraoperative hemorrhage, as can collateral vessels that have resulted from years of cyanosis. At the same time, knowledge of substernal great vessels may lead some surgeons to expose the femoral vessels prior to sternotomy to facilitate emergency femoro-femoral bypass should the need arise.

Before implantation can occur, it is sometimes necessary to normalize recipient anatomy, for instance, in the case of bilateral cavopulmonary anastomoses. Any extra procedures that are anticipated must be allowed for when planning the operation in order to synchronize the prepared recipient and the arrival of the organ, thus avoiding long ischemic times.

ABO incompatibility

Compared with adult transplantation, the prospective donor pool of hearts suitable for infant recipients is small. Infants with blood group O have a further reduced donor pool. This imbalance has prompted advances in transplanting across blood groups – the so-called ABO-incompatible transplant. In adults, heart transplants across ABO blood groups have occurred only by mistake, with high rates of both hyperacute rejection and mortality.

In contrast to mature adult immune systems, however, infants have very low levels of isohemagglutinins, allowing the possibility of transplanting an organ of blood type B, say, into a recipient of type A. In 1996, Lori West led the team that performed the first intentional heart transplant across an ABO incompatibility. The recipient was a 25-day-old infant with hypoplastic left heart syndrome of blood group O who received an organ of blood group AB. During cardiopulmonary bypass, plasma exchange was performed until the levels of isohemagglutinins were non-detectable. In the paper reporting the first 10 ABO-incompatible transplants, rates of mortality, rejection, and morbidity were equivalent to those of ABO-compatible transplants, with two deaths and one other graft loss unrelated to ABO activation. It is thought that donor-specific B-cell elimination results in immunological tolerance in recipients of ABO-incompatible hearts. In order to ensure the ongoing success of the graft, future transfusion of blood products must occur according to strict criteria (Table 13.1). The exact age and level of isohemagglutinins that are acceptable for ABO mismatch transplant are unclear, but an isohemagglutinin dilution of 1:16 is used at our center as a cut-off value, and few such transplants have been performed over the age of 2 years.

Lymphocytotoxic antibodies

Another problem in pediatric transplantation is the presence of pre-existing HLA antibodies, which have been linked to increased hyperacute, cellular, and humoral rejection and increased mortality post-transplant. There are several factors that cause the formation of such antibodies. However, most antibodies are formed in response to blood products (particularly white cells and platelets) or homograft tissue. Thus prior HLA sensitization is much more common in children who have undergone surgery for congenital heart disease, or those who have required

Table 13.1 Required blood groups for transfusion after ABO-incompatible pediatric heart transplantation

Donor blood group	Recipient blood group	Indicated plasma	Indicated red cells	Indicated platelets
AB	O	AB	O	AB
B	O	AB or B	O	AB or B
A	O	AB or A	O	AB or A
AB	B	AB	O or B	AB
A	B	AB	O or B	AB
AB	A	AB	O or A	AB
B	A	AB	O or A	AB

mechanical support. For children on longer term mechanical support, the "prophylactic" use of supplements of iron, folic acid, and erythropoietin may avoid blood transfusion.

When a patient is sensitized, a prospective cross-match between donor and recipient serum prior to transplantation would be the perfect solution, but it is time-consuming, which limits the geographical area from which a sensitized recipient can receive an organ. Alternatively, it is possible to test antibodies against specific HLA antigens, thereby facilitating a "virtual" cross-match once a potential donor has been found. Although this will not be as specific as a prospective cross-match, it has been used safely in both adult and pediatric transplantation.

It is also possible to reduce the level of HLA antibodies prior to transplantation. Strategies for de-sensitization include intravenous immunoglobulin, methotrexate, mycophenolate mofetil (MMF), cyclophosphamide, and rituximab, and newer monoclonal antibodies to plasma cells, to lower the level of panel reactive antibodies prior to transplantation. However, there has not been uniform success with these strategies, and there is often a limited window of low antibody levels in which transplantation can be performed. This has led some North American centers to transplant across the HLA barrier using intra-operative plasma exchange and post-operative plasmapheresis with other antibody-reducing strategies. Results are still at a preliminary stage, but it appears that primary graft failure can often be avoided, and although antibody-mediated rejection is common, it may resolve with possible accommodation to the antibody. The long-term consequences of this strategy are as yet unknown.

Immunosuppression

It does appear that acute cellular rejection, in particular that associated with hemodynamic compromise, is becoming less common. This may be the result of newer drugs and increased experience. Over the last decade or so, there has been a gradual shift toward using induction therapy in pediatric heart transplantation, with current levels at about 60%. Antithymocyte globulin remains the preferred agent in children, although the proportion of centers using an interleukin-2 receptor antagonist such as basiliximab is increasing. Basiliximab may be more effective given prior to bypass and organ implantation, and its more selective action is felt by some to cause less of the problems associated with "over-immunosuppression," such as post-transplant lymphoproliferative disorder (PTLD) and cytomegalovirus (CMV).

Maintenance therapy is most commonly a combination of a calcineurin inhibitor (CNI) and cell cycle inhibitor. Tacrolimus (TAC) has become the CNI of choice in 58%, taking over from cyclosporine (CyA) at least in part due to the latter's unwanted side-effect profile of hirsutism and gingival hypertrophy, which can lead to problems with compliance in pediatric patients. Cell cycle inhibitors are used by 80% in the first year, with MMF the most common, being used in 59% of children; approximately one third of all patients are prescribed it in combination with TAC. This figure is slightly less than the equivalent value in adults, approximately half of whom are taking TAC and MMF in combination.

Steroids still hold a place in pediatric practice, particularly in the first year post-transplant, and in the treatment of rejection. The proportion of patients using steroids is slightly less than in adults, with 55% of children taking prednisolone at 1 year; by 5 years post-transplant, this figure has fallen to less than 40%.

Renal disease

Chronic use of CNI induces renal dysfunction. This is clearly crucial in pediatrics, where patients are still young and hopeful of a second heart transplant when the first one eventually fails. Nephrotoxicity can be reduced by using lower levels both early post-transplant and later in the recipient's course. The main pediatric use of sirolimus (SRL) and everolimus (EVL) has been in children with impaired renal function after transplant, along with reduced doses of CNI. Others have used CNI regimes. The latter may be associated

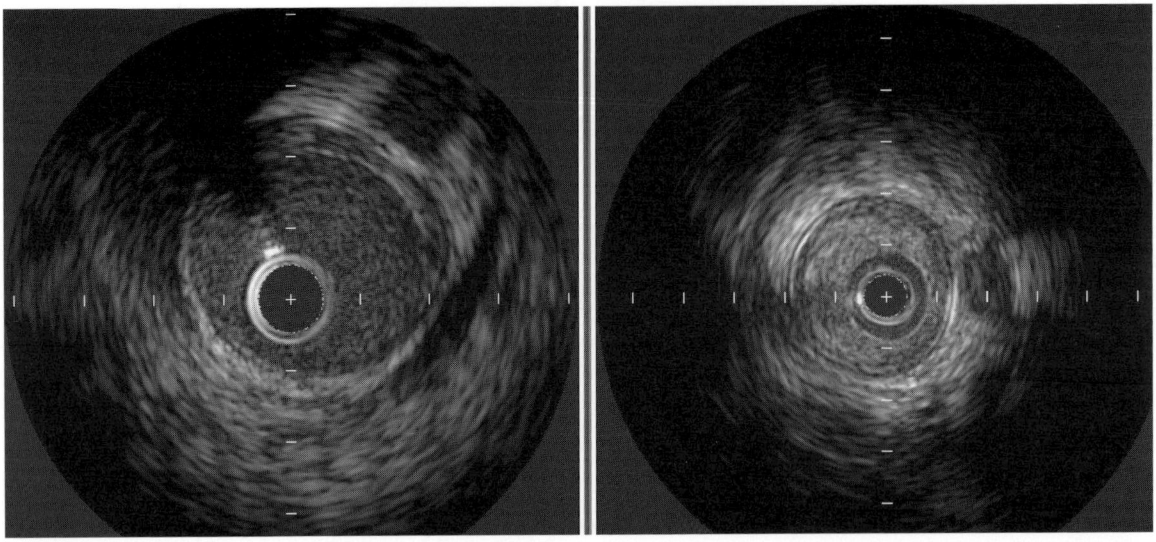

Figure 13.1 Intravascular ultrasound images of the left anterior descending coronary artery of the same patient taken 1 and 2 years post-transplant. The figure on the left shows a relatively healthy artery, with good lumen size, and only a small amount of intimal thickening in the upper left quadrant. The figure on the right shows the effective lumen now decreased to only slightly larger than the ultrasound probe, with the rest of the artery replaced by grossly thickened intima. The patient had clinically significant CMV disease during the period between the images.

with an increased risk of rejection, and greater surveillance with biopsy and non-invasive testing are needed.

Lymphoma

Unlike adult transplant medicine, pediatric transplant teams do not have to deal with a wide range of malignancies after transplant. Even skin malignancies are uncommon in children, but this does not preclude the need for sun protection and surveillance. The main malignancy in children after transplant is lymphoma. Usually, this is a B-cell lymphoma and is triggered by Epstein-Barr virus (EBV). Surveillance using quantitative polymerase chain reaction for the virus may give early warning of incipient lymphoma, and many teams will reduce immunosuppression when viral loads are high. The risk of lymphoma appears greater in children that seroconvert after transplant. The site of the lymphoma varies, but is often in the gut (typically associated with a low albumin), lungs (where chronic chest infections may be wrongly diagnosed), or tonsils. Tissue diagnosis is usually needed. Treatment is similar to that of PTLD in the adult and may involve reduction of immunosuppression, with rituximab increasingly used in the initial stages. Treatment may escalate to conventional chemotherapy, and even specific T cells have been generated to destroy the EBV-associated B cells.

Cardiac allograft vasculopathy

Like adults, the major obstacle to late patient survival in pediatric heart transplantation is cardiac allograft vasculopathy (CAV), an accelerated form of obliterative cardiovascular disease (Figure 13.1). CAV causes considerable morbidity and mortality, affecting approximately 50% of patients 5 years post-transplant. It is the leading cause of death in children more than 3 years post-transplant. As it is accompanied by remodeling and compensatory luminal dilatation in the early phases, it may best be diagnosed with intravascular ultrasound rather than conventional angiography. However, because this technique is not widely available in children, it is likely that the prevalence of the disease has been underestimated. Moreover, once a diagnosis of CAV has been made, graft survival is limited to 50% at 2 years. It is thus the greatest limitation on long-term outcome and remains the most pressing problem for transplant programs worldwide. The cause remains unknown, but conventional risk factors such as smoking, hypertension, diabetes, hypercholesterolemia, and obesity are less of a problem in pediatrics than in adults. In children, chronic viral infection such as CMV and recurrent acute or chronic cellular rejection appear important. It does seem that chronic inflammation is important in the development of CAV.

Current treatment is severely limited. The use of statins has been shown to improve outcome after transplantation in adults, and pravastatin has been safely used in children including infants with few problems. Pravastatin has the advantage of not interfering with cytochrome p450 and thus CNI. Reversal of CAV is much harder, although SRL is thought to have useful anti-proliferative properties. Ultimately, however, many patients with CAV face the prospect of re-transplantation relatively soon after diagnosis. In the pediatric age group, it is the most common indication for re-transplantation, making up just over half of all re-transplants.

Psychological, developmental, and behavioral issues

Ultimately, the success of individual transplants and the program as a whole depends on well-informed, psychologically stable and motivated patients. In pediatric transplant, these are even more vital, as the advent of adolescence often magnifies any psychological stressors. The prevalence of behavioral problems in post-transplant children is over 25%, a frequency that exceeds that of children following conventional cardiac surgery. Moreover, the effects of such problems, in particular non-compliance with immunosuppression, are potentially more serious. It is therefore of paramount importance to make psychological and social assessments of potential recipients prior to transplant and try to address any issues that may arise.

Cognitive development of children following cardiac transplant is obviously an important outcome variable. Many studies have tried to evaluate accurately the impact of transplantation. In general, the transplant group has mean mental and psychomotor scores at the low end of the normal range. Many factors are postulated as causes for this discrepancy between the transplant and healthy population, including hospitalization, missed school, cardiopulmonary bypass, and the side effects of post-transplant drugs. Encouragingly, the vast majority of pediatric heart transplant recipients should look forward to reintegrating fully into normal schooling and social activities.

Adherence to post-transplant medication regimes is not universally high among childhood recipients, and it is commonly cited as a cause of acute rejection and death, particularly among teenagers. Early recognition of clues to non-compliance, for instance wildly variable immunosuppressant levels and erratic lifestyles (including school avoidance and irregular sleeping patterns) must be taken seriously, and causes to the root problems must be addressed. Addressing concerns over the cosmetic side effects from medication and more convenient medicine regimes may help.

Ultimately, psychological and behavioral difficulties must be considered on an individual basis. A coordinated multi-disciplinary approach to any problems, involving medical and nursing teams both at the transplant center and locally, must be undertaken when problems arise and include the family doctor, school teachers and nurses, family members, and teams of specialists such as social workers and special educational providers when necessary.

Outcomes

The overall survival for children following transplantation has steadily increased throughout the history of the subspecialty. The ISHLT data show half-life for patients aged 11–17 years of 11.3 years and those aged 1–10 years of 15.5 years. Despite transplantation in infancy having a higher early mortality, half-life is excellent at 18 years. The highest rate of graft loss in all age groups was seen in the first 6 months post-transplant. With improvements in surgical expertise and immediate postoperative intensive care, there has been a very marked reduction in early deaths and significantly reduced deaths from acute rejection in the first 12 months. Survival after the first 12 months, however, has largely plateaued, creating roughly parallel survival curves from year 2 onwards.

Our figures from Great Ormond Street (London, United Kingdom) illustrate the improvements in outcome in more detail and largely mirror experience from the registry (Figure 13.2). Overall survival has increased over time, with patients undergoing transplant in the recent eras having a much

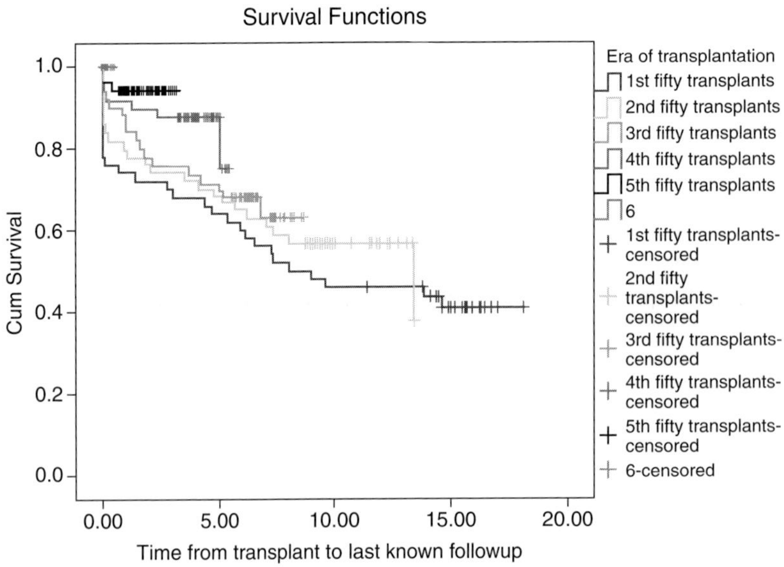

Figure 13.2 Survival of pediatric patients after heart transplantation at Great Ormond Street Hospital, London, United Kingdom.

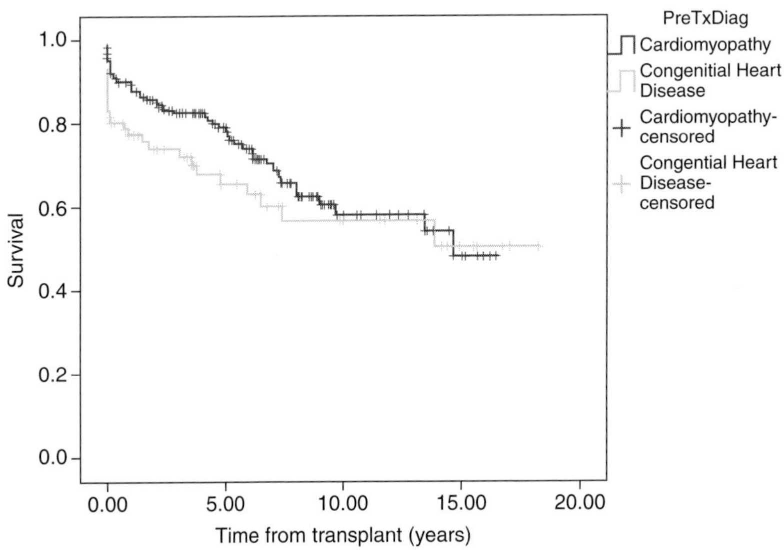

Figure 13.3 Comparison of the survival of patients with cardiomyopathy and congenital heart disease.

better survival, particularly in the first 6 months post-transplant.

Diagnosis has an important bearing on survival post-transplant. Over the 20 years of the transplant program at Great Ormond Street, those patients undergoing transplant for congenital heart disease fared less well than children with cardiomyopathy (Figure 13.3). However, on closer scrutiny, it is easy to see that the difference in survival between these two groups is largely due to an early attrition of approximately 20% in the CHD group, and that conditional survival of patients who have survived 1 year is similar between the groups.

Further reading

Canter CE, Shaddy RE, Bernstein D, *et al.* Indications for heart transplantation in pediatric heart disease: a scientific statement from the American Heart Association Council on Cardiovascular Disease in the Young; the Councils on Clinical Cardiology,

Cardiovascular Nursing, and Cardiovascular Surgery and Anesthesia; and the Quality of Care and Outcomes Research Interdisciplinary Working Group. *Circulation* 2007; **115**: 658–76.

Kirk R, Edwards LB, Aurora P, *et al.* Registry of the International Society for Heart and Lung Transplantation: Twelfth Official Pediatric Heart Transplantation Report-2009. *J Heart Lung Transplant* 2009; **28**: 993–1006.

Lamour JM, Kanter KR, Naftel DC, *et al.* The effect of age, diagnosis, and previous surgery in children and adults undergoing heart transplantation for congenital heart disease. *J Am Coll Cardiol* 2009; **54:** 160–5.

Mangat J, Carter C, Riley G, Foo Y, Burch M. The clinical utility of brain natriuretic peptide in paediatric left ventricular failure. *Eur J Heart Fail* 2009; **11**: 48–52.

Pollock-BarZiv SM, den Hollander N, Ngan BY, *et al.* Pediatric heart transplantation in human leukocyte antigen sensitized patients: evolving management and assessment of intermediate-term outcomes in a high-risk population. *Circulation* 2007; **116**: I172–8.

West LJ, Pollock-Barziv SM, Dipchand AI, *et al.* ABO-incompatible heart transplantation in infants. *N Engl J Med* 2001; **344**: 793–800.

Chapter 14

Recipient selection

J.S. Parmar

Key points

- Critical organ shortage makes careful patient selection essential.
- Patients should be New York Heart Association class III–IV with a median survival of < 2 years.
- The best outcomes are in recipients with single-organ failure.
- Complex patients should be discussed with transplant centers early.
- Infections with hepatitis B virus, hepatitis C virus, human immunodeficiency virus, and highly resistant bacteria are relative contraindications.
- Pulmonary rehabilitation prior to listing for transplant is essential.

The low number of donated lungs and heart–lung blocks means that careful patient selection remains critical to ensure the best utilization of a scarce resource. This chapter focuses on how to select patients who will gain maximum benefit from lung transplantation (LT). In the first part of this chapter, general considerations and exclusions pertaining to all potential recipients are outlined, and in the second half the focus is on disease specific guidance for the major recipient groups: chronic obstructive pulmonary disease (COPD), cystic fibrosis (CF), idiopathic pulmonary fibrosis (IPF), and idiopathic pulmonary arterial hypertension (IPAH).

Background

Transplantation of cardiothoracic organs is a therapeutic option for a large variety of end-stage cardiorespiratory diseases. As LT carries a moderate early operative risk to the patient (5–10% mortality in first 30 days), it is a clinical imperative to ensure that all other therapeutic options are fully explored prior to considering this as a treatment option.

An acceptable risk profile will vary from patient to patient and will depend on the overall clinical picture. However, in general, when considering who to refer, the patient should have a chronic disorder causing single-organ failure with a predicted 2-year survival from the organ failure of less than 50%. Most potential recipients with this severely limited prognosis will be in at least New York Heart Association (NYHA) class III or IV. Patients with this severity of disease are often very limited and suffer with a poor quality of life. This combination of poor prognosis and poor quality of life make the operative risks more acceptable.

Although the ideal LT candidate is a patient who has single-organ failure with no associated comorbidities, very few potential recipients fall into this ideal category, and most will have associated or independent medical issues. It is critical that these conditions, if present, should have an independent prognosis for survival of at least 5 years, as the median survival for lung transplant recipients is 5.7 years. When considering who to refer for consideration of LT, there are a few absolute contraindications, which would be impediments to consideration of LT (Table 14.1). In addition there are a number of comorbidities, which can impact on recipient suitability.

Absolute contraindications

With the improving outcomes achieved over the last 20 years in the field of LT, there is an increasing desire to re-examine clinical scenarios that were initially considered to be absolute contraindications. An example of this is the transplantation of patients who

Organ Transplantation: A Clinical Guide, ed. A.A. Klein, C.J. Lewis, and J.C. Madsen. Published by Cambridge University Press.

Table 14.1 Contraindications to consideration of lung transplantation

Incurable chronic extrapulmonary infection
Malignancy
Any other medical condition with a prognosis < 5 years
Active substance addiction or abuse within the last 6 months
Untreatable psychiatric or psychological condition
History of non-compliance with medical therapy
Absence of a reliable or consistent social support system
Significant chest wall or spinal deformity
Severely limited functional status with poor rehabilitation potential
Colonization with highly resistant or virulent bacteria, fungi, or mycobacteria
Obesity, defined as a BMI > 30 kg/m^2, or severe cachexia, defined as BMI < 18 kg/m^2
Corticosteroid therapy > 15 mg/day
Severe gastroesophageal reflux with dysmotility

are ventilator-dependent. Previously, this state had been associated with poor outcomes, but with increasing experience, patients may undergo transplantation from either ventilator-based or extracorporeal membrane oxygenation (ECMO)–based respiratory support with reasonable outcomes. However, even with these improvements, there remain certain conditions that are still considered to be absolute contraindications. The presence of chest wall deformity that would militate against successful surgery is a clear example of this. Coexisting viral infections with hepatitis B virus (HBV), hepatitis C virus (HCV), and human immunodeficiency virus (HIV) have been considered absolute contraindications to LT. However, experience with these particular infections is growing in other solid organ transplants so that some centers have listed and performed LT on a small number of patients with these infections. Evidence of severe, untreatable second organ damage or failure is an absolute contraindication, unless it is feasible to perform a combined transplant. An example of this is the presence of severe concurrent liver disease in a CF patient with end-stage bronchiectasis. In this situation, isolated organ transplantation may result in decompensation in the other failing organ and thus a poor outcome. However, combined synchronous lung–liver transplantation from the same donor may provide a viable alternative.

Chronic infections, both pulmonary and extrapulmonary, are a cause of major morbidity and mortality in potential LT recipients and can be impediments to listing. The presence of a chronic infection affecting an extrapulmonary site, which is not curable prior to transplantation, is an absolute contraindication, because immunosuppression will exacerbate the infection.

Pulmonary infections with highly resistant bacteria have been shown to have poorer outcomes in comparison with non-infected patients. For instance, patients with CF who are colonized with *Burkholderia cenocepacia* have been shown to have a very poor outcome and thus are not generally currently considered candidates for LT. Similarly, patients who are recurrently colonized with atypical mycobacteria who fail to clear on medical therapy have a high rate of re-infection and are thus not considered to be good candidates. This is particularly important in patients who are colonized with fast-dividing atypicals (*Mycobacteria kansasii or Mycobacteria abscessus*) who are at risk of systemic dissemination.

The presence of fungus in the native lungs can cause problems after LT and will need careful assessment in each individual. The presence of large cavities, pleural involvement, and highly resistant fungi may be a contraindication. As this is an area in which experience is limited, it is prudent to discuss each patient on a case-by-case basis with the local transplant team.

Over the last few years there has been an increasing recognition of the importance of gastroesophageal reflux disease (GERD) as a cause of chronic rejection (obliterative bronchiolitis). For this reason, patients who have severe reflux associated with esophageal dysmotility are not considered for LT.

The presence of a malignancy is still considered an absolute contraindication, as most are exacerbated by long-term immunosuppression. Although each case should be considered on its merits, a disease-free interval of at least 5 years is recommended for most major malignancies. The one exception to this guidance is the presence of limited cutaneous malignancies that can be treated with local excision. In this particular situation, the disease-free period can be reduced to 2 years.

Cigarette smoking remains the number one cause of lung disease worldwide. Smoking-related lung injury is significantly greater in transplanted lungs than in native lungs. For this reason, recipients are required to demonstrate a period of complete abstinence of at least 6 months prior to listing for LT. A similar approach is also used for patients who have a history of illicit drug abuse. Periodic testing of the urine for toxicology will help to confirm abstinence.

Comorbidities

As highlighted previously, the presence of comorbidities outside of the failing respiratory system are important considerations that can impact patient outcomes. Each individual comorbidity may not be a significant concern in isolation; however, if there are multiple comorbidities, then the total impact on the survival of the patients will need to be assessed. Although the number of possible comorbidities is limitless and specific guidance on each and every situation is impossible, the most frequently occurring are considered in detail next.

Compliance

The transplanted lung remains vulnerable to acute rejection throughout the lifetime of the graft. The risk of rejection is highest in the first 6 months but remains high if the recipient develops low levels of immunosuppression. In view of this, a previous history of poor compliance with treatment is a significant concern for any patients being considered for LT. Careful assessment and re-enforcement of the message of absolute compliance with immunosuppression is a key requirement.

Rehabilitation

The general condition of the patient needs to be sufficient robust to be able to cope with the severe stresses that the process of transplantation places on the recipients. Potential recipients are encouraged to maintain as higher level of activity as possible and to undertake some form of regular exercise every day. Patients with severe musculoskeletal deconditioning are poor candidates for LT and if possible should be optimized prior to referral. Pulmonary rehabilitation can be extremely useful in helping to train patients in how best to exercise within the very limited confines of their pulmonary reserve. It is useful for all patients who are being considered as potential candidates to have had at least one course of pulmonary rehabilitation. Six-minute walk tests can be a useful metric for determining the level of deconditioning and any improvement after pulmonary rehabilitation.

Corticosteroid usage

Many respiratory patients are given high-dose steroids as part of their treatment regime. This is particularly true in IPF patients. High-dose steroids affect healing generally but in particular the healing of the bronchial anastomosis. Early experience in this area demonstrated a higher rate of dehiscence of the bronchial anastomosis and concomitant mortality in patients who are on high doses. Thus the preference is for patients to be on the lowest dose tolerable, ideally below 15 mg per day of prednisolone.

Gastroesophageal reflux disease

Many of the potential recipients have respiratory diseases that have been shown to be exacerbated by coexistent GERD. The highest frequency of GERD has been described in CF and IPF patients. All recipients are screened with barium swallows and 24-hour pH studies. If there is significant reflux, patients are advised that this is a risk factor for early obliterative bronchiolitis and that it will need careful follow-up and probable further surgery. The procedure of choice is a Nissan's fundoplication, which has been shown to improve outcomes.

Psychosocial assessment

The whole transplant process from referral through to the long-term follow-up involves a series of emotional highs and lows. For both the referring and transplant team, this can present dilemmas, as there is a delicate balance between offering the patient hope and the realistic expectation of LT. Many patients find the uncertainty that the transplant process encompasses extremely difficult. These situations require a large degree of mental strength and fortitude to cope with the fluxes. Although there is no solution to these difficulties, patients who are well supported by friends and families appear to fare better. When necessary, formal evaluation and ongoing support by psychiatric or psychological services may be invaluable.

Age

Age is an independent risk factor for outcome post LT, with outcomes declining with rising age, in particular over the age of 60 years. Although there is no absolute age cut-off and each patient is considered on his or her clinical merit, age associated with other comorbidities may be an absolute contraindication. For guidance, we will consider patients up to the age of 55 years for combined heart and lung transplant, up to 60 years for bilateral LT, and up to 65 years for a single LT. However, robust individuals without comorbidities who are outside this age will also be considered in some centers.

Osteoporosis

Osteoporosis (OP) in the general population is a risk factor for spontaneous bone fractures. Patients with chronic respiratory disease appear to be more vulnerable to OP than the general population. This increased vulnerability is likely to be multi-factorial; however, significant contributing factors include use of long-term oral corticosteroids, chronic immobility, and in CF patients, malabsorption of vitamin D. The prevalence of OP in waiting list recipients has been estimated at between 29–43%, and a much higher high rate of fractures is seen after LT in comparison with other solid organ transplants.

Although there are a variety of methods to assess bone density, the best established is dual-energy X-ray absorptiometry (DEXA), and using this method, osteoporosis is defined as a T-score of less than −2.5. Using the World Health Organization (WHO; FRAX) scale, it is possible to estimate the risk of fracture for an individual. This tool can be very helpful in establishing risk profiles. Most units will regard severe or symptomatic osteoporosis with T-score of less than −3.5 as a relative contraindication. Some patients benefit from treatment with intravenous bisphosphonates to try and improve their bone density.

Body mass index

Extremes of body weight are associated with poorer outcomes after LT. Lower body mass indices (BMI) of less than 18 are associated with poor nutritional status and can lead to poor outcomes due to poor post-surgical rehabilitation. Higher BMIs of greater than 30 present surgical challenges that may translate into poorer outcomes and the development of late weight-associated comorbidities.

Pneumothorax

Patients with advanced respiratory disease due to the structural damage to the lung are very vulnerable to the development of pneumothoraces. As a result of the underlying disease, a conservative approach may not be successful, and these patients may require more aggressive intervention. For patients who are potential recipients, this may make explantation of the native lungs difficult. Although it is impossible to give categorical advice for these patients as general principle, it is advisable to ensure that the least disruptive intervention, pleural abrasion rather than pleurectomy, is performed that will provide adequate resolution of the pneumothorax but may allow the potential explantation of the lungs at the time of transplantation.

Disease-specific guidance

COPD accounts for approximately 40% of LTs performed, with CF and IPF accounting for 20% each. IPAH accounts for approximately 5% of recipients. As these indications form the major bulk of patients, specific clinical considerations in these groups are discussed in Table 14.2.

COPD

COPD patients are the largest single group of patients referred for consideration of LT. Deciding on which patients to refer for assessment can be difficult. Some of the useful clinical indicators to assess for are low baseline lung function (forced expiratory volume in 1 second [FEV_1] <25 % and transfer coefficient for carbon monoxide [TLCO] <20% of predicted), especially if this is associated with resting hypercapnia and or hypoxia ($PaCO_2 > 6.0$ kPa, $PaO_2 < 8$ kPa), the clinical syndrome of Cor Pulmonale, or the presence of secondary pulmonary hypertension on echocardiography (estimated pulmonary systolic artery pressure > 40 mmHg). Frequent exacerbations associated with a rapid decline in lung function and/or the requirement for intensive care admission are useful pointers for referral for LT.

The BODE index (body mass index, airflow obstruction, dyspnea, and exercise capacity), although not validated in this specific group, can be useful to assess the probability of prognostic benefit from LT (Table 14.3). A BODE score of >7 may indicate a patient who would gain benefit from LT. Although these measures may help to identify some patients, it is important to consider the quality of life of the individual, as this is a potent consideration in COPD patients.

Table 14.2 Disease-specific guidance

	Disease			
	COPD	CF	IPF	IPAH
Lung function	$FEV_1 < 25\%$ TLCO < 20%	$FEV_1 < 30\%$ FVC < 40%	VC < 60% TLCO < 50%	Coexisting lung disease
Oxygen	$PaCO_2 > 6$ kPa $PaO_2 < 8$ kPa	$PaCO_2 > 6.5$ kPa $PaO_2 < 7.5$ kPa	Resting hypoxemia Early desaturation on exercise	$PaO_2 < 8$ kPa Overnight desaturation (mean < 90%)
Other	BODE > 7 ITU admissions Frequent exacerbations Secondary PH Poor quality of life	Hemoptysis > 240 ml Pneumothorax Rapid decline Weight loss Frequent exacerbations Nasal ventilation Small diabetic females ITU admissions	RAP > 15 mmHg Rapid decline Secondary PH	RAP > 15 mmHg Mixed venous sats < 60% MPAP > 50 mmHg CO < 2 l/min Failure of medical therapy

Cystic fibrosis

Potential recipients with CF benefit from being looked after in dedicated CF units where they are carefully followed up. Patients who have low lung function ($FEV_1 < 30\%$ predicted or forced vital capacity [FVC] < 40% predicted) should be considered for transplantation. In addition, any patients who have rapidly declining lung function with increased frequency of infective exacerbations should have the possibility of LT raised. These may be associated with changes in oxygen requirement and possibly the requirement for non-invasive ventilation ($PaCO_2 > 6.5$ kPa, $PaO_2 < 7.5$ kPa). Both of these should independently prompt consideration of referral for LT. The development of severe hemoptysis (>200 ml) or recurrent pneumothoraces is associated with a poor prognosis, and patients with these complications should be referred for consideration. A specific group of patients at high risk of rapid decline are young female diabetic patients, and they should be referred early for consideration.

Table 14.3 Calculation of body mass index, degree of airflow obstruction and dyspnea, and exercise capacity (BODE) index

	Points on BODE index			
	0	1	2	3
FEV_1 (% of predicted)	>65	50–64	36–49	<35
6 minute walk (m)	>350	250–349	150–249	<150
Dyspnea score (4 most severe)	0–1	2	3	4
Body mass index	>21	<21		

IPAH

Over the last 5 years, there has been a dramatic improvement in the range of therapies available for treatment of IPAH patients. This has resulted in an improvement in the median survival for most patients. A rare subset of patients with pulmonary venoocclusive disease and pulmonary capillary hemangiomatosis do not respond to pulmonary vasodilator therapy and should be referred for LT early. The clinical consequences of progressive IPAH are all the features of right ventricular (RV) failure. These are manifest as progressive fall in exercise tolerance (NYHA class III–IV, 6-minute walk test < 350 m), syncopal episodes, increasing peripheral edema and ascites, hemoptysis, and chest pains. In addition, patients who are deteriorating despite increasing pulmonary vasodilator therapy should be referred for LT. Right heart catheter measurements can be very helpful in helping to determine the patients who should be referred.

IPF

IPF is the commonest of all the diffuse parenchymal lung diseases. It is unfortunately associated with a very poor prognosis and is largely unresponsive to current therapies. Although large strides have been made in understanding the pathophysiology of IPF, LT remains the only therapy that has been shown to offer prognostic benefit. Unfortunately, IPF patients also have the highest mortality on the transplant waiting list. Early referral of patients with IPF is imperative to ensure that patients have a reasonable prospect of transplantation. Of particular concern are patients with rapidly changing lung function, e.g., a fall in FVC of more than 10% in 6 months and TLCO of $<$ 39% predicted. Resting hypoxemia (saturations $<$ 88%) and early desaturation on 6-minute walk testing are adverse prognostic signs and merit referral for transplantation. The presence of secondary pulmonary hypertension may allude to a different diagnosis but may reflect the severity of the underlying lung disease. Its presence is an additional marker of disease severity and should merit referral.

Selection for heart–lung transplantation

The success of single and bilateral lung transplantation has improved so that combined heart–lung transplant has fewer indications. In addition, urgent status heart (and in some countries, lung) transplant recipients has limited the availability of heart–lung blocks so that very few procedures are performed in the current era. In the 1990s, congenital heart disease with secondary pulmonary hypertension (Eisenmenger syndrome) was the most frequent indication (approximately 30%). Other complex congenital heart defects have also been treated successfully with heart–lung transplantation, including univentricular heart with pulmonary atresia, truncus arteriosus, and hypoplastic left heart syndrome, although palliation or repair of complex congenital lesions is now preferred due to improved survival. In patients with simple cardiac defects, repair of the defect combined with single or bilateral lung transplantation is a potential option. Primary pulmonary hypertension with right heart failure accounted for approximately 25% of combined heart–lung transplants, although now bilateral lung transplantation is the preferred option. CF remains an indication for which right heart failure is thought unlikely to recover or domino transplantation is feasible. Ischemic heart disease with end-stage lung disease and cardiac failure with fixed moderate to severe pulmonary hypertension (systolic pulmonary artery pressure $>$ 75–80 mmHg, pulmonary vascular resistance $>$ 5 Wood units, or TPG $>$ 15 mmHg) remain indications for combined heart–lung transplantation, although survival is inferior to that of heart transplant alone.

Conclusions

Lung transplantation offers prognostic benefit and an improvement in the quality of life for carefully selected patients. In the current era there remains a critical shortage of donor organs, and thus unfortunately, recipient selection remains extremely important. As expertise increases, previous contraindications may be re-examined, and patients who were previously considered unsuitable may now be given the opportunity of LT. The inherent complexity of these patients means that proscriptive inclusion and exclusion criteria will not cover every situation, and thus where there is any doubt over a patient's suitability, early discussion with the transplant team is advised.

Further reading

Dolgos S, Hartmann A, Isaksen GA, *et al.* Osteoporosis is a prevalent finding in patients with solid organ failure awaiting transplantation – a population based study. *Clin Transplant* 2010; **24**: E145–52.

D'Ovidio F, Singer LG, Hadjiliadis D, *et al.* Prevalence of gastroesophageal reflux in end-stage lung disease candidates for lung transplant. *Ann Thorac Surg* 2005; **80**: 1254–60.

Fisher AJ, Verleden GM, Massard G. *Lung Transplantation European Respiratory Monograph 45*. Sheffield, United Kingdom: European Respiratory Journals Ltd., September 2009.

Iacono A, Groves S, Garcia J, Griffith B. Lung transplantation following 107 days of extracorporeal membrane oxygenation. *Eur J Cardiothorac Surg* 2010; **37**: 969–71.

Orens JB, Estenne M, Arcasoy S, *et al.* International guidelines for the selection of lung transplant candidates update–a consensus report from the Pulmonary Scientific Council of the International Society for Heart and Lung Transplantation. *J Heart Lung Transplant* 2006; **25**: 745–55.

Chapter 15

Living donor lobar lung transplantation

Hiroshi Date

Key points

- Bilateral living donor lung transplantation in which two healthy donors donate their right or left lower lobes is an alternative to cadaveric transplantation.
- The most common procedure involves a right lower lobectomy from a larger donor and a left lower lobectomy from a smaller donor.
- Right-sided donors are more likely to have a perioperative complication than left-sided donors, probably secondary to right lower and middle lobe anatomy.
- Pulmonary arterial hypertension is not a contraindication to living donor lung transplantation.
- Although only two lobes are transplanted, living donor transplantation seems to be associated with less frequent primary graft failure than cadaveric transplantation.

Living donor lobar lung transplantation (LDLLT) was developed at the University of Southern California (USC) to offset the mismatch between supply and demand for those patients awaiting cadaveric lung transplantation. A single donor was used initially; however, the results of single lobe transplantation were not satisfactory. Therefore, bilateral LDLLT in which two healthy donors donate their right or left lower lobes (Figure 15.1) was developed. As of 2010, LDLLT has been performed in approximately 350 patients worldwide. The survival of LDLLT appears to be better than that of cadaveric transplantation.

Surgical technique

The most common procedure involves a right lower lobectomy from a larger donor and a left lower lobectomy from a smaller donor. After induction of general anesthesia, donors are intubated with a left-sided double-lumen endotracheal tube. The donors are placed in the lateral decubitus position and a posterolateral thoracotomy is performed though the fifth intercostal space. Fissures are developed using linear stapling devices. The pericardium surrounding the inferior pulmonary vein is opened circumferentially. Dissection in the fissure is carried out to isolate the pulmonary artery to the lower lobe and to define the anatomy of the pulmonary arteries to the middle lobe in the right side donor and to the lingular segment in the left side donor. If the branches of middle lobe artery and lingular artery are small, they are ligated and divided. Intravenous prostaglandin E1 may be administered to decrease systolic blood pressure by 10–20 mmHg. Five thousand units of heparin and 500 mg of methylprednisolone are administered intravenously. After placing vascular clamps in appropriate positions, the division of the pulmonary vein, the pulmonary artery, and bronchus are carried out in this order. On the back table, the lobes are flushed with preservation solution (such as ET-Kyoto solution) both antegradely and retrogradely from a bag approximately 50 cm above the table. Lobes are gently ventilated with room air during the flush.

Recipients are anesthetized and intubated with a single-lumen endotracheal tube in children and with a left-sided double-lumen endotracheal tube in adults. The "clamshell" incision is used, and both chest cavities are entered through the fourth intercostal space. Pleural and hilar dissections are performed as much as possible. The ascending aorta and the right atrium are cannulated after heparinization, and patients are placed on standard cardiopulmonary bypass (CBP). After bilateral pneumonectomy, the right lower lobe

Organ Transplantation: A Clinical Guide, ed. A.A. Klein, C.J. Lewis, and J.C. Madsen. Published by Cambridge University Press.

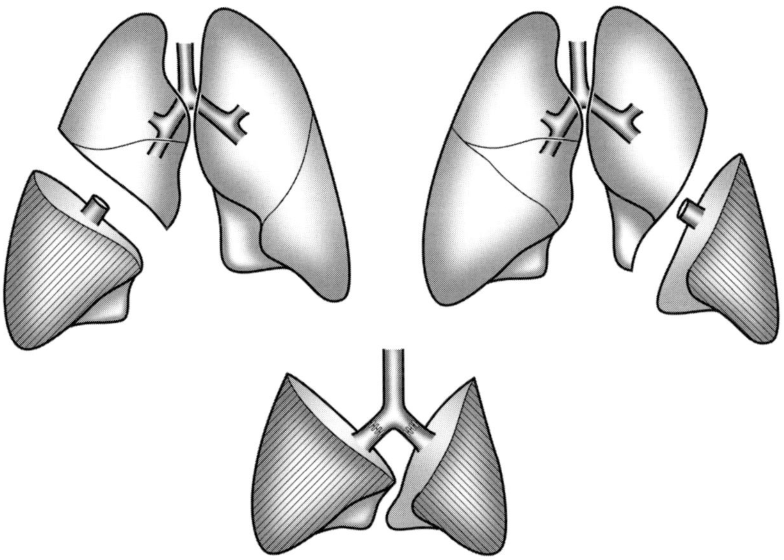

Figure 15.1 Bilateral living donor lobar lung transplantation. Right and left lower lobes from two healthy donors are implanted in a recipient in place of whole right and left lungs, respectively.

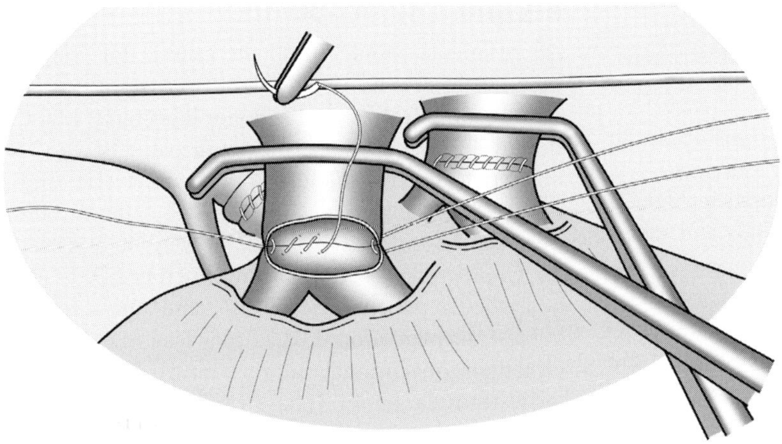

Figure 15.2 Right lower lobe implantation. The bronchus, the pulmonary vein, and the pulmonary artery are anastomosed consecutively. The venous anastomosis is conducted between the donor inferior pulmonary vein and the recipient superior pulmonary vein.

implantation is performed, followed by the left lower lobe implantation. The bronchus, the pulmonary vein, and the pulmonary artery are anastomosed consecutively. The venous anastomosis is conducted between the donor inferior pulmonary vein and the recipient superior pulmonary vein (Figure 15.2). Just before completing the bilateral implantations, 500 mg to 1 g of methylprednisolone is given intravenously, and nitric oxide inhalation is initiated at 20 ppm. After both lungs are reperfused and ventilated, CPB is gradually weaned and then removed. Three surgical teams are required in LDLLT, and they communicate closely to minimize graft ischemic time.

Donor selection, size matching, and outcome

Although immediate family members (relatives within the third degree or a spouse) have been the only donors in our institution, other institutions have accepted extended family members and unrelated individuals. Eligibility criteria for living lobar lung donation at Kyoto University are summarized in Table 15.1.

Potential donors should be competent, willing to donate free of coercion, medically and psychosocially suitable, and fully informed of risks, benefits, and alternative treatment available to the recipient. In our institution, potential donors are interviewed at least three

Table 15.1 The eligibility criteria for living lung donation (Kyoto University)

Medical criteria
Age 20–60 years
ABO blood type compatible with recipient
Relatives within the third degree or a spouse
No significant past medical history
No recent viral infection
No significant abnormalities on echocardiogram and electrocardiogram
No significant ipsilateral pulmonary pathology on computed tomography
Arterial oxygen tension ≥ 80 mmHg (room air)
Forced vital capacity, forced expiratory volume in 1 second ≥ 85% of predicted
No previous ipsilateral thoracic surgery
No active tobacco smoking
Social and ethical criteria
No significant psychiatric disorders
No ethical issues or concerns about donor motivation

times to provide them with multiple opportunities to ask questions, reconsider, or withdraw as a donor.

Because only two lobes are implanted in LDLLT, appropriate size-matching between donor and recipient is important. We have previously proposed a formula to estimate the graft forced vital capacity (FVC) based on the donor's measured FVC and the number of pulmonary segments implanted. Given that the right lower lobe consists of five segments, the left lower lobe of four, and the whole lung of 19, total FVC of the two grafts is estimated by the following equation.

$$\begin{aligned}&\text{Total FVC of the 2 grafts}\\&\quad = \text{Measured FVC of the right donor} \times 5/19\\&\qquad + \text{Measured FVC of the left donor} \times 4/19\end{aligned}$$

When the total FVC of the two grafts is more than 45–50% of the predicted FVC of the recipient (calculated from a knowledge of height, age, and sex), we accept size disparity regardless of the recipient's diagnosis.

It has been reported that patients receiving lobes whose combined resultant total lung capacity (TLC) was anticipated to be more than 80% of the recipient's predicted TLC had a 5-year survival of 57% compared with 26% in those who did not. Three-dimensional computed tomography (CT) volumetry has been recently introduced in LDLLT following wide use in living donor liver transplantation.

The Vancouver Forum Lung Group has summarized the world experience of approximately 550 living lung donors. Sixty percent of the live lung donors have been male, 76% have been related to the recipient, and 24% were unrelated. There has been no reported perioperative mortality of a lung donor. Approximately 4% of live lung donors have experienced an intraoperative complication that included the necessity of a right middle lobe sacrifice. Approximately 5% of them have experienced complications requiring surgical or bronchoscopic intervention. Right-sided donors may be more likely to have a perioperative complication than left-sided donors, probably secondary to right lower and middle lobe anatomy.

Recipient selection

All recipients should fulfill the criteria for conventional cadaveric transplantation. Because of possible serious complications in the donor lobectomy, LDLLT should be reserved for critically ill patients who are unlikely to survive the long wait for cadaveric lungs. In our LDLLT experience (n = 60), 36 patients (60%) were bed bound and seven (12%) were on a ventilator. Controversy exists regarding whether LDLLT can be applied to patients already on a ventilator or requiring re-transplantation. LDLLT may lead to better survival than conventional cadaveric lung transplantation for re-transplantation. It has been reported that perioperative mortality of re-transplantation is only 7.7% in patients who had LDLLT versus 42.3% in the cadaveric group.

In the United States, because only two lobes are transplanted, cystic fibrosis represents the most common indication for LDLLT, as these patients are usually small in body size. The distribution of diagnoses is different in Japan, where cystic fibrosis is a very rare disease. Bronchiolitis obliterans, interstitial pneumonia, and idiopathic pulmonary arterial hypertension are the three major indications in Japan (Table 15.2). LDLLT appears possible despite pulmonary hypertension; in fact, mean pulmonary artery pressure has been shown to decrease by discharge in transplanted patients, validating the functional capacity of the two lobes to handle the entire cardiac output in these recipients.

Table 15.2 Recipient indication for LDLLT (n = 60)

Bronchiolitis obliterans	16
Interstitial pneumonia	16
Idiopathic pulmonary arterial hypertension	15
Bronchiectasis	5
Lymphangioleiomyomatosis	4
Cystic fibrosis	1
Eisenmenger syndrome	1
Emphysema	1
Eosinophilic granuloma	1

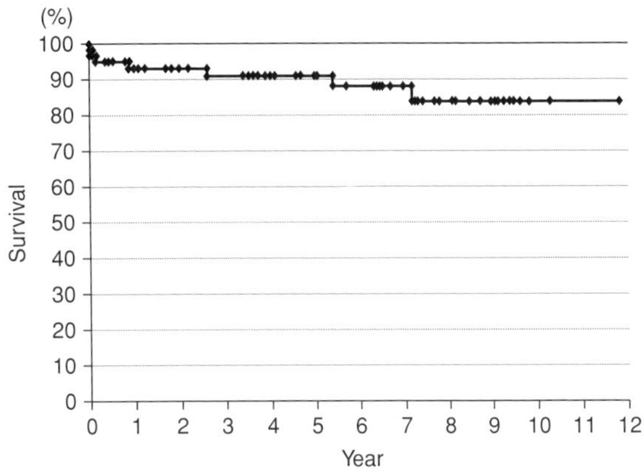

Figure 15.3 Survival after living donor lobar lung transplantation (n = 60). The 5- and 10-year survivals were 91% and 84%, respectively.

Postoperative management of the recipient

The patient is usually kept sedated and ventilated for at least 3 days to maintain optimal expansion of the implanted lobes. Fiberoptic bronchoscopy should be performed regularly to assess donor airway viability and suction any retained secretions. Bedside postoperative pulmonary rehabilitation is initiated as soon as possible.

Postoperative immunosuppression usually consists of triple-drug therapy with cyclosporine (CyA) or tacrolimus (TAC), azathioprine (AZA), or mycophenolate mofetil (MMF) and corticosteroids without induction. Acute rejection should be diagnosed on the basis of radiographic and clinical findings without transbronchial lung biopsy because the risk of pneumothorax and bleeding after transbronchial lung biopsy may be greater after LDLLT. Because two lobes are donated by different donors, acute rejection is usually seen unilaterally. Early acute rejection episodes are characterized by dyspnea, low-grade fever, leukocytosis, hypoxemia, and diffuse interstitial infiltrate on chest radiograph. A trial bolus dose of methylprednisolone 500 mg is administered, and clinical signs are carefully observed.

Recipient outcome

There are only three groups that have reported recipient outcome. The USC group recently published their 10-year experience of 123 LDLLT recipients, including 39 children. In their series, re-transplantation and mechanical ventilation were identified as risk factors for mortality. One, 3- and 5-year survival rates were 70%, 54%, and 45%, respectively. The St. Louis group reported similar results in 38 pediatric LDLLT recipients. We recently published institutional results in 30 LDLLT recipients. Five- and 10-year survival rates were 91% and 84% in 60 LDLLT recipients, respectively (Figure 15.3).

The question of whether two pulmonary lobes can provide sufficient long-term pulmonary function and clinical outcome to recipients is debated. The USC group has reported that LDLLT provides comparable intermediate and long-term pulmonary function and exercise capacity to bilateral cadaveric lung transplantation in adult recipients surviving more than 3 months after transplantation.

Comparison with cadaveric lung transplantation

The current availability of cadaveric donor lungs has not been able to meet the increasing demand of potential recipients in most counties. The recent change by the Organ Procurement and Transplantation Network in the United States to an urgency/benefit allocation system for cadaveric donor lungs in patients 12 years and older has most recently led to a marked decline in LDLLT. However, in countries where such an allocation system does not exist, LDLLT is still a relatively common procedure. For example, the average waiting time for a cadaveric lung is more than 3 years in Japan, hence the requirement for LDLLT.

In general, the ischemic time for LDLLT is much shorter than cadaveric transplantation. Although only two lobes are transplanted, LDLLT seems to be associated with less frequent primary graft failure. We believe that using a "small but perfect graft" is a great advantage in LDLLT.

Experienced centers have recently reported the incidence of bronchial complications in cadaveric lung transplantation to be about 5%. Contraindications to cadaveric lung transplantation include current high-dose systemic corticosteroid therapy because it may increase airway complications, although low-dose pre-transplantation corticosteroid therapy ($\leq$20 mg/day of prednisone) is acceptable. Various factors, such as short donor bronchial length, high blood flow in the small grafts implanted, and well-preserved lung parenchyma with short ischemic time, may contribute to better oxygen supply to the donor bronchus, resulting in excellent bronchial healing in LDLLT.

Bronchiolitis obliterans syndrome (BOS) has been the major obstacle after cadaveric lung transplantation. LDLLT may be associated with a lower incidence of BOS, especially in pediatric patients. Transplanting two lobes obtained from two different donors appears to be beneficial in the long term, because the contralateral unaffected lung may function as a reservoir in case of unilateral BOS.

Further reading

Barr ML, Belghiti J, Villamil FG, *et al.* A report of the Vancouver Forum on the care of the live organ donor. Lung, liver, pancreas, and intestine data and medical guidelines. *Transplantation* 2006; **81**:1372–87.

Date H, Aoe M, Sano Y, *et al.* Improved survival after living-donor lobar lung transplantation. *J Thorac Cardiovasc Surg* 2004; **128**: 933–40.

Date H, Kusano KF, Matsubara H, *et al.* Living-donor lobar lung transplantation for pulmonary arterial hypertension after failure of epoprostenol therapy. *J Am Coll Cardiol* 2007; **50**: 523–7.

Shoji T, Bando T, Fujinaga T, Date H. Living-donor single-lobe lung transplant in a 6-year-old girl after 7-month mechanical ventilator support. *J Thorac Cardiovasc Surg* 2010; **139**: e112–13.

Starnes VA, Bowdish ME, Woo MS, *et al.* A decade of living lobar lung transplantation. Recipient outcomes. *J Thorac Cardiovasc Surg* 2004; **127**: 114–22.

Sweet SC. Pediatric living donor lobar lung transplantation. *Pediatr Transplantation* 2006; **10**: 861–8.

Chapter 16

Surgical procedure

Faruk Özalp, Tanveer Butt, and Stephan V.B. Schueler

Key points

- Bilateral lung transplantation has evolved into a routine procedure and is the most frequently performed method. Combined heart–lung transplant has been in decline internationally, with negligible overall numbers now reported annually.
- The surgical incision is not only center-specific, but also surgeon-specific. Some centers advocate smaller incisions to minimize trauma and allow faster postoperative recovery; however, there is limited evidence in this area of practice.
- Cardiopulmonary bypass is often avoided for both single and bilateral lung transplantation; however, clamping of the pulmonary artery leading to significant increase in pulmonary artery pressure, right atrial distension, and desaturation or hypercapnia should prompt its use.
- The technique of lung donation after cardiac death has been established successfully in recent years, thereby avoiding damage to donor organs by the effect of brainstem death and expanding the donor pool.

Since the early series of successful lung transplantation in the 1980s, it has become clear that this treatment method offers the best outcome for patients with deteriorating end-stage lung disease and who are unresponsive to conventional therapy. Over the past two decades, some adjustments have been made regarding recipient and donor selection, treatment of rejection, maintenance immunosuppression, and, importantly, the selection of the surgical procedure. The evidence for these changes is based on case series and information gathered from large international registries rather than on randomized controlled trials (RCTs), in particular, the registry of the International Society for Heart and Lung Transplantation (ISHLT).

Although single lung transplantation (SLT), bilateral lung transplantation (BLT), and combined heart–lung transplantation (HLT) have all been proven to be successful for the appropriate recipient, based on the information from the registries, some of these procedures have undergone considerable modification over time. Overall, BLT has evolved into a routine procedure and is the most frequently performed method of the three, whereas HLT has been in decline internationally, with negligible overall numbers now reported annually.

Single lung transplantation

Traditionally SLT has been the procedure of choice in patients with non-infective end-stage lung disease such as chronic obstructive pulmonary disorder (COPD); idiopathic pulmonary fibrosis (IPF); and rare conditions such as α_1-antitrypsin deficiency, sarcoidosis, and pulmonary vascular disease. However, in recent years, there has been a clear shift toward BLT for these patients because the overall outcome has improved and the long-term beneficial impact of BLT on quality of life and exercise capacity has become more apparent.

Technique

Different incisions are used for SLT. Most common is the posterolateral thoracotomy; less frequent are anterolateral thoracotomy and median sternotomy, which are usually used if CPB has to be employed. The selection of the surgical incision is not only

Organ Transplantation: A Clinical Guide, ed. A.A. Klein, C.J. Lewis, and J.C. Madsen. Published by Cambridge University Press.

center-specific but also surgeon-specific. Furthermore, some centers advocate smaller incisions to minimize trauma and allow faster postoperative recovery; however, there is limited evidence since the numbers are small and RCTs are not available.

After anaesthesia and tracheal intubation with a double-lumen tracheal tube, the patient is secured on the table in the lateral position. The tracheal tube position is re-checked, as it can be displaced by this maneuver. Skin preparation is carried out on the chest, abdomen, and ipsilateral groin.

For posterolateral thoracotomy, a curved incision is made from the mid-axillary line around the inferior angle of the scapula, and the pleural space is entered through the fifth intercostal space. Any adhesions are dissected, avoiding trauma to phrenic and vagal nerves, and the hilar structures are exposed.

The pulmonary artery and veins and the main bronchus are identified, dissected, and encircled with tapes. Before dividing the artery and the veins, it is important to decide whether cardiopulmonary bypass (CPB) has to be used to allow safe implantation of the new lung. Therefore, a vascular clamp is placed on the main pulmonary artery (PA) for 10 minutes and the hemodynamic and respiratory stability is assessed. Significant increase of PA pressures, right atrial distension, and desaturation or hypercapnia should prompt the use of CPB. Cannulation for right SLT is either through the right femoral vessels or via the thoracotomy using the ascending aorta and the right atrium. In left SLT, arterial cannulation is performed, either via the left femoral artery or the descending aorta, and the main pulmonary artery is used as the venous return.

The extraction of the lung continues with clamping and division of the PA followed by the pulmonary veins, which are isolated outside the pericardium, ligated and divided. The main bronchus is then dissected just to the level above the upper lobe bronchial takeoff. The PA is further dissected off the surrounding tissue, ensuring a sufficient length for the anastomosis. For the purpose of orientation, the first branch is marked for alignment with the donor PA.

Using a running 4/0 monofilament suture, the bronchus is anastomosed first, avoiding extensive dissection of adjacent recipient tissue that could jeopardize bronchial healing. In earlier series, a combination of a running suture for the membranous part of the bronchus and interrupted figure-of-eight sutures for the cartilaginous part was used in order to prevent bronchial ischemia; however, a number of reports have demonstrated similar or better results using continuous suture alone.

A Satinsky clamp is placed across the ligated pulmonary veins to facilitate the suture of the left atrium. On the right side, it is beneficial to dissect into the inter-atrial groove, which allows more secure placement of the clamp. The bridge between the upper and lower vein is cut, creating a single left atrial cuff. Both cuffs are carefully aligned and a continuous 4/0 monofilament suture is used for anastomosis. The suture is left untied to allow de-airing via this route later on. The PA is anastomosed with a running 5/0 monofilament suture and the first branch of the recipient PA is used for appropriate alignment. This is crucial to avoid kinking or twisting of the anastomosis. After meticulous de-airing via the left atrial suture line, the clamps are taken off and the donor lung is reperfused in a controlled fashion by gradual release of the PA clamp over 10 minutes. Lungs are ventilated with room air.

If CPB is used, a PA vent can decompress the RV, allowing a bloodless field that facilitates an open PA anastomosis without the need for a clamp. This also allows easier alignment of the vessels. If the left atrial cuff is very short, CPB facilitates the heart to be fibrillated or even cardiopleged to facilitate an open surgical anastomosis. After completion of the anastomoses, transesophageal echocardiography (TEE) examination of the left atrial anastomosis allows exclusion of a pressure gradient. Bronchoscopy can clear the airway and can help to identify any suture line problems. The chest is closed in standard fashion over apical and basal drains.

Bilateral lung transplantation

The number of BLTs (otherwise known as bilateral sequential single-lung transplant) is now on the rise because of improved outcomes, exercise capacity, and quality of life. Initially this procedure was considered to be more suitable for patients with infective lung diseases such as cystic fibrosis (CF) or bronchiectasis, making the new SLT at risk of cross-contamination. Nowadays, patients with COPD and IPF who traditionally would have received SLT are increasingly considered for BLT.

The question of whether there is evidence for or against the use of CPB for BLT seems to be unanswered. Avoiding CPB has the well-known advantage of evading complications such as increased inflammatory response and coagulopathy. In our own experience, however, these complications seem to have no effect on outcomes. The use of CPB may have significant advantages throughout the whole procedure, including hemodynamic stability, better access in patients with dense adhesions, better management in technically challenging situations, and the possibility of controlled reperfusion of the transplanted lung.

The preferred surgical incision for BLT is a bilateral transverse thoracotomy joint across the middle, best known as a "clamshell" incision. Bilateral thoracotomy through the fourth intercostal spaces is performed and the sternum divided after ligation both of the internal thoracic arteries.

Alternatively, a median sternotomy is advocated, particularly in patients in whom adhesions are not anticipated, e.g., emphysema patients. However, access to hilar structures especially on the left side can be limited. The advantages of a median sternotomy are better wound healing and pain control.

After gaining access to the mediastinum and systemic heparinization, the pericardium is opened, the ascending aorta and the right atrium are cannulated for CPB, and the dissection of both hilar structures is commenced. Special care is taken to prevent recurrent laryngeal, phrenic, and vagal nerve injury. The inferior pulmonary ligaments are divided and the hilar structures prepared for lung extraction as for SLT. Once the lungs are mobilized and hilar dissection is completed, CPB can be commenced. A pulmonary vent is placed for a bloodless field. Both lungs are resected with meticulous hemostasis, especially in the posterior hilum, as access to this area is very restricted once the lung is implanted. In case of infected lung disease, a thorough washout of the thoracic cavity is carried out to reduce the risk of contamination due to transection of the main bronchi.

The preparation of the donor lungs and implantation process are the same as for SLT. If no CPB is used, the recipient lung with the worse function is implanted first. But if CPB is used, the sequence seems more related to surgeon preference.

Cold gauze packs are put on the posterior wall of the thoracic cavity before the donor lung is placed inside. Once both lungs are implanted and de-airing is completed, a period of 30 minutes of controlled reperfusion is commenced in order to ameliorate lung injury. During this period of reperfusion, a mean PA pressure of 15–20 mmHg should not be exceeded.

CPB can be weaned off and the cannulae removed. After hemostasis and placement of apical and basal chest drains on each side, the chest is closed using two or three wires for the sternum and pericostal Vicryl sutures for the ribs.

Echocardiographic assessment of the left atrial and PA suture lines to exclude flow-limiting narrowing of the lumen is important, as is flexible bronchoscopy to assess the bronchial anastomosis before leaving the operating theatre. Broncho-alveolar lavage samples of donor lung are analyzed for unknown donor bronchial infection.

Combined heart–lung transplantation

Depending on the recipient diagnosis, the removal of the heart and both lungs can be quite challenging. In patients with congenital heart disease and cyanosis, there are large mediastinal collaterals requiring careful dissection and ligation. In addition, the chance of damage to the phrenic, recurrent laryngeal, and vagus nerves is significant. Through a median sternotomy and wide opening of the pleural spaces, some of the anterior part of the pericardium is removed. Preserving the lateral walls of the pericardium together with the phrenic nerve prevents the heart from slipping into the left chest. Incision of the pericardium posterior to the phrenic nerve at the hilum is performed to allow the donor lungs to pass through later on.

Cannulation for CPB is achieved using the ascending aorta and both the inferior vena cava (IVC) and superior vena cava (SVC) with tapes around for sealed occlusion. CPB is commenced and body temperature is lowered to 28°C. The ascending aorta is dissected off the PA and cross-clamped. Routine cardiectomy is carried out by dividing the IVC and SVC, ascending aorta, PA, and left atrium, leaving the left atrial cuff within the pericardium. The left-sided phrenic nerve is freed by a horizontal incision anterior to the pulmonary veins. Pulmonary ligaments are divided and hilar structures dissected on both sides. Pulmonary vessels are ligated and the main bronchus is stapled, with care taken to avoid injury to the vagus and recurrent laryngeal nerves. Intrapericardial remnants of the left atrium and pulmonary artery are removed. Only a small portion of PA at the level of the ligamentum arteriosum is left intact to save the recurrent laryngeal nerve. The pericardium at the superior mediastinum is opened and the distal trachea dissected and stapled just above the carina. The trachea will not be opened until the donor organs are prepared for implantation. Before placing the donor organs inside the chest cavity, meticulous hemostasis, especially of the posterior mediastinum, is secured, and a thorough washout is performed.

The heart–lung block is trimmed and brought into the operative field and the lungs are passed into the pleural spaces through gaps created below the phrenic nerves. Alternatively the organ block can be placed anterior to the phrenic nerves. This minimizes the risk of nerve damage and allows easier hemostasis. The chest is irrigated with cold saline solution.

Tracheal anastomosis is performed first using continuous 4/0 monofilament suture and after trimming the donor trachea to just one cartilaginous ring above the carina. The recipient trachea is transected just above the carina. The donor aorta is then anastomosed using a 4/0 monofilament suture. After meticulous de-airing, the aortic cross-clamp can be released and the two caval anastomoses performed while the heart is being re-perfused. Alternatively, the IVC anastomosis can be carried out with the cross-clamp in place and with suction catheter in the right atrium for a bloodless field. Then the SVC anastomosis can be performed without a cross-clamp.

The lungs are re-perfused and ventilated gently with room air and reduced tidal volume for 20–30 minutes. The patient is re-warmed and weaned from CPB, followed by de-cannulation. Two chest drains are placed in each chest cavity. After meticulous hemostasis, the sternotomy is closed as usual.

Lung transplantation from donation after cardiac death

After intensive animal research and clinical experience gained from kidney and liver donation, the technique of lung donation after cardiac death (DCD) has been established successfully in recent years.

Damage to donor organs is aggravated by the effect of brainstem death in donation after brain death (DBD) by the inflammatory response, release of catecholamines, hemodynamic instability, and metabolic and neuroendocrine derangement, resulting in organ injury. Avoiding brainstem death and its detrimental effects is an attractive alternative. However, this requires a different logistical approach to lung preservation, as the organ will have to go through a period of warm ischemia without significant antegrade circulation via the PA or the bronchial arteries. There is good evidence that the lung parenchyma can survive for up to 2 hours without ventilation or circulation if the lung is inflated at the time of circulatory arrest on account of oxygen still being present in the alveoli.

Proper organ assessment of DCD lungs is difficult due to a lack of information in such donors. For instance, the differential pulmonary vein gases, which are often crucial in decision making about the viability of donor lungs, is not available in this scenario. Thus the assessment is subjective and done mainly by visual inspection and palpation of the lungs. This clearly requires significant lung transplant experience.

After cardiac arrest and a "hands-off" period, bronchoscopy is performed. Rigid bronchoscopy is preferred for adequate removal of secretions. The trachea is then re-intubated and ventilation commenced with inspired oxygen of 30%. This is all carried out while the abdominal surgeons are in the process of performing laparotomy and inserting perfusion cannulae for kidney and liver harvesting.

Median sternotomy is performed; pericardium and pleural cavities are widely opened. The lungs are assessed visually for compliance, atelectasis, tumor, edema, consolidation, or any other abnormality. The PA is incised and any clot is removed by suctioning. Low-potassium dextran solution is infused antegrade into the PA, and the left atrial appendage is incised to allow efflux of the preservation solution. To augment hypothermia, topical cold saline is poured onto the lung surface. Uniform distribution of the preservation solution is essential for adequate protection. After completion of perfusion, the lungs are removed as usual. Retrograde flush through the pulmonary veins enhances protection and helps to further remove clots in the PA. If there is any doubt about the organ quality, very recent studies suggest that further assessment of the lungs on the ex-vivo lung-perfusion apparatus is a valuable adjunct tool for assessing the suitability of DCD lungs prior to implantation.

Further reading

Aigner C, Jaksch P, Seebacher G, *et al.* Single running suture – the new standard technique for bronchial anastomoses in lung transplantation. *Eur J Cardiothorac Surg* 2003; **23**: 488–93.

Gammie JS, Cheul Lee J, Pham SM, *et al.* Cardiopulmonary bypass is associated with early allograft dysfunction but not death after double-lung transplantation. *Thorac Cardiovasc Surg* 1998; **115**: 990–4.

Garfein ES, McGregor CC, Galantowicz ME, *et al.* Deleterious effects of telescoped bronchial anastomosis in single and bilateral lung transplantation. *Ann Transplant* 2000; **5**: 5–11.

Hlozek C, Smedira NG, Kirby TJ, *et al.* Cardiopulmonary bypass for lung transplantation. *Perfusion* 1997; **12**: 107–12.

Macchiarini P, Ladurie FL, Cerrina J, *et al.* Clamshell or sternotomy for double lung or heart-lung transplantation? *Eur J Cardiothorac Surg* 1999; **15**: 333–9.

Pochettino A, Bavaria JE. Anterior axillary muscle-sparing thoracotomy for lung transplantation. *Ann Thorac Surg* 1997; **64**: 1846–8.

Chapter 17

Management during surgery

David Ip and Peter Slinger

Key points

- Thoracic epidural analgesia should be considered in all cases, but may be most safely sited postoperatively.
- A left-sided double-lumen endotracheal tube is preferred in all cases except left-sided single lung transplant when a right-sided double-lumen tube may be better.
- Dynamic hyperinflation may occur in severe obstructive lung disease, leading to decreased venous return and circulatory collapse.
- Right ventricular failure may be encountered at induction of anesthesia, after commencing one-lung ventilation, during manipulation of the hilum, at pulmonary artery clamping, after reperfusion, and with severe early graft dysfunction.
- Inhaled aerosolized prostacyclin is an alternative to inhaled nitric oxide; it is less expensive and does not require a bulky delivery system.

Preparation

Patient assessment

The broad categories of end-stage lung disease requiring lung transplantation (LT) are suppurative, obstructive, restrictive, and pulmonary vascular. They each lend themselves to different potential complications during anesthesia and thus require slightly different management strategies.

The nature of transplantation surgery is that it is unpredictable and emergent. Hence the preoperative work-up of transplant recipients must be thoroughly performed in advance, with appropriate updating of clinical data and investigations while on the waiting list. Specific information required includes patient height and current weight; results from latest pulmonary function test; trans-thoracic echocardiography; left heart catheterization if appropriate; lung perfusion scan, which gives information on which lung will better tolerate one-lung ventilation (OLV); presence of antibodies to the donor; and current blood tests.

In addition to the usual anesthetic issues of aspiration risk, airway assessment, comorbidities, medications, and adverse reactions, assessment on the day of surgery focuses on the current illness state and amount of deterioration since investigations were performed, as the patient's physical state may be significantly worse than investigations may suggest.

Premedication

Normal medications that need to be continued include bronchodilators, antibiotics, and pulmonary vasodilators. If the patient is receiving intravenous prostaglandins, it is continued until cardiopulmonary bypass (CPB) is initiated. Immunosuppression regimes commence pretransplantation and vary between institutions. Broad-spectrum antibiotics are given for prophylaxis, but for patients with suppurative lung disease or a current chest infection, the choice of antibiotics will be determined by the actual or suspected microbiological burden. The microbiological burden of the donor is also taken into account. Due to the lack of respiratory reserve, sedation outside of the operating room is not recommended and should only be given with extreme caution, as it may easily precipitate a cardiorespiratory arrest due to hypoxemia, hypercarbia, or increased pulmonary vascular resistance (PVR) resulting in acute right ventricular (RV) failure.

Organ Transplantation: A Clinical Guide, ed. A.A. Klein, C.J. Lewis, and J.C. Madsen. Published by Cambridge University Press.

Thoracic epidural analgesia

Adequate postoperative analgesia is important to facilitate extubation. Thoracic epidural analgesia (TEA) provides superior analgesia compared with systemic opioids; however, special problems and risks with preoperative epidural insertion need to be considered in the LT population. First, in the event of a bloody tap, the risk of an epidural hematoma is magnified with subsequent full heparinization for CPB. Timely decompression may be delayed due to prolonged surgery and inability to elicit clinical signs in the sedated and intubated patient. Second, the benefit of TEA is shortened or lost if tracheal extubation is delayed due to other complications. Therefore, patients should be selected carefully based on risk and benefit discussions. Alternatives are to have the epidural inserted postoperatively in an awake or lightly sedated patient prior to tracheal extubation or only if systemic multi-modal analgesics are inadequate. For single-sided surgery, paravertebral catheter insertion is an alternative to TEA.

Monitoring and vascular access

Vascular access comprises a large peripheral intravenous (IV) cannula, a pulmonary artery (PA) catheter sheath with side port, a multi-lumen central line, and an arterial cannula. Mandatory monitoring includes five-lead electrocardiography; pulse oximetry; invasive measurement of arterial, central venous, and PA pressures; urine output via an indwelling catheter; temperature; capnography; spirometry; and anesthetic agent gas analysis.

Other options include depth-of-anesthesia monitoring, cerebral oximetry using transcutaneous near infrared spectroscopy, continuous arterial blood gas monitoring, continuous cardiac output, and mixed venous oximetry.

Transesophageal echocardiography

There is no consensus about routine use of intraoperative transesophageal echocardiography (TEE) during LT for assessing surgical anastomotic sites. It is useful for evaluation of pulmonary hypertension, RV dysfunction, and suspicion of a patent foramen ovale. It provides useful information about left and right heart preload, left ventricular (LV) and RV function, regional wall motion abnormalities, and intracardiac air, especially when used in situations of hemodynamic instability. It may also identify intracardiac thrombus and other unexpected abnormalities. In the case of unexplained or refractory hypoxemia, it can detect the presence of intracardiac shunting.

Induction

The induction of anesthesia is one of the most critical periods, and the surgeon and perfusionist must be present and prepared to urgently perform sternotomy and initiation of CPB in the event of severe cardiorespiratory instability. In the patient with little or no cardiorespiratory reserve, cardiovascular collapse can be precipitated by many factors. These include hypoxia, hypercarbia, the reduction of endogenous sympathetic drive, drugs causing myocardial depression or vasodilatation, and the commencement of positive pressure ventilation of the lungs causing reduction of systemic venous return and increased RV afterload.

Therefore, the hemodynamic goals of induction of anesthesia are to preserve systemic vascular resistance (SVR), myocardial contractility, and avoidance of any increase in PVR. This can usually be achieved with a titrated narcotic-based induction consisting of 0.05–0.1 mg/kg of midazolam, 5–10 μg/kg of fentanyl, and judicious doses of propofol followed by a muscle relaxant. Other induction regimes have also been described. In patients with high aspiration risk, gastric acid lowering premedication and cricoid pressure during induction with suxamethonium or high-dose rocuronium is used. A non-titrated rapid-sequence induction is rarely justifiable due to the risk of hemodynamic collapse. Ketamine is an alternative and ideal choice of induction agent in patients with severe pulmonary hypertension.

With the exception of a left-sided single lung transplant in which a right-sided double-lumen endotracheal tube may be better, a left-sided double-lumen endotracheal tube is preferred for all other cases. Use of a bronchial blocker through a single-lumen tube is an alternative, but a double-lumen tube allows increased surgical flexibility, irrigation of the divided bronchus, differential ventilation after the graft is reperfused, and faster lung isolation. The double-lumen tube is changed to a single-lumen tube at the end of surgery before leaving the operating room. Doing this under direct vision or preferably using a tube exchange catheter is recommended, as airway edema and swelling can occur during the course of the operation. Loss of the airway in this situation

Table 17.1 Disease-specific intraoperative anesthetic considerations

Recipient pathology	Intraoperative complications
Emphysema (COPD, α_1-antitrypsin deficiency)	Hypotension with positive-pressure ventilation due to auto-PEEP.
Cystic fibrosis	Profuse thick secretions. Difficult to maintain baseline $PaCO_2$ with positive pressure ventilation. Small stature, often difficult access in chest for surgeon.
Idiopathic pulmonary fibrosis	May have associated diseases (e.g., scleroderma). Often older with coronary artery disease. May have severe pulmonary hypertension. May not tolerate one-lung ventilation and may require CPB.
Primary pulmonary hypertension	Cardiovascular collapse secondary to hypotension on induction. Always require CPB.
Bronchoalveolar carcinoma	Profuse watery secretions

has occurred with disastrous outcomes. The anesthetic considerations specific to recipient pulmonary pathology are shown in Table 17.1.

Obstructive lung disease

This group includes patients with chronic obstructive pulmonary disease (COPD) and α_1-antitrypsin deficiency, and bronchiolitis obliterans syndrome presenting for re-transplantation. Patients with obstructive lung disease may undergo a single or bilateral LT. The majority of this group will have smoking-related emphysema and so may have coexisting cardiovascular disease.

A preinduction arterial blood gas is required for baseline $PaCO_2$. There is an increased risk of pneumothorax with positive pressure ventilation and central line insertion. Cor pulmonale may exist with increased PVR, elevated PA pressure, and right heart dysfunction. These patients already have a reduced venous return to the left heart with reduced LV end-diastolic volume, reduced stroke volume, and reduced cardiac output compared with normal patients. A longer expiratory time is required to prevent dynamic hyperinflation, further reduction in venous return, and circulatory collapse. Disconnecting the endotracheal tube (ETT) and allowing lung deflation will permit venous return to the heart and restore blood pressure if this is the cause of hypotension. These patients have a high level of intrinsic positive end expiratory pressure (PEEP), and external PEEP is usually not required and may in fact cause hyperinflation, increase shunt, and reduce PaO_2. A large alveolar dead space makes the end tidal CO_2 underestimate the $PaCO_2$ by an unpredictable amount. Frequent correlation to arterial blood gases is required. It is appropriate to ventilate the patients to their baseline $PaCO_2$.

Restrictive lung disease

This group includes patients with idiopathic pulmonary fibrosis, connective tissue disease, and drug- or radiation-induced parenchymal lung disease. Ventilating these patients can be difficult. To obtain adequate tidal volumes, peak inspiratory pressures exceeding 40 cm H_2O may be required. This is tolerated especially if bilateral lung transplantation (BLT) is planned. Volume-controlled ventilation allows better control of tidal volumes, and some ventilators may not allow pressure control ventilation mode to exceed 40 cm H_2O. These patients benefit with some PEEP. An intensive care unit–level ventilator may be required if the ventilator on the anesthesia delivery unit is not adequate. Pulmonary hypertension is common and can be severe. Elderly patients with end-stage restrictive lung disease are one subgroup in whom the long-term outcomes from SLT are equivalent to those from BLT.

Suppurative lung disease

The majority of these patients have cystic fibrosis (CF), but may also include patients with non-CF bronchiectasis. At induction, a single-lumen tube is inserted to allow a fiberoptic bronchoscope with a large working channel to perform adequate pulmonary toilet. The single-lumen tube is then changed to a double-lumen tube. Aggressive airway toileting is required during surgery as lung manipulation can squeeze purulent alveolar secretions into the large conducting airways.

Intraoperative ventilation of CF patients can be extremely difficult and may require high airway pressures and relatively large volumes to maintain the patient's preoperative PaCO2. For chronically hypercapnic patients, if CPB is required, we try to maintain the PaCO2 during CPB at the patient's normal preinduction baseline. Due to multi-resistant organisms, some CF patients require consultation with infectious diseases or microbiology specialists to determine appropriate antibiotic cover.

Pulmonary hypertension

In the context of patients with pulmonary hypertension presenting for lung transplantation, the cause may be (1) idiopathic, (2) associated with lung disease or hypoxia (pulmonary fibrosis, COPD), or less commonly, (3) associated with connective tissue disease and (4) intracardiac shunt with Eisenmenger physiology. It may also be seen post-transplantation in primary graft dysfunction.

In patients with severe pulmonary hypertension and right heart failure, it is advisable to have central venous access and the pulmonary artery catheter floated into position prior to induction because these patients may become hemodynamically compromised with induction of anesthesia and need inotropic or vasopressor support. Preinduction surgical femoral cannulation under local anesthesia for cardiopulmonary bypass should be considered for very high-risk patients.

Maintenance of anesthesia

Patients undergoing LT feature prominently in studies of intraoperative awareness. Care must be taken to ensure that these high-risk patients receive adequate amounts of anesthetic agents. Maintenance of anesthesia by propofol infusion, inhalational anesthetic agent, or both have been described. Nitrous oxide is avoided due to its deleterious effect on PVR. The theoretical advantage of a total IV technique is less inhibition of hypoxic pulmonary vasoconstriction, although this does not translate to a clinically significant increase in PaO_2 when less than 1.0 MAC of inhalational anesthetic is used. There is also less myocardial depression and smoother transition to CPB if required. The advantage of an inhalational technique is bronchodilatation, especially in patients with reversible obstructive airways disease. A disadvantage is the slower wash-in of the anesthetic due to the limited minute volume encountered in some of these patients.

OLV is better tolerated in the lung with greater perfusion. The shunt fraction is greater compared with OLV in the decubitus position due to the lack of benefit of gravity. The strategies of managing hypoxia on OLV are listed in Table 17.2. Severe respiratory acidosis (pH < 7.2) can be problematic, and strategies employed to increase alveolar minute volume may ultimately be unsuccessful, therefore requiring CPB.

Table 17.2 Treating hypoxia during one-lung ventilation

Increase FiO_2 to 1.0
Resume two-lung ventilation
CPAP or O_2 insufflation to non-ventilated lung
Optimize PEEP to ventilated lung
Expediting surgical ligation of ipsilateral pulmonary veins and arteries to reduce shunt fraction

Temperature monitoring and active warming is required, as hypothermia worsens pulmonary hypertension, coagulopathy, and risk of arrhythmias. We routinely use both upper- and lower-body forced-air heating blankets. Magnesium sulphate (2 g) is infused to try to prevent arrhythmias.

Repeated hilar manipulation and cardiac compression lead to reduced cardiac output and hypotension. Vasopressor support is invariably required to maintain adequate perfusion pressure. Optimizing fluid status is important, but excessive fluid therapy is to be avoided as the graft is susceptible to pulmonary edema. Finding evidence to recommend one type of fluid over another is difficult due to multiple confounding factors and small series of patients; however, the volume of intraoperative gelatin-based colloid given has been associated with worse postoperative oxygenation and delayed extubation.

Single versus bilateral LT

Most patients with end-stage parenchymal lung disease can get symptomatic improvement with SLT. Suppurative lung disease is a contraindication for SLT. Although SLT allows more patients to undergo transplantation by splitting pair of lungs between two patients, case-control studies have shown BLT to be an independent factor in improved long-term survival. Potential therapeutic benefits of BLT include a reduction in alveolar damage during reperfusion, improved pulmonary compliance and mechanics, and the avoidance of native lung pathology.

Cardiopulmonary bypass

In institutions that do not use CPB routinely, planned CPB is used when patients have severe pulmonary hypertension, require a concomitant cardiac procedure such as repair of intracardiac shunt, or require plasmapheresis due to human leukocyte antigen (HLA) mismatch and presence of HLA antibodies against the donor. In unplanned cases, the decision to use CPB is made if the patient (1) does not tolerate OLV (either hypoxia or refractory hypercarbia), (2) does not tolerate clamping of a PA (RV failure), or (3) has other refractory hemodynamic instability. If high PA pressures do not fall after the first side is reperfused, CPB may also be commenced to protect the graft from pulmonary hypertension, which can contribute to primary graft dysfunction. CPB is required if the patient already is dependant on extracorporeal membrane oxygenation (ECMO) or the Novalung interventional lung assist device, although some centers consider this a contraindication to LT due to potentially poorer outcomes. In our adult practice, two thirds of cases are done without CPB. In the cases in which CPB is used, two thirds are elective, and one third is for specific intraoperative problems, most commonly hemodynamic instability.

Warm (37°C) beating heart CPB is routinely used unless a concomitant cardiac procedure is also performed. Bypass times are often prolonged, so a centrifugal pump offers some advantage over a continuous flow roller pump. Venous drainage may often be impaired by severe surgical manipulation of the heart and hilum; therefore, vigilance is required, and flows may often need to be temporarily reduced to prevent complete emptying of the reservoir. Bicaval cannulation provides less interruption of venous return than single two-stage atrial cannulation.

Reperfusion and ventilation of the first side commences while still on CPB to limit the warm ischemic time of the graft. Major coagulopathy is invariably present after coming off prolonged CPB, so platelets and fresh-frozen plasma should be available if coagulopathy after reversal of heparinization is present. An antifibrinolytic is routinely given. We use Tranexamic acid (30 mg/kg load and 16 mg/kg infusion until the end of CPB).

The advantages of CPB are hemodynamic stability and that it allows controlled reperfusion of grafts. Disadvantages of CPB are hemolysis and activation of proinflammatory cascades that increase the risk of lung injury. It also increases the need for transfusion of blood products due to hemodilution, coagulopathy, and platelet dysfunction. Use of CPB has been associated with a longer period of postoperative mechanical ventilation, more pulmonary edema, and increased early mortality, although this is controversial.

RV failure

RV failure can be precipitated by an acute increase in afterload or ischemia due to either prolonged hypotension or air embolism. This is encountered at induction, after commencing OLV, during manipulation of the hilum, at PA clamping, after reperfusion, and with severe early graft dysfunction. RV afterload reduction is the primary treatment goal. Also important are preserving coronary perfusion and biventricular inotropic support. Basic things such as correcting acidosis, hypoxia, hypercarbia, hypothermia, minimizing ventilation pressures, and undoing the precipitating event (if possible) should not be overlooked. Inotropes most commonly used are phosphodiesterase inhibitors (e.g., milrinone), norepinephrine, and epinephrine.

Stages of surgery

Dissection and removal of native lung

This may be difficult and prolonged if extensive pleural adhesions are present. This is more likely in patients with previous thoracic surgery or restrictive or suppurative lung disease. Significant blood loss may occur. For BLT performed off pump, if there is a significant perfusion asymmetry, the lung with the lower perfusion is transplanted first. Testing the hemodynamic consequences of dividing the PA by pinching it off temporarily is advised, as the RV can acutely fail.

Anastomosis of donor lung

Surgical access to the hilum and atrium requires retraction on the heart, causing intermittent periods of hypotension and low cardiac output. Communication between anesthetist and surgeon is critical. The circulation usually requires support with vasopressor agents. Some degree of fluid expansion may be required to optimize preload, although caution should be exercised because low-pressure pulmonary edema in the grafts may occur if excessive fluid has been given.

Reperfusion of graft

This is a busy period which that often requires an extra set of hands to deal with differential lung ventilation and cardiovascular emergencies at the same time. Before tying the final stitch of the atrial anastomosis, the graft is de-aired through an opening in the atrial anastomosis. This is done by inflating the lung to a sustained pressure of 15–20 cm H_2O and partially releasing the PA clamp. The atrial clamp is then released to de-air the atrial cuff before the final knot is tied. At this point, hypotension may occur due to several causes. There are sometimes leaks in the vascular anastomosis that need to be controlled by placing further sutures. A significant amount of blood loss may rapidly occur in the interim, requiring prompt intravascular volume replacement. Temporary myocardial stunning occurs because the initial venous return to the left atrium is cold and contains ischemic metabolites, and treatment with a small bolus of epinephrine or calcium is often required to improve myocardial contractility. Coronary artery air embolism may also occur. This is usually seen in the right coronary artery as it is uppermost in the supine position. ST depression or elevation may be seen in the inferior leads and, if treated with vasopressor agents, is usually transient.

The PA clamp is slowly released over a 10-minute period, limiting initial flows to the vascular bed of the graft, which has been shown to reduce primary graft dysfunction. To reduce lung injury, initial ventilation to the graft should be with a low inspired oxygen concentration (FiO_2), low peak inspiratory pressures of 15–20 cm H_20, and a positive end expiratory pressure of 5 cm H_20. The respiratory rate is initially set to 8–10 breaths per minute. The other lung requires 100% oxygen, most easily given via a self-inflating bag. Once the PA clamp is fully released, ventilation settings need to be adjusted to ensure adequate minute ventilation and CO_2 removal, and the FiO_2 titrated to a safe level of oxygen saturation. For the first side of an off-pump BLT, the new graft needs to support the ventilatory requirements of the patient while the contralateral side is operated on. For patients on CPB, ventilation is continued on the initial settings, and restriction of venous cannula drainage by partial clamping allows some RV ejection to perfuse the graft. This is titrated to a PA pressure of 10–15 mmHg.

Primary graft dysfunction

Primary graft dysfunction (PGD) is a devastating complication akin to acute lung injury due to the transplantation process. It has been reported to occur in up to 25% of LTs and increases both short- and long-term mortality. It may manifest immediately following reperfusion during surgery and can occupy a spectrum of mild self-limiting disease to fulminant respiratory failure. Other features encountered in the operating room are poor respiratory compliance, high PVR, and pulmonary edema.

Nitric oxide

Inhaled nitric oxide (iNO) in the range of 10–40 parts per million (ppm) may be used in established PGD to treat severe hypoxia or elevated PA pressures. NO increases cyclic guanosine monophosphate, which relaxes smooth muscle. It improves ventilation/perfusion matching and decreases PA pressure by selectively vasodilating pulmonary vasculature in ventilated portions of the lung. The effect is transient, with rebound pulmonary hypertension seen during weaning, and survival benefit has not been shown, but its use may help stabilize the patient sufficiently during this turbulent period. Prophylactic use of iNO has not been shown to prevent PGD. Disadvantages of iNO include the potential for methemoglobinemia and cytotoxicity from free radical production. NO oxidizes to nitrogen dioxide and other higher oxides that are pulmonary toxic. Therefore, specialized monitoring and delivery systems need to be used, which contributes to the very high cost.

Prostaglandins

Inhaled aerosolized prostacyclin (PGI_2) is an alternative to iNO. It is less expensive and does not require a bulky delivery system. Commercial PGI_2 "Epoprostenol" is reconstituted in sterile glycine, diluted with normal saline according to body weight, and aerosolized via a "low-flow" nebulizer that delivers 8 ml/hr of solution with a driving flow rate of 2 L/min to give a typical dose of 50 ng/kg/min. Relatively large doses are required due to the inefficiency of aerosolized particles reaching the alveoli. A continuous nebulizer is required due to the short half-life of epoprostenol. A small amount of literature in the use of PGI_2 for primary graft dysfunction shows equivalence in lowering PA pressures, improving oxygenation, and lack of systemic side effects compared with iNO. There are no studies that show long-term outcome in this setting. Prostaglandins administered IV are rarely used in the acute setting due to their systemic effects causing hypotension and non-selective pulmonary vasodilatation that may worsen intrapulmonary shunt and oxygenation.

Further reading

Christie JD, Van Raemdonck D, de Perrot M, *et al.* Report of the ISHLT Working Group on Primary Lung Graft Dysfunction Parts I to VI. *J Heart Lung Transplant* 2005; **24**: 1451–500.

Lee JC, Jason D, Christie JD. Primary graft dysfunction. *Proc Am Thorac Soc* 2009; **6**: 39–46.

McIlroy DR, Pilcher DV, Snell GI. Does anaesthetic management affect early outcomes after lung transplant? An exploratory analysis. *Br J Anaesth* 2009; **102:** 506–14.

Subramaniam K, Yared JP. Management of pulmonary hypertension in the operating room. *Semin Cardiothorac Vasc Anesth* 2007; **11**: 119–36.

Chapter 18

Postoperative care and early complications

Vlad Vinarsky and Leo C. Ginns

Key points

- The major challenge of postoperative fluid management following lung transplantation is to minimize pulmonary edema while maintaining optimal cardiac function.
- Immunosuppression protocols are usually divided into three broad categories: induction, maintenance, and treatment of rejection.
- Primary graft dysfunction, the major cause for morbidity and mortality in the early postoperative period, is diagnosed when acute and hyperacute rejection, infection, venous anastomosis complication, and cardiogenic pulmonary edema have been excluded.
- Lung transplant recipients' increased susceptibility to infections frequently requires prompt treatment with anti-microbials and lowering of the net level of immunosuppression.

Over the last several decades, lung transplantation (LT) has become a viable option for a number of end-stage lung diseases. Heart–lung transplantation (HLT) remains one alternative for select patients with end-stage cardiopulmonary disease, although its use is infrequent. In the annual report on heart and lung transplantation in 2009, the International Society for Heart and Lung Transplantation (ISHLT) received reports of only 75 HLT recipients compared with 2708 LTs performed in 2007. Similarly, only 29 HLTs were performed in the United States in 2009, in contrast to 1661 lung transplants performed during the same period. There has been a growing preference for single-lung transplantation (SLT) and bilateral-lung transplantation (BLT) over HLT, especially with the recognition that LT alone can be performed even in the setting of severe right heart failure. The postoperative management of HLT recipients is similar to that of SLT and BLT patients. Furthermore, the level of immunosuppression and the majority of the early postoperative complications, including acute rejection and infection, are related to the lung allograft rather than the cardiac allograft. For these reasons, this chapter focuses on postoperative management and early complications of LT.

Postoperative management

After transplantation surgery, patients are transferred to the intensive care unit, usually with a single-lumen endotracheal tube in situ. Universal precautions, including hand washing, masks, and gloves, are indicated. An isolation room with HEPA-filtration of ambient air may limit the incidence of fungal infections from extrinsic sources in transplant patients.

Ventilation

Ventilator management in most cases follows standard postoperative practice. The FiO_2 is adjusted to maintain a PaO_2 greater than 65 mmHg. Significant barotrauma due to increased airway pressure or excessive tidal volume is uncommon after LT, and higher airway pressures may have a beneficial effect in minimizing postoperative pulmonary edema. Weaning the patients from the ventilator requires appropriate management of postoperative pain. A functional thoracic epidural catheter is useful (in the absence of coagulopathy), although intravenous (IV) opiates via a patient-controlled analgesia approach may be useful after the patient achieves a conscious state, followed by transition to oral medications. Anti-inflammatory

Organ Transplantation: A Clinical Guide, ed. A.A. Klein, C.J. Lewis, and J.C. Madsen. Published by Cambridge University Press.

pain medications should be avoided because of added nephrotoxicity with the peri-operative antimicrobial and immunosuppressive medications. Tracheal extubation is carried out when the patient has a normal mental status and has achieved a reasonable rate of ventilation and spontaneous tidal volume. Early tracheal extubation in the operating room may be possible, especially following SLT in chronic obstructive pulmonary disease (COPD) patients, depending on institutional experience and expertise. Good bronchopulmonary hygiene with frequent endotracheal aspiration of secretions and physiotherapy is crucial in achieving and maintaining extubation in transplant recipients.

Patients with emphysema who undergo SLT require special attention to airway pressures and the compliance difference between the allograft and the native lung. Hyperinflation of the native lung will progressively interfere with ventilation of the allograft and can result in compromise of cardiac filling. Efforts to control hyperinflation of the native lung include lower levels of positive end expiratory pressure (PEEP; 1–3 cmH_2O). Positioning of the patient with the native lung down may further increase impedance of that hemithorax and limit hyperinflation, although increased blood flow to the native lung induced by this maneuver may require adjustment of ventilatory parameters in order to maintain satisfactory gas exchange. In rare circumstances, when marked edema has occurred in the allograft, independent lung ventilation using a double-lumen endotracheal tube may be needed. In such cases, more rapid ventilation of the allograft with smaller tidal volumes, using PEEP and higher inspiratory flow rates, will provide carbon dioxide clearance, whereas ventilation of the native lung at very low rates, with standard volumes and no PEEP, will maintain oxygenation but minimize hyperinflation. Early tracheal extubation after SLT in COPD may decrease the risk of native lung hyperinflation.

Pulmonary hypertension

Patients with severe pulmonary hypertension who undergo LT are managed differently because they have a unique postoperative physiology. The right ventricle (RV) in these patients has been conditioned to generate peak systolic pressures against a markedly elevated PVR. Following LT, an abrupt near-normalization of the PVR occurs, accompanied by improved ventricular hemodynamics. With minimal catecholamine stimulation, as seen upon awakening from anesthesia or weaning from a ventilator, the RV generates a peak systolic pressure similar to that required pre-operatively. The resultant abrupt rise in PA pressure, in combination with increased vascular permeability and the absence of lymphatic continuity, can cause rapid fluid accumulation in the donor lung and lead to labile oxygenation and hemodynamics following transplantation. Preemptive treatment for this condition involves maintaining a high degree of sedation, or even muscular paralysis, in the first 3 to 5 days postoperatively. This approach minimizes catecholamine stimulation during the time in which ischemia and reperfusion injury in the allograft is resolving. Minimizing other provocations to RV output, such as hypercarbia or hypoxia, within the first few days of following transplantation is also beneficial. Following this period, patients are cautiously awakened and standard ventilator weaning can proceed while closely monitoring cardiac output, blood gases, and pulmonary artery (PA) pressures. In some cases, additional measures such as low dose beta-blockade to diminish myocardial contractility or IV anxiolytic therapy may be required in the presence of significant hemodynamic abnormalities. Other strategies to control pulmonary edema and resultant hypoxia in the setting of pulmonary hypertension include fluid restriction and judicious use of higher PEEP. Inhaled nitric oxide (iNO) as well as intravenous or inhaled prostacyclin can be employed in select cases.

Fluid management and hemodynamics

Regarding postoperative fluid management, there is often a tension between the need to maintain sufficient left atrial filling pressure for adequate cardiac output and the desire to minimize pulmonary edema. As noted above, the effects of ischemia–reperfusion injury and lymphatic discontinuity all contribute to a tendency toward pulmonary edema in the lung graft. PA pressures and pulmonary wedge pressures need to be kept as low as possible postoperatively without compromising ventricular preload and cardiac output. Achieving this goal requires continuous hemodynamic monitoring and accurate intake-output measurements during this early postoperative period in order to make the necessary adjustments in rates of fluid administration, inotrope, pressors, and diuretic therapy. Most patients have an increase in total body water immediately postoperatively but may be relatively intravascularly depleted. Although the optimal fluid for volume replacement remains unknown, it is common practice to use colloid over crystalloid and to transfuse with red blood cells to a relatively higher hemoglobin goal (up to 10 mg/dl) in LT recipients.

For most patients, the effects of a reduction in pulmonary vascular resistance (PVR) almost immediately following LT results in improved RV and secondarily left ventricle (LV) performance. Some inotropic support may be warranted, however, in patients who have preexisting RV hypertrophy, particularly when pressure overload of the RV occurs during the implantation procedure or following CPB. These cases require inotropic stimulation with a selective phosphodiesterase III inhibitor milrinone, a pure beta-receptor agonist such as dobutamine, or a balanced alpha and beta agent such as dopamine or norepinephrine in order to optimize cardiac output in the face of a reduced preload relative to the preoperative state.

Preoperative renal dysfunction may further complicate fluid management postoperatively. A low cardiac output state, prolonged central venous hypertension, and the chronic use of nephrotoxic antibiotics or diuretics prior to transplantation may have adverse effect on glomerular filtration rate. The liberal use of diuretic therapy is helpful in the postoperative management of these patients. After stabilization and tracheal extubation of the LT recipient, ongoing loss of lean body mass occurs for patients in a postoperative stress state. At this point, daily recording of body weight is useful in assessing fluid balance. Weight loss of up to 10% of pre-operative lean body mass is typical in the first 4 weeks following LT. Continued use of diuretic therapy is usually required during this period in order to maintain a non-edematous state.

Anti-microbial therapy

Prophylaxis against Gram-positive organisms in combination with broad-spectrum antibiotics to provide appropriate coverage for organisms identified preoperatively from the sputum of the recipient is required. Recipients, who have been recently hospitalized and exposed to drug-resistant bacterial pathogens or those with cystic fibrosis (CF) will require additional coverage for *Pseudomonas*. For CF patients, ongoing surveillance of sputum flora and determination of antibiotic sensitivities is important in the period prior to transplantation in order to develop an appropriate multidrug anti-microbial regimen for peri-operative use. The addition of inhaled antimicrobial therapy, either tobramycin or colistin, can have additive effects in the management of *Pseudomonas* in these patients. Postoperative antimicrobial coverage should be modified if pathogens are identified in the sputum of the donor that are not already covered by the recipient-specific regimen. Duration of treatment is dictated, in part, by the clinical appearance of the bronchial anastomosis and by the microbiology recovered from donor cultures or serial bronchoscopy examinations of the allograft.

Routine prophylaxis for fungal organisms is useful when preoperative recipient sputum cultures have demonstrated the presence of *Aspergillus* at any time preceding the transplant procedure, when there has been evidence of heavy overgrowth of yeast (e.g., *Candida*) in the donor sputum culture or when cytolytic induction immunosuppression is used. Some centers continue to use fungal prophylaxis for all recipients after LT. Aerosolized amphotericin B, fluconazole, and itraconazole have the most published experience for prophylactic use. If the recipient has severe structural lung disease such as bronchiectasis and *Aspergillus* or heavy growth of *Candida* is identified in the sputum preoperatively, the patient is treated with IV lipid formulation of amphotericin B followed by oral voriconazole for an extended period of time, even in the absence of evidence of invasive or disseminated fungal infection. Duration of therapy is guided by surveillance bronchoscopy results.

Pneumocystis jiroveci (*carinii*) pneumonia in LT patients has been virtually eliminated by the routine use of trimethoprim-sulfamethoxazole beginning 1 week postoperatively. Alternative treatments recommended for patient with sulfa allergy include atovaquone, dapsone, and aerosolized pentamidine. Sulfa desensitization is frequently possible in such patients and is often recommended given the efficacy of sulfa prophylaxis against *P. jiroveci* and its broad spectrum against a range of additional organisms (e.g., *Toxoplasma gondii*, *Listeria* spp, *Nocardia* spp, *Streptococcus pneumoniae*).

The incidence of herpes simplex infection, including mucosal ulceration and pneumonitis, has been eliminated by the routine use of acyclovir prophylaxis after lung transplantation. Cytomegalovirus (CMV) infection, however, remains an important problem following lung transplantation. The incidence of CMV infection following lung transplantation is related to the preoperative CMV status of both the donor (D) and the recipient (R). A discordant CMV status between the donor and the recipient may result in either primary infection of the donor lungs by the recipient (in the case of D–/R+) or in the more serious circumstance of primary systemic CMV infection (in the case of D+/R–). In either case, without CMV prophylaxis, the incidence of acute and chronic rejection and of mortality is higher in mismatched patients than among patients in whom CMV status is concordant. The use of ganciclovir and valganciclovir prophylaxis decreases the incidence of primary disease and improves the outcome of CMV-disparate lung transplants. Prophylactic ganciclovir therapy should be resumed whenever immunosuppression is augmented to treat episodes of acute rejection in CMV-discordant patients. In some centers, CMV-negative recipients who receive lung from CMV-positive donors also are treated with CMV hyperimmune globulin, given their high risk of developing severe disease.

Nutrition

Maintaining optimal nutrition in the postoperative period is essential and may improve operative outcomes. Most patients can resume oral intake following tracheal extubation, although dietary consultation should be obtained to assess the adequacy of caloric intake. Energy and protein needs specifically after LT have not been quantified; however, energy requirements in postsurgical patients and in other transplant patients are estimated at 1.35–1.75 times basal energy expenditure, and protein requirements are predicted to be 1.3–2.5 g of protein per kilogram of body weight. Frequently, because of poor appetite and slow recovery, the addition of liquid nutritional supplements will be needed to meet these caloric requirements. If the patient is unable to resume an oral diet due to prolonged ventilatory support or any postoperative complication that prevents eating, enteral alimentation via a nasogastric feeding tube is preferred, although IV total parenteral nutrition may be required. Specialty diets may be recommended if hyperglycemia, hypertension, or hyperkalemia develops as a result of side effects of immunosuppressive medications, including high-dose steroids and calcineurin inhibitors (CNIs).

Patients with CF often have a malabsorptive syndrome that will require resumption of preoperative pancreatic enzyme supplementation. CF patients are also prone to both gastroparesis and meconium ileus equivalent, both of which may be avoided by the use of promotility agents and a cathartic bowel regimen.

Immunosuppression

The induction of a state of relatively non-specific immunosuppression by pharmacological means has been the key to successful LT. Specific, permanent tolerance of the allograft without the need for chronic medications would be ideal, but this is presently not possible. As a result, although the current regimens lead to satisfactory control of most acute rejection processes, the combined side-effects of these medications and their incomplete ability to control chronic rejection in the lung account for the major long-term morbidity and mortality associated with LT. Immunosuppression regimens depend on experience and preference of each institution, and protocols vary widely among LT programs. In general, the protocols are divided into three broad categories: induction, maintenance, and treatment of rejection.

Most patients receive induction immunosuppression despite the lack of evidence for this treatment post-LT in clinical trials. The percentage of patients who received induction has increased steadily from 24% in 1997 to 62% in 2008. Although polyclonal anti-thymocyte globulin (ATG) or anti-lymphocyte globulin (ALG) dominated cytolytic therapy in 1997, over the last decade, the interleukin-2 receptor (IL-2R) agents (basiliximab, daclizumab), CD52 agents (alemtuzumab), and muromonab-CD3 (OKT3) are being used more frequently as induction immunosuppression.

No standard protocol exists for the timing of initiation or the regimen of maintenance immunosuppression therapy following LT. However, virtually all centers use a three-drug regimen for maintenance that includes an anti-proliferative agent, an anti-metabolite, and a steroid. Historically, this regimen consisted of cyclosporine (CyA), azathioprine (AZA), and a low-dose prednisone. Recently, tacrolimus (TAC) has replaced CyA and mycophenolate mofetil (MMF) has replaced AZA in most regimens. Close drug level monitoring is necessary in the early period after transplantation and when any possible drug interaction is likely.

Early complications of LT

Early complications of LT can be classified into four broad categories: complications of the surgery itself, re-implantation response and primary graft dysfunction (PGD), immunologic complications including rejection, and organ-specific complications of the immunosuppressive agents used to prevent rejection, including direct side effects of the medication and infection.

Complications of the operation itself

In the first 2 weeks following LT, the greatest cause of morbidity and mortality are complications due to the transplant operation itself. These early complications include those related to the LT operation specifically, such as airway anastomotic complications, and those complications related to thoracic surgical operations generally. The latter include pain, phrenic nerve dysfunction, retained bronchial secretions and mucous plugging, atelectasis, pneumonia, persistent air leaks, tension and non-tension pneumothoraces, hemorrhage, respiratory failure, and cardiac and hemodynamic complications. Therapies of certain of these general thoracic surgical complications must be modified for the LT recipient. For example, concern about healing of the airway anastomosis limits endotracheal suctioning to the airways proximal to the anastomosis. Retained bronchial secretions and mucous plugging distal to the anastomosis are treated instead with frequent therapeutic flexible bronchoscopies in the early postoperative period.

Major technical complications following LT have become increasingly rare with improvements in operative technique and peri-operative management. PA obstruction can occur as a result of anastomotic stenosis, kinking, or extrinsic compression. Persistent pulmonary hypertension and unexplained hypoxemia may be evident in these cases. Left atrial anastomotic obstruction can also occur due to faulty anastomotic technique or due to extrinsic compression by clot or pericardium. This problem results in more severe abnormalities than PA obstruction, including marked pulmonary hypertension and ipsilateral pulmonary edema. Diagnostic methods for theses vascular anastomotic complications include routine intra-operative measurements of anastomotic gradients and transesophageal echocardiography, which is particularly helpful in assessing the left atrial anastomosis. Postoperatively, diagnostic measures include contrast angiography and ventilation/perfusion scanning.

Reimplantation response and PGD

The re-implantation response has been defined broadly as a triad of worsening gas exchange, decreased lung compliance, and alveolar and interstitial infiltrates, typically most extensive in perihilar regions. This syndrome develops in the immediate post-transplant period, usually within the first 72 hours. In its mildest form, it remains extremely common, occurring in the majority of patients to some degree. The most severe form of re-implantation response represents PGD. The syndrome of PGD is the leading cause of death early after lung transplantation, accounting for nearly 30% of mortality in the first 30 days. PGD is characterized by diffuse alveolar damage on pathology, but the pathogenesis of the disease and the risk factors that determine the degree of lung injury remain largely unknown. Importantly, PGD remains a diagnosis of exclusion, and one must consider other diagnoses that could lead to the same clinical presentation. The differential diagnosis includes hyperacute and acute rejection, infection, venous anastomosis complication, and cardiogenic pulmonary edema.

Treatment of re-implantation response and PGD is supportive with mechanical ventilation, diuretics, and fluid restriction as tolerated. The typical course of mild re-implantation response is marked by progressive clearing of the infiltrates to complete resolution within several days to several weeks. However, patients with PGD, marked by severe hypoxemia refractory to conservative management, require prolonged mechanical ventilation, and they are treated like patients with acute respiratory distress syndrome (ARDS). General principles of supportive care in these patients include protective lung ventilation strategies with lower tidal volumes to target lower plateau pressures, and fluid restriction with tolerance of some degree of renal dysfunction. Development of ARDS unilaterally in an SLT recipient can make the ventilatory requirements of the transplanted lung differ dramatically from those of the remaining native lung. When there is marked compliance difference between the native lung and the lung graft, independent lung ventilation using double-lumen endotracheal tube, as mentioned previously, should be considered.

iNO has been used clinically to treat cases of established PGD with refractory hypoxemia or markedly elevated PA pressure. Extracorporeal membrane oxygenation (ECMO) can be instituted using arteriovenous (VA) routes in order to provide optimal gas exchange and allow decompression of the pulmonary circulation. Alternatively, venovenous (VV) ECMO avoids the complete diversion of pulmonary arterial flow from the anastomosis and the graft, which may be critical in the setting of disrupted bronchial artery circulation. The ECMO approach is guided by the center's experience, and treatment success of PGD with both VA and VV approaches have been reported. Despite all of these maneuvers, PGD remains the most common serious early complication of LT with a high rate of mortality.

Pleural complications

Pleural space complications are quite common after LT. Pneumothorax may occur on either side of a lung graft or on the side of a native lung. Pneumothoraces that arise from the lung graft are of greatest concern because of the possibility of airway dehiscence communicating with the pleural space. Flexible bronchoscopy is indicated for diagnostic purposes in patients presenting with this rare complication. In most cases, placement of a chest tube with re-expansion of the allograft will limit the process. More commonly, pneumothorax is the result of rupture of a bullous lesion in an emphysematous native lung after SLT. Conservative management with intercostal tube drainage is indicated. Occasionally, pneumothoraces will be noted after BLT when a significant size discrepancy exists between the donor lungs and the recipient thorax. In these cases, the space will resolve spontaneously over a short period of time, and specific interventions are not required.

Hemothorax caused by traumatic lesions during surgery is a potential complication of all thoracic surgical procedures. The underlying pulmonary disease of the LT recipient frequently leads to the formation of dense pleural adhesions and hypertrophy of the bronchial circulation. These changes may promote hemorrhage following the removal of the recipient's native lung(s). Any degree of hemorrhage that occurs can be exacerbated by the anticoagulation necessary for cardiopulmonary bypass, which is required during some transplant operations. The incidence of major hemothorax may be reduced by the use of a transverse, or "clamshell," incision rather than a median sternotomy in BLT recipients, which allows better visualization of the pleural surface and posterior mediastinum.

Pleural effusions are common after LT, particularly when a large size discrepancy exists between donor lungs and the thorax. Continued chest tube drainage following the primary procedure is not indicated as a preventive measure for these effusions and may actually lead to secondary infection and empyema. Management of these effusions is conservative, with diuretic therapy and dietary salt restriction. Invasive measures, such as thoracentesis or tube drainage, are indicated only for effusions complicated by a delayed pneumothorax, enlarging effusions, or for large effusions that persist for more than 4 weeks postoperatively.

Empyema is uncommon after LT. It is seen most frequently when a persistent pleural space due to a prolonged air leak, a chronic effusion, or an incompletely expanded lung is secondarily infected, usually with sputum flora. Management is initially conservative, with tube drainage and antibiotic therapy. However, when the etiologic agent has a limited antimicrobial sensitivity (*Burkholderia cepacia* or *Aspergillus*), more aggressive measures such as transposition of muscle flaps or limited thoracoplasty to obliterate the space may be indicated. Chylothorax has been reported after LT as well.

Early airway complications

The door to successful LT was opened by the demonstration that wrapping the airway anastomosis with a protective flap of well-vascularized tissues, such as intestinal omentum, can provide an adequate blood supply for healing. However, interruption of the normal bronchial blood supply to the anastomotic site still makes it the most vulnerable site for airway complications. There is surgeon and center variation about the anastomosis technique. Omentopexy and other tissue wraps are employed less frequently, whereas the use of telescoping anastomosis and end-to-end anastomosis with bronchial artery revascularization has grown. The surgical technique influences the type of possible airway complications. For example, unlike an end-to-end anastomosis, telescoping anastomosis that involves intussusception of the donor bronchus into that of recipient may decrease the incidence of early airway dehiscence but may increase the incidence of later airway stenosis.

Early airway anastomotic complications include necrosis, dehiscence, and anastomotic infection. Necrosis varies from mild and asymptomatic to severe and life-threatening. Severe necrosis and bronchial dehiscence present with difficulty weaning from the ventilator, pneumomediastinum, subcutaneous emphysema, pneumothorax, and persistent air leak. Anastomotic necrosis is diagnosed by direct visualization with bronchoscopy, although computed tomography scanning can often identify dehiscence on the basis of bronchial wall defects and irregularities. Relative devascularization of the anastomosis also makes it particularly more susceptible to infections. Anastomotic granulation tissue can also interfere with the clearance of secretions from the distal lung and can serve as a nidus for colonization by pathogens. For these reasons, significant granulation tissue should be excised by rigid bronchoscopy or laser excision, sometimes repeatedly until healing is complete.

Cardiovascular and hemodynamic complications

Both peri-operative myocardial infarction and cardiac arrests have occurred in LT recipients, though relatively infrequently. More common cardiac and hemodynamic complications are atrial arrhythmias and episodes of systemic hypotension. Postoperative atrial arrhythmias, including atrial fibrillation and flutter, are not unexpected given that atrial clamps are applied intraoperatively and that some handling of the heart is inevitable. They occur in up to 40% of patients, and most convert spontaneously or with medical therapy limited to several weeks, making the need for DC cardioversion infrequent.

Systemic hypotension requiring vasopressor and inotropic support is common in the first week following transplantation. The hemodynamic profile seen typically includes severely depressed systemic vascular resistance with a normal or diminished cardiac index. This complication has been associated with re-implantation response. Postoperative hemodynamic instability also has been common in patients with underlying pulmonary hypertension. In the first week post-transplant, minimal activity, suctioning, or pain can cause wide swings in the PA pressures in these patients, which can result in episodes of systemic hypotension or hypertension, as well as oxygen desaturation.

Venous thromboembolism (VTE), including deep venous thrombosis and pulmonary embolism, is a common diagnosis in all postoperative patients. VTE is a frequent complication of LT, with several studies consistently reporting an incidence of 20–30%. Approximately one fifth of VTE events occur in the first 30 days after transplantation. Many of the clots are associated with IV central catheters in the upper extremities. Other risk factors for VTE after LT include older age and diabetes.

Gastrointestinal complications

The incidence of early and late gastrointestinal (GI) complications in LT recipients substantially exceeds that observed in patients undergoing non-transplantation thoracic surgery. Delayed gastric emptying is extremely common after LT. Gastroparesis may be related to vagus nerve injury during transplantation and can be exacerbated by medications. This complication can lead to gastroesophageal reflux disease, malnutrition, malabsorption of anti-rejection medications, and recurrent aspiration of gastric contents into the allograft. Biliary pathology such as cholelithiasis and choledocholithiasis, as well as pancreatitis are frequent later manifestations of GI complications of LT, often related to direct toxicities of immunosuppressive medications.

GI complications may present atypically. Transplant patients may fail to manifest the usual symptoms and signs of intra-abdominal pathological processes due to their immunosuppressive medications, which reduce their ability to mount inflammatory responses. This can result in delays in diagnosis and lead to poorer outcomes. For this reason, a high index of suspicion and liberal use of diagnostic studies has been recommended in evaluating abdominal complaints post-transplant. Additionally, pretransplant GI imaging to identify pre-existing abdominal conditions can be extremely helpful in post-transplant management.

A GI complication unique to patients with underlying CF is the development of a meconium ileus equivalent. In this syndrome, inspissated intestinal contents in the distal ileum and proximal colon cause small bowel obstruction, presenting with pain, distension, constipation, and bilious vomiting. The syndrome is likely related to malabsorption due to the exocrine pancreatic insufficiency commonly occurring in CF patients. Preventive strategies center around the resumption of supplemental pancreatic enzymes as soon as bowel function permits. Some centers also add N-acetylcysteine to the enteral feedings of these patients.

Renal complications

Nephrotoxicity remains one of the most common long-term complications of anti-rejection medications. However, the renal toxicity of post-transplant medications can become apparent within the first hospitalization after LT. Calcineurin inhibitor (CNI) toxicity in LT recipients may be exacerbated by multiple other drugs and require CNI dose adjustment, e.g., furosemide, amphotericin B, ganciclovir, acyclovir, trimethoprim-sulfamethoxazole, and the aminoglycosides. Similar to with other organ transplants, other early renal complications after LT requiring treatment include hypertension, hypomagnesemia, and hyperkalemia.

Rejection following LT

Hyperacute rejection has been documented following LT in a number of case reports. Acute cellular rejection after LT is characterized by lymphocyte-predominant inflammatory infiltrate around blood vessels and/or airways. This syndrome of acute rejection is rare in the immediate post-transplantation period prior to hospital discharge, likely because of the relatively high level of immunosuppression that normally follows lung transplantation. Symptoms of acute rejection include non-productive cough, dyspnea, and fatigue, although a number of people with rejection can be asymptomatic. Signs of rejection include fever, rales and wheezes on exam, hypoxia, and a fall in forced expiratory volume in 1 second (FEV_1). Radiographic findings associated with acute rejection are non-specific, including septal line thickening, new pleural effusions, and new or increased air-space disease. When acute rejection is suspected early after transplantation, infection must be excluded, since infection and rejection can occur simultaneously and can be confused even histologically. The treatment of allograft rejection depends on severity and clinical setting. Treatment protocols also vary according to different centers but are similar to those described in other transplanted organs (Chapter 3).

Early infections

The rate of infectious complications is higher in LT patients than in recipients of other solid organs, accounting for more than 20% of mortality in the first 30 days following LT. There are multiple factors contributing to this higher infection rate. First, the possibility of organ donation is established by donors' brain death, and hence donors are intubated and mechanically ventilated. This exposes donor lungs to aspiration, airway colonization, and parenchymal infections. Second, LT recipients are commonly intubated for longer periods of time after their operation than other solid organ transplant recipients, further increasing their risk of pneumonia. Third, the lung allografts, like the bowel, are unique among organ transplants in that they are exposed continuously to the external environment, and consequently, to potential pathogens. Finally, two important pulmonary defense mechanisms, the cough reflex and mucociliary clearance, are impaired in transplanted lungs. All of these factors increase LT patients' susceptibility to pulmonary infections and, in fact, the lung is the site of the majority of their post-transplant infections.

Bacterial infections

The majority of infections in LT recipients are caused by bacteria, and the most common bacterial infections in these patients are pneumonia. Bacterial pneumonias occur most frequently in the early postoperative period, although the incidence has decreased with routine antibiotic prophylaxis against any potential pathogens isolated during the first 7–10 days. Gram-negative bacilli are the most common causative organisms, although Gram-positive bacteria including methicillin-resistant *Staphylococcus aureus* (MRSA) have become important pathogens as well. Clinically, these infections present with fever, new or increased radiographic infiltrates, and the presence of a new or newly predominant organism by sputum Gram stain and culture. The diagnosis frequently is confirmed by bronchoscopy. Patients are treated with culture-directed antibiotics for 2–4 weeks, often accompanied by a modest reduction in immunosuppression. When a limited spectrum of antimicrobial sensitivity is available, the use of aerosolized antimicrobial therapy in additional to intravenous therapy may be helpful.

Potential host sources of contamination of the respiratory tract should be evaluated, particularly in patients with CF. Chronic sinus infection is common among CF patients and may act as a source of contamination of the lower respiratory tract. Gastroesophageal reflux is common in both CF and COPD patients and can lead to recurrent aspiration pneumonia in dependent regions of the lung. Elevation of head of bed and administration of pro-motility agents, in addition to acid suppression with proton pump inhibitors, will control the reflux in most cases. After an SLT, the native lung may become the site of pneumonia or a lung abscess. Standard therapy is recommended in the early post-transplant setting, although a focal structural abnormality may require surgical removal if it becomes the source of recurrent infection. Transplant patients are susceptible to infections with bacterial pathogens in sites other than the lungs. This includes catheter infections, wound infection, and *Clostridium difficile* colitis.

CMV and other viral infections

CMV is a chief opportunistic infection in LT recipients and the second most frequent infection in these patients overall. CMV disease in the lung transplant recipient can result from either (1) reactivation of a latent CMV infection acquired by the recipient prior to transplant, or (2) transmission of CMV to the recipient following transplant, from either the donor lung or transfused blood products, resulting in a new primary infection. The frequency of CMV disease, therefore, depends on whether the recipient and donor carry latent CMV, which is determined by the presence or absence of antibodies to CMV. Post-transplant infections are most frequent in recipients positive for CMV antibodies, indicative of prior CMV exposure, regardless of CMV status of donor. CMV infections in these patients are felt to be due to re-activation of their own latent infections, due to their immunosuppressive therapy. However, CMV infections are most severe in recipients negative for CMV antibodies who receive lungs from CMV-positive donors. CMV infections in these patients are felt to be due to primary infections with the virus transmitted from the allograft, which has been documented to occur in renal transplant recipients. Primary infections have been associated with more severe manifestations of disease, and higher mortality rates, than re-activation of latent infections. CMV and other viral infection are extremely rare in the first few weeks after transplantation, especially with the use of ganciclovir prophylaxis.

Herpes simplex virus (HSV) can cause necrotizing tracheobronchitis or esophagitis, and less frequently, pneumonitis in the early weeks post-transplant, but these infections have become uncommon with the widespread use of prophylactic acyclovir or ganciclovir. Epstein-Barr virus (EBV) may cause fever, malaise, pharyngitis, and adenopathy in LT patients, and contribute to development of PTLD. Respiratory syncytial virus (RSV) has been implicated in a broad spectrum of respiratory illness in lung and other solid organ transplant recipients, ranging from isolated rhinitis to fatal ARDS. RSV hyperimmune globulin and aerosolized ribavirin have been used to treat these infections, with successful outcomes.

Fungal infections

Fungal infection in the LT recipient is relatively rare, especially early after surgery. Candidemia can occur due to critical illness and recent surgery. *Candida albicans* may also cause invasive pneumonia following LT. The fungal source is usually the donor trachea.

Aspergillus species are the most common cause of fungal infections following LT, although they occur usually several months after the transplantation. *Aspergillus* may present as part of the resident flora of the recipient or it may cause an invasive infection, either an ulcerative tracheobronchitis involving the anastomosis and airways or a disseminated illness with pneumonitis and fungemia. *Aspergillus* airway colonization is not uncommon after LT, and in most cases is transient. Invasive *Aspergillus* disease, in contrast, is less common but frequently fatal. An ulcerative tracheobronchitis due to *Aspergillus* involving the anastomotic site and large airways also has been described and appears to be highly specific to LT and HLT. Unfortunately, symptoms are often minimal or absent in these infections initially, which can lead to a delay in diagnosis. Consequently, fungal infections are frequently disseminated at the time of recognition and are associated with high mortality rates. Some centers routinely use galactomannan antigenemia and beta-D-glucan assays to screen for invasive fungal infections such as aspergillosis, although the data on the use of these tests are limited. Beta-D-glucan assay, in particular, must be interpreted with caution because of false-positive results due to a variety of antibiotics.

Although sputum colonization may be treated with an azole or inhaled amphotericin B, such therapy rarely is able to clear the airways of fungus. In the absence of symptoms, a specific anatomical abnormality or radiographic changes suggesting pneumonitis, most patients with sputum colonization can be managed without specific antifungal therapy. When invasive *Aspergillus* infection is identified, therapy with treatment dose of voriconazole is required. Furthermore, during any infection in the LT recipient, including fungal infection, lowering the net level of immunosuppression should be considered.

Further reading

Augoustides JG, Watcha SM, Pochettino A, Jobes DR. Early tracheal extubation in adults undergoing single-lung transplantation for chronic obstructive pulmonary disease: pilot evaluation of perioperative outcome. *Interact Cardiovasc Thorac Surg* 2008; **7**: 755–8.

Bhorade SM, Stern E. Immunosuppression for lung transplantation. *Proc Am Thor Soc* 2009; **6**: 47–53.

Christie JD, Edwards LB, Aurora P, *et al.* The Registry of the International Society for Heart and Lung Transplantation: Twenty-sixth Official Adult Lung and Heart-Lung Transplantation Report – 2009. *J Heart Lung Transplant* 2009; **28**: 1031–49.

Lee JC, Christie JD. Primary graft dysfunction. *Proc Am Thorac Soc* 2009; **6**: 39–46.

Paul S, Escareno CE, Clancy K, *et al.* Gastrointestinal complications after lung transplantation. *J Heart Lung Transplant* 2009; **28**: 475–9.

Chapter 19

Long-term management and outcomes

Paul Corris

Key points

- Although the outcomes of lung transplantation lag behind those of other solid organs, clear evidence of a survival benefit exists for this procedure for patients with advanced lung disease as a whole.
- The long-term management of patients following lung transplantation should focus on the general medical health of the patient as much as monitoring of the graft, with particular emphasis on tight control of hypertension, diabetes, dyslipidemia, and renal function.
- Bronchiolitis obliterans syndrome remains the major barrier to improved longer term outcomes, though progress has been made in the approach to therapy. A subset of such patients with evidence of neutrophilic inflammation respond well to azithromycin.
- Viral, fungal, and bacterial infections remain common after lung transplantation, with the majority being due to common community pathogens rather than opportunists.
- The incidence of malignancy is increased following lung transplantation with skin cancers and post-transplant lymphoproliferative disorder most common

Successful lung transplantation (LT) requires a substantial continuous commitment from the patient and lifelong adherence to immunosuppressive medication. Patients are required to attend post-transplant clinics and undergo frequent testing to monitor graft status, drug levels, renal/hepatic function, glucose, and lipids. Although there remains a strong focus on monitoring the status of the lung graft, long-term outcomes are also directly dependent on trying to minimize the side effects of immunosuppression and careful attention to the function of other organs. LT is associated with higher rates of acute rejection than other solid organ transplantation, necessitating higher levels of immunosuppression. Moreover, the lung is also at greater risk of injury due to direct exposure to insults including pathogens and inorganic particles. This injury may increase the immunogenicity culminating in allograft rejection.

The nephrotoxicity associated with calcineurin inhibitors (CNIs) is well recognized, and a balance must be struck in deciding on the target level of drug between preventing episodes of acute rejection and maintaining renal function. Virtually all grafts are subject to a lifelong threat of rejection, and patients will generally require maintenance triple immunosuppressive therapy comprising CNI, cell-cycle inhibitor, and corticosteroid.

Patients beyond 6 months after transplantation will generally be seen at three monthly intervals. At each clinic visit, blood tests, chest radiograph, and lung function (forced expiratory volume in 1 second [FEV_1], forced vital capacity [FVC], forced expiratory flow 25–75% [FEF25–75%]) are performed. Some transplant centers perform surveillance bronchoscopy with lavage and transbronchial biopsy to detect indolent asymptomatic infection/or rejection up to the first year.

Long-term surveillance

Lungs

History, clinical examination, sequential lung function, and imaging provide the cornerstone of

Organ Transplantation: A Clinical Guide, ed. A.A. Klein, C.J. Lewis, and J.C. Madsen. Published by Cambridge University Press.

surveillance of the lungs following transplantation. Monitoring lung function has been shown to be particularly effective, and many units train recipients to perform home-based daily spirometry and self-report sustained falls in FEV_1. The development of new signs on physical examination such as crackles, squeaks, and a pleural effusion mandate further elucidation of cause. A detailed commentary on the lung-specific complications following transplantation follows in this chapter, and this should be used to drive the investigation plan and management. Shared care protocols with effective communication should be organized in patients who live at a distance from the transplant center to ensure that local follow-up includes monitoring of the lung function and imaging.

Patient

It has been increasingly realized that improved outcomes depend on careful review of the whole patient as well as monitoring of the lungs, and that careful management of general medical issues such as detection and control of systemic hypertension is very important. As a consequence, it is important that the long-term management and follow-up of such patients includes an ordered review. Systemic hypertension, renal dysfunction, dyslipidemia, and hyperglycemia are common complications and need careful monitoring and control via optimization of treatment. Hypertension is usually managed using angiotensin-converting enzyme (ACE) inhibitors or calcium channel blockers initially, and it is important to check on renal function and potassium levels shortly after commencement of the former. Statin therapy is required in the vast majority of patients to control lipids, and new onset diabetes may occur in up to 30% of recipients. Glycemic control should follow usual guidelines to prevent complications in the long term and commonly requires insulin.

Renal dysfunction that progresses with time is commonly seen as a consequence of CNI-based immunosuppression and mandates regular monitoring of estimated glomerular filtration rat, proteinuria, and drug levels at least at three monthly intervals. Finally physical examination of the patient is important, with specific emphasis on skin and lymph node regions, since skin cancers and post-transplant lymphoproliferative disorder (PTLD) are common and increase with time following LT.

Maintenance immunosuppression

Tacrolimus (TAC) is now the most commonly used calcineurin inhibitor, with mycophenolate mofetil (MMF) the most used anti-metabolite initiated post-LT. Several small single-center studies have suggested a trend toward reduced acute rejection episodes in LT patients treated with MMF and the potential for less long-term development of malignancy. Nearly all centers continue to use corticosteroid at a low maintenance dose ($\leq$10 mg per day), with fewer than 5% of patients weaned from this therapy. There are no controlled studies of steroid withdrawal in lung transplantation. The exact role of mammalian target of rapamycin (mTOR) inhibitors is not fully evaluated following lung transplantation; however, several studies suggest that they can be used to replace CNI in patients with renal dysfunction. For further details, see Chapter 3.

Although it is possible to establish a maintenance dose of immunosuppressive drugs using target drug levels, in practice the intensity of immunosuppression for any individual is often determined by clinical course. The optimal level of immunosuppression after LT can be perceived as a compromise between an acceptable number of acute rejections, the number of infections, and other complications of therapy, including blood count and renal function. The two largest biopsy studies have demonstrated that acute rejection is most prevalent in the first 6 months. Overall the data suggest that with target cyclosporine (CyA) levels of 200–400 ng/ml in the first 6 months after transplantation, approximately 50% of patients can expect to have at least one episode of acute rejection.

The monitoring of immunosuppression by using infection as a surrogate marker is both intuitively and practically more difficult than the monitoring of rejection. Epstein-Barr virus (EBV) polymerase chain reaction (PCR) monitoring of viral load has been proposed as a surrogate marker of immunosuppression and can be used to reduce the level of immunosuppression if an increase in the EBV copy load is measured. The majority of transplant physicians, however, simply monitor the frequency of viral, bacterial, and fungal infections, and as in a patient with deteriorating renal function, a non-rejecter with frequent infections may have their target drug levels reduced.

Therapeutic drug monitoring

CyA

Therapeutic drug monitoring using trough levels has been used since the start of lung transplantation programs. Studies in LT recipients have shown that C2 monitoring (CyA level at 2 hours post-dose) is the best single time point predictor of an abbreviated area under the concentration curve. Initial C2 levels should be between 1000–1500 ng/ml; after 6 months, the target level can be reduced to below 1000 ng/ml.

TAC

A recent comprehensive review has suggested that target trough levels should be between 10–25 ng/ml in the first 2 weeks, 10–20 ng/ml up to 3 months, and 10–15 ng/ml thereafter. In practice, however, these levels may be associated with worsening renal function, and moreover, full randomized trials of TAC have employed lower maintenance ranges.

Cell-proliferation inhibitors (sirolimus and everolimus)

Although these agents are not nephrotoxic in their own right, they do amplify the nephrotoxicity associated with CNI therapy. As a rule of thumb, the dose of CyA should be reduced by 50% if these drugs are added, with a target trough level of 50–80 ng/ml. Drug levels of sirolimus and everolimus should be kept between 3–8 ng/ml, as there is evidence of a lack of efficacy in levels of less than 3 ng/ml and increased toxicity in levels above 8 ng/ml.

Longer term management issues post-transplantation

Infection (also see Chapter 4C)

Infections are the commonest cause of morbidity and mortality at any point after LT, and the incidence of infection is higher in LT recipients compared with the recipients of any other solid organ. The combination of higher levels of immunosuppression and direct exposure to the external environment provides a plausible reason. Other predisposing conditions include denervation with impaired mucociliary clearance, reduced cough, and injury to the bronchial mucosa. Studies have also demonstrated that hypogammaglobulinemia may also occur, particularly in transplant recipients for emphysema receiving MMF therapy, and this should be excluded in a patient with regular bacterial infections.

Bronchial infections predominate, and the development of a cough productive of sputum positive for *Pseudomonas aeruginosa* may be the first sign of the development of chronic graft dysfunction, predating the development of bronchiolitis obliterans syndrome (BOS) by many months. Both common community viral and bacterial infections occur seasonally, and frequent infection has been associated with the development of BOS. Lower respiratory infections including pneumonia are also common and usually caused by regular community-associated viruses (e.g., influenza, parainfluenza, respiratory syncytial virus, adenovirus) and bacteria (e.g., *Streptococcus pneumoniae* and *Haemophilus influenza*) rather than opportunist infections despite immunosuppression. Two notable exceptions to this rule comprise cytomegalovirus (CMV) and *Pneumocystis jiroveci.* LT recipients are more susceptible to infection with intracellular bacteria such as *Legionella* spp and mycobacteria.

Pseudomonal infection is particularly troublesome in the context of chronic allograft dysfunction due to BOS. The onset of pseudomonal infection in the sputum or lavage should prompt the commencement of nebulized therapy such as colimycin on a twice-daily basis to reduce the colonizing load of bacteria in the lung, and this may be required on a permanent basis if colonization occurs.

Treatment of community-acquired lower airway respiratory tract infections or pneumonia should be as per guidelines for such infections in general; however, one must avoid the use of macrolide antibiotics without a reduction in CNI dosage and close monitoring of levels since there is a danger of precipitating acute renal failure. In practice, these antibiotics should be avoided as first-line agents.

A patient presenting with a diagnosis of pneumonia should be treated urgently with antibiotic therapy to cover both typical and atypical community bacteria, with appropriate culturing of blood, sputum, and pleural effusion if present. Urine should be sent for antigenemia. The antibiotics can subsequently be tailored by the microbiological results. A patient who is failing on this approach after 48 hours and in whom no positive microbiological diagnosis is forthcoming should undergo bronchoscopy and bronchoalveolar lavage with transbronchial biopsy.

Viral infection

Respiratory viral infections can occur at any time post-transplantation and, in common with the non-transplant population, occur seasonally. They can range from causing a mild coryzal illness to severe fulminant infection and are often complicated by secondary bacterial infections. Seasonal flu vaccination is recommended for all LT recipients.

CMV is the commonest viral pathogen isolated in the postoperative period and remains problematic post-transplantation despite surveillance monitoring and prophylaxis. Presentation with CMV disease can be variable with organ-specific features (e.g., lung, GI tract, CNS, or retina) or a non-specific, insidious presentation with symptoms of lethargy and malaise and low-grade temperature. Leukopenia may be present on blood tests. Disease typically occurs in the first 3 months, but it may be delayed by prophylaxis. Diagnosis is by CMV PCR detecting a significant elevation in viral DNA copies or observation of characteristic CMV viral inclusion bodies on tissue biopsy. Treatment is with intravenous (IV) ganciclovir or a 2-week course of valganciclovir (dose-titrated against renal function) depending on the degree of viremia. Relapse rates of 60% in primary infection and 20% in previously exposed recipients have been reported.

Fungal infection

Candida and *Aspergillus* account for the majority of fungal infections. Colonization is frequent, with a combined incidence of up to 85%, though the prevalence will vary considerably from center to center and depend on local environment and changes in environment. Any perturbation of surrounding soil associated with new buildings, for example, will lead to an increase in environmental *Aspergillus* spores.

Aspergillus is often asymptomatic and detected on surveillance bronchoscopy and lavage. True invasive *Aspergillus* infection is estimated at approximately 5% of LT recipients, with only 3% of those colonized progressing to invasive disease. However, *Aspergillus* colonization has been linked to airway complications such as bronchial stenosis.

The spectrum of presentation includes asymptomatic colonization, necrosis, ulceration at the anastomosis, invasive pulmonary disease, and systemic fungal sepsis. Systemic aspergillosis carries a high mortality of up to 75%. Voriconazole is the current treatment of choice, but care must be taken to reduce CNI doses and monitor levels because azole antifungal agents interact leading to an increase in CNI levels, which can rapidly become toxic and lead to acute renal failure.

Infection with *Pneumocystis jiroveci* was previously significant, but with the introduction of lifelong prophylaxis in the form of co-trimoxazole (Septrin), the incidence and morbidity has dramatically decreased.

Acute cellular rejection and surveillance biopsies

Acute allograft rejection is common, with most patients experiencing more than one episode in the first year. Though it is most commonly seen within the first 3 months, later presentation is also seen and should alert one to the possibility of poor adherence to immunosuppression. Acute rejection can be identified on lung biopsies obtained via transbronchial biopsy (TBBx) at fiberoptic bronchoscopy. Many transplant centers perform regular bronchoscopy and TBBx in addition to spirometry in the first year to enable early diagnosis and treatment of asymptomatic rejection, with the aim of preserving graft function and protecting against BOS. The role of surveillance TBBx remains controversial, with some centers advocating its usefulness and others declaring it an unjustified risk.

Acute rejection can be asymptomatic or present with low-grade fever, lethargy, dyspnea, and/or small pleural effusion on chest radiograph associated with a drop in pulmonary function. FEF 25–75% is a more sensitive marker of lung function and may fall before a decrease in other lung function values. Classification is according to histological criteria found on TBBx and ranges from none (A0) to severe (A4) (International Society for Heart and Lung Transplantation [ISHLT]) (Table 19.1).

Rejections grade A2 or above are usually treated with IV methylprednisolone (10 mg/kg) followed by tapering dose of augmented oral prednisolone (initially 1 mg/kg). Recurrent episodes of rejection and lymphocytic bronchiolitis are risk factors for chronic allograft rejection and dysfunction, with acute rejection being the single most important risk factor for the development of BOS. Treatment options for steroid-resistant cellular rejection include T-cell ablation with anti-thymocyte globulin or similar medications. Total lymphoid irradiation has been shown to be effective at controlling the frequency of rejection when drug-based immunosuppression has failed.

Table 19.1 Pathologic grading of lung rejection (ISHLT)

Category	Grade	Meaning	Appearance
A acute rejection	0	None	Normal lung parenchyma
	1	Minimal	Inconspicuous small mononuclear, perivascular infiltrates
	2	Mild	More frequent, more obvious, perivascular infiltrates. Eosinophils may be present.
	3	Moderate	Dense perivascular infiltrates, extension into interstitial space. Can involve endotheliosis, eosinophils, and neutrophils.
	4	Severe	Diffuse perivascular, interstitial and air-space infiltrates with lung injury. Neutrophils may be present.
B airway inflammation (lymphocytic bronchiolitis)	0	None	No evidence of bronchiolar inflammation
	1R	Low grade	Infrequent, scattered, or single-layer mononuclear cells in bronchiolar submucosa
	2R	High grade	Larger infiltrates of larger and activated lymphocytes in bronchiolar submucosa. Can involve eosinophils and plasmacytoid cells.
	X	Ungradeable	No bronchiolar tissue available

Non-cellular antibody-mediated rejection associated with the deposition of complement-activating antibody in the lung should also be considered in a patient failing to respond to steroid therapy and requires treatment directed toward B and plasma cells. The development of both donor-specific and non-HLA antibodies and subsequent development of BOS remains to be fully elucidated. Plasmapheresis, IV immunoglobulin G, and rituximab therapy has been advocated as effective treatment for acute antibody-mediated rejection, and patients who develop antibodies should probably receive MMF.

Chronic allograft dysfunction (BOS) (see also Chapter 4A)

BOS is characterized by progressive airflow obstruction and is a clinical diagnosis defined by a persistent, irreversible drop in pulmonary function (FEV_1, FVC, FEF25–75%) supported by radiological findings on high resolution CT, such as bronchial dilatation, tree in bud appearance, and mosaicism with air trapping, best seen in expiratory images. BOS is a diagnosis of exclusion and can be formulated only when other causes of drop in FEV_1 (i.e., acute rejection, infection, and bronchial anastomotic stricture) have been excluded by bronchoscopy, bronchoalveolar lavage (BAL), and TBBx. Clinically there may be squeaks found on auscultation. If alternative causes of reduced lung function are present, then they must be treated, and if the reduction in lung function persists, a final diagnosis of BOS can be made.

BOS is now the major limiting factor reducing long-term survival and quality of life after LT and remains a challenging problem despite improvements in other aspects of care. BOS affects up to 50–60% of patients surviving more than 5 years and is ultimately responsible for more than 30% of all deaths 3 years post-transplantation. The timing of onset is highly variable, ranging from months to years, with a median time from transplantation to diagnosis of 16–20 months. It also results in significantly reduced health-related quality of life, with more than 80% of patients being functionally limited 2 years after diagnosis.

The histological lesion of chronic rejection is obliterative bronchiolitis (OB), characterized by loss of epithelium, an increase in fibrosis, and eventual occlusion of the bronchiole by intraluminal granulation tissue. The mechanism is thought to be due to repeated injury and inflammation that causes airway epithelial damage and loss, resulting in an exaggerated healing response and fibro-proliferation involving myofibroblasts. BOS can be patchy in distribution and is not invariably seen on TBBx, despite a typical functional decline. Positive histology is not required to make a diagnosis (Table 19.2).

Recently the importance of detecting early, subclinical BOS before irreversible fibroproliferative disease has become established has been recognized, and a new stage of BOS 0-p has been added. This uses FEF 25–75% in addition to FEV_1 to diagnose loss of function. In established disease, patients experience repeated symptomatic infection followed by persistent colonization with organisms such as pseudomonas

Table 19.2 Severity criteria for BOS (ISHLT)

Stage	Spirometry
BOS 0	FEV_1 > 90% baseline, FEF25–75 > 75% baseline
BOS 0-p	FEV_1 81–90% baseline, FEF25–75 < or equal to 75% baseline
BOS 1	FEV_1 66–80% baseline
BOS 2	FEV_1 51–65% baseline
BOS 3	FEV_1 < or equal to 50% baseline

Baseline FEV_1: average of the two highest FEV_1 measurements obtained more than three weeks apart post transplantation without preceding bronchodilator therapy.

Table 19.3 Risk factors for development of BOS

Alloimmune	Non-alloimmune	
Recurrent acute rejection (A2 or above)	Primary graft dysfunction	Ischemic-reperfusion injury
Lymphocytic bronchiolitis on BAL	Viral infections	CMV pneumonitis community respiratory virus
HLA mismatching	Bacterial infection	Pseudomonas
Anti-HLA antibodies	Gastric reflux Airway ischemia Medication non-compliance Older donor age, prolonged graft ischemic time	

and aspergillus. It is unclear whether pseudomonas infection is a risk factor for development of BOS or simply a representation of damaged airways that are prone to colonization.

The rate of progression of disease can also be variable, including (1) sudden onset and acute deterioration followed by rapid decline of lung function; (2) initial acute deterioration in lung function followed by a plateau and prolonged period of stability; and (3) insidious onset with slow, progressive decline in lung function. Acute onset occurring early after surgery is associated with a worse prognosis. There are many risk factors both hypothesized and proven for developing BOS (Table 19.3).

Alloimmune-dependent risk factors

Alloimmune risk factors include number and severity of episodes of acute rejection, lymphocytic bronchiolitis, and HLA mismatching. Acute rejection is the most significant risk factor for development of chronic rejection. In multivariate analysis, three or more episodes of A2 grade or above acute rejection was strongly associated with the development of BOS. Late episodes of acute rejection are also associated with subsequent development of BOS. Lymphocytic bronchitis/bronchiolitis has been shown to be a risk factor for BOS independently of acute perivascular rejection.

Non–alloimmune-dependent risk factors

CMV pneumonitis is a recognized risk factor for BOS. Other viral and bacterial infections have also been implicated, as well as gastroesophageal reflux, medication non-compliance leading to low immunosuppression levels, and airway ischemia and injury. Primary graft dysfunction has also been shown to increase the risk.

Gastroesophageal reflux disease

Gastroesophageal reflux disease (GERD) is common after LT (65–70%) due to a combination of medication-induced gastroparesis and damage to the vagal nerve during surgery, causing delayed gastric emptying and altered lower esophageal sphincter function. Post LT, many asymptomatic patients are found to have GERD, as measured by 24-hour pH studies. Denervation of the lungs reduces the cough reflex, and the likelihood of silent aspiration is increased. This continuous micro-aspiration of gastric contents and bile acids may promote chronic inflammation, airway damage, and bacterial infection/colonization, all of which may predispose to BOS. GERD has been demonstrated to be a reversible cause of allograft dysfunction, and fundoplication has been shown to improve pulmonary function and improve survival in patients with graft dysfunction and reflux in uncontrolled studies, but this requires confirmation.

Treatment of BOS

Azithromycin is already used in the treatment of bronchiectasis, pan-bronchiolitis, and cystic fibrosis (CF) due to its anti-inflammatory and immunomodulatory effects. Studies to date have been on small numbers but have shown promising results using thrice weekly dosing at 250 mg or 500 mg once daily, with responders showing significant improvement in FEV_1. Response appears to be better in patients with higher levels of neutrophils on BAL and those who started treatment earlier post-transplantation. Randomized controlled trials to substantiate this effect are ongoing. Two phenotypes of allograft dysfunction have been proposed, given the apparent reversibility of a previously designated irreversible condition: (1) classic BOS, which does not respond to azithromycin and is associated with a BAL neutrophilia less than 15%; and (2) neutrophil-associated reversible airways disease, which is at least reversible in part with azithromycin and associated with a BAL neutrophilia greater than 15%.

Other treatments for BOS with uncontrolled studies suggesting benefit include cytolytic therapy, photophoresis, total lymphoid irradiation (TLI), cyclophosphamide, and methotrexate. TLI has been used with benefit in very small numbers of patients and has been shown to significantly slow the rate of decline of FEV_1, with some patients gaining lung function. Potentially TLI may have its role in rapidly deteriorating patients not responding to azithromycin.

There is uncontrolled evidence suggesting that switching patients to TAC from CyA slows the rate of decline in patients with BOS. Increasing maintenance immunosuppression is ineffective and generally leads to increasing problems with infection. Preventing infection may be an important strategy, but has not been formally examined in a clinical trial.

Post-transplant lymphoproliferative disorder

LT has the highest reported incidence of post-transplant lymphoproliferative disorder (PTLD; 4–10%) which is thought to be due to the higher degree and duration of immunosuppression needed to prevent rejection (further detail in Chapter 4A). The incidence of PTLD is highest in the first year, when it is usually polyclonal and responsive to reduced immunosuppression. Later disease is commonly monomorphic and has a clinical course resembling that of diffuse large B-cell lymphoma. Patients acquiring EBV infection from the donor are at highest risk of developing PTLD. World Health Organization classification of PTLD is shown in Table 19.4.

Diagnosis can be difficult, and a high index of suspicion is needed for diagnosis due to the varied clinical and histological presentation. Symptoms include malaise, sweats, and weight loss, or may be due to the site and extent of disease, e.g., lymphadenopathy. The commonest extranodal sites involved after LT are the allograft (69–89%) and the GI tract (20–34%). Excisional biopsies should be obtained wherever

Table 19.4 World Health Organization (WHO) classification of PTLD

Category	Subtype
Early lesions	Reactive plasmacytic hyperplasia
Polymorphic	Polyclonal or monoclonal
Monomorphic	Diffuse large B-cell lymphomas Burkitt's/ Burkitt's-like lymphoma Plasma cell myeloma
T-cell lymphomas	Peripheral T-cell lymphoma
Others	Hodkgin's disease-like Plasmacytoma-like Myeloma

possible for histology, including immunohistology and determination of EBV status.

Survival is variable, with some centers quoting 25–60% survival rates. Factors predicting a poor outcome are performance status 3 or 4 at the time of diagnosis, late presentation following transplantation, monomorphic disease, and CNS and allograft involvement.

Initial treatment for polymorphic EBV-positive disease is reduced immunosuppression, and approximately 25–50% of patients respond to reduction alone. No clear benefit has been shown for antiviral therapy. More than 90% of PTLD after solid organ transplant is CD20 positive, defining a role for anti-CD20 antibodies (rituximab), which have been associated with complete remission. Response rates with rituximab are around 60%, which is similar to cyclophosphamide, doxorubicin, vincristine, and prednisone (CHOP) chemotherapy given in the context of more aggressive, CNS disease or those failing to respond to rituximab.

Nephrotoxicity

CNIs are nephrotoxic and have a deleterious effect on kidney function. This is in addition to the insults to renal function in the peri-operative period, such as hypotension, sepsis, and medications. It is not unusual for patients to need a period of ultrafiltration or hemodialysis in the immediate postoperative period. Ninety-one percent of patients exhibit a decrease in renal function at 6 months post-transplantation. The presence of hypertension post-transplantation has been linked to more severe renal dysfunction requiring aggressive blood pressure control with ACE inhibitors or angiotensin receptor blockers. Factors worsening

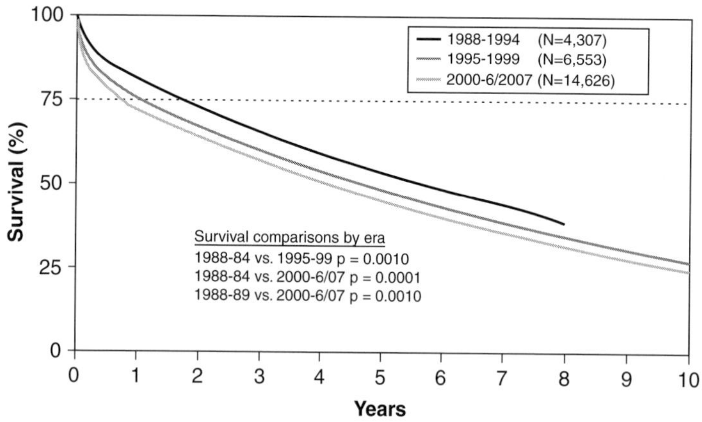

Figure 19.1 Adult lung transplantation, survival by era (transplants: January 1988 – June 2007). From *J Heart Lung Transplant* 2009; 28: 989–1049. Reproduced with permission from the International Society for Heart and Lung Transplantation.

chronic renal failure include hypertension, hyperlipidemia, and diabetes mellitus.

Skin and other cancers

The commonest malignancy after LT is skin cancer, with approximately 8% of patients developing this after 5 years and 18% at 10 years. Other non-PTLD solid malignancies are seen in 6% and 14%, respectively. Patients should be advised to undergo yearly skin checks and always wear sun block outdoors.

Osteoporosis

Osteoporosis is an important cause of morbidity post-transplantation and has the potential to compromise outcome after LT due to poor mobility and pain secondary to fractures. The frequency of osteoporosis is increased after LT due to the use of long-term immunosuppressive medication, particularly steroids, occurring on top of already demineralized bone due to chronic disease and prolonged immobility pre-transplantation. Studies have shown that patients lose approximately 5% of bone density within the first transplant year, with a post-transplantation osteoporosis prevalence of 78% and fracture rate of 18%. Patients should have bone scans at 3–5 yearly intervals following transplantation, and osteopenia or osteoporosis should be treated with bisphosphonates and calcium supplementation.

Drug-induced diabetes mellitus and dyslipidemia (metabolic syndrome)

The reported incidence of diabetes mellitus after LT is 24.3% at 1 year post-transplantation and 33.5% at 5 years. Dyslipidemia is virtually universal in patients other than those with CF and statin therapy is required. Indeed, there is some evidence to support the role of statin therapy as an anti-inflammatory agent in LT leading to improved outcomes.

Venous thromboembolism

The incidence of venous thromboembolism is 8–29% after LT. The factors responsible are not well understood; however, concomitant infection, immobility, and immunosuppression all contribute. It is therefore important to consider pulmonary embolism as a cause of breathlessness in a patient presenting acutely with this symptom post-transplantation.

Outcomes

LT is now a proven treatment option for carefully selected patients with end-stage lung disease, such as CF, interstitial lung diseases, pulmonary arterial hypertension, and emphysema. The procedure is performed to provide survival benefit, alleviate symptoms, and to improve quality of life. Though outcomes continue to lag behind those of other solid organs, the current mean actuarial 5-year survival rate is 50% according to the ISHLT database (Figure 19.1). Individual centers report 5-year survival rates of up to 75%. The increased survival rate over the last few years is mainly due to a better operative and peri-operative outcome, thanks to improved surgical techniques, peri-operative anesthetic, and intensive care management. Careful longer term surveillance and management as described previously has also contributed. Chronic allograft dysfunction or chronic rejection,

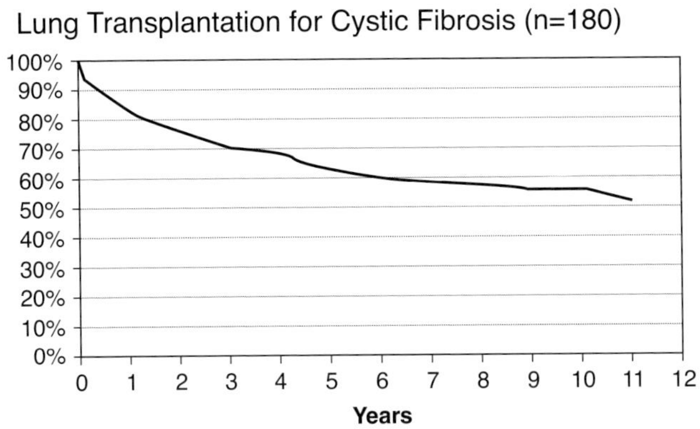

Figure 19.2 Actuarial survival after lung transplantation for cystic fibrosis, Newcastle Freeman Hospital.

histologically diagnosed as OB, remains the leading cause of morbidity and of late mortality after LT, which accounts for up to 30% of all deaths between 3 and 5 years after the transplantation procedure. Although the prevalence of OB/BOS after LT has not changed significantly, remaining at 40–50% 5 years after transplantation, some patients now respond to therapy, which may explain why patients with this condition live longer. Better understanding and use of immunosuppression together with an appreciation of the need to monitor and control general health has improved longer term care of recipients.

Survival rates do vary according to transplant procedure, era, patient age, and underlying diagnosis, and young patients with CF in particular have excellent outcomes (Figure 19.2). Several centers report 10-year survival rates in excess of 50%. Pooled data suggest better long-term outcomes and an improved health-related quality of life for younger patients with emphysema undergoing BLT.

A survival benefit following transplantation has been shown for advanced pulmonary disease as a whole, but there is some debate in the literature over patients with advanced COPD. Studies following LT in general have reported significant improvements in all domains of health-related quality of life following transplantation, and the majority of long-term survivors are living independent lives, with many when it is feasible returning to full-time education or employment.

Further reading

Belperio JA, Weigt SS, Fishbein MC, Lynch JP. Chronic lung allograft rejection: Mechanisms and therapy. *Proc Am Thorac Soc* 2009; **6**: 108–21.

Christie JD, Edwards LB, Aurora P, *et al.* The Registry of the International Society for Heart and Lung Transplantation: Twenty-sixth Official Adult Lung and Heart-Lung Transplantation Report. *J Heart Lung Transplant* 2009; **28**: 989–1049.

Iverson M, Corris PA. Immunosuppression. *Eur Respir Mono* 2009; **45**: 147–68.

Kotloff RM, Ahya VN. Medical complications of lung transplantation. *Eur Resp J* 2009; **22**: 334–42.

Yates B, Murphy DM, Forrest IA, *et al.* Azithromycin reverses airflow obstruction in established bronchiolitis obliterans syndrome. *Am J Resp Crit Care Med* 2005; **172**: 772–5.

Chapter 20

Pediatric lung transplantation

Stuart C. Sweet and Samuel Goldfarb

Key points

- Pediatric lung transplantation presents many unique challenges compared with adult lung transplant and is a viable therapy for infants, children, and adolescents with end-stage pulmonary parenchymal and vascular disease.
- Survival after pediatric lung transplantation has improved over the past decade; however, long-term survival rates remain well below those of heart and other solid organ transplants.
- Ongoing challenges remain regarding ensuring that patient selection decisions and allocation systems maximize survival and/or quality-of-life benefit.
- Increased competition for organs due to increased numbers of adults undergoing lung transplantation will require innovative strategies to ensure that children have equal opportunity for transplant.

The first human lung transplantation (LT) was performed by Hardy in 1963; however, it was not until the early 1980s that challenges related to rejection and healing of the airway anastomoses were successfully overcome. Interest in offering such potential life-saving interventions to children was kindled by success in adults; the first pediatric LT was performed at the University of Toronto in 1987. Now into a third decade, LT and heart–lung transplantation (HLT) have become accepted therapies for end-stage pulmonary disease in children. As of June 2009, 1400 LT and more than 500 HLT in pediatric recipients have been reported to the Registry for the International Society for Heart and Lung Transplantation (ISHLT). After dropping from more than 80 in the late 1990s to below 70 in the early 2000s, the number of pediatric LTs per year has risen steadily and exceeded 100 for the first time in 2008 (Figure 20.1). Interestingly, the steady increase likely reflects increases outside the United States, as the number of transplants performed there has remained steady in recent years.

Elsewhere in this volume, the details of all aspects of LT from an adult perspective, including patient selection, surgical techniques, early and late complications, and outcomes, have been covered (Section 3, Chapters 14–19). This chapter addresses aspects of LT that are unique to infants, children, and adolescents.

Indications/contraindications

The primary diagnoses leading to LT in the pediatric age group are cystic fibrosis (CF), making up more than 50% of the population, and pulmonary hypertension, either idiopathic or related to congenital heart disease.

A detailed breakdown of diagnoses for which children are considered for LT is shown in Figure 20.2, grouped by age at time of transplantation. In children younger than 1 year, the most frequent diagnoses are those seen primarily in children (pulmonary hypertension associated with congenital heart disease, pulmonary vein stenosis, and rarely, alveolar capillary dysplasia) or unique to children (pediatric interstitial lung disease syndrome disorders, including diseases of surfactant metabolism such as surfactant protein B and C mutations and ABCA3 transporter mutations). CF becomes the most common indication in patients 6–11 years of age. In the 12–17 year group, nearly 70% of pediatric LTs are performed in patients with CF. In the most recent decade, the relative percentage of children with primary pulmonary hypertension requiring LT has diminished significantly, largely because of

Organ Transplantation: A Clinical Guide, ed. A.A. Klein, C.J. Lewis, and J.C. Madsen. Published by Cambridge University Press.

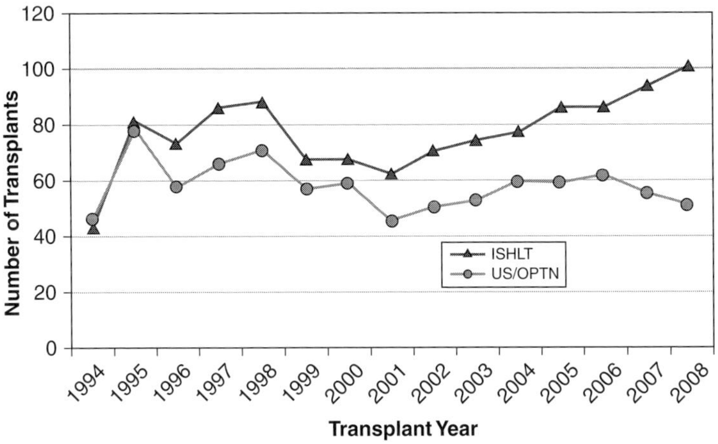

Figure 20.1 Number of pediatric lung and heart–lung transplants performed each year internationally (International Society for Heart and Lung Transplantation [ISHLT]) and in the United States (Organ Procurement and Transplantation Network [OPTN]).

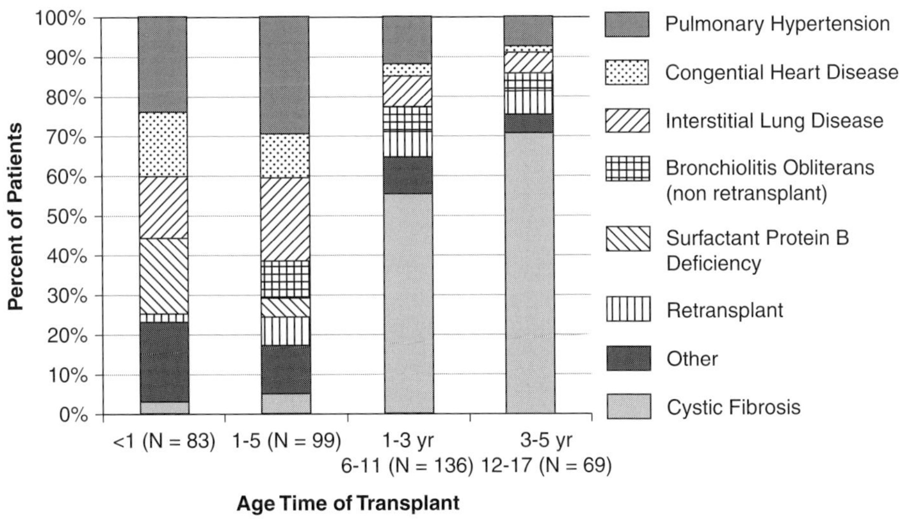

Figure 20.2 Indications for pediatric lung transplantation.

the introduction of effective medical therapies including prostaglandins (epoprostenol), phosphodiesterase inhibitors (bosentan), and sildenafil. In contrast, in spite of a steady increase in the median survival for CF, the relative percentage of CF as the diagnosis leading to pediatric lung transplant has not changed appreciably in recent years.

Contraindications for LT in children generally parallel those in adults and are described in detail in Chapter 14. These include malignancy within the last 2 years, sepsis, multi-organ failure, active tuberculosis, acquired immune deficiency syndrome, hepatitis B or C, severe neuromuscular disease, and documented refractory non-adherence to a medical regime.

There are several pediatric-specific aspects to the list of relative contraindications. Children, particularly infants, are more likely than adults to require mechanical ventilation at referral or prior to LT. Although mechanical ventilation is a significant risk factor for morbidity and mortality in adults and older children, the impact on infants is less clear. Therefore, ventilator use is generally not considered a contraindication in infants and older children unless associated with systemic infection.

Because the majority of children referred for LT have CF as their underlying diagnosis, organisms harbored in their airways may raise concerns. In general, colonization with multi- or pan-resistant

Table 20.1 Indications for and timing of pediatric lung transplantation

Specific disease	Timing of referral
Surfactant deficiencies	Patients with SPB deficiency and ABCA3 deficiency with refractory respiratory failure should be referred immediately. Patients with SPC deficiency and less severe forms of ABCA3 deficiency may respond to medical therapy and should be referred when unrelenting progression of disease develops.
Idiopathic pulmonary hypertension	Patients who present in NYHA class III or IV or have evidence of right heart failure should be referred immediately. Patients who fail to respond adequately to vasodilator therapy should also be referred.
Eisenmenger syndrome	When the trajectory of PH appears to be worsening with impaired exercise tolerance and worsening quality of life
Other pulmonary vascular disorders (pulmonary vein stenosis, alveolar capillary dysplasia)	These patients should be referred immediately since they typically do not respond to medical management and are at risk for sudden death.
Cystic fibrosis	Patients with percent predicted FEV_1 values less than 30%, frequent hospitalizations, and refractory hypoxemia or hypercapnia should be referred for transplant.
Bronchopulmonary dysplasia	Patients with recurrent or severe episodes of respiratory failure or evidence for progressive pulmonary hypertension
Diffuse parenchymal lung disease	Patients without evidence for systemic disease that could affect outcome should be referred early.

ABCA3: ATP-binding cassette subfamily A member 3 gene; FEV_1: forced expiratory volume in 1 second; NYHA: New York Heart Association Classification; PH: pulmonary hypertension; SPB: pulmonary associated surfactant protein B. Adapted from Faro *et al.*, 2007.

Pseudomonas aeruginosa is not felt to pose increased risk. However, *Burkholderia cepacia* complex, particularly *B. cenocepacia* and a related organism (*B. gladioli*), carries significant risk. Interestingly, infection with either one of the two so-called epidemic strains common in the United States (strain PHDC and the Midwest clone) are associated with better survival when compared with infection with non-epidemic strain. In general, *B. cenocepacia* colonization remains an absolute contraindication to LT at a significant percentage of pediatric centers.

Finally, non-adherence can be a particularly challenging in pediatrics, as often the child's parents share significant responsibility for following the medical regimen. In this situation, care must be taken to minimize the risk that denying a child the opportunity for transplant will be perceived to be a punishment for his or her parents. In many centers, such psychosocial risks become a significant contraindication only when other medical risk factors are present or the child and family demonstrate inability to meet a set of agreed upon expectations for care and follow-up.

Once listed, determining the appropriate time to accept organs becomes the next challenge. Ideally, based on the trajectory of illness in spite of optimal medical therapy, patients are deemed ready to accept organs when they are at significant risk of dying without an LT. Although in some cases, such as surfactant protein B deficiency or alveolar capillary dysplasia, this is a straightforward decision, in other cases, such as surfactant protein C deficiency, the unpredictable natural history of the disease process makes this decision difficult (Table 20.1). Even in the case of CF, for which a significant body of modeling work exists, controversy exists regarding whether pediatric LT for CF confers a survival benefit. In this setting of limited predictive data, variable disease course, and unique diagnoses, most pediatric centers use multiple factors, including diminished waiting list survival estimates (when available), worsening growth and nutrition status, increased frequency of hospitalizations, and potential for significant improvement in overall quality of life as components of the decision to accept organs.

Allocation

Decisions regarding the timing of transplantation are also influenced by the efficacy of the underlying allocation system (see Chapters 40 and 41). In the United States, legislative guidance for organ allocation systems include a directive to "recognize the differences in health and in organ transplantation issues between children and adults throughout the system and adopt criteria, polices, and procedures that address the unique health care needs of children." For this reason, and because end-stage organ dysfunction can significantly impair growth and development, US transplant allocation systems give priority to children. Also, due to steady increases in the number of adults receiving LT, children face increased competition with adults for organs (this situation may explain the finding that the ratio of transplants to waiting list deaths in pediatric candidates remains higher than that in adults). For these reasons, preferential allocation of lungs from pediatric donors to pediatric recipients was included in the Lung Allocation System (LAS), introduced in 2005, which allocates lungs to candidates over 12 years of age based on a combination of transplant benefit and medical urgency. The LAS models include several indicators of disease severity, including forced vital capacity (FVC), body mass index, serum creatinine, presence of diabetes, 6-minute walk test distance, supplemental oxygen requirement, serum carbon dioxide levels, need for assisted ventilation, functional status, and presence of pulmonary hypertension. More recently, a mechanism to reduce waiting list mortality for LT candidates younger than 12 years of age was implemented. The new system stratifies younger patients based on objective medical urgency criteria and distributes organs from donors under 12 years of age over a much greater distance before offering them to older children or adults. Taken together, these changes to lung allocation in the United States have significantly reduced the duration of waiting time required to receive deceased donor lungs and thus increased the frequency of "urgent" referrals, particularly of children and adolescents with respiratory failure, some with unknown etiology. Because, apart from infants, LT from mechanical ventilation poses increased risk, and the child's level of illness usually precludes an effective psychosocial evaluation, most centers have been extremely selective regarding accepting this group of patients for LT evaluation.

Surgical procedure and complications

The LT and HLT procedures performed in pediatric recipients are essentially the same as those used in adults and described in Chapter 16. Size matching of organs is based primarily on donor height, and to a lesser extent weight, with donors within 25% above or below the recipient height considered acceptable.

The main difference in surgical technique relates to the increased use of bypass. Because some studies have suggested that cardiopulmonary bypass (CPB) is an independent or contributing factor for primary graft dysfunction (PGD), most adult centers attempt to perform lung transplantation without CBP by using dual-lumen endotracheal tubes to allow single-lung ventilation (see Chapter 17). Because dual-lumen tubes are not widely available or utilized in pediatric settings, CPB is used in most pediatric LT. There is some evidence that CBP does not carry additional risk of PGD in pediatric recipients, based on a single-center comparison of the incidence of PGD in a large number of pediatric and adult LT recipients.

The vast majority of pediatric LT recipients receive two lungs; for those with CF and other suppurative diseases, the decision is based on the infection risk. For the remainder, the decision is generally dictated by a desire to provide as much healthy tissue as possible to balance the potential that the lungs will not grow commensurate with the patient and/or develop chronic allograft dysfunction. When HLT is a consideration, the choice typically hinges on whether irreversible left ventricular failure is present. In congenital heart disease, where concomitant repair will be required, LT (as opposed to HLT) is often considered in order to limit the potential for cardiac allograft complications.

Because of the relative scarcity of donors under the age of 12 years, younger pediatric candidates are more likely to be considered for technical LT variants than adolescents or adults. Historically there have been two approaches used. In the first, initially reported by Starnes and colleagues, a lower lobe from each of two living donors, serves as one lung for the recipient. Living donor lung transplantation (LDLT) has been used most often in children and adults with CF with an unexpected and rapid progression of their disease. Few centers offer LDLT because the procedure requires significant resources and the donor lobectomy carries significant risk (see Chapter 15).

Another area of technical variation involves reducing the size of lungs procured from larger (often adolescent or adult) deceased donors. Lung size may be reduced by lobectomy (most commonly involving the right middle lobe or lingula), resection of a tissue wedge by a linear stapling device, transplant of a single lobe, or split LT (where two smaller "lungs" are created from a single deceased donor lung). Case series suggest that outcomes in recipients of reduced-size transplant are comparable to those of recipients of full-sized grafts in adults.

Although the smaller airways and vasculature of children raise the possibility of a higher frequency of anastomotic complications, this has not been documented. A systematic review of airway complications in a large pediatric center found similar frequencies of complications in pediatric age group as compared with adults.

Management challenges

The post-transplant management of pediatric LT recipients is guided by the strategies used in adults (see Chapter 18). A consortium of pediatric LT programs has developed a consensus approach to immunosuppression, including tacrolimus, mycophenolate mofetil, and prednisone. For this consortium, induction remains a center-specific decision with 60–80% of recipients receiving some form of induction, usually an interleukin-2 receptor antagonist. Most pediatric centers perform surveillance biopsies.

However, several important challenges exist for pediatric recipients. Perhaps the most important relates to the diagnosis of bronchiolitis obliterans syndrome (BOS). Although spirometric measurement of forced expiratory volume in 1 second (FEV_1) and forced expiratory flow (FEF) 25–75% are necessary for the clinical diagnosis of BOS, children under 4 years of age are generally not able to perform spirometry, and results are not considered reliable until 6 years of age. Using external compression vests, infant pulmonary function testing can provide information regarding the presence of airflow obstruction, but requires specialized equipment and experience. Because they require anesthesia, however, such tests cannot be performed with the same frequency as conventional spirometry. Moreover, BOS criteria do not exist for parameters obtained using infant pulmonary function testing. For older children, because spirometric parameters are proportional to height, the most recent BOS grading scheme revision recommends that percent predicted values, rather than absolute measurements, be used for calculating the BOS score. This approach has yet to be validated. Thus, for infants and to lesser extent older children, diagnosis of chronic allograft dysfunction by pulmonary function criteria is problematic.

Transbronchial biopsies (TBBx) are also more challenging in pediatrics, particularly in infants and toddlers. Due to limitations imposed by airway size, endoscopes used for bronchoscopy in young children have a suction channel 1.2 mm in diameter (compared with 2.0 mm or greater for larger scopes). Although smaller forceps that fit into these channels are available, in practice, obtaining sufficient tissue for diagnosis of rejection is often quite difficult. More importantly, adequate airway tissue is rarely present in such biopsies to allow assessment of airway inflammation ("B" grade) or BOS grade. For this reason, establishing a histological diagnosis of chronic lung allograft dysfunction in infants and young children often requires performing an open lung biopsy. When sufficient pulmonary function information is not available to establish a BOS diagnosis and biopsies are non-diagnostic, many pediatric centers rely more heavily on imaging modalities such as ventilation/perfusion scanning and inspiratory/expiratory high-resolution CT scanning to assess for the presence of airflow obstruction and guide decisions regarding obtaining open lung biopsies before initiation of therapy for chronic allograft dysfunction.

For children, therapeutic challenges also exist. Many newer medications, including immunosuppressant and anti-infective agents, do not have a pediatric license. Most do not include the liquid forms required for young children. Liquid preparations must be specially prepared by the pharmacist and may have a short shelf life. Thus for patients not residing near a pediatric medical center, they may be difficult to readily obtain. Moreover, absorption and pharmacokinetic data for infants and children may not exist, making dosing decisions for drugs with narrow therapeutic indices more complex. Finally, generic preparations for many of the primary immunosuppression agents have recently become or will soon become available. The potential variations allowed by the generic approval process add another dimension of complexity to the therapeutic decision making for pediatric LT recipients.

Finally, infections pose greater risk in children, particularly infants. Young children may not have completed their primary immunization series by the time they undergo transplantation. The efficacy of immunization in the setting of immunosuppression is unclear. Although there is some evidence that live viral vaccines may be safely administered after transplant, most centers remain reluctant to give live viral vaccines. For other infectious agents, particularly

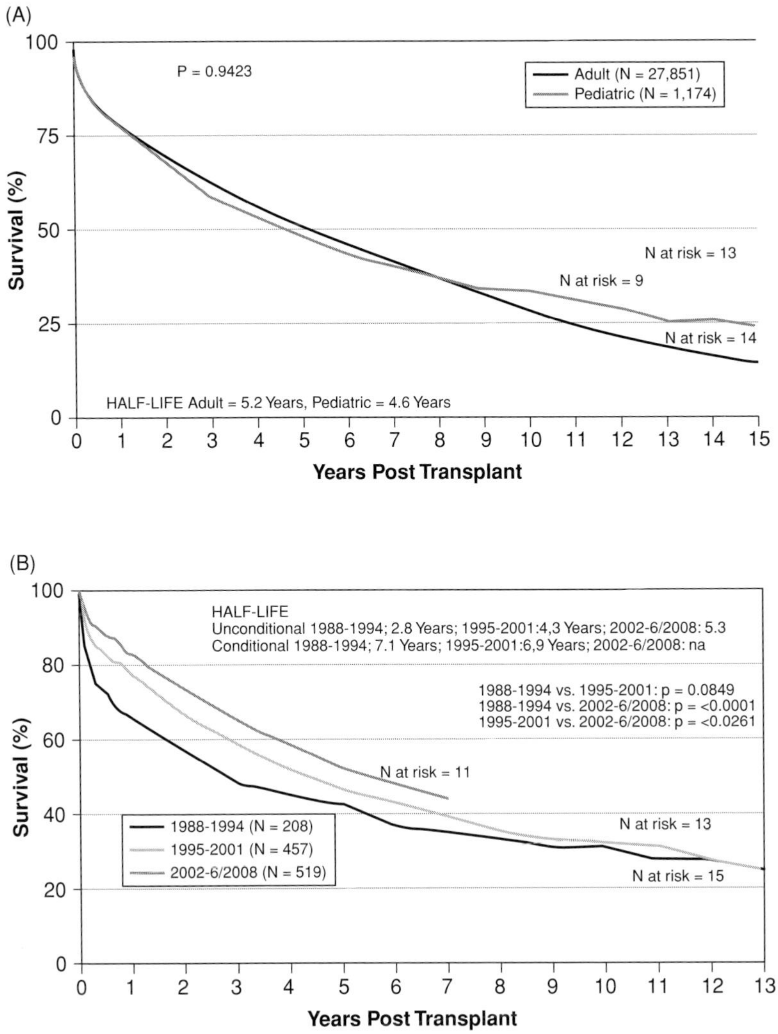

Figure 20.3 (A) Survival after pediatric compared with adult lung transplant. (B) Survival after pediatric lung transplant, stratified by era of transplant. Figures modified, with permission, from Aurora *et al.*, 2010.

respiratory pathogens, children are often immunologically naive. Thus it is not surprising that respiratory viral infections (RVI) have been shown to effect outcome in children. In an international, multi-center retrospective study of pediatric LT recipients, RVI was an independent risk factor for 1-year mortality (hazard ratio = 2.6), with younger age identified as one of the risk factors for RVI.

Although the impact of cytomegalovirus (CMV) in LT has been significantly reduced by the availability of ganciclovir, children are more likely to be CMV negative and thus have higher risk for CMV complications. Indeed, CMV was associated with increased mortality within the first post-transplant year in pediatric LT recipients. Adenovirus and paramyxoviruses including parainfluenza and respiratory syncytial virus can cause significant lung injury or mortality. Many centers treat these viruses aggressively with cidofovir and ribavirin, respectively. Lastly, respiratory fungal infections were identified as a risk factor for mortality in a retrospective, multi-center study of pediatric LT recipients.

In addition to direct effects of infection, the incidence of post-transplant lymphoproliferative disorder (PTLD) in pediatric LT recipients is higher than that in adults. Elevated quantitative polymerase chain reaction (PCR) for Epstein-Barr virus (EBV) has been shown to be a sensitive and somewhat specific marker for PTLD; most centers monitor this test on a regular basis. When EBV PCR is elevated, positron emission tomography can be a sensitive and specific test to identify PTLD. Other morbidities associated with

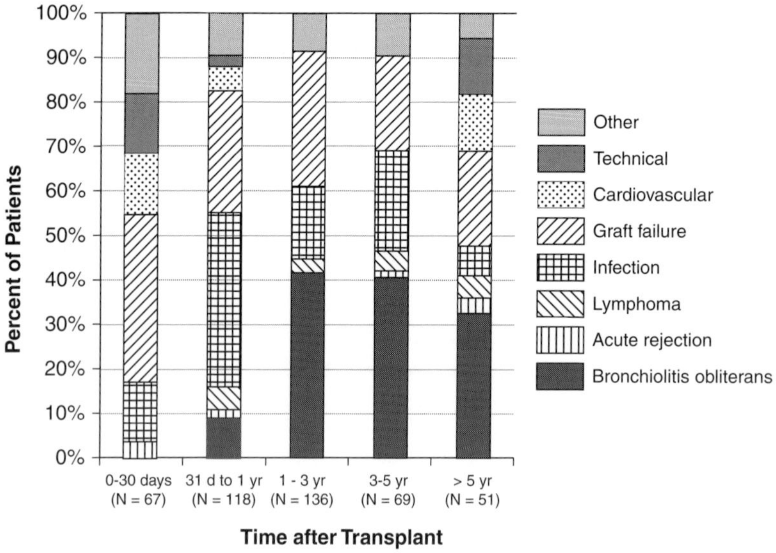

Figure 20.4 Causes of death after pediatric lung transplant. Data adapted from Aurora *et al.*, 2010.

LT, in particular end-stage renal disease and diabetes, occur with similar frequency to that of adults.

Outcomes

In spite of the challenges outlined above, pediatric LT recipients have survival comparable to that of adults (see Chapter 12 and Figure 20.3A), with median survival in the most recent ISHLT registry report of 4.6 years. Outcomes for pediatric recipients have demonstrated improvement in the most recent cohort (Figure 20.3B). This era effect is due primarily to reduction in early mortality; the era effect disappears when comparison is conditional on survival of at least 1 year.

One-year mortality risk, in addition to the era effect noted above, was increased in patients on the ventilator at the time of transplant (relative risk [RR] = 3.73) and lower in patients receiving bilateral lung transplantation (RR = 0.40). One-year mortality risk was also lower in centers performing more than five transplants per year. Five-year mortality risk again includes an era effect as well as being on a ventilator prior to transplant (RR = 2.69). However, one large single center found no mortality risk associated with ventilator use in infants. Younger children had lower 5-year mortality than adolescents, typically ascribed to poor adherence in adolescence, but the fact that infants appear to have a lower incidence of acute rejection and BOS may also play a role.

Re-transplant accounts for roughly 7% of pediatric LT, compared with only 2.5% in adults. The frequency of re-transplantation has increased recently, perhaps as a result of the new allocation system in the United States. However, outcomes are worse for re-transplant patients in both adults and children, with only 37% 5-year survival in the most recent ISHLT cohort.

Causes of death after pediatric LT are depicted in Figure 20.4. Graft failure and infection are important causes of death in the first year after transplant. In the first 30 days after transplant, surgical complications are an important cause of death, with a slightly higher rate than in adults (13.4% versus 8.2%). After the first 30 days and before a year post-transplant, infection from any cause accounts for roughly 40% of deaths. Infection remains an important cause of death throughout the follow-up period, but by 1–3 years after transplant, BOS becomes the leading cause of death, accounting for nearly 40% of the mortality. This is a somewhat higher frequency than in adults, where BOS is responsible for roughly 25% of deaths beyond the first year. This difference can be accounted for by the larger percentage of deaths in adults from non-PTLD malignancies and "other" causes.

Poor long-term outcomes in adolescents may be one reason why more pediatric LTs are not being performed, particularly in the United States. Most reports ascribe this to poor adherence in the teenage population, as medical non-adherence appears to be more common in pediatric LT recipients. Yet other mechanisms, including the impact of hormonal changes associated with puberty, have not been fully explored.

Nonetheless, adherence is a significant area of focus during the assessment of candidates pretransplant and is an important consideration post-transplant. Most pediatric transplant practitioners have encountered adolescents who developed graft failure after choosing to stop taking their immunosuppressant medications.

Further study of adherence in pediatric transplant is needed. Literature regarding objective measures of adherence, identification of non-adherence risk factors, and potential interventions is limited. One area of particular interest is care transition. Transplant candidates and recipients undergo several transitions during their experience during the process of diagnosing the underlying disease leading to transplant, with new care providers often introduced. Another care team is encountered after referral to the transplant center, usually followed by relocation to the transplant center to await transplant. After a successful transplant, patients return home a few months later and often need follow-up with new pediatric subspecialty care providers. Outside of the medical arena, adolescence is a prolonged period of transition during which increased independence is attained, particularly when attending college or university. This process places increased responsibility for adherence on the adolescent/young adult patient. Unfortunately, maturity and judgment don't always develop commensurate with independence. Depression, anxiety, and adjustment disorders may also play a role in this process; all are comorbidities associated with chronic disease in the adolescent population. The CF patient registry reports an incidence of these problems of 5–17%, with increasing frequency in older teenagers. Depression rates in general in patients pretransplant can be as high as 20%. Thus access to mental health services for treatment of depression is a critical aspect of pretransplant care. Moreover, because transplantation does not guarantee cure for anxiety or adjustment or depressive disorders, transplant care providers must be cognizant of persistence or recurrence of these problems post-transplant. Finally, transition of care to an "adult" transplant center occurs (usually between the ages of 18 and 21 years), often with expectations for minimal parental involvement in the care process. The latter transition may be associated with reduced adherence. Thus research exploring risk factors for ineffective care transition and possible intervention to better prepare patients for these transitions is needed.

Growth

Growth is an important outcome measure unique to pediatrics, as growth and developmental delays are a significant side effect of end-stage organ failure. Although growth rates improve following LT, patients may not attain normal height due to the suppressive effect of immunosuppressant medications, primarily corticosteroids. This is an additional reason (beyond infection risk) that most transplant programs attempt to reduce dosage of immunosuppressant medications, particularly corticosteroids, as soon as possible after transplant. Growth hormone has been used following transplant, but there are theoretical concerns about the risk of triggering rejection and one report of negative impact. Steroid-free immunosuppression regimens are being explored with some success in kidney, liver, and heart transplantation, but have not been reported in pediatric LT.

Data regarding growth after pediatric LT is limited. A single-center study found the overall rate of somatic growth was roughly 64% of the predicted values. Some patients in that study who were doing well more than 4 years post-transplant achieved growth parameters in the normal range. Thus with careful reduction in immunosuppression, adequate growth can occur. Growth of the transplanted lungs is another unique outcome measure for pediatric LT. Although studies using immature animals showed that lung tissue growth can occur after LT, similar invasive studies are not possible in humans, and non-invasive assessment of lung growth is difficult. Spirometry volumes (i.e., FEV_1 and FVC) following LT may be in the normal range in infants and older children. Diffusing capacity of carbon monoxide (DLCO) is a better measure of lung growth, as it assesses surface area for gas exchange. However, DLCO does not appear to increase in pediatric recipients of cadaveric and living donor transplants. Unfortunately, DLCO is not readily measurable in the infant population. Finally, airway growth, as measured by serial imaging studies, has been demonstrated in a small retrospective study. Thus further study is required to clarify whether growth of lung tissue occurs after pediatric transplant.

Transplant benefit/quality of life

Most transplant physicians and surgeons would agree that the primary goal of LT is to prolong life. Moreover, allocation systems and clinical decision making regarding the timing of transplantation tend to focus on providing lungs for transplant when death without transplant is likely. As noted above, recent changes to the system for allocation of lungs in the United States has been modified to incorporate predicted survival benefit in the prioritization process. This change may be particularly important for pediatrics, as a recent study suggested that children with CF who underwent transplantation in the United States under the prior system did not achieve a survival benefit. The study findings are contrary to previous findings from the United Kingdom, where a different allocation system was used and was subject to other methodologic criticisms. Nonetheless, the study reinforced the concept that in decisions regarding benefit of transplantation, quality of life (QoL) must be considered, ideally with objective measures. Unfortunately, literature systematically evaluating QoL either before or after pediatric LT are limited. Although the QoL and survival in adult LT recipients was better than candidates who remained on the waiting list, extrapolation to children and adolescents must be approached cautiously, and measures of childhood development must also be included. Although in the most recent ISHLT registry report, 80% of children surviving 7 years after LT had no activity limitation, published research investigating QoL in pediatric LT recipients has largely been descriptive and contains limitations regarding study design and methodology. Nonetheless, one study suggests that children may experience psychological difficulties and an impaired QoL after transplant. It is also worth emphasizing that assessments of QoL may be affected by the child's baseline capabilities prior to transplant and their expectations after transplant. Systematic assessment of QoL and developmental impact of transplant on pediatric recipients remains an underexplored area of pediatric LT.

Future considerations

It is hoped that improved outcomes will lead to increased focus on growth and development in pediatric LT recipients. Long-term side effects, particularly renal dysfunction, also require further attention. Understanding how to minimize the effects of transplantation and immunosuppression on pediatric LT recipients is critical. Moreover, identifying the etiologies responsible for and providing interventions to improve poor outcomes in the adolescent population remains an important area for study.

Removing BOS as the primary barrier to long-term survival continues to be a priority in LT research. In pediatrics, as few centers perform enough transplants each year to adequately power outcome studies, uniform treatment strategies and multi-center collaborations will help to identify strategies for earlier diagnosis and allow assessment of treatment efficacy. A key research opportunity may be exploring the reduced incidence of rejection and BOS in the naive but developing immune system of infants.

In spite of these obstacles, nearly 2000 LTs and HLTs have been performed in children during the last three decades, giving these patients a chance for long-term survival. Although recent improvements in outcome for children with CF and pulmonary hypertension will hopefully reduce the number of children needing LT, those who do should continue to benefit.

Further reading

Aurora P, Edwards LB, Kucheryavaya AY, *et al.* The Registry of the International Society for Heart and Lung Transplantation: thirteenth official pediatric lung and heart-lung transplantation report. *J Heart Lung Transplant* 2010; **29**: 1129–41.

Faro A, Mallory GB, Visner GA, *et al.* American Society of Transplantation executive summary on pediatric lung transplantation. *Am J Transplant* 2007; **7**: 285–92.

Elizur A, Faro A, Huddleston CB, *et al.* Lung transplantation in infants and toddlers from 1990 to 2004 at St. Louis Children's Hospital. *Am J Transplant* 2009; **9**: 719–26.

Wells A, Faro A. Special considerations in pediatric lung transplantation. *Semin Resp Crit Care Med* 2006; **27**: 552–60.

Chapter 21

Recipient selection

Alex Gimson

Key points

- The selection process in the liver transplant context entails making a life and death decision that has the potential of saving the life of an individual but, inevitably, doing so at the expense of denying a life-saving organ to another.
- The practice of candidate selection and organ allocation is predicated on two fundamental ethical principles: justice and utility.
- The most commonly used scoring system for estimating prognosis is the Model for End-Stage Liver Disease, which is derived from serum creatinine, bilirubin, and international normalized ratio.
- The Milan criteria for selecting patients with hepatocellular carcinoma for transplantation require the presence of a single mass lesion ≤ 5 cm in diameter or up to five lesions that are all ≤ 3 cm, in the absence of evidence of extrahepatic disease or radiological evidence of vascular invasion.
- Patients with alcoholic liver disease are usually excluded from transplantation if they show clinical or histological evidence of active alcoholic hepatitis or evidence of return to drinking after full professional assessment and advice.

The ultimate objective of candidate selection for liver transplantation is to offer it to those who are sufficiently sick to justify the risks of the procedure but not too sick to benefit from it. Important progress has been made in recent years toward devising selection as well as allocation criteria based on more objective and evidence-based definitions of candidate disease severity, transplant outcome, and organ quality.

A stringent process of selection of appropriate candidates for liver transplantation is necessary for a number of reasons. First, liver grafts are a finite, precious resource as a result of the wide discrepancy between the supply of and demand for all deceased organs in general and absence of life-sustaining therapy in patients with end-stage liver disease in particular. Thus the selection process in the liver transplant context entails making a life and death decision that has the potential of saving the life of an individual but, inevitably, doing so at the expense of denying a life-saving organ to another. Second, not all patients with end-stage liver disease would necessarily derive a survival benefit from the procedure, and those who would may not necessarily benefit equally. Third, a thorough assessment of potential liver transplant candidates is required to disentangle liver-related extrahepatic manifestations, which may be considered indications for transplantation, from extrahepatic disease that would contraindicate the procedure. Examples include the need to exclude fixed chronic obstructive or restrictive pulmonary disease in patients with suspected hepatopulmonary syndrome; dementia and other neurodegenerative and psychiatric disease in patients with chronic encephalopathy; malignancy of the colon and biliary tree in patients with primary sclerosing cholangitis; surreptitious alcohol intake in patients with end-stage alcoholic liver disease; and underlying malignancy in patients with Budd-Chiari syndrome.

In addition to the need to be stringent, the candidate selection process for liver transplantation should ideally be evidence-based, transparent, objective, time-efficient, standardized, and multi-disciplinary, comprising hepatologists, liver transplant surgeons, anesthetists, transplant nurse coordinators, dieticians,

Organ Transplantation: A Clinical Guide, ed. A.A. Klein, C.J. Lewis, and J.C. Madsen. Published by Cambridge University Press.

dentists, social workers, and, where appropriate, specialists from other disciplines, including psychiatrists.

Although the principles of candidate selection and organ allocation are generic, important differences in their application exist between different health care systems as a result of differences in the degree of mismatch between the demand for and supply of donor liver organs, legislative framework, availability of alternative forms of organ donation (e.g., live donor and splits), type of health economy, and prevalent cultural norms. In addition, the selection criteria should be subject to regular review and modification as the relevant evidence base continues to evolve.

This chapter is confined to deceased organ transplantation in adults and does not discuss live donor or pediatric selection and allocation. In liver transplant practice, a distinction needs to be made between the process of *selection* of appropriate candidates for transplant, which is the main focus of this chapter, and that of organ *allocation* for those candidates who have been placed on the waiting list for the procedure. Both of these processes are underpinned by similar considerations with respect to the relevant clinical end points and ethical standpoints, each of which will be briefly discussed next.

Clinical end points

The outcome of liver transplantation can be defined by a number of end points. Although patient survival, defined as the length of time between the dates of transplant and death or last known follow-up, has historically been the most important and commonly utilized end point, graft survival, defined as the time interval between transplant and graft loss (as a result of death or graft failure requiring re-transplant surgery), represents another key outcome measure. Another important end point that incorporates the "intention-to-treat" principle is transplant benefit, which is a measure of life-years gained, taking account of survival while waiting for transplantation as well as thereafter. Arguably, assessment of transplant benefit to guide decision making in this setting of candidate selection and organ allocation should ideally be based on graft rather than patient survival. since it is the life-saving potential of one liver graft that is usually under consideration. Other important but less commonly used outcomes include improvement of quality of life or functional status; quality-of-life–adjusted survival, cost-effectiveness, resource utilization (e.g., duration of hospital and/or intensive care stay and blood transfusion requirements); and morbidity indicators (e.g., incidence of vascular and biliary complications, renal dysfunction, sepsis, and immunosuppression-related malignant disease).

Ethical standpoints

The practice of candidate selection and organ allocation is predicated on two fundamental ethical principles: justice (or equity) and utility (or efficiency). The principle of justice stipulates that liver organs should be prioritized according to the degree of an individual's *need* for transplant, thereby ensuring that those with equal needs can have equity of access to this scarce resource. A number of scoring systems have been utilized to predict the survival of patients with end-stage liver disease (Table 21.1), a surrogate for need for transplantation. A need-based system would therefore prioritize patients according to their projected survival without transplant, irrespective of their post-transplant outcome.

In contrast, the principle of utility mandates that candidate selection and organ allocation prioritize patients with the greatest survival prospects after undergoing transplant, thereby maximizing the overall absolute (rather than net) life-saving utility of this finite resource. Thus a purely utilitarian system would select and subsequently rank transplant candidates according to their anticipated post-transplant outcome, regardless of their survival prospects in the absence of this procedure.

In liver transplantation practice, incorporating those two ethical principles is not always straightforward because patients with the greatest need for transplantation (the sickest) are often also those most likely to succumb from it. However, a sensible compromise can be achieved by utilizing the principle of transplant benefit in both candidate selection and organ allocation decisions, thereby prioritizing organs according to the difference in survival prospects with and without transplant or, in other words, the number of life-years gained by undergoing transplant.

Although the outcome of selection and allocation decision making based on the principles of medical need may intuitively be considered similar to that of a benefit-based system, since most of the variability in survival benefit is usually determined by differences in survival without, rather than with, transplant, current evidence suggests that many of the candidates

Table 21.1 Clinically useful prognostic scores for selection of chronic liver disease candidates for liver transplantation

	Points assigned		
Parameter	**1**	**2**	**3**
Ascites	Absent	Slight	Moderate
Bilirubin	<2 mg/dl (<34.2 micromol/liter)	2–3 mg/dl (34.2 to 51.3 micromol/liter)	>3 mg/dl (>51.3 micromol/liter)
Albumin	>3.5 g/dl (35 g/liter)	2.8–3.5 g/dl (28–35 g/liter)	<2.8 g/dl (<28 g/liter)
Prothrombin time Seconds prolonged INR	 <4 <1.7	 4–6 1.7–2.3	 >6 >2.3
Encephalopathy	None	Grade 1–2	Grade 3–4

A total score of 5–6 is considered grade A (well-compensated disease); 7–9 is grade B (significant functional compromise); and 10–15 is grade C (decompensated disease).
1. MELD score: $MELD = 10 \times [0.957 \times \log_e (\text{creatinine in mg/dl}) + 0.378 \times \log_e(\text{bilirubin mg/dl}) + 1.120 \times \log_e (\text{INR}) + 0.643]$
2. UKELD score: $UKELD = (5.395 \times \log_e (\text{UKELDINR}) + 1.485 \times \log_e (\text{creatinine in mmol/L}) + 3.130 \times \log_e (\text{bilirubin in micromol/liter}) - [81.565 \times \log_e (\text{sodium in mmol/L})] + 435$
3. Child-Pugh score: Modified Child-Pugh classification of severity of liver disease

selected for transplantation by need-based systems have in fact no demonstrable survival benefit from the procedure. However, although the development of an accurate model for predicting liver transplant benefit remains to be accomplished, indirect implementation of the principle of transplant benefit in the selection of liver transplant candidates is feasible by excluding those with survival prospects without transplantation, as judged by currently available need-based prognostic scoring systems (e.g., Model for End-Stage Liver Disease [MELD], United Kingdom Model for End-Stage Liver Disease [UKELD], Child-Pugh score) that exceed the observed or predicted 1- or 3-year survival after transplantation.

The role of public preferences in formulating liver transplant selection and allocation criteria is also controversial. On the one hand, it is the public that ultimately both funds transplantation and provides organ donors, and any transplant selection and allocation system should therefore command public confidence. On the other hand, basing allocation decisions on public preferences can be problematic because those preferences tend to adversely prejudice patients whose disease is perceived as being self-inflicted and are therefore regarded by most philosophers as unethical.

Conceptually, the selection of liver transplant candidates is best considered in four distinct, albeit not mutually exclusive, contexts: chronic liver disease, variant syndromes (including hepatocellular carcinoma), acute liver failure, re-transplantation, and multi-organ transplantation (most commonly simultaneous liver–kidney grafting). Each of those settings will be discussed in the following sections.

Candidate selection in chronic liver disease

Disease severity scores

The allocation of donor livers to transplant candidates has been the subject of considerable public health policy debate in much of the Western world in general and the United States in particular.

For many years, the main tool for estimating survival without transplant has been the modified Child-Pugh score (Table 21.1), which was originally developed to predict the survival prospects of patients undergoing porto-systemic shunt surgery. In addition, disease-specific prognostic models for primary biliary cirrhosis, primary sclerosing cholangitis, hepatitis C virus (HCV) cirrhosis, and alcoholic cirrhosis have been developed but are used less commonly.

However, the use of the Child-Pugh score in the setting of candidate selection and organ allocation has proved contentious for several reasons. First, the categorical nature of both the overall score (stratifying patients in three prognostic groups) and the format of some of its components (prothrombin time, albumin, bilirubin) effectively ascribes prognostic value to what are arbitrary thresholds and assigns patients with potentially diverse prognoses to the same risk group. Furthermore, the inclusion in the Child-Pugh score of two variables that cannot be objectively defined (severity of ascites and encephalopathy) has exposed it to criticism of subjectivity and vulnerability to manipulation. Lastly, the Child-Pugh score had never been developed or validated in the setting of candidate selection or liver allocation before its use for this purpose.

Increasing dissatisfaction with successive inequitable liver organ allocation policies, based on the Child-Pugh score, led to the adoption in 2002 of a new evidence-based continuous scoring system that accurately predicts prognosis among patients with end-stage liver disease as the basis for the US national allocation system of donor livers. This essentially medical need–based scheme is based on the Model for End-Stage Liver Disease (MELD, Table 21.1), which is a mathematical formula derived from three objective, readily available, and reproducible laboratory parameters (serum creatinine, bilirubin, and international normalized ratio [INR] of prothrombin time). The MELD score, which had originally been developed to predict the mortality of patients with end-stage liver disease undergoing transjugular intrahepatic portosystemic shunting and subsequently proved an accurate predictor of 3-month mortality of wait-listed US liver transplant candidates, can be calculated using a hand-held computer and has values ranging between 6 and 40, with adjustment made for those receiving renal support (serum creatinine set to 4 mg/dl) or warfarin anticoagulation (INR capped at 2.5). A number of modifications to the MELD score have since been proposed (see below), but none is currently implemented in practice.

Similarly, a continuous mortality risk score, the United Kingdom Model for End-Stage Liver Disease (UKELD) score, was developed and validated for end-stage chronic liver disease candidates awaiting liver transplantation in the United Kingdom (Table 21.1). This score is calculated from the serum bilirubin, INR, serum creatinine, and serum sodium concentrations and was shown to outperform MELD in predicting mortality on the UK liver transplant waiting list.

Disease-severity selection criteria (Table 21.2)

Although no formal "minimal listing" criteria for liver transplant candidates currently exist in the United States, the evidence suggests that only those with MELD scores greater than 14 derive a survival benefit at 3 years after transplantation, and those with low MELD scores (with a threshold that remains to be determined) should not therefore be listed for the procedure.

In the pre-MELD era, minimal listing criteria for liver transplant candidates in the United States formally stipulated the presence of Child-Pugh score of $\geq$7 which corresponds to a projected 1-year mortality rate in the absence of transplantation of $\geq$ 10%.

In the United Kingdom, current listing guidelines stipulate that chronic liver disease candidates should only be selected for transplant if their projected 1-year mortality in the absence of the procedure, as estimated by UKELD, exceeds the observed 1-year mortality post-transplant among such patients in the United Kingdom. This currently equates to a mortality rate of 9% or more, which corresponds to a UKELD score >49.

Table 21.2 Commonly used selection criteria for liver transplantation for candidates with benign end-stage chronic liver disease

MELD score > 14 or
UKELD score > 49 or
Child-Pugh score $\geq$ 7 (i.e., Child's class B or C)
and
Predicted 5-year post-transplant survival of >50% (subjectively judged on the basis of absence of absolute contraindications and/or combinations of relative contraindications or markers of adverse post-transplant survival)

Variant exceptional diagnoses

The use of generic mortality scoring models such as MELD and UKELD to guide candidate selection and/or organ allocation decision making is not appropriate for all patients with chronic liver disease. Such "variant syndromes," also referred to as exceptional diagnoses or MELD exceptions, are recognized in the United Kingdom and United States selection and allocation systems as valid indications for transplant that may merit selection and/or additional priority for the procedure beyond that dictated by the UKELD and MELD scores, respectively (Table 21.3). Some of those diagnoses are automatically granted such status, whereas others currently require formal approval by a peer-review system in the form of a National Appeals Panel in the United Kingdom or a Regional Review

Table 21.3 Commonly used criteria for selection for liver transplantation for patients with variant syndromes

Variant syndrome	Selection criteria
1. Diuretic-resistant ascites	International Ascites Club grade 3 ascites (massive abdominal distension) with current imaging documenting the presence and severity of ascites and UKELD/MELD scores are below the required criteria for listing *and* ≥2 of the following additional criteria: ≥3 therapeutic paracenteses (≥ 2 l each) in last 60 days. ≥2 episodes of spontaneous bacterial peritonitis with supporting documentation (ascitic polymorphonuclear granulocyte count ≥250 or positive culture) Previous transjugular intrahepatic portosystemic shunt Ascites unresponsive or intolerant to maximum doses of diuretics (i.e., spironolactone 400 mg/day and furosemide 160 mg or equivalent) ≥2 therapeutic thoracenteses Serum sodium ≤125 mEq/l
2. Hepatopulmonary syndrome	The presence of intrapulmonary shunting as evidenced by echocardiographic appearance of microbubbles in the left heart ≥ cycles after venous injection of agitated saline and alveolar-arterial oxygen gradient of ≥ 2 Kpa (or ≥ 2.7 kPa if older than 64 years) in the setting of liver disease and/or portal hypertension.
3. Chronic hepatic encephalopathy	Confirmed by EEG or trail-making tests with at least two admissions in 1 year or requirement for endotracheal intubation for airway protection due to exacerbations of encephalopathy that have not been manageable by standard therapy.
4. Persistent and intractable pruritus	Pruritus consequent on cholestatic liver disease that is intractable after therapeutic trials, which might include cholestyramine, ursodeoxycholic acid, rifampicin, ondansetron, and naltrexone, and after exclusion of psychiatric comorbidity that might contribute to the itch.
5. Familial amyloidosis	Biopsy-proven evidence of amyloid deposition and documentation of the most common TTR gene mutations in the absence of significant/debilitating cardiac involvement (on the basis of ventricular wall thickness, ejection fraction, arrhythmias, and New York Heart Association class), malnutrition or autonomic neuropathy (assessed by the polyneuropathy disability score).
6. Primary hyperlipidemias	Homozygous familial hypercholesterolemia with absent LDL receptor expression and LDL receptor gene mutation.
7. Polycystic liver disease (PLD)	Patients should meet the following criteria: Satisfy criteria for massive PLD (total cyst:parenchyma ratio >1) and have a complication of the PLD that is likely to resolve after liver transplantation Are not candidates for, or have disease that has failed to respond to, non-transplant interventions for relief of symptoms; malnutrition may be considered a primary contraindication to non-transplant surgery. Have clinically significant manifestations of liver disease that can be attributed to massive PLD, which may include cachexia, ascites, portal hypertension (variceal bleeding), hepatic venous outflow obstruction, biliary obstruction, cholestasis, or recurrent cyst infection. Have severe malnutrition (assessment made on the basis of hypoalbuminemia or decreased lean body mass). Have serum albumin < 2.2 mg/dl. Have lean body mass reflected by decreased midarm circumference, measured in the non-dominant arm midway between the acromion and the olecranon process: <23.1 cm in female patients and <23.8 cm in male patients.
8. Portopulmonary hypertension	Defined as the occurrence of a combination of pulmonary hypertension (mean pulmonary artery pressure >25 mmHg as estimated by right heart catheter), raised pulmonary vascular resistance (>240 dynes/sec/cm^{-5}) and normal (≤15 mmHg) pulmonary capillary wedge pressure and/or transpulmonary gradient of >10–12 mmHg in the setting of evidence of portal hypertension. Patients must have demonstrated a mean pulmonary artery pressure less than 50 mmHg, and those with a mean pulmonary artery pressure of >35 mmHg who have demonstrated evidence of significant response (mean pulmonary artery pressure <35 mmHg and PVR of <400 dynes/sec/cm^{-5} in the presence of a satisfactory RV function) to a 12-week trial of pulmonary arterial hypertension therapy (iloprost, sildenafil, or bosentan).
9. Uncommon hepatic tumors	Examples include carcinoid tumors that are limited to the liver, hepatic epithelioid hemangioendotheliomas (even with extrahepatic spread), and hepatic adenomas in the setting of glycogen-storage disease.
10. Small for size syndrome	Defined as meeting 4 of the following 6 criteria: >5 days after living donor liver transplantation; serum bilirubin concentration ≤10 mg/dl in the absence of rejection or common duct obstruction; bile duct ischemia (leak); INR ≤1.5; significant ascites as noted on clinical exam; biopsy with centrilobular ballooning, necrosis, and cholestasis.

(*cont.*)

Table 21.3 *(cont.)*

Variant syndrome	Selection criteria
11. Recurrent cholangitis	Patients who have ≥2 culture-proven bacteremias within a 6-month period or who have septic complications of bacterial cholangitis and no underlying correctable dominant lesion. Bacteremia should be non-iatrogenic (unrelated to a procedure such as recent endoscopic retrograde cholangiogram or transhepatic cholangiogram) and should occur in a patient who does not have a biliary tube or stent; in addition, these bacterial cholangitic episodes should occur in patients who have been treated with antibiotic therapy that has failed to suppress these septic episodes.
12. Cholangiocarcinoma	As part of a research study protocol including the administration of neoadjuvant therapy before transplantation, and operative staging to exclude patients with regional hepatic lymph node metastases, intrahepatic metastases, and/or extrahepatic disease and the following criteria: Candidates must satisfy diagnostic criteria for hilar CCA: malignant-appearing stricture on cholangiography and biopsy or cytology results demonstrating malignancy, carbohydrate antigen 19–9 >100 U/ml, or aneuploidy. The tumor should be considered unresectable on the basis of technical considerations or underlying liver disease (e.g., PSC). If cross-sectional imaging studies (CT scan, ultrasound, MRI) demonstrate a mass, the mass should be <3 cm. Intra- and extrahepatic metastases should be excluded by cross-sectional imaging studies of the chest and abdomen at the time of initial exception and every 3 months before score increases. Regional hepatic lymph node involvement and peritoneal metastases should be assessed by operative staging after completion of neoadjuvant therapy and before LT. Endoscopic ultrasound-guided aspiration of regional hepatic lymph nodes may be advisable to exclude patients with obvious metastases before neoadjuvant therapy is initiated. Transperitoneal aspiration or biopsy of the primary tumor (either by endoscopic ultrasound, operative, or percutaneous approaches) should be avoided because of the high risk of tumor seeding associated with these procedures.
13. Heriditary hemorrhagic telangiectasia	Complicated by intractable high-output heart failure, biliary sepsis, and intrahepatic hemorrhage.
14. Portal hypertensive bleeding	Refractory variceal bleeding can be defined as acute severe variceal bleed requiring >6 units in 24 hours or >2 units per day over 3 days, airway intubation and the insertion of a Minnesota or Blakemore tube, in spite of optimal endoscopic treatment, coagulation support, and pharmacologic management and where is either ineffective or contraindicated. Chronic recurrent variceal or portal hypertensive gastropathy bleeding can be defined as the requirement of more than 2 units of blood transfusion per week for more than 6 weeks in a patient with a TIPS or if TIPS is contraindicated and lack of response to endoscopic and pharmacological treatment.

EEG: electroencephalogram; LDL: low-density lipoprotein; TIPS: transjugular intrahepatic porto-systemic shunt; UKELD: United Kingdom Model for End-Stage Liver.

Board in the United States. Given the relatively small volume of such cases and often subjective nature of non-mortality end points, the selection and allocation criteria for patients with variant syndromes (particularly those without hepatocellular carcinoma) are inevitably less well-developed, less objective, and less evidence-based than those used for other patients with chronic liver disease.

Patients with exceptional diagnoses can be grouped into at least three broad categories:

1. Those for whom there are good reasons to believe that longer waiting time for a transplant would not necessarily compromise their transplant-free short-term survival prospects but would have a significantly deleterious impact on their survival prospects after the procedure. Examples of such diagnoses include hepatocellular carcinoma (see below), familial amyloid polyneuropathy, primary oxalosis, hepatopulmonary syndrome, and portopulmonary hypertension.
2. Diseases for which the pretransplant mortality risk may not be reliably estimated by MELD/UKELD alone. Examples include HCV/human immunodeficiency virus coinfection and total intestinal failure requiring concurrent small bowel transplantation.
3. Diseases or syndromes that may merit selection, but not necessarily prioritization, for transplant on the grounds of poor liver disease-related quality of life in the absence of high mortality risk without transplant. Examples include patients with chronic liver disease and refractory pruritus,

chronic or relapsing hepatic encephalopathy, and recurrent cholangitis.

Candidate selection for hepatocellular carcinoma

Most liver transplant programs have adopted the Milan criteria for selecting patients with hepatocellular carcinoma (HCC) for transplantation. These require the presence of a single mass lesion ≤ 5 cm in diameter or up to five lesions that are all ≤ 3 cm in the absence of evidence of extrahepatic disease or radiological evidence of vascular invasion. Lesions between 5 and 7 cm in diameter may be considered after demonstration of favorable tumor biology. In addition, the presence of clinical, radiological, or histological evidence of cirrhosis and/or portal hypertension is an additional prerequisite for transplantation in most selection schemes since resection or ablation is usually considered more appropriate for non-cirrhotic, or even some compensated cirrhotic, patients who otherwise satisfy the above criteria.

Although histological proof is only occasionally required, radiological assessment by means of ultrasonography, computed tomography, magnetic resonance imaging, and (in borderline cases) hepatic angiography is usually used to establish the diagnosis, size, and number of focal liver lesions. The radiological diagnosis of HCC requires evidence of lesion congruity and both arterial enhancement and portal venous phase washout on at least two radiological imaging modalities with the size being assessed by the widest dimensions on either scan. Biopsy evidence of HCC and/or markedly elevated alpha-fetoprotein level are additional selection criteria in patients with inconclusive radiological evidence of HCC. In addition, chronic liver disease candidates who have a rising alpha-fetoprotein level ≥ 500 ng in the absence of imaging evidence of HCC may be listed for liver transplantation in the United States.

Notwithstanding these criteria, however, 20% of patients undergoing liver transplantation for HCC in the United States in the MELD era exhibit no explant evidence of HCC. The fibrolamellar variant of HCC is not constrained by these size and volume criteria for transplant, although, given the absence of cirrhosis, resection is considered more appropriate in most such cases.

There has been increasing recognition in recent years that the Milan criteria may be too restrictive, excluding from transplant many patients with potentially curable disease. Expansion of the HCC selection criteria by adoption of those of the University of California, San Francisco (a single-tumor nodule ≤ 6.5 cm; or three or fewer tumors, the largest being < 4.5 cm with the sum of the total tumor diameters equaling < 8 cm) or the more recently proposed "up-to-seven criteria" (a single nodule ≤ 7 cm; two nodules with each ≤ 5 cm; three nodules with each ≤ 4 cm; four nodules with each ≤ 3 cm; five nodules with each ≤ 2 cm) has been shown to be associated with a 5-year graft survival exceeding 50%.

Candidate selection in patients with acute liver failure

The process of selection for patients with acute liver failure presents clinicians with the unique challenge of the need for prompt assessment and decision making while carefully balancing the risks of death and progression to non-transplantable disease with the potential for recovery in the absence of a transplant. Acute liver failure patients are given the highest priority for donor organs in almost all allocation systems. The selection criteria in patients with acute liver failure in the United States, United Kingdom, and much of the Western world are predicated on those developed by King's College Hospital (Table 21.4). These criteria differ according to the underlying etiology (depending on whether or not it is related to acetaminophen ingestion) and use easily obtainable parameters. The MELD score may also be of prognostic utility in these cases.

The Clichy criteria, which are commonly used in France and a number of Northern European countries, stipulate that a transplant is necessary in patients with grade 3 or 4 encephalopathy and a factor V level $< 20\%$ in those younger than 30 years of age or $< 30\%$ if older than 30 years of age. These criteria are rarely used elsewhere as a result of the limited availability of factor V assay, uncertain applicability to patients with non–hepatitis B virus (HBV) acute liver disease, and scarce evidence of reproducibility in validation studies.

Candidate selection for re-transplantation and simultaneous liver and kidney transplantation

Both candidate selection and organ allocation in the setting of re-transplantation are compounded by

Table 21.4 Selection criteria for patients with acute liver failure

Category 1: Etiology: Acetaminophen poisoning – pH < 7.25 more than 24 hours after overdose and after fluid resuscitation
Category 2: Etiology: Acetaminophen poisoning – coexisting prothrombin time > 100 seconds or INR > 6.5, serum creatinine > 300 mmol/l or anuria, and grade 3 or 4 encephalopathy
Category 3: Etiology: Acetaminophen poisoning – serum lactate more than 24 hours after overdose, > 3.5 mmol/l on admission or > 3.0 mmol/l after fluid resuscitation
Category 4: Etiology: Acetaminophen poisoning – any two of the criteria from category 2 with clinical evidence of deterioration (e.g., increased ICP, $FiO_2 \geq 50\%$, increasing inotrope requirements) in the absence of clinical sepsis
Category 5: Etiology: Seronegative hepatitis, hepatitis A, hepatitis B, or an idiosyncratic drug reaction; prothrombin time > 100 seconds or INR > 6.5, and any grade of encephalopathy
Category 6: Etiology: Seronegative hepatitis, hepatitis A, hepatitis B, or an idiosyncratic drug reaction; any grade of encephalopathy, and any three from the following: unfavorable etiology (idiosyncratic drug reaction, seronegative hepatitis), age > 40 years, jaundice-to-encephalopathy time > 7 days, serum bilirubin >300 mmol/L, prothrombin time > 50 seconds, or INR > 3.5
Category 7: Etiology: Acute presentation of Wilson's disease or Budd–Chiari syndrome; combination of coagulopathy and any grade of encephalopathy
Category 8: Hepatic artery thrombosis on days 0–21 after liver transplant
Category 9: Early graft dysfunction on days 0–7 after liver transplant with at least two of the following: AST > 10|000 IU/l, INR > 3.0, serum lactate > 33 mmol/l, absence of bile production
Category 10: Any patient who has been a live liver donor who develops severe liver failure within 4 weeks of the donor operation

AST: aspartate aminotransferase; Fio2: inspired oxygen concentration; ICP: intracranial pressure; INR: international normalized ratio.

unique clinical and ethical dilemmas. In practice, patient beneficence and the consequences of suboptimal organ utilization or technical reasons for graft failure are often more pressing considerations in re-transplant decision making than mitigating concerns about compromising graft utility as a result of inferior survival and risk of disease recurrence. In general, patients with irreversible graft failure should ideally be listed for re-transplantation at a lower degree of disease severity than that warranting primary transplantation, given the poor outcome of re-transplanting sick recipients, risk of accelerated disease progression in the absence of re-transplantation, and underestimation of mortality by scoring systems such as MELD among re-listed candidates. It has therefore been argued that re-transplant candidates in the United States are underserved by the MELD-based allocation system and that such candidates need to be given additional priority points, as is the case currently with HCC, to maximize graft utility.

Similarly, judging the appropriateness of liver transplantation concurrently with another organ, usually a kidney, presents transplant professionals with a difficult challenge.

On the one hand, for example, offering simultaneous liver and kidney transplantation to patients with hepatorenal syndrome could constitute an inappropriate use of a scarce resource given the high probability of post-transplant recovery of native renal function, high risk of post-transplant mortality in the setting of increased recipient disease severity, and high quality of kidney grafts utilized in liver–kidney transplants. On the other hand, published data showed that impaired renal function has an adverse impact on both pre- and post-liver transplant survival; that dual transplantation is associated with superior rejection-free kidney allograft but not patient survival compared with a sequential kidney-after-liver procedure; that combined transplantation confers patient and liver allograft survival benefit over solitary liver transplantation only among those requiring long-term (>3 months) dialysis; and that equivalent kidney allograft survival to that after solitary kidney transplantation can only be achieved if dual transplantation is restricted to patients on long-term dialysis with MELD scores less than 23.

A recent consensus conference in the United States has concluded that Regional Review Boards should determine listing for simultaneous liver and kidney transplantation, as with other MELD exceptions, with automatic approval for (1) end-stage renal disease with cirrhosis and symptomatic portal hypertension or hepatic vein wedge pressure gradient ≥ 10 mmHg; (2) liver failure and chronic kidney disease with a measured glomerular filtration rate ≤ 30 ml/min; (3) acute kidney injury or hepatorenal syndrome with creatinine $\geq$ 2.0 mg/dl and dialysis $\geq$ 8 weeks; and (4) liver failure and chronic kidney disease with renal histology demonstrating > 30% glomerulosclerosis or 30% fibrosis. Similar criteria are now used in the United Kingdom.

Rarely, patients with heart and liver failure will be considered for combined heart–liver or heart–lung–liver transplant. Indications include heart failure with cirrhosis, hemochromatosis, and cystic fibrosis. The short-term mortality is higher than that of each transplant procedure alone, but the long-term outcome is similar to that of heart or liver transplant alone. Selection should be done in conjunction with Regional Review Boards or similar organizations.

Contraindications and delisting criteria

The relative sparseness of published evidence in this area makes it difficult to define the degree of disease severity that renders liver transplantation a futile undertaking. In addition, several other recognized recipient risk factors for post-transplant mortality need to be taken in to account, and, although none proscribes transplantation, accumulation of these risk factors or extremes thereof is, in practice, deemed a bar to the procedure, particularly if they are considered predictive of less than 50% 5-year survival after transplantation.

These factors include advancing age (although no specific age limitation to successful liver transplantation has been identified), diabetes, ischemic heart disease, renal dysfunction, requirement for renal support, requirement for mechanical ventilation, malnutrition, morbid obesity, extensive portal venous system thrombosis, advanced encephalopathy, previous upper abdominal surgery, prior transplant, poor functional status, hyponatremia, and higher serum potassium. Importantly, there is no good evidence that liver disease severity (e.g., assessed by MELD) per se, however extreme, predicts transplant futility.

Current guidelines for selection of patients with alcoholic liver disease usually exclude those with clinical or histological evidence of active alcoholic hepatitis, history of repetitive episodes of non-adherence to medical care, evidence of return to drinking after full professional assessment and advice, and history of current or consecutive illicit drug misuse (except occasional cannabis use).

Most centers' selection guidelines require at least 6 months of recorded abstinence before offering a liver transplant to patients with alcoholic liver disease. Nevertheless, there is no robust evidence base to support this practice. Allowing sufficient time for any potential improvement in liver function with abstinence that might allow transplantation to be avoided is very important. Thus assessment of the prognosis for sobriety should also be based on the patient's insight, social support, and the presence of psychological comorbidity. Active cigarette smoking is also a contraindication in some transplant centers because of recognized increased transplant morbidity and mortality. Methadone usage is not necessarily a contraindication but requires careful analgesic management both before and after transplantation.

Few transplant systems have formulated standardized de-selection criteria for patients already listed for transplant. Indeed, the evidence suggests a lack of agreement among US transplant programs regarding which cases should be removed from the waiting list due to a change in clinical status. In practice, however, patients are de-selected for one of the following reasons: (1) if their clinical status sufficiently improves or, in the case of those with HCC or other exceptional diagnoses, progresses to a point whereby they cease to meet the criteria on which their original selection for the procedure was based; (2) if they develop one of the above absolute contraindications while on the waiting list; (3) if their clinical status deteriorates to an extent whereby they would be deemed unlikely to survive the procedure. Determination of this point is heavily subject to clinical judgment but, in practice, is guided by the accumulation of the above-mentioned adverse risk factors.

Further reading

Neuberger J, Gimson A, Davies M, *et al.* Selection of patients for liver transplantation and allocation of donated livers in the UK. *Gut* 2008; **57**: 252–7.

Steinman T, Becker B, Frost A, *et al.* Guidelines for the referral and management of patient's eligible for solid organ transplantation. *Transplantation* 2001; **71**: 1189.

United Network for Organ Sharing (UNOS). Allocation of livers. Available at: www.unos.org.

Wiesner R, Lake JR, Freeman RB, Gish RG. Model for End Stage Liver Disease (MELD) exception guidelines. *Liver Transpl* 2006; **12**(Suppl 3): S128–36.

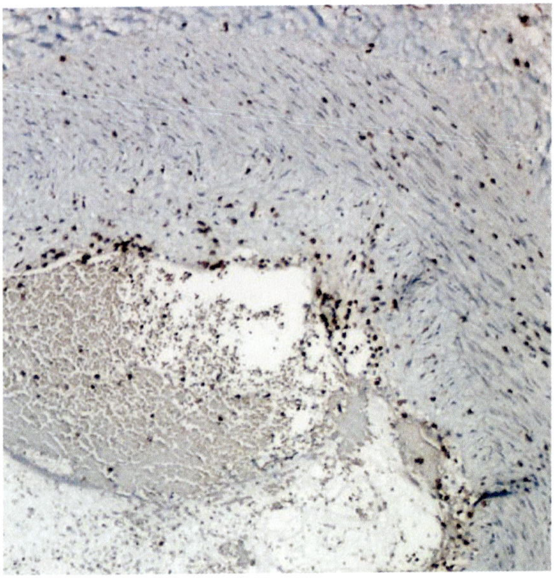

Figure 4B.1 Chronic, active TA can be identified by the inflammatory infiltrate that is typically under the endothelium and accompanied by intimal fibrosis. This artery from a renal allograft shows T cells within an arterial wall and focally lifting the endothelium of an affected vessel stained for CD3 by immunohistochemistry. Antibody also may play a role in the pathogenesis of TA, as shown in experimental studies.

(A) (B)

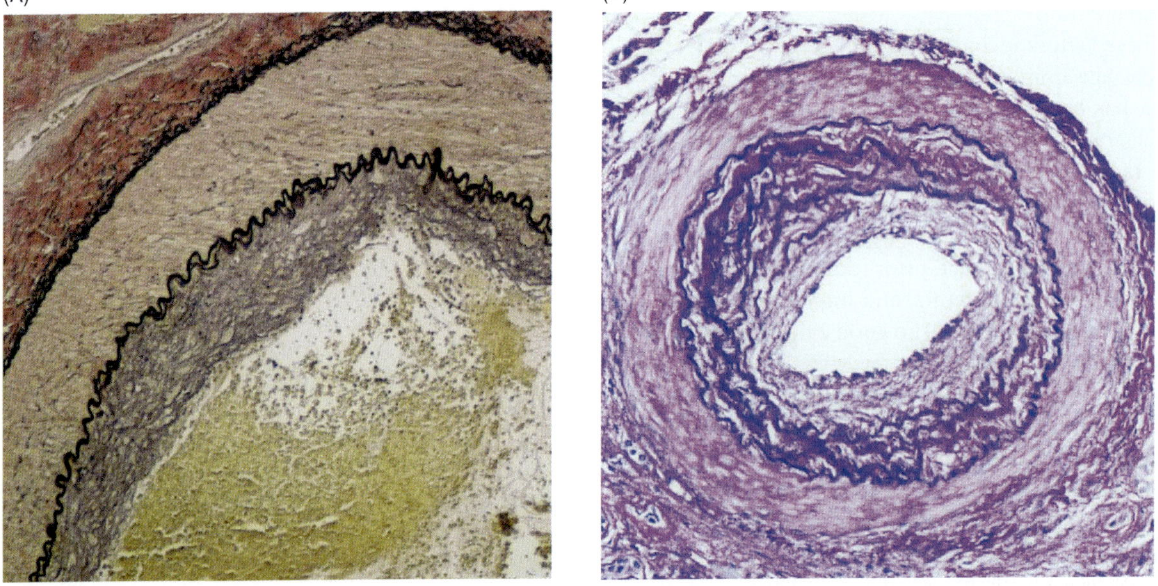

Figure 4B.2 Contrasting appearances of TA and non-immunologic arteriosclerosis can be appreciated in sections stained for elastic fibers. (A) An artery from a renal allograft with TA shows intimal fibrosis without an increase in elastic fibers and with infiltrating inflammatory cells. (B) An artery from a native kidney with arteriosclerosis shows duplication of the elastic lamina, termed *fibroelastosis*, and few inflammatory cells. A and B, Weigert elastic stain.

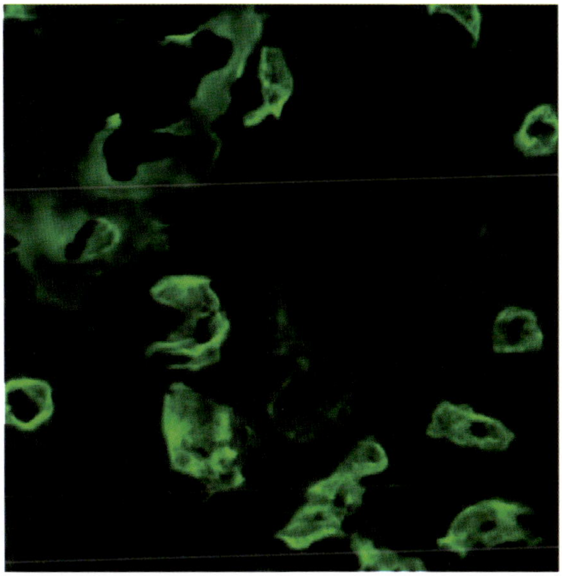

Figure 4B.3 In chronic antibody-mediated rejection CHR, C4d is deposited in peritubular capillary walls, as shown in this immunofluorescence micrograph of an allograft kidney cryostat section stained with anti-C4d monoclonal antibody. CHR is well documented in the kidney but not yet in other organs, although it probably exists.

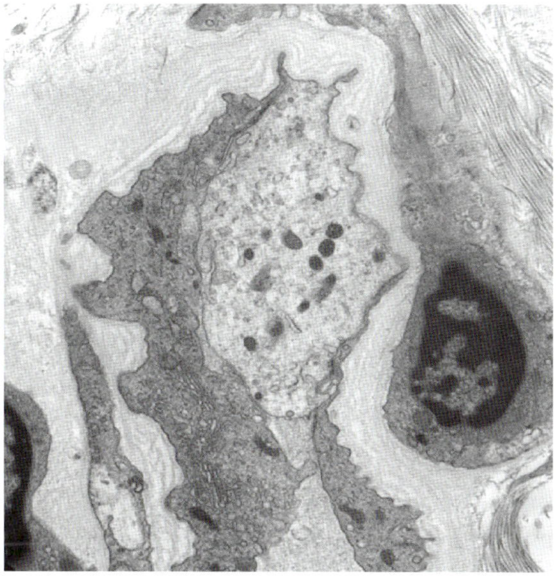

Figure 4B.4 In CHR, multi-lamination of peritubular capillary walls occurs in renal allografts, best shown by electron microscopy. This is a manifestation of repeated episodes of endothelial injury and repair mediated by antibodies. Similar changes occur in glomerular capillaries, where it is termed *transplant glomerulopathy*.

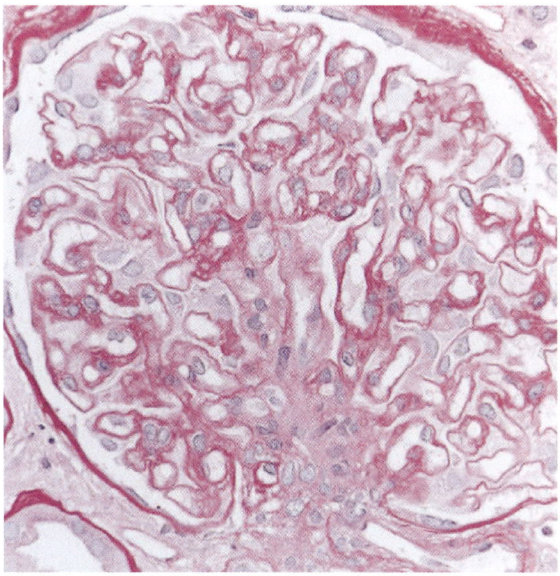

Figure 4B.5 Transplant glomerulopathy (TG) is defined by duplication of the glomerular basement membrane, easily appreciated when severe by light microscopy in sections stained with PAS. This is highly associated with circulating anti-donor antibodies and deposition of C4d. However, the pattern of injury can be due to other causes, such as thrombotic microangiopathy.

(A) (B)

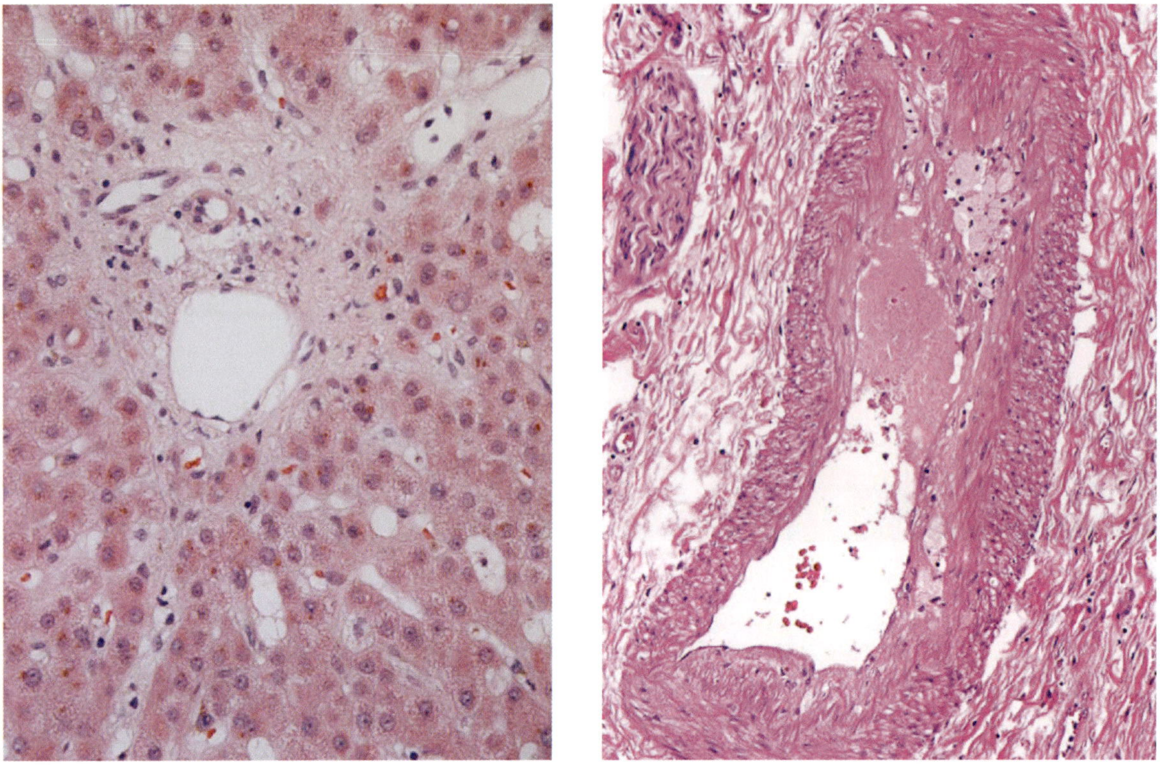

Figure 4B.6 Chronic rejection in the liver affects bile ducts and vessels. (A) In vanishing bile duct syndrome, a manifestation of chronic rejection in the liver, there is loss of bile ducts in portal tracts with associated cholestasis. (B) Chronic allograft vasculopathy in an hepatic artery shows prominent foam cells in the intima. Foam cells, which are macrophages filled with lipid, are characteristic of chronic rejection and are probably related to hyperlipidemia. Photomicrographs courtesy of Dr. V.A. Marcus, McGill University (A) and A.J. Demetris, University of Pittsburgh (B).

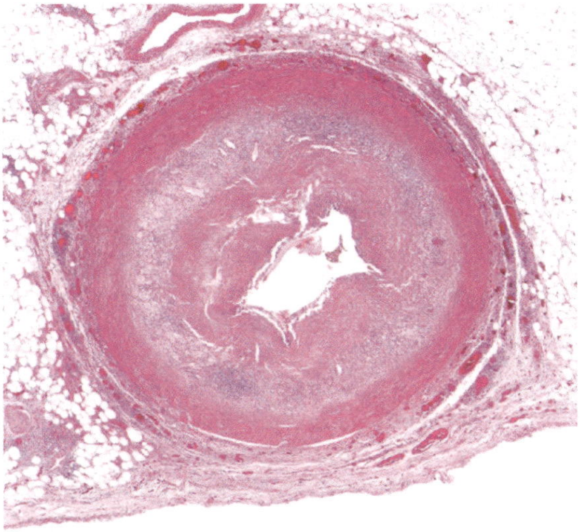

Figure 4B.7 Chronic rejection in heart allografts is generally best appreciated in angiographic studies, such as intravascular ultrasound, because the diagnostic lesion is in the small-to-large arteries not typically sampled in endomyocardial biopsies. TA is manifested in the heart by the same features as in other organs, namely, concentric intimal fibrosis leading to luminal stenosis and eventual occlusion with intramural chronic inflammation, as shown in this explant sample (Courtesy of Dr. J.R. Stone, Massachusetts General Hospital).

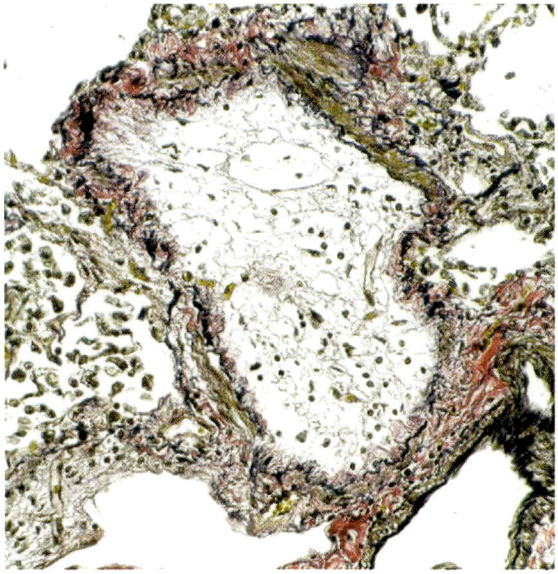

Figure 4B.8 In addition to TA, chronic rejection in the lung results in edematous myofibroblastic obliteration of a bronchiolar lumen, termed *obliterative bronchiolitis*, which can be identified in biopsies and has characteristic effects on pulmonary function (Courtesy of Dr. E.J. Mark, Massachusetts General Hospital).

Chapter 22

Living donor liver transplantation

Koji Hashimoto, Cristiano Quintini, and Charles Miller

Key points

- Living donor liver transplantation has been a major area of development in the field for the last two decades.
- Major technical and physiological advances have made this technology the standard of care in parts of the world where deceased donor options are rare or non-existent.
- In most Western countries where the majority of liver transplantation is performed with deceased donor grafts, the decision to use a living donor rather than wait for a deceased donor graft is a complicated ethical and surgical conundrum.
- The combination of concern for donor safety and the possible availability of a deceased donor graft has limited the expansion of adult-to-adult living donor liver transplantation in the West.

The idea of donating part of the liver from a living donor was conceived and described in the late 1960s, but it took more than 20 years to implement clinically. In December 1988, Raia and colleagues attempted the first living donor liver transplantation (LDLT) on a 4-year-old boy who died 6 days after the transplant. In July 1989, the first successful LDLT was performed by Russell Strong in Australia; a pediatric patient received a left lateral segment (segments II and III) from his mother. This was followed by the first successful LDLT of a child in the United States by Cristoph Broelsch at the University of Chicago; their team performed 20 cases in the ensuing 12 months.

Theoretically, LDLT has the potential of supplying an unlimited number of liver grafts, but its practical application is mitigated by the ethical principle of *primum non nocere* – first do no harm. Living organ donation is the only field in medicine in which a healthy person undergoes a major surgical procedure without presenting a pathological condition and in which the only aspiration of the patient is to benefit another human being. Therefore, the initial era of LDLT involved only adults donating a small portion of their liver to small pediatric recipients, thus maximizing donor safety. But with ever-increasing success and experience, living donor technology was gradually applied in the adult setting. The first successful application of adult-to-adult LDLT was performed in 1993 in Japan by Makuuchi using the left lobe rather than the right lobe, again due to concerns about donor safety and the known morbidity and mortality associated with right hepatic lobectomy. This was successful, but its application was limited by the theoretical and actual amount of liver tissue needed by the recipient. As the demand for this life-saving therapy has increased, surgeons have been forced to utilize the larger right lobe, especially when the donor is smaller than the recipient. However, donor morbidity and mortality remains a major issue, and the significant risk of donor harm or death must always be borne in mind by both the transplant team and the donor and their relatives.

Indications

The indications for LDLT are the same as that for deceased donor transplantation (see Chapter 21). Careful selection of both donor and recipient is crucial in preventing donor complications and optimizing recipient outcomes. Poor survival rates have been

Organ Transplantation: A Clinical Guide, ed. A.A. Klein, C.J. Lewis, and J.C. Madsen. Published by Cambridge University Press.

reported in LDLT involving recipients with very high Model for End-Stage Liver Disease (MELD) scores. In Western countries or where there are significant cadaveric donor programs, the candidate for a potential LDLT is listed for donation after brain death (DBD) liver transplantation. Because a patient with a high MELD score is more likely to receive a DBD organ in a timely fashion, LDLT in the United States is now mainly applied to adult patients with lower MELD scores who, for a variety of reasons such as encephalopathy, large tumor, or other unusual complications, are disadvantaged and do not fair well with the MELD system. In addition, living donor options should not be used for indications that result in only short-term gains for the recipient.

Special recipient indications

Hepatocellular carcinoma

Hepatocellular carcinoma (HCC) patients usually have less portal hypertension and lower chemical MELD scores. Furthermore, the shorter waiting time can reduce the risk of drop-out from transplant waiting list due to tumor progression. The Adult-to-Adult Living Donor Liver Transplantation Cohort Study (A2ALL) group revealed that LDLT recipients had a shorter waiting time compared with DBD liver transplantation (LT) recipients (160 versus 469 days), but a higher rate of HCC recurrence within 3 years (29% versus 0%) than classical transplant recipients. However, it is still controversial whether LDLT accelerates the recurrence of HCC.

Although HCC was once the major indication for LDLT in the United States, with the introduction of the MELD system and the priority given to patients with HCC, most patients can receive a DBD graft within 3 months, thus making the use of LDLT far less important.

Hepatitis C

An early study from Spain suggested that hepatitis C virus (HCV) recurrence is more severe after LDLT. One possible explanation is that the regenerating liver is more susceptible to HCV infection; a hypothesis based on early in vitro studies. However, more recent studies suggest that there is no difference in HCV recurrence. Because of the high chance for recurrent disease after any type of transplant, patients with HCV cirrhosis are best managed by avoiding early transplantation, thus negating one of the most beneficial aspects of LDLT.

Donor evaluation

The aim of the donor evaluation is to assess whether the donor is medically and psychologically suitable for living donation. Equally important is to identify anatomical conditions that could increase donor risks and jeopardize either donor or recipient recovery.

Donor selection criteria vary slightly among different programs. In the United States, to avoid a conflict of interest, the evaluation of the donor is conducted by a designated donor advocacy team, which independently assesses donor candidacy. During the evaluation, the donor is educated regarding the risks of the procedure. This includes discussion of the morbidity and mortality rates reported in the medical literature, as well as outcomes of the surgeons who will perform the operation. The donor has the right to withdraw his willingness to donate right up to the time of surgery. Normally the donor should be completely healthy, between 18 and 55 years of age, and have a clear and established relationship with the recipient. The donor and recipient should be blood group identical or compatible.

The first step of the evaluation begins with a thorough medical history and physical examination. Particular emphasis is placed in the psychosocial evaluation of the potential donor. The donor should make the decision voluntarily, without any coercion and any direct or indirect financial gain deriving from the donation. An extensive lab profile and serologic tests complete the first step of the evaluation. If the donor is deemed to be a good candidate from a medical and psychosocial perspective, then the next step is to assess the anatomical and surgical aspect. Recent advances in the three-dimensional reconstruction of the liver using multi-phase computed tomography (CT) scans has contributed to a precise non-invasive mapping of the most important vascular structures, allowing for a preoperative simulation of the graft procurement (Figure 22.1). The type of graft (left lateral segment, left lobe, right lobe) is determined by the donor liver anatomy and by the recipient size and severity of disease. Biliary imaging can be performed with contrast-enhanced CT imaging or by endoscopy. At the end of the evaluation process, only 30–40% of aspiring donors will be considered good candidates for donation.

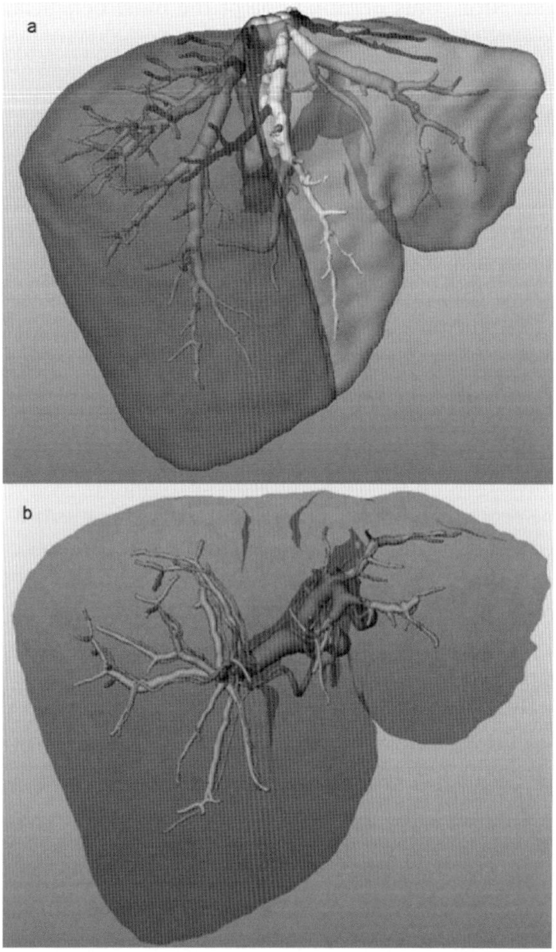

Figure 22.1 Three-dimensional reconstruction of the liver using multi-phase CT scan.

Donor operation and type of liver grafts

In order to understand the type of grafts used in LDLT, it is important to define two concepts: the future liver remnant (FLR) and the graft-to-recipient body weight ratio (GRWR). The FLR is the proportion of the whole donor liver that is estimated to remain after the donation. An FLR of 30–35% is considered a safe and acceptable lower limit under which donation should not be attempted due to the higher risk of developing postoperative liver insufficiency or failure. The GRWR is the ratio between the donor graft weight and the recipient body weight. The lower limit of graft acceptability is considered to be approximately 0.6–0.8%; however, many transplant programs like to have a GRWR of at least 1% to give a margin of safety to the recipient in case of certain specific technical complexities. A GRWR below 0.6–0.8% increases the chance of developing postoperative liver insufficiency known as small-for-size syndrome (SFSS). Donor safety is the primary concern; therefore, the ideal graft is the one that leaves a donor an FLR above 35% and at the same time provides a graft with an adequate size with respect to the recipient.

Familiarity with the liver anatomy is essential for safe performance of LDLT. The liver can be divided into two lobes (right and left). Each lobe can be further divided into four segments. The left lobe consists of segments I–IV; the right lobe consists of segments V–VIII. Each segment is independent from a functional stand point and relies on one arterial and portal venous inflow (segmental branch of the hepatic artery and portal vein). The venous outflow is different, as both lobes share drainage via the middle hepatic vein (MHV); this anatomical detail has created an extensive literature regarding the appropriate partition of the MHV to either the donor or recipient. A clear understanding of the biliary duct anatomy is critical in preventing complications in both donor and recipient. There are essentially three types of grafts that can be considered in LDLT (Figure 22.2); the left lateral segment (segments II and III), the left lobe (segments I–IV), and the right lobe (segments V–VIII). The smallest graft is represented by the left lateral segment, which usually represents 20–25% of the total liver volume. This graft is reserved for pediatric recipients. The left lobe, which usually represents 30–40% of the total liver volume, is usually offered to teenagers or small adults. Finally, the right lobe, which represents about 60–70% of the total liver volume, is reserved for the remainder of the adult population. This is the largest graft, and although it offers the most consistent results in the recipient, it is also the one that is associated with the highest morbidity and mortality in the donor.

Donor complications

Despite donor safety being of paramount importance in LDLT, finite morbidity and mortality rates have been reported worldwide. The mean rate of complications for left lateral segment, left lobe, and right lobe living donor hepatectomy in the most experienced centers are, respectively, approximately 15%, 25%, and 35%. These remain very high despite a

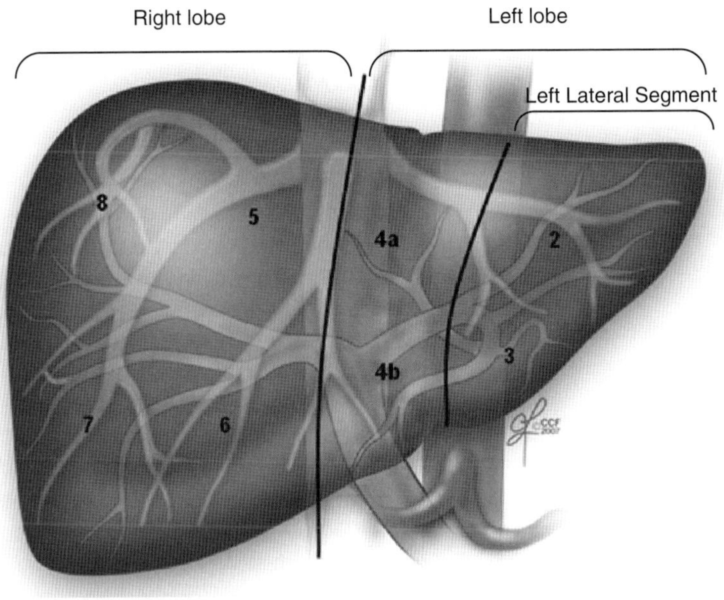

Figure 22.2 Diagram of the liver anatomy; the liver can be divided into two lobes (right and left). Each lobe can be further divided in four segments. The left lobe consists of segments I–IV; the right lobe consists of segments V–VIII.

number of improvements in surgical technique and patient care, which must always be borne in mind when considering LDLT as a treatment option. It is important to report these complications according to the Clavien system, which scores them according to five categories of severity (Table 22.1). Despite this, reported complications vary significantly among different programs, possibly due to different experience or reporting methodology. Biliary complications represent the most frequent source of morbidity occurring in 5–25% of these patients. Vascular complications are rare, but accompanied by significant morbidity and mortality (5–7%). The complication rate is directly correlated to the amount of parenchyma removed from the donor, although complications associated with anesthesia and postoperative recovery (deep vein thrombosis, pulmonary embolism, etc.) have been reported. The overall donor mortality rate is approximately 0.1% for left lobe donation and 0.5% for right lobe donor hepatectomy. This remains high and must be discussed closely with donors and their family when considering LDLT and during the consent process.

Table 22.1 Classification of complications according to the Clavien system

Grade 1	Any deviation from the normal postoperative course without the need for pharmacological treatment or surgical, endoscopic, and radiological interventions. Allowed therapeutic regimens are drugs as antiemetics, antipyretics, analgesics, diuretics, electrolytes, and physiotherapy. This grade also includes wound infections opened at the bedside.
Grade 2	Complications requiring pharmacological treatment with drugs other than such allowed for grade 1 complications. Blood transfusions and total parenteral nutrition are also included.
Grade 3	Complications requiring surgical, endoscopic, or radiological intervention.
Grade 3a	Intervention not under general anesthesia.
Grade 3b	Intervention under general anesthesia.
Grade 4	Life-threatening complications (including central nervous system complications) requiring intensive care unit stay.
Grade 4a	Single-organ dysfunction (including dialysis).
Grade 4b	Multi-organ dysfunction.
Grade 5	Death of the patient.

Recipient operation

The hepatectomy is performed preserving the retrohepatic vena cava. Intraoperative hemodynamic studies are emerging in recent years as a tool to guide implantation technique and inflow modulation. Severe portal hypertension may in fact be responsible for graft congestion and dysfunction associated with SFSS. To combat this problem, various forms of inflow modulation such as portosystemic shunts, splenectomy, splenic artery ligation, and infusion of vasoactive agents have been described as promising tools to avoid SFSS in marginal-sized grafts.

One of the most important technical aspects of LDLT is optimization of venous outflow. The graft is placed in an orthotopic position. The hepatic vein anastomosis should take into consideration the final position of the graft and the anatomical adjustments in the first month post-transplantation, when the partial graft usually doubles its size. Venous outflow reconstructions are very common when using right lobes as opposed to left lateral segments and left lobes, which most commonly present with a single common outflow.

After completing the hepatic vein anastomosis, the portal vein anastomosis is performed and the graft is reperfused. The arterial anastomosis is often performed using loop magnification or the microscope due to the small caliber of the vessel. The duct-to-duct biliary reconstruction is performed whenever possible using the recipient bile duct. This decreases the biliary complication rate, is easier to perform, and provides endoscopic access to the duct in case of complications. When multiple ducts are presents, the biliary reconstruction is usually achieved by mean of a hepato-jejunostomy with a Roux-en-Y limb.

Recipient outcomes

Graft and patient survivals

For children, graft and patient survivals are comparable or better for LDLT than deceased donor grafting. In a large series from Kyoto University, 5-year graft and patient survivals were 81% and 82%, respectively. Similar survival rates have been observed in other Asian, European, and US centers.

In general, adult patients undergoing LDLT have lower MELD scores than those undergoing DBD LT, so direct comparisons of post-transplant survival may be misleading. On the other hand, when analyzed on an intent-to-treat basis from the time of evaluation, the A2ALL group found a significant advantage for those recipients receiving living donor grafts. Most of the advantage was due to the avoidance of death on the waiting list.

In Asia, where the number of DBD is extremely limited, LDLT has been performed even in patients with very advanced liver failure. In contrast, those patients are rarely considered as candidates for LDLT in Western countries because such patients are listed as high urgency and have the best chance of receiving an organ from a DBD in a timely fashion. Even considering this disadvantage, the long-term survival in adult LDLT is satisfactory.

Left lobe versus right lobe

Information regarding the comparison between left lobe and right lobe grafting is very limited. Although favorable outcome of LDLT using left lobe graft has been reported in adult recipients, many transplant centers still routinely use right lobe grafts. This practice best ameliorates the issue of graft size inherent in the fact that right lobe represents 60–70% of whole liver volume, whereas the left lobe provides only 30–40%. The larger graft is more likely to provide at least 40% of the recipients' standard liver volume, be able to meet the patient's metabolic demands, and withstand the hyperdynamic splanchnic flow seen in adult cirrhotics.

In determining whether a donor liver can provide sufficient hepatocyte function, it is important to estimate the functional capacity of the graft. This estimate is known as "functional graft size" and is a composite function of actual graft size modified by severity of the recipients' condition, the degree of portal hypertension, and the degree to which a graft's outflow might be impaired. In using left lobe grafts, actual graft size may not always exceed the 40% of standard liver volume threshold. Even in such cases, left lobe grafts have excellent venous outflow and can provide adequate functional mass in patients with low MELD score and/or little portal hypertension. However, if small left lobe grafts are used for patients with high MELD score or with severe portal hypertension, the risk of graft failure is very high. Thus careful donor and recipient selection clearly affects the outcome. In addition, inflow modifications to reduce portal flow have also been beneficial when using left lobe grafts.

Recipient complications

Small-for-size syndrome

In adult-to-adult LDLT, recipients have a risk of early postoperative graft failure that is separate and distinct from primary non-function seen in deceased donor grafting. This graft dysfunction is known as *small-for-size syndrome* (SFSS) and is characterized by progressive cholestasis, intractable ascites, coagulopathy, and renal failure. SFSS typically results in a reduction of graft survival rate and may increase recipient mortality. The pathogenesis of SFSS is multifactorial and has not been completely elucidated. Small graft size has been shown to be related to SFSS; however, actual graft size does not always reflect functional liver mass as described previously. In general, when GRWR is less than 0.8% or graft volume is less than 40% of a recipient's standard liver volume, the risk of SFSS becomes higher.

The severity of liver disease and recipient status along with severe portal hypertension also affects the risk of SFSS. Portal hyperperfusion to the small graft induces shear stress and sinusoidal injury as well as vasospasm in the hepatic artery. Although MELD score does not accurately reflect the severity of liver disease for all liver transplant candidates, patients with a lower MELD score tend to have a lower risk of developing SFSS. Thus patient selection plays a crucial role in regard to graft and patient outcomes.

In the case of portal hyperperfusion in the small graft, inflow modification of the portal vein is essential. To reduce portal vein flow, a pharmacological approach may be beneficial. Beta-blockers and somatostatin have been used in an attempt to attenuate portal hyperperfusion. Surgical approaches include splenic artery ligation, splenectomy, and portocaval shunt. The application of these approaches should be based on intraoperative measurement of portal vein flow and pressure. Ideally, portal vein flow should be less than 2 ml/min/g (liver weight). According to a recent report from Kyoto University, portal vein pressure less than 15 mmHg is related to better outcome. The major concern with portocaval shunt is the steal phenomenon of the portal flow to the systemic circulation, which may jeopardize graft regeneration and function. When this occurs, the shunt must be closed. Assuring perfect venous outflow is equally as important as appropriate portal inflow in avoiding SFSS. In the left lobe graft, venoplasty between left and middle hepatic veins is useful to increase the diameter of graft venous orifice. In the right lobe graft, drainage of middle hepatic vein tributaries is crucial to prevent congestion of the anterior segment. When the inferior right hepatic vein is greater than 5 mm in diameter, reconstruction of this vein to vena cava is strongly recommended.

Biliary complications

Biliary complications are the most common cause of significant recipient morbidity and come in two varieties: early bile leaks and late biliary strictures. The incidence of biliary complications has decreased over time, but it is still higher than that of DBD liver transplantation. Because right lobe grafts often have multiple bile ducts, they are associated with a higher rate of biliary complications than the left lobe graft, which almost always has only a single duct to reconstruct. In recent years, most centers prefer duct-to-duct reconstruction to hepato-jejunostomy because it is less time-consuming, is associated with a lower incidence of early bile leaks, and allows easy postoperative access to examine the bile duct endoscopically.

Bile leaks typically originate from either the anastomotic site or cut surface of the liver graft. They are diagnosed when biliary drainage is seen from the abdominal drain or the patient develops fever, abdominal pain, and abnormal liver function tests. In most cases, this complication can be managed by percutaneous drainage and biliary stenting. If left untreated, bile leaks can lead to sepsis and graft dysfunction. If infection occurs, antibiotic treatment in addition to drainage will be necessary.

Biliary anastomotic strictures are usually caused by local ischemia at the anastomotic site. Stricture causes elevated liver function tests with or without biliary dilatation. It usually can be managed with a biliary stent placed endoscopically or percutaneously and rarely requires surgical revision. Biliary complications secondary to hepatic artery complications are resistant to these interventions, and re-transplantation may be required.

Vascular complications

The concept of post-transplant vascular complications in LDLT is not different from DBD liver transplantation. Hepatic artery thrombosis (HAT) is a catastrophic complication with high risk of biliary necrosis and graft loss. The incidence of HAT has significantly decreased from 25% in the 1990s to less than 10% in the last 10 years. This improvement has been achieved by the introduction of microsurgical techniques in hepatic artery anastomosis. Frequent monitoring with duplex ultrasonography is very useful for early detection of HAT. Urgent thrombectomy and revascularization are sometimes effective to prevent devastating biliary complications. However, most recipients with early HAT experience intrahepatic biliary strictures and bilomas, which can cause biliary sepsis. Despite efforts at graft salvage, these patients have a high risk of graft failure and mortality.

The incidence of portal vein thrombosis ranges from 2–6%; it is also a devastating complication after LDLT. Risk factors include small graft size, presence of portal vein thrombus at the time of LDLT, and use of vein grafts for portal vein reconstruction and the presence of large porto-systemic shunts. Early diagnosis with duplex ultrasonography is key to reduce graft loss and mortality. Thrombectomy and revascularization is the gold standard for portal vein thrombosis; however, new interventional techniques including percutaneous thrombolysis and suction thrombectomy have been reported.

Hepatic outflow obstruction is a serious complication after LDLT. The main causes of the obstruction are a twist of the hepatic vein anastomosis or rotation of the graft and compression of the anastomosis after graft regeneration. Appearance of monophasic wave form and disappearance of triphasic wave form is diagnostic in duplex ultrasonography. Venoplasty and stent placement are effective to avoid graft failure. The long-term efficacy and patency of these intravascular stents need to be evaluated.

Rejection (LDLT versus DBD LT)

Kidney transplant recipients from living donors experience a lower incidence of acute and chronic rejection compared with those from deceased donors. This might be a consequence of shorter ischemic time and better graft quality, as well as an immunological advantage due to human leukocyte antigen (HLA) matching between biologically related individuals. This finding is less obvious in LDLT. The overall rates of acute rejection in LDLT are 47–68% in children and 11–33% in adults. According to a retrospective study from the A2ALL group, however, biopsy-proven acute rejection occurred in 27% of LDLT for adult recipients, which was comparable to recipients from deceased donors (27%). Comparative rates of acute rejection have also been reported in children. However, the rates of steroid-resistant rejection and chronic rejection are lower in LDLT for children.

Recent topics in LDLT

Dual graft

Up to 25% of living donors are not suitable for right lobe donation due to a proportionately large right lobe (>70% of total liver volume). In these cases, the FLR after right lobectomy will be less that 30%, which leads to an unacceptably high risk of donor morbidity and mortality. To reduce the donor risk and obtain sufficient liver volume for an adult recipient, two small grafts from two different living donors can be transplanted into the single recipient. There may be many different graft combinations used, such as two left lateral segments, two left lobes, a left lobe and small right lobe, or a small right lobe and a left lateral segment graft. The purpose is to keep the donor risk index as small as possible for each donor while providing adequate functional liver mass to the recipient. Common complications in dual-graft recipients are biliary anastomotic stricture and outflow obstruction of the hepatic vein. Although dual-graft LDLT is accepted in Asian countries, it has not become widely used in the West.

ABO-incompatible LDLT

Liver transplantation across the ABO blood type barrier is usually not done except in emergent situations when an ABO-compatible donor is not available. ABO-incompatible LT is associated with a high risk of antibody-mediated rejection, infectious complications, and vascular thrombosis resulting in poor graft and patient survivals. Immunomodulation is key to minimizing complications. In Japan, the utilization of ABO-incompatible donors is not just a rescue therapy; it is an extended routine application if no compatible donors are available. According to the Japan Study Group for ABO-Incompatible Transplantation, this technique was started for pediatric recipients in the early 1990s and was recently extended to adult patients.

Interestingly, recipient age is a major determinant of graft and patient survival in ABO-incompatible LDLT. The 5-year survival rate of infants (<1 year old) is 85%, which is comparable to ABO-compatible LDLT. In contrast, the 5-year survival rate of adults (>16 years old) is only 52%. ABO-incompatible LDLT can be considered as a standard treatment for pediatric patients when no other identical or compatible donor is available. For adult patients, ABO-incompatible LDLT is still a challenge. The recent improvement in survival rates justifies continuing ABO-incompatible LDLT for adults in particular areas where living donors are realistically the only source of liver grafts.

Paired liver donor exchange program

Another approach to avoid ABO incompatibility between donor and recipient is paired donor exchange. Paired kidney donor exchange programs have successfully increased organ availability in many countries since 1986 and are currently functioning as a valuable tool for patients with ABO-incompatible donors. A liver donor exchange program was implemented in Korea in 2003 and Hong Kong in 2009. At the Asan Medical Center in Seoul, 16 donor–recipient pairs (eight pair sets) were involved in an exchange program from 2003 to 2009. Operations were performed on an elective basis in 12 and on an emergency basis in 4. After exchange, all pairs were ABO-identical or ABO-compatible. The 5-year graft and patient survival rates were 93.8%. Although there are logistical, ethical, religious, cultural, and mathematical issues limiting availability of paired donor programs, recipients with no suitable donors can benefit from this modality, and the results are far better than those achieved with ABO-incompatible grafts.

Further reading

Akamatsu N, Sugawara Y, Tamura S, Imamura H, Kokudo N, Makuuchi M. Regeneration and function of hemiliver graft: right versus left. *Surgery* 2006; **139**: 765–72.

Barr ML, Belghiti J, Villamil FG, *et al.* A report of the Vancouver Forum on the care of the live organ donor: lung, liver, pancreas, and intestine data and medical guidelines. *Transplantation* 2006; **81**: 1373–85.

Fan ST (eds). *Living Donor Liver Transplantation.* Hong Kong: Takungpao Publishing, 2007.

Fisher RA, Kulik LM, Freise CE, *et al.* A2ALL Study Group. Hepatocellular carcinoma recurrence and death following living and deceased donor liver transplantation. *Am J Transplant* 2007; **7**: 1601–8.

Gruessner RWG, Benedetti (eds). *Living Donor Organ Transplantation.* New York: McGraw-Hill, 2008.

Hwang S, Lee SG, Moon DB, *et al.* Exchange living donor liver transplantation to overcome ABO incompatibility in adult patients. *Liver Transpl* 2010; **16**: 482–90.

Chapter 23

Surgical procedure

Simon J.F. Harper and Neville V. Jamieson

Key points

- A successful liver transplant requires a number of procedures, including donor hepatectomy, preparation of the donor liver, recipient hepatectomy, and implantation of the liver graft.
- The cold ischemic time of the liver (period between cold perfusion and reperfusion with recipient blood) should not be more than 16 hours and ideally less than 12 hours.
- The recipient hepatectomy is frequently the most difficult part of the transplant procedure, described by Starzl as "the bloodiest and most stressful experience in a surgeon's life."
- If there is hemodynamic instability during the anhepatic phase, veno-venous bypass is instigated via the femoral vein (usually via the saphenous vein) to an internal jugular or subclavian line in the neck, with or without a combined portal bypass limb.
- Reperfusion of the liver is often the most dangerous part of the transplant procedure, and close communication between surgeon and anesthetist is crucial.

Liver transplantation is life-saving but remains one of the most challenging surgical procedures undertaken. The unique anatomical and physiological properties of the liver and the profound pathological changes associated with liver disease were long thought to render transplantation impossible. The first human liver transplant was performed by Starzl in 1963 on a 3-year-old girl with biliary atresia; the patient unfortunately succumbed to massive intra-operative hemorrhage. Successful liver transplantation, without early mortality, was not achieved until 1967, such was the formidable challenge it presented. Now long established as a standard treatment for fulminant liver disease, the liver transplant operation is still a major undertaking for both patient and surgeon alike. However, continuous refinement of all aspects of the procedure over nearly 50 years has contributed greatly to the excellent outcomes now available to increasing numbers of patients with liver disease. A successful liver transplant relies on the effective execution of several component procedures, frequently involving several surgeons; fundamentally these are the donor hepatectomy, preparation of the donor liver, recipient hepatectomy, and implantation of the liver graft.

Donor procedure

The donor procedure represents the first crucial step in a liver transplant and should be performed by an experienced retrieval surgeon, aiming to preserve the donor liver in optimal condition (discussed further in Chapter 5).

Donor hepatectomy in donors after brainstem death

In procurement from donation after brain death (DBD) donors, unlike donation after cardiac death (DCD) donors, maintenance of cardiac output after confirmation of death allows a significant proportion of dissection to be performed prior to cold perfusion with preservation solution ("warm dissection"). This has the distinct advantage that important structures are much easier to identify and can be prepared with greater precision, minimizing organ damage and shortening dissection after perfusion ("cold dissection"), during which suboptimal cooling of the organs may occur. It is suggested by some surgeons that only

Organ Transplantation: A Clinical Guide, ed. A.A. Klein, C.J. Lewis, and J.C. Madsen. Published by Cambridge University Press.

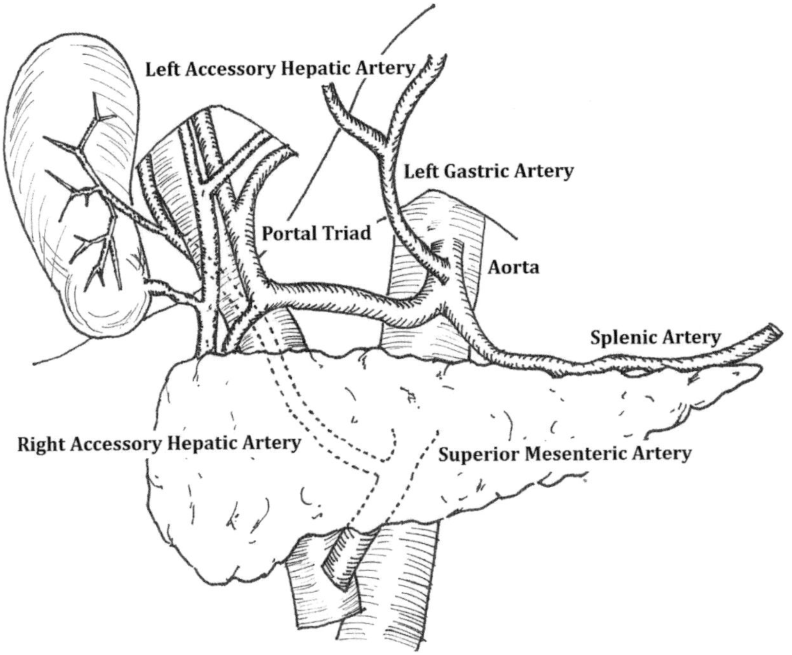

Figure 23.1 Anatomy of accessory hepatic arteries. The left accessory or replaced hepatic artery arises from the left gastric and traverses the lesser omentum to enter the left lobe of the liver. The right accessory or replaced hepatic artery arises from the SMA near its origin and runs behind the pancreas and portal triad before entering the posterolateral aspect of the hilum of the liver.

minimal warm dissection should ever be undertaken, however, arguing that a prolonged laparotomy in the context of major pathophysiological changes associated with brainstem death may cause organ injury. With this later approach, an en bloc technique, as commonly used in DCD donation (see next section), is usually employed for organ extraction, reserving delicate hilar dissection to the back table, thus minimizing risk of injury. There is little robust evidence to support either approach, and surgeons frequently vary the extent of warm dissection undertaken depending on factors such as donor instability, aberrant donor anatomy, and donor obesity.

A midline laparotomy and sternotomy is performed and can be extended using transverse abdominal incisions to maximize surgical access. A full exploratory laparotomy is undertaken to exclude intra-abdominal sepsis or malignancy, and any suspicious lesions are biopsied and sent for urgent histological analysis. Early assessment of liver quality is performed, in particular the degree of steatosis and, in cases of donor death secondary to trauma, exclusion of liver injury.

Dissection commences with mobilization of the right colon, duodenum, and small bowel leftward and superiorly (the Cattell-Braasch maneuver) to expose aorta and inferior vena cava (IVC). The aorta is encircled at this early stage in preparation for cannulation to allow rapid perfusion in the case of sudden donor instability or cardiopulmonary arrest. The inferior mesenteric vein (IMV) is then prepared if it is to be used for perfusion of the portal system. In combined liver–pancreas procurement, IMV cannulation is usually avoided, as the increased portal pressure can cause pancreatic edema and compromise perfusion. In this scenario, early division and direct cannulation of the portal vein during cold dissection is performed instead, allowing both portal perfusion of the liver and adequate drainage of the pancreas.

The liver is mobilized by dividing the falciform and left triangular ligaments. The lesser omentum is then divided, taking care to exclude a left replaced or accessory hepatic artery, present in approximately 10% of donors. If identified, the left accessory artery is preserved by dissecting the left gastric artery, from which it arises, from the lesser curve of the stomach, leaving it and the common hepatic artery (if present) with a common inflow at the celiac trunk (Figure 23.1).

The liver hilum is dissected to identify structures of the portal triad and exclude or preserve a replaced or accessory right hepatic artery. The common hepatic artery is traced from the origin of the gastroduodenal artery (GDA) to the celiac axis, where the splenic artery is identified. The common bile duct (CBD) is found on the right edge of the portal triad, ligated distally, and divided. Hilar dissection above the level of the GDA and extensive peri-ductal dissection is avoided to protect the fragile blood supply to the CBD.

The portal vein is then encircled and adjacent tissue carefully inspected for the presence of a right accessory/replaced hepatic artery arising from the origin of the superior mesenteric artery (SMA; Figure 23.1). If present, the vessel must be traced along its course behind or within the pancreas in preparation for careful preservation during hepatectomy. Extensive dissection at this stage, particularly intra-pancreatic, is often best avoided by excising a "cuff" of pancreatic parenchyma during the cold dissection (to be removed on the bench) or in the case of combined pancreatic retrieval, removal of liver and pancreas en bloc for back table separation. This approach can also be used in the rare anatomical variant in which the common hepatic artery arises from the SMA.

Preparation for cold-phase hepatectomy is completed by slinging the supraceliac aorta behind the divided right crus, systemic heparinization of the donor, and cannulation of aorta and IMV. The supraceliac aorta is then clamped, perfusion with preservation fluid commenced, venting performed via atrium or IVC, and crushed ice instilled into the peritoneal cavity. A total volume of 5–6 liters of preservation solution is infused via portal and systemic cannulae, aiming to observe clearing of the vented effluent. It is very important that the cold-phase hepatectomy is timely to minimize the interval between core cooling with preservation fluid infusion and effective external cooling in the organ transport carrier. Mobilization should therefore be started during perfusion by dividing the suprahepatic IVC and the diaphragm well clear of the ligamentous attachments of the liver to release the right lobe. On completion of perfusion, the portal vein is transected and the hepatic artery dissected back to the aorta leaving a patch around the celiac trunk, preserving the left gastric in the case of a left accessory artery. A right accessory artery is preserved as described above, usually maintaining a stump of SMA, although a common patch with the celiac trunk can also be used. The donor hepatectomy is completed by dividing the infrahepatic IVC above the renal veins and transecting the adherent right adrenal gland, thereby avoiding capsular injury to the liver.

Donor hepatectomy in donors after cardiac death

In DCD retrieval, a rapid technique after immediate perfusion and cooling is employed. After confirmation of death and a stand-off period, usually 5 minutes, rapid laparotomy and iliac artery or aortic cannulation and perfusion is performed. Instillation of crushed ice, thoracotomy for atrial venting and aortic cross clamp, division and direct cannulation of the portal vein, and division and saline flushing of CBD must follow in rapid succession. After adequate perfusion, donor hepatectomy is most rapidly and safely performed en bloc with the pancreas, assuming the presence of accessory hepatic arteries and avoiding the need for any further in situ hilar dissection. The major attachments of the liver are divided as described for DBD donors, ensuring the left gastric artery is dissected away from stomach and preserved with the organ block. The anterior surface of the pancreas is exposed by dividing the greater omentum, short gastric vessels, the transverse mesocolon, and the root of the small bowel mesentery. The head of the pancreas is mobilized by full Kocherization and stapled transection of the pylorus and proximal jejunum. The tail of the pancreas is elevated medially using the spleen as a "handle" or can be transected if not for transplantation. The resection is completed by dividing the SMA flush with the aorta and continuing superiorly to create an aortic patch at the celiac ostium.

Benchwork preparation of the liver for transplantation

Preparation of the liver for transplantation is usually performed following a period of efficient cooling in an ice box and transportation (if required) to the recipient center. The cold ischemic time (period between cold perfusion and reperfusion with recipient blood) should not be more than 16 hours and ideally less than 12 hours. When possible, the recipient hepatectomy should be commenced simultaneously with liver procurement and transportation to allow much shorter cold ischemic times. This is particularly pertinent in the context of DCD donation, where detrimental effects of warm and cold ischemia are potentially compounding. Prior to implantation, the IVC is dissected clear of surrounding tissue ensuring that both atrial and diaphragmatic muscle is removed, as fibrotic changes within this may contribute to post-implantation caval stenosis. Care must also be taken to avoid injury to the main hepatic veins, which can have a significant extra-parenchymal component, and to ligate phrenic veins, which are a troublesome source of bleeding on reperfusion. The portal vein and hepatic artery are dissected free of surrounding tissue and reconstructed if required (discussed below); the bile duct is left undisturbed. At this stage, reduction or splitting of the graft for two recipients can be performed. The technical details of split liver transplantation for both adult and pediatric grafts are discussed in Chapters 22 and 26.

Recipient procedure

Recipient hepatectomy and caval anastomosis

The preoperative preparation of potential recipients for liver transplantation is discussed in detail in Chapter 24. Once under anesthesia, central and peripheral venous access is obtained and arterial cannulation and catheterization performed. The patient is draped, leaving access to chest, abdomen, and groins, and a cell-saver system is prepared. An inverted "L," Mercedes Benz, or rooftop incision is made in the right upper quadrant, and an exploratory laparotomy is performed. The recipient hepatectomy is frequently the most difficult part of the transplant procedure, described by Starzl as "the bloodiest and most stressful experience in a surgeon's life." Intra-abdominal varices can be extremely large, friable, and associated with torrential hemorrhage, which can start with cavernous cutaneous tributaries at the initial skin incision. The surgeon must often strike a difficult balance between acceptable control of hemorrhage and adequate rate of progression through the procedure, in the knowledge that both variceal dilatation and coagulopathy will rapidly improve following implantation.

The hepatectomy begins with division of the left triangular ligament, falciform ligament, and lesser omentum before moving to the hilum. In direct contrast to the donor hepatectomy, the dissection is focused high up in the hilum to obtain maximal length of vessels for anastomosis. The common hepatic artery is ligated and divided at its bifurcation, as this can often be split to form a patch for the arterial anastomosis. The CBD is divided at a similar level, again keeping peri-ductal dissection to a minimum. The portal vein is then encircled and remaining periportal tissue (predominantly lymphatics) divided, ensuring that an accessory right hepatic artery is not missed. The infrahepatic vena cava is then dissected and encircled, often requiring division of the right adrenal vein.

Mobilization of the liver continues with division of the right triangular ligament and separation of the bare area of the liver from the retroperitoneum, exposing the retrohepatic IVC on the right side. The ongoing dissection around the IVC then depends on the elected management of graft caval outflow, which can be approached with three different techniques: "classical" caval replacement, "piggyback," or cavocavoplasty (Figure 23.2). In a "classical" liver transplant, complete retrocaval dissection is performed and the supra and infra-hepatic vena cava cross-clamped, allowing resection of the liver and intrahepatic vena cava en bloc (Figure 23.2A). The main disadvantage of this technique is the marked decrease in venous return during the anhepatic phase, which can lead to profound hemodynamic instability. It is therefore essential that a "test" cross-clamp be performed prior to hepatectomy. If instability is observed or expected, venovenous bypass is instigated via open cannulation of the femoral vein (usually via the saphenous vein) in the groin connected by a roller pump–driven circuit to an internal jugular or subclavian line in the neck, with or without a combined portal bypass limb. In early canine and human liver transplantation, with the absence of experienced anesthetic care, the introduction of bypass massively reduced operative mortality. However, it is now recognized that the majority of patients can tolerate caval cross-clamp without bypass, avoiding the associated risks of vascular injury, pulmonary thromboembolism, and air embolus.

The "piggyback" and cavocavoplasty techniques almost completely obviate the need for bypass, as the liver is dissected from the vena cava, leaving the latter in situ without the need for cross-clamping and interruption of venous return. This technically challenging maneuver, first performed by Calne in Cambridge, United Kingdom, involves careful separation of liver and vena cava starting caudally with the division of the numerous tributaries draining the caudate lobe until only the three main hepatic veins remain. In the "piggyback" technique, the three veins are cross-clamped and, after excision of the liver,

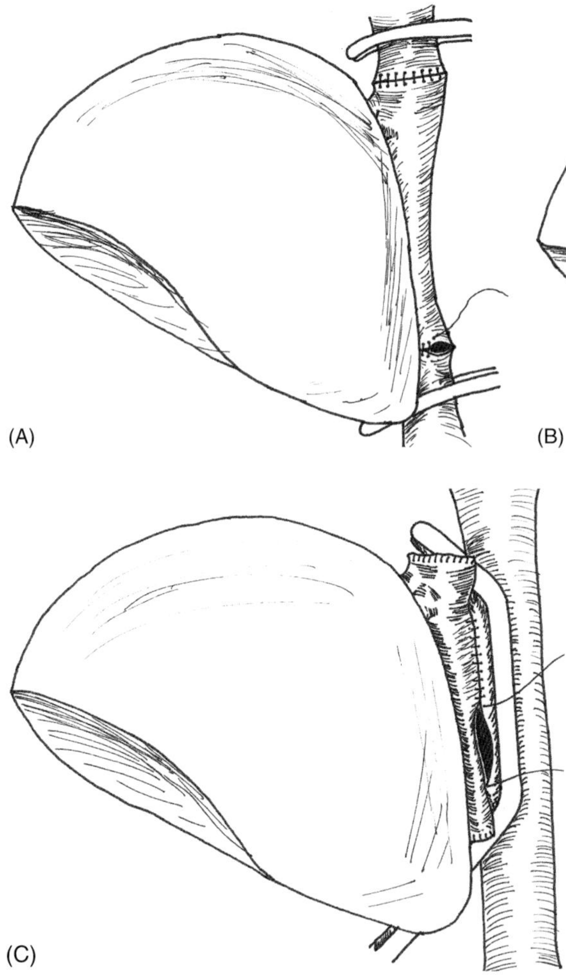

Figure 23.2 Techniques for caval anastomosis. (A) The classical caval replacement involves complete excision of recipient intrahepatic vena cava en bloc with the explanted liver, which is then replaced by donor cava using upper and lower end-to-end anastomoses. (B) The "piggy back" technique requires preservation of recipient vena cava and cross-clamping of the main hepatic veins, which are opened into a single orifice for anastomosis to the top end of the donor vena cava. (C) The cavocavoplasty is performed by joining donor and preserved recipient vena cavae via longitudinal venotomies following closure of both ends of the donor vena cava.

opened into a single orifice for anastomosis to the top end of the donor vena cava (the bottom end being closed off; Figure 23.2B). In a cavocavoplasty, the recipient hepatic veins are stapled or sutured closed at hepatectomy, as are the ends of the donor vena cava, and donor and recipient vena cavae are anastomosed together via symmetrical longitudinal venotomies (Figure 23.2C). Despite the advantages of the cava-preserving techniques, the classical approach remains very useful, particularly in offering maximal tumor clearance in transplantation for hepatocellular carcinoma and rapidity of hepatectomy in the unstable patient. Furthermore, in severely distorted cirrhotic livers, particularly with significant compensatory caudate lobe hypertrophy, the risks associated with caval preservation may outweigh the potential benefits.

Portal venous anastomosis

On completion of the caval anastomosis, the portal venous and hepatic arterial anastomoses are performed. It is common practice to complete the portal anastomosis first and reperfuse the liver prior to the arterial anastomosis in order to minimize secondary warm ischemic time (the time in which the liver is removed from ice but not yet reperfused). However, these anastomoses can be performed in reverse or both completed prior to reperfusion, the argument being that portal perfusion alone may allow organ

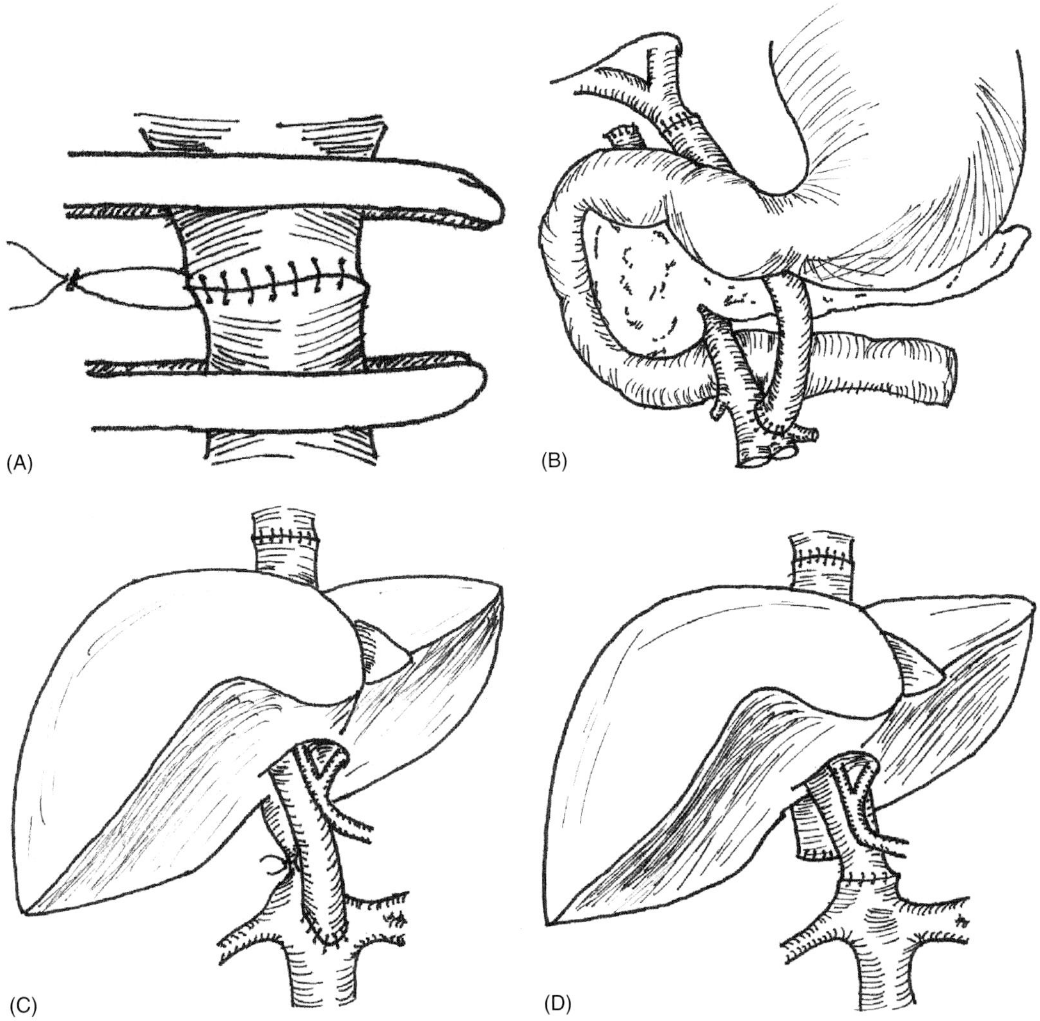

Figure 23.3 Techniques for portal inflow to the transplanted liver. (A) The simple portal vein anastomosis is performed with a continuous suture, and it is crucial that a "growth factor" is left to allow for significant expansion at the anastomosis on reperfusion. (B) In cases of portal vein thrombosis with minimal SMV involvement, an anti-pancreatic jump graft between SMV and donor portal vein using donor iliac vessels can be created. In cases of more extensive SMV involvement, a portocaval hemitransposition can be performed by end-to-side (C), or by end-to-end (D) anastomosis of recipient vena cava to donor portal vein.

warming in the context of suboptimal oxygenation, particularly of the biliary tree. The portal anastomosis usually involves simple end-to-end apposition of donor and recipient portal veins, although this must be done with technical precision. The correct final length of the portal vein is essential, and accurate estimation is facilitated by placing packs between the unperfused liver and diaphragm during the anastomosis, thus simulating the increased size of the graft observed following reperfusion. If the vein is too short, excessive tension causes tearing of the thin-walled vein, and an overlong portal vein is prone to kinking and thrombosis. It is also very important that on completion of the continuous suturing for the anastomosis, the knot is tied several centimeters from the vein to allow a "growth factor" on reperfusion and prevent a dumbbell-shaped anastomotic narrowing (Figure 23.3A). Alternatively, tying of the final knot can be delayed until after release of clamps and complete filling of the vein.

The greatest challenge when performing the portal venous anastomosis is the presence of portal vein thrombosis (PVT), which was originally an absolute contraindication to liver transplantation, but is now part of standard practice. Despite advances in surgical techniques, PVT at transplantation is still associated with a high risk of re-thrombosis, graft loss, and mortality. The difficulty in creating adequate portal inflow is compounded by severe portal hypertension and variceal formation, marked peri-portal fibrosis, and previous porto-systemic bypass procedures that frequently require reversal. The extent of PVT governs the management and has been classified by Yerdel into four grades. Grade 1 and 2 PVT describes thrombus in the portal vein with no more than minimal involvement of the superior mesenteric vein (SMV), causing less than or greater than 50% occlusion, respectively. In the majority of these cases, thrombectomy and/or excision of the affected vein with primary anastomosis to distal portal vein or proximal SMV can be performed. A similar approach can on occasion be applied to grade 3 PVT (complete PV occlusion extending to the proximal SMV), although exploration and thrombectomy behind the pancreas should be avoided due to risk of significant bleeding, pancreatic injury, and pancreatitis. In such cases, drainage of the SMV proximal to the occlusion is best achieved by using a jump graft to the donor portal vein fashioned using donor iliac vessels (Figure 23.3B). In grade 4 PVT (extensive SMV thrombosis) and grade 3 PVT in which a bypass is not possible, portal inflow can sometimes be derived from large collateral vessels and donor portal anastomosis to left gastric, right gastroepiploic, splenic, right or middle colic, pericholedochal, and renal veins have been described. In the absence of adequate collaterals, the options remaining are cavoportal hemitransposition, in which the lower end of the transected recipient IVC is anastomosed to the graft portal vein instead of the lower vena cava, and multi-visceral transplantation (Figures 23.3C and 3D).

Hepatic artery anastomosis

The dominant recipient hepatic artery, whether common or accessory, is prepared and used for the arterial anastomosis. In the donor artery, the common anastomotic sites are the origin of the celiac trunk with aortic patch or branch patches using the left gastric or GDA. In the recipient, branch patches using the hepatic artery bifurcation or at origin of the GDA are most frequently employed. In the situation in which poor inflow or vascular disease prevents use of a GDA patch in the recipient hepatic artery, more proximal exploration along the common hepatic artery is usually not helpful. The best option in such cases is formation of an aortic conduit running from an anastomosis on the front of the infra-renal aorta, via a carefully created retropancreatic tunnel, to the graft hepatic artery (Figure 23.4A). The ideal conduit is usually both donor iliac vessels joined end-to-end or a segment of donor thoracic aorta, avoiding prosthetic grafts as far as possible.

In the presence of variations in donor arterial anatomy, a right accessory artery is most commonly prepared for implantation by anastomosing a short trunk of SMA, with right accessory artery attached, between the celiac trunk and the recipient hepatic artery (Figure 23.4B). Alternatively, the accessory artery can be anastomosed to a branch on the common hepatic trunk (usually the GDA or splenic artery), again creating a single anastomosis to the recipient artery (Figure 23.4C). On occasion, the celiac trunk and SMA (with right accessory artery) can be kept on a single aortic patch and anastomosed together, particularly when employing an aortic conduit. A left accessory hepatic artery is usually easily managed, providing the liver has been retrieved correctly. In most cases, anastomosis using the donor celiac patch is performed allowing inflow into both the main hepatic artery and left hepatic artery via the left gastric without need for reconstruction (Figure 23.4D). In uncommon cases when the celiac trunk is unusable or the left accessory has been damaged beyond simple repair, reconstruction is performed by joining the end of the accessory or adjoining left gastric to another celiac artery branch (e.g., splenic artery or GDA).

Reperfusion and bile duct anastomosis

Reperfusion of the liver is often the most dangerous part of the transplant procedure, and close communication between surgeon and anesthetist is crucial. Prior to reperfusion, it is essential that the liver is flushed of potassium-rich preservation fluid to avoid significant risk of arrhythmia or cardiac arrest. This is performed using a cold colloid infusion via the portal vein just before completion of the caval

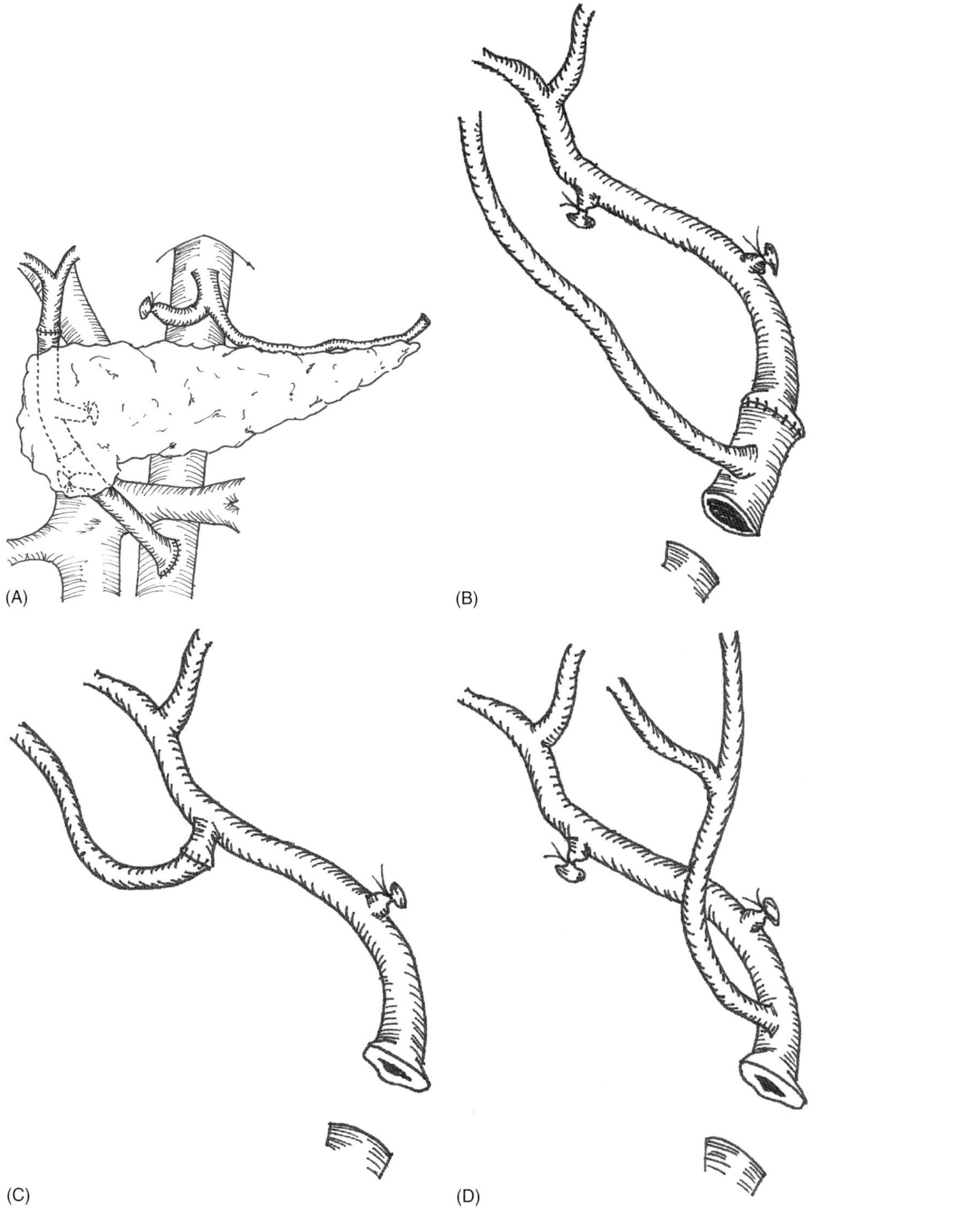

Figure 23.4 Techniques for hepatic arterial anastomosis. (A) In the absence of adequate inflow from the recipient coeliac axis, a conduit from the infrarenal aorta to the donor hepatic artery can be created, most commonly using both donor iliac arteries anastomosed together. In the presence of a right accessory artery an attached segment of SMA can be anastomosed to the coeliac aortic patch (B), or the accessory vessel can be anastomosed to a branch of the celiac trunk (the GDA shown here) (C). The left accessory artery is perfused by preserving the left gastric artery from which it arises. (D)

anastomosis and/or using a blood flush on reperfusion, allowing loss of 300–500 ml of blood via the caval anastomosis prior to closure and release of caval clamps. Despite this precaution, profound hypotension may occur on reperfusion due to the combination of a marked systemic ischemia–reperfusion response and significant blood loss.

Once stability of the patient and meticulous hemostasis has been established, occasionally taking several hours, the bile duct anastomosis is performed. The standard technique involves apposition of donor and recipient ducts with minimal preparatory dissection to preserve blood supply. The supply to the cut ends comes from three fine vessels running longitudinally along the duct surface, and so interrupted suture placement is used to minimize its disruption, aiming to avoid local ischemia and anastomotic dehiscence or stenosis. Alternatively, the donor bile duct can be anastomosed to a Roux-en-Y loop of jejunum via a small enterotomy, again using interrupted suturing. The most common indications for the latter technique are transplantation for primary sclerosing cholangitis, re-transplantation, donor/recipient duct size discrepancy, and concern over recipient duct viability.

The transplant is completed by thorough hemostasis, confirmation of adequate graft perfusion, placement of drains to the hilum and suprahepatic space, and closure. The patient is then transferred to intensive care or high-dependency setting for close postoperative monitoring.

Further reading

Busuttil R, Klintmalm G. *Transplantation of the Liver*. Philadelphia, PA: Saunders, 2005.

Calne R. *Liver Transplantation: the Cambridge-King's College Hospital Experience*. (2nd Edition). Orlando, FL: Grune and Stratton, 1987.

Humar A, Matas A, Payne W. *Atlas of Organ Transplantation*. London: Springer, 2006.

Molmenti E, Klintmalm G. *Atlas of Liver Transplantation*. Philadelphia, PA: Saunders, 2002.

Starzl T. *The Puzzle People: Memoirs of a Transplant Surgeon*. Pittsburgh, PA: University of Pittsburgh Press, 1992.

Chapter 24

Peri-operative care and early complications

John Klinck and Andrew J. Butler

Key points

- Severe liver disease affects all organ systems, and comorbidity is common.
- The transplant procedure is marked by cardiovascular instability, major hemorrhage, and important electrolyte, acid–base, and hemostatic disturbances.
- Marginal grafts are increasingly used, increasing the risk of postoperative complications.
- Bleeding is usually due to transections in the complex mesh of portosystemic collateral veins; therefore, fluid management, portal hyperemia, and blood loss may be linked.
- The most important early complications are primary non-function, hepatic artery thrombosis, and bleeding.

The peri-operative and early postoperative management of the liver transplant recipient presents a formidable challenge. This chapter outlines the pathophysiology of liver disease as it affects patient selection and management in the peri-operative period and key aspects of anesthetic, surgical, and early postoperative care.

Preoperative assessment

Pathophysiology and relevant comorbidity

Chronic liver disease is associated with portal hypertension, impaired hepatic synthetic function, malnutrition, peripheral and pulmonary microvascular shunting, renal impairment, and encephalopathy. Life-threatening complications are common, including variceal hemorrhage and sepsis from bacterial peritonitis or pneumonia. Common pathophysiological disturbances and their management in the peri-operative period are summarized in Table 24.1.

Cardiovascular

Cardiovascular function in liver failure is characterized by a disturbance of microcirculatory function causing arteriovenous shunting, increased cardiac output, and abnormal blood volume distribution, in proportion to the severity of the underlying hepatic disease. Central blood volume is reduced, inducing increased sympathetic and hormonal vasoconstrictor activity. Despite this, splanchnic blood volume and flow are increased. Subtle functional and structural changes occur in the heart, now described as cirrhotic cardiomyopathy. These include impaired responses to increased preload and afterload and conduction abnormalities. Left atrial enlargement, mild left ventricular (LV) hypertrophy, and diastolic dysfunction are common echocardiographic findings.

Patients with alcoholic cirrhosis, amyloidosis, or Wilson's disease may have overt cardiomyopathy. Any evidence of significant cardiac disease must be taken seriously in view of the major insults imposed during and after surgery. Patients with known ischemic heart disease (IHD) or peripheral or cerebrovascular disease should be considered for coronary angiography. Significant coronary disease and/or global LV dysfunction probably contraindicate transplant.

The approach to patients without known IHD but with risk factors (age $>$ 55 years, diabetes, hypertension, smoking, obesity) is more controversial. Non-invasive stress imaging (dobutamine stress echo or myocardial perfusion scan) followed by coronary angiography is costly and will identify occult disease

Organ Transplantation: A Clinical Guide, ed. A.A. Klein, C.J. Lewis, and J.C. Madsen. Published by Cambridge University Press.

Table 24.1 Preoperative disorders and peri-operative management in the liver transplant recipient

System	Disorder	Peri-operative management
Cardiovascular: systemic and splanchnic	Increased cardiac index Reduced central and increased splanchnic blood volumes Impaired diastolic function Cardiomyopathy (esp. alcohol, amyloid, Wilson's, hemochromatosis) Autonomic neuropathy (mild in cirrhosis, marked in amyloid)	Balance preload and vasoconstrictors (see text) If renal or cardiac dysfunction consider piggyback or veno-venous bypass TEE Pacing wire if amyloid polyneuropathy
Cardiovascular: pulmonary	Portopulmonary hypertension (PA mean > 25, PVR > 250)	Preop right heart catheter if Doppler PA sys > 40 (to differentiate from high-flow state and overload) Defer transplant and treat if PA mean > 35 or RV dilated or impaired Intra-operative PA catheter (± TEE) essential if pulmonary hypertension suspected
Respiratory	Restrictive defect (ascites) Pleural effusion Flow-related or anatomical intrapulmonary shunting (hepatopulmonary syndrome) Non-cardiogenic pulmonary edema (fulminant hepatic failure) Obstructive airways disease (esp. cystic fibrosis, α_1-antitrypsin deficiency) Interstitial lung disease (primary biliary cirrhosis).	$FiO_2 \geq 0.5$ Drain large effusion early intra-operatively (beware re-expansion pulmonary edema, especially at reperfusion) Cautious use of PEEP
Renal	Hepatorenal syndrome (prerenal failure from splanchnic "steal") Acute tubular necrosis from sepsis Tacrolimus/cyclosporine-related renal impairment Renal tubular acidosis	Preoperative hemodiafiltration if K+ > 5.5 Maintain arterial pressure Consider intraoperative pressor (norepinephrine or vasopressin) Anhepatic, mannitol
Electrolytes/metabolic	Hyponatremia, hypomagnesemia, hyperkalemia, metabolic acidosis, and hypoglycemia in fulminant liver failure	Defer transplant if high surgical risk and Na < 122; treat hyperkalemia if preanhepatic > 5.0 or rapid anhepatic rise; – MgSO4 if any arrhythmia; consider tris-buffer, hemodiafiltration if acidosis severe; close monitoring and treatment of hypo/hyperglycemia
Hematological/coagulation	Reduced/defective synthesis of Vitamin K-dependent clotting factors Low-grade DIC ± hyperfibrinolysis Anemia, thrombocytopenia (hypersplenism and marrow depression) Platelet dysfunction Note impaired synthesis of anticoagulant factors may preserve hemostasis	Consider prophylactic tranexamic acid if high risk and no prothrombotic history Assess coagulation clinically before treatment (cannulation sites, surgical field): treat clinical coagulopathy according to TEG and laboratory data (blood products, antifibrinolytic, protamine). Maintain normothermia. If intractable coagulopathy consult hematologist and consider FVIIa by local protocol.
Central nervous system	Encephalopathy Cerebral edema	Avoid/minimize benzodiazepines; in fulminant liver failure with grade III/IV encephalopathy consider ICP monitoring and maintain cerebral perfusion pressure >60 mmHg (norepinephrine), ± mannitol/hypertonic saline/thiopental to control ICP.

DIC = disseminated intravascular coagulation; ICP = intracranial pressure.

in many (5–27%). However, few patients are suitable for revascularization, and there is no evidence of better outcomes. Screening on the basis of clinical assessment (including exercise tolerance) and resting echocardiography alone is more cost-effective but will occasionally miss occult disease that (rarely) might have been treated.

Like IHD, valvular aortic stenosis is increasingly seen in older patients referred for liver transplantation and remains an important cause of peri-operative death. Mild functional mitral, tricuspid, and aortic regurgitation are frequently found on echocardiography but are usually attributable to the hyperdynamic state.

Pulmonary

Pulmonary hypertension is seen in up to 20% of adult liver transplant candidates and is usually identified by transthoracic echocardiography. In most cases it is caused by LV overload (high cardiac output in the presence of diastolic dysfunction) and is not true portopulmonary hypertension. This condition is pathologically indistinguishable from primary pulmonary hypertension and occurs in less than 4% of adult candidates. Peak echo-Doppler pulmonary artery (PA) pressure greater than 40 mmHg should be investigated by PA catheterization to measure mean PA pressure, pulmonary capillary wedge pressure (PCWP), and pulmonary vascular resistance (PVR). Mean PA pressure greater than 35 mmHg with a high PVR ($>$240 dyn s/cm^5) has a reported 50% peri-operative mortality, approaching 100% if greater than 50 mmHg or if associated with right ventricular (RV) dysfunction. Effective treatments are available (sildenafil, bosentan, iloprost) and appear to reduce peri-operative risk. In most patients, pulmonary hypertension resolves after transplant.

Hepatopulmonary syndrome is characterized by marked pulmonary shunting and orthostatic arterial desaturation (orthodeoxia) in the absence of intrinsic pulmonary disease. It is associated with portal hypertension and presents a spectrum of severity, affecting up to 33% of transplant candidates, about 4% severely. The most common pathophysiological feature is the "perfusion–diffusion" defect of high flow through diffusely dilated pulmonary capillaries. Arteriovenous malformations identifiable on computed tomography (CT) pulmonary angiogram are an uncommon cause. Contrast echocardiography is a sensitive screening tool and also serves to exclude right-to-left shunt at the atrial level. A preoperative PaO_2 less than 50 mmHg or radiolabeled macroaggregated albumin uptake in the brain greater than 30% are associated with increased 90-day mortality, although this is not prohibitive. In our unit, oxygen dependency, age greater than 50 years, and the presence of other major comorbidity would probably contraindicate transplant. Although intra-operative problems with oxygenation are rarely observed, weaning from mechanical ventilation may be prolonged, and these patients are more vulnerable to sepsis and other post-transplant complications.

Obstructive airways disease, usually related to smoking but occasionally to familial emphysema or alpha-1 antitrypsin deficiency, is seen in up to 18% of adults presenting for liver transplant. Recurrent chest infections may be a feature, but history and clinical signs are often minimal. Flow-volume measurements show an obstructive pattern, often mixed with the restriction of vital capacity seen in massive ascites. There are no data on its effect on liver transplant outcome. Forced expiratory volumes in 1 second (FEV_1) as low as 30% of predicted are associated with good outcomes in young recipients with cystic fibrosis (CF), but in older patients, values below 40–50% in the absence of pleural effusion or ascites require a cautious approach.

Other causes of respiratory impairment include ascites and hydrothorax, poorly controlled asthma, aspiration, and pulmonary infection. Primary biliary cirrhosis is occasionally associated with interstitial lung disease, which causes disproportionate dyspnea and a restrictive defect on pulmonary function testing,

Coagulation defects are often identified in laboratory screening tests, and reduced concentrations of Vitamin K–dependent clotting proteins are well-documented. However, liver disease has complex effects on hemostasis and on the balance between pro- and anti-hemostatic processes, and these measurements may not predict bleeding. Prothrombin time (PT) or international normalized ratio, activated partial thromboplastin time, and platelet count all highlight procoagulant functions, whereas the effects of anti-coagulant proteins, such as protein C and anti-thrombin, are not measured. Similarly, although platelet numbers and function may be reduced, high levels of factor VIII and von Willebrand factor in cirrhosis may compensate. The fibrinolytic system is also affected, as both pro- and anti-fibrinolytic factors may be decreased in cirrhosis. The net effect of these imbalances is unpredictable, and sensitivity of the coagulation system to factors promoting both bleeding and thrombosis is probably increased. Routine preoperative administration of fresh-frozen plasma, platelets, and other products is no longer commonly practiced, and treatment may be better based on clinical findings, such as bleeding from puncture sites, oozing in the operative field, or failure of shed blood to form clots.

Hematological

Anemia is common, from impaired hematopoiesis, gastrointestinal bleeding, or hypersplenism. Varices should be treated and overt iron deficiency corrected, but transfusion is only carried out for active bleeding or in the presence of symptoms clearly attributable to low hemoglobin.

Metabolic

Hyponatremia may be caused by diuretic therapy, secondary hyperaldosteronism, and other poorly understood renal abnormalities. It predicts worse outcome, with or without transplant. Rapid increases in plasma sodium in the peri-operative period, associated with transfusion, carry a significant risk of central pontine myelinolysis and long-term neurological disability. Many centers suspend patients from the transplant waiting list when values fall below 122–125 mmol/l and attempt correction. Patients with Na $<$ 122 mmol/l are considered on an individual basis according to the risks of major operative blood loss. Factors such as anemia, re-transplant, portal vein thrombosis, and extended criteria donor may favor deferral in the patient with plasma sodium below this threshold.

Preoperative hyperkalemia is uncommon but should be treated aggressively, since fatal intra-operative hyperkalemic arrest, usually at reperfusion of the liver, still occurs. It may be associated with renal failure, treatment with spironolactone, or transfusion. Preoperative values above 5.5 mmol/l should be treated with hemofiltration, continued into the intra-operative phase if it does not fall to less than 5.0 mmol/l.

Renal

Renal impairment develops easily because of underlying circulatory and hormonal disturbances. Overtreatment with diuretics is a common cause, and acute tubular necrosis may be seen in patients with acute hepatic failure or sepsis associated with spontaneous bacterial peritonitis or chest infection. Hepatorenal syndrome, a form of prerenal failure occurring in the absence of clinical hypovolemia or intrinsic renal disease, is also common. This may respond to vasopressor treatment combined with volume loading and resolves after transplantation. Renal impairment is a strong predictor of increased mortality.

Nutritional

Nutritional impairment is severe in up to 30% of patients, resulting from anorexia, malabsorption, impaired protein synthesis, and chronic catabolism. Nutritional reserve is further depleted by accelerated catabolism during infection and surgery. Poorer outcomes are seen in low body mass index (BMI) patients, and most centers would not list at BMI less than 15. BMIs above this value but with low measured nutritional indices (e.g., grip strength, triceps skin-fold thickness, mid-upper arm circumference $<$ fifth percentile) are common but are not regarded as contraindications to transplant. BMI less than 18.5 associated with other major comorbidities would be regarded as potentially prohibitive. Calorie, protein, and vitamin supplementation is essential.

Morbid obesity (BMI $>$ 35) is increasingly common in patients presenting for liver transplantation. It is known to affect intensive care unit length of stay and long-term outcomes but is not regarded as prohibitive in most centers. An abdominal ("apple-shaped") pattern of obesity affects surgical access, peri-operative respiratory parameters, and ventilator weaning much more than a pelvic ("pear-shaped") pattern, although this has not been formally investigated. Marked abdominal obesity (BMI $>$ 40) in the presence of one or more major comorbidities would contraindicate transplant in many units.

Acute liver failure with multi-organ failure

Special problems are encountered in patients with multi-system failure caused by fulminant hepatic failure, primary non-function of a liver graft, or terminal decompensation in chronic liver failure. These patients usually have severe coagulopathy and encephalopathy. Non-cardiogenic pulmonary edema, renal insufficiency, and/or sepsis may also be present. Raised intracranial pressure is commonly seen in fulminant hepatic failure with encephalopathy and may rapidly progress to fatal brainstem compression if untreated. Intracranial pressure monitoring is advocated in this setting, although hemorrhagic complications, occasionally fatal, occur, and no consensus on the balance of risks has emerged. Paralysis, ventilation, and 30-degree head-up tilt are essential, supplemented by mannitol and pentobarbital if needed. Moderate hypothermia is now used in many units to control severe intracranial hypertension. Continuous veno-venous hemofiltration may be needed to correct hyperkalemia and control metabolic acidosis.

Sepsis may be difficult to diagnose in this context, as many of its clinical manifestations are mimicked in terminal hepatic decompensation. However, fever, hypotension, and dependence on vasopressors clearly suggest its presence, and the risks of proceeding with transplantation at this stage may be prohibitive.

Intra-operative care

Immediate preoperative preparation

Full multi-system assessment should be performed before listing for transplantation, and the patient reviewed when a donor liver becomes available. It is important to exclude untreated infection (e.g., incipient bacterial peritonitis or bronchopneumonia), hyperkalemia, and severe hyponatremia. If unusual risks are identified, a discussion between the attending anesthesiologist, hepatologist, and surgeon is essential. Although cold ischemia times should be kept be as short as possible, retrieval times and liver preservation techniques typically allow adequate time for assessment and intervention. The patient's usual proton pump inhibitor should be given, along with antibiotic prophylaxis according to local protocol.

Ten units of blood are routinely cross-matched, and at least 20 additional group-specific units should be available if needed. Predictors of transfusion requirement include preoperative anemia, renal impairment, and previous transplant. Fresh-frozen plasma and platelets must be available because of the possibility of coagulopathy during surgery.

Anesthetic technique

Careful preoxygenation and a rapid-sequence induction (or modified) are recommended. A nasogastric tube and urinary catheter are placed. Maintenance with fentanyl, remifentanil, or sufentanil given with air/oxygen/desflurane or isoflurane are common techniques. The choice of muscle relaxant is arbitrary, with most units using atracurium or cis-atracurium. Short-acting agents are advocated as many patients can be awakened soon after surgery.

Vascular access

Large-bore intravenous access is vital. Two peripheral lines are dedicated to transfusion. A triple-lumen catheter and PA catheter introducer can both be placed in the right internal jugular vein under ultrasound guidance. It is our practice to place two 5F cannulae alongside these in the right internal jugular vein. These may be used as reserve volume-infusion lines or re-wired to 10F size for use in the return limb of a venovenous bypass circuit (see below). The femoral route is usually avoided because the cava is clamped intra-operatively, and these vessels may be needed for venovenous bypass. Subclavian cannulation has a higher risk of arterial hematoma and pneumothorax and in our unit is now performed only under ultrasound and fluoroscopic guidance in an angiography suite.

Monitoring

Radial or femoral arterial and central venous pressure monitoring are essential, whereas PA catheters are used routinely in most centers. Radial artery pressure monitoring may underestimate aortic pressure in hypotensive states, especially when vasopressors are used, and should be interpreted with caution. PA pressure and thermodilution cardiac output measurements help in the assessment and management of hypotension, which may arise unpredictably because of changes in venous return, altered systemic vascular resistance (SVR), and cardiac or embolic events. A PA catheter is essential if pulmonary hypertension is present or suspected.

Cardiovascular monitoring is further enhanced by the use of transesophageal echocardiography (TEE), which gives continuous if subjective information on ventricular function and an immediate diagnosis of embolization of air or thrombus. A history of variceal bleeding is a contraindication for TEE.

Measurement of arterial blood gases, sodium, potassium, glucose, lactate, ionized calcium, and hematocrit should be performed at frequent intervals, at least hourly during the initial and closing phases of the operation and more often during the anhepatic period.

Coagulation monitoring practices vary widely. In most centers, routine coagulation screening tests, including PT, partial thromboplastin time, fibrinogen, and platelet count, are supplemented by thromboelastography (TEG). Despite poor agreement with conventional laboratory coagulation tests, TEG provides a prompt global assessment of coagulation function, and targeted sample treatment also allows demonstration of heparin effect and platelet function. However, as outlined above, abnormal results in both conventional and TEG testing are poorly correlated with visually apparent coagulopathy (oozing in the surgical field and/or lack of visible clot), and their main value may be to indicate the appropriate treatment when coagulopathy is a clinical problem. Bedside (point-of-care) monitors are also available but, again, often reflect clinical coagulation poorly in the setting of liver disease.

Blood replacement and fluid management

Blood product use during liver transplantation has declined over the last 20 years. The current median red cell requirement is to 2–5 units, with a substantial proportion of recipients avoiding blood products altogether. Refinement in surgical techniques, better understanding of hemostasis, and improved anesthetic management have all contributed.

Because bleeding during liver transplantation is not usually caused by problems with the major anastomoses, but more often by transections in the complex mesh of portosystemic collateral veins, fluid management, portal hyperemia, and blood loss may be linked. Patients with cirrhosis and portal hypertension have splanchnic hypervolemia, which volume loading increases. They also have smaller increases in cardiac output with fluid infusion, so the larger volumes needed to improve systemic perfusion may have a disproportionate effect on portal venous pressure and flow. Aggressive administration of crystalloid and colloid may also have a more detrimental effect on clotting, since factor levels are low.

Thus the conventional approach of administering blood products preemptively and optimizing cardiac output by generous fluid loading has been questioned. Indeed, fluid restriction with vasopressor infusion during the dissection and anhepatic phases has been associated with very low blood product use. On the other hand, volume restriction requires liberal use of vasopressors and risks systemic and especially renal hypoperfusion. The optimal approach to volume management remains to be determined.

The choice of fluid is controversial. Albumin appears to be safe and has no effects on coagulation apart from dilution, but is costly. Gelatin solutions are inexpensive and have been used in high volumes in liver recipients in Europe for many years, but are more allergenic. Hydroxyethyl starch solution (HES 130/0.4) has been reported to be safe in terms of effects on renal function and coagulation. This was well tolerated in a recent series of liver recipients, but effects of high-infusion volumes are unknown. A balanced electrolyte preparation of this is under development, reducing chloride ion load, which may reduce metabolic acidosis.

When surgical bleeding occurs, many now accept a hemoglobin transfusion threshold of 7.0 g/dl (hematocrit 20–22). Transfusion at a higher value may be prudent in renal impairment, given the sensitivity of renal oxygen consumption to hemoglobin concentration in experimental models.

Management of coagulopathy

New concepts in the interpretation of coagulation tests in liver disease, outlined above, should be considered in intra-operative management. Further changes imposed by the procedure include dilution, pathological fibrinolysis, effects of synthetic colloids, and release of heparinoids and inflammatory mediators from the graft. Prophylactic antifibrinolytic (tranexamic acid) is used selectively in many units.

Treatment of established coagulopathy is guided by monitoring (see below). In the presence of fibrinolysis or heparin effect, an anti-fibrinolytic or protamine can be given. Otherwise, platelets, fresh-frozen plasma, and cryoprecipitate remain the mainstay of treatment, with frequent assessment of the surgical field to minimize the number of units given. Although data in liver recipients are limited, factor concentrates, including fibrinogen and prothrombin preparations, appear safe and effective and are increasingly used to treat established coagulopathy. Normothermia and a pause in the procedure (after full reperfusion) to allow the liver to recover from surgical handling may also help.

Recombinant factor VIIa (eptacog alpha activated) has controlled intractable bleeding in patients with complex acquired coagulation defects, but two randomized trials have failed to show efficacy when the drug is given prophylactically. There is no consensus on the role of this costly treatment, and most centers use it on specialist advice according to local protocol.

A growing number of case reports indicate that hypercoagulability and thromboembolism may cause serious or fatal complications during liver transplant. The incidence of pulmonary thromboembolism or intracardiac thrombus formation has been estimated at 1–1.5%. Hypercoagulability is demonstrable on TEG and other tests in a significant number of liver recipients, particularly those with primary sclerosing cholangitis and HCC, but its importance as a cause of intra-operative thrombosis is unclear. Thromboembolism may occur at any stage of the procedure, and mortality is high (up to 68% in one series). Aggressive therapy with thrombectomy or thrombolysis has been successful in some cases. TEE should permit immediate diagnosis.

Autotransfusion techniques are widely used and safe, but effects on coagulation and even on total use of bank blood are still unproven. Cell-salvage may be contraindicated in patients with hepatic malignancy and when enteric contamination of the peritoneum has occurred.

Electrolyte and acid–base changes

The infusion of large volumes of blood products and reperfusion of the donor liver cause marked changes in plasma biochemistry. Plasma sodium is subnormal in many recipients and tends to increase during surgery. Rises of more than 12 mmol/l in 24 hours have been associated with pontine myelinolysis and neurological injury. In susceptible patients this may happen with smaller increases, and this has been well-described in liver recipients. Avoiding sodium bicarbonate, minimizing use of citrated blood products, and washing of bank blood may attenuate this increase.

Plasma potassium increases on reperfusion of the liver. Many anesthetists give 5–10 ml of calcium chloride at reperfusion to reduce the risk of hyperkalemia-induced ventricular tachycardia or fibrillation. In most patients redistribution follows within seconds, and a progressive decrease is subsequently seen. However, pre-existing renal failure, residual beta-blockade, and a relatively large, fatty, or ischemic donor liver may be associated with prolonged and life-threatening hyperkalemia.

Hyperkalemia may also complicate rapid transfusion, especially in the presence of renal impairment. Plasma potassium concentration in stored blood increases with storage time and may be greater than 20 mmol/l. Potassium concentration should be checked frequently when transfusion is rapid and donor units washed in the cell saver whenever hyperkalemia is anticipated. An increase in potassium concentration of greater than 0.5 mmol/l between successive measurements or a value above 5.0 mmol/l at any time should prompt washing of all further donor units. Values above 5.0 mmol/l during the dissection or anhepatic phases should be treated aggressively with furosemide and glucose-insulin. Nebulized or intravenous salbutamol and sodium bicarbonate should also be considered. As at reperfusion, any ECG changes associated with hyperkalemia should be treated with calcium chloride.

Trisodium citrate in transfused blood and plasma depresses ionized calcium, which should be maintained to preserve myocardial function. Calcium chloride is given if hypotension occurs in the presence of a depressed ionized calcium value. A less marked effect is seen on magnesium concentrations, although supplementation in the absence of either arrhythmia or availability of rapid measurement is not routine.

Metabolic acidosis is usually absent or minimal initially, unless there is renal impairment, but becomes increasingly apparent during the procedure. Transfused blood introduces a substantial quantity of exogenous lactic acid into the circulation, whereas liver lactate and urea metabolism are impaired. Acid metabolites associated with venous stasis in the portal and lower body circulations, as well as those that accumulate in the new liver during storage, are released into the general circulation on reperfusion, causing a further increase in acidosis. A poorly functioning liver fails to metabolize lactate, and worsening lactic acidosis is a typical sign of graft failure.

Acidosis is usually treated with modest hyperventilation. The place of sodium bicarbonate in the management of acidosis remains controversial. Evidence that global circulatory function is impaired by moderate metabolic acidosis is slight, whereas detrimental effects on oxygen delivery and intracellular pH and plasma lactate associated with bicarbonate therapy have been described. Alternative buffers producing less or no carbon dioxide, including dichloroacetate and tris-buffer, may be of value but remain to be fully assessed.

If liver and cardiovascular function are adequate after reperfusion, there is a tendency for metabolic acidosis to clear. Potassium may be needed in the early postoperative period when reuptake by the grafted liver can cause hypokalemia

Glucose control

In most patients blood glucose is normal before operation but increases during the procedure because of administration of acid–citrate–dextrose blood and stress-related insulin resistance. Hypoglycemia, although seen preoperatively in patients with fulminant hepatic failure, is rarely observed intra-operatively, even when normal hepatic glucose release is interrupted during the anhepatic and early reperfusion phases. Recent literature has highlighted the association between poor glucose control and adverse outcomes in the peri-operative and critical care settings, but a clear causal relationship has not been established, and hypoglycemia is a significant hazard when tight control is attempted, especially in the unconscious patient. Insulin infusions have been advocated to moderate blood glucose values and prevent hyperkalemia, ranging from 2–10 units per hour. Blood glucose and electrolyte checks, at least hourly, are essential.

Cardiovascular changes

Surgical bleeding presents the greatest threat, and it is essential that blood lost can be replaced rapidly at any point during the procedure (see Chapter 23). Cardiac filling may be impaired during the dissection phase by intermittent obstruction of venous return during surgical manipulation of the liver or by direct compression of the diaphragmatic surface of the heart. Anesthetic agents and hypocalcemia will amplify these effects. Interpretation of filling pressures may be difficult during the dissection phase, since caval obstruction is variable and may coexist with true hypovolemia. Observation of the surgical field and communication with the surgeon are vital when there is uncertainty about the cause of reduced venous return. The response to clamping of the inferior vena cava (IVC) for hepatectomy and to unclamping when the grafted liver is reperfused depends on several factors. The most important of these is whether the cava is side-clamped for a piggyback implantation or cross-clamped for the conventional method.

Cross-clamping of the cava at hepatectomy produces a marked (40–50%) decrease in central venous pressure and cardiac output. SVR increases, but a decrease in blood pressure is expected. Provided cardiac filling pressures and contractility are maintained, frank hypotension (systolic < 80 mmHg) is unusual. Although the need for veno-venous bypass is usually predetermined by other factors (discussed below), when its use is not planned, many teams perform a trial clamping of the IVC to assess the patient's ability to maintain an adequate systemic blood pressure. Once the liver is removed, lower filling pressures are accepted as long as the arterial blood pressure is satisfactory. Over-transfusion at this stage, more likely when bypass is not used since higher filling pressures are needed to maintain cardiac output, may result in high filling pressures following unclamping. This may have adverse effects on RV function, gas exchange, and hepatic blood flow.

When a piggyback technique or venovenous bypass is used, the decrease in cardiac output is usually less (20–30%). Arterial pressure is well maintained, although this depends on the flows obtained through the bypass circuit. Nonetheless, a progressive decline in cardiac output occurs during the anhepatic phase, and both bypass and the piggyback technique fall short of maintaining a normal circulatory state, reflected in worsening metabolic acidosis.

Reperfusion of the transplanted liver is usually associated with reduced heart rate, contractility, and peripheral vascular tone. Portal unclamping releases desaturated blood from the obstructed portal circulation, which mixes with cold, potassium-rich preservation fluid in the new liver and enters the systemic circulation. Slowing of the heart and hyperkalemia are common, and asystole, tachyarrhythmia, and ventricular fibrillation are sometimes seen. Blood pressure decreases in almost all patients because of arteriolar vasodilatation and transient myocardial depression. These changes may be caused by inflammatory mediators from the ischemic liver, by peptides released during splanchnic stasis, or by reflex vasodilatation. In most patients, blood pressure and cardiac output are restored within minutes. In some, typically those with a marginal graft or pre-existing vasopressor dependency, recovery takes longer, and sustained vasopressor support is needed. This has been described as the "post-reperfusion syndrome." In patients undergoing urgent re-transplantation for graft non-function or infarction, or in whom unrecognized sepsis has supervened, hypotension and acidosis after unclamping may be progressive and irreversible.

Transient pulmonary hypertension may be seen at reperfusion, as central blood volume increases. PCWP is raised and the TPG is normal (<15 mmHg). Pre-existing pulmonary hypertension is usually diagnosed by echocardiography at the time of referral, but is occasionally found only on placement of the PA catheter for transplant. If it is true portopulmonary hypertension (PVR > 240 dyn s/cm^5, TPG > 15 mmHg), the risks of proceeding need to be balanced against those of deferring transplant in favor of treatment. If severe (mean PA pressure > 50 mmHg, or RV dysfunction), peri-operative mortality approaches 100%, and the operation should not proceed. If moderate (35–50 mmHg), a trial of treatment with prostacyclin and/or inhaled nitric oxide is advocated, ideally monitored by TEE. It may be reasonable to proceed if right heart function is well maintained, especially if the patient responds to vasodilator therapy.

Veno-venous bypass

Veno-venous bypass is a pumped extracorporeal shunt taking blood from the femoral and (sometimes) portal vein to the axillary or internal jugular vein, intended to decompress the portal system and maintain venous return during the anhepatic phase. Heparin-bonded tubing and non-occlusive pumps allow its use without systemic heparinization. Use has declined as use of the piggyback technique has become more widespread, and because many centers have demonstrated good results without it. It is now used selectively in most liver transplant programs and in some units never.

Advocates of bypass cite physiological advantages during the final stages of dissection and during the anhepatic period, at least when the implantation technique involves full clamping of the cava. These include decompression of the portal, lower caval, and renal venous systems and maintenance of cardiac output, thus preserving splanchnic and renal blood flow. Hemodynamic stability and systemic acidosis are improved, and control of surgical bleeding is easier because venous pressure in portosystemic collaterals is reduced. However, evidence that bypass improves results is lacking, and a comprehensive evaluation of its complications has yet to be published.

The most serious hazards of bypass are perforation of central vessels during insertion of large-bore percutaneous catheters, and embolization of air or thrombus, all of which have caused fatalities. Body temperature decreases during bypass unless a heat exchanger is used, which may carry an added risk of thromboembolism. Local complications at access sites also occur, including nerve injury, hematoma, lymphocele, and infection. Most units now reserve the technique for patients most likely to gain from its use. Indications may include severe portal hypertension, renal or cardiac impairment, marked metabolic acidosis or vasopressor dependency, and hypotension on trial clamping of the cava.

Respiratory function

Changes in respiratory function caused by liver disease have been described above. Further respiratory problems arising during surgery are not common. Rapid arterial oxygen desaturation occurs easily after induction of anesthesia, even after pre-oxygenation, since functional residual capacity is often reduced by ascites or hydrothorax. Pulmonary edema presents a more important hazard. Over-transfusion can occur because of the highly variable rate of blood loss. Plasma oncotic pressure is reduced and some patients appear to have abnormal vascular permeability, especially after reperfusion and if graft function is poor. Intra-operative drainage of a large pleural effusion (hepatic hydrothorax) is routine but can cause re-expansion pulmonary edema, which may only present after reperfusion. Atelectasis, tension pneumothorax, and pulmonary embolism may occur intra-operatively but are rare. Patients with the hepatopulmonary syndrome and CF present few problems intra-operatively, although in those with severe pulmonary shunting, postoperative ventilation and oxygen dependency may be prolonged.

Renal function

Intra-operative changes in renal function are related to marked alterations in cardiac output and renal blood flow. Urine flow is diminished and markers of renal injury are raised during caval clamping, when cardiac output is reduced and renal venous pressure acutely raised. This response may be attenuated when veno-venous bypass or a piggyback implantation is used. Pre-existing renal impairment, prolonged hypotension, and high transfusion volumes are associated with a high risk of post-operative renal failure. No measures have yet been shown to prevent intra-operative renal injury, although a rationale for the use of low-dose vasopressors including vasopressin and norepinephrine exists, given the pathophysiology of the hepatorenal syndrome. However, concerns about the effects of these on perfusion of the newly implanted liver remain.

Early postoperative care and complications

Management of liver transplant recipients between transplantation and discharge is usually undertaken by a multi-disciplinary team that includes

Table 24.2 Diagnosis and management of early postoperative complications

Complication	Risk factors	Diagnosis	Management
Bleeding	Previous surgery Severe portal hypertension Poor graft function	↑Drainage ↓ Blood pressure ↓ Hemoglobin	Transfuse, correct coagulation, re-explore
Primary non-function	Marginal or NHB donor, steatosis Long cold or warm ischemic times Revascularization problems	↑ Lactate ↑ K+ Acidosis Coagulopathy Oliguria MOF	MOF support, urgent re-transplant (consider hepatectomy once donor identified)
Hepatic artery thrombosis	Primary sclerosing cholangitis Small artery or complex arterial anatomy,	Doppler US, CT, or direct angiography to confirm Liver enzymes may not rise	Early thrombectomy or revision; urgent re-transplant if graft failure
Bile leak	↑ warm ischaemia: delayed arterialization NHB donor Donor duct too long	Bile in drains (drain bilirubin > serum); perihilar collection on US or MRI	Repair (Roux loop drainage)
Rejection	> 5–7 days post-transplant	↑ ALT and bilirubin Pyrexia Biopsy	Pulsed prednisolone
Sepsis	> 5–7 days post-transplant Debilitated patient Atelectasis/pneumonia Recent pulsed steroid	↑ WBC and CRP Tachycardia Hypotension Delirium Oliguria Acidosis	HDU/ICU monitoring, volume resuscitation, cultures (blood, drains, intravascular catheters, wound, sputum, urine); antibiotics; USS/MRI for collections
Deterioration of graft function (after 5–7 days)	Rejection Sepsis Bile leak Compromised arterial inflow	Identify cause as above (imaging ± biopsy, septic screen)	Treat cause as above

ALT: alanine aminotransferase; CRP: C-reactive protein; MOF: multi-organ failure; NHB: non–heart-beating; US: ultrasound; WBC: white blood cell count.

intensivists, hepatologists, and transplant surgeons. Recipients (and their grafts) are heterogeneous, and the postoperative course is highly variable. Frequent adjustment of immunosuppression, anticoagulation, antimicrobial treatment, and prophylaxis are all required, and much of this can be protocol-driven. The formulation of a set of protocols that are regularly reviewed and modified is essential to high-quality, co-coordinated care. Complications are summarized in Table 24.2. The most important early complications are primary non-function, hepatic artery thrombosis, and bleeding. Biliary leaks, rejection, and sepsis tend to occur after the first 5–7 days.

Intensive care unit care

Most liver recipients are transferred to the intensive care unit (ICU) for postoperative care. Tracheal extubation in the operating room or within a few hours of admission to ICU is usually possible, but this depends on recipient comorbidity, complexity of the surgery, and especially adequate initial graft function. To be extubated, the patient must be awake, hemodynamically stable, and normothermic, with good gas exchange and no bleeding or major acidosis. Measures such as 30-degree head up tilt while ventilated (semi-sitting once extubated) and regular tracheal toilet/physiotherapy may reduce pulmonary atelectasis and subsequent infection. Adequate analgesia and exercises to encourage deep breathing and coughing are also important. The use of modest positive end-expiratory pressure (PEEP) while ventilated and non-invasive positive pressure ventilation after tracheal extubation may be considered and do not appear to compromise hepatic venous flow.

Non-cardiogenic pulmonary edema (acute respiratory distress syndrome) is an infrequent complication, but occurs in the setting of massive transfusion, graft non-function or infarction, and fulminant sepsis or rejection. It is managed with mechanical ventilation with small tidal volumes, PEEP, and increased inspired oxygen sufficient to prevent systemic hypoxemia. Significant hepatic hydrothorax can be drained transdiaphragmatically at the time of surgery, and recurrence large enough to need a pleural drain is uncommon. Prophylactic antibiotics for 24–48 hours are routine in most units.

Primary non-function

Primary non-function is often first apparent in the operating room, manifest by coagulopathy, persistent hyperkalemia, acidosis, hyperlactatemia, hypotension, and oliguria. These worsen in the early postoperative period, accompanied by hypoglycemia, anuria, deteriorating gas exchange, and circulatory collapse. Urgent re-transplantation may be life-saving, but these patients deteriorate rapidly and may become too sick to withstand the procedure. Some groups perform total hepatectomy once a suitable replacement organ has been identified, which may stabilize the patient, but clear indications and evidence are lacking.

Hepatic artery thrombosis

The patient should have a Doppler ultrasound study within 24 hours and at least daily afterward to confirm hepatic arterial and portal venous flow. Absence of either should prompt urgent angiography and thrombectomy or revision. Vascular thrombosis may not result in immediate biochemical changes and may otherwise be missed when early intervention could save the graft. The highly variable vascular anatomy of the liver and the variety of vascular reconstruction techniques may make imaging difficult to interpret, so a diagram for the radiologist is essential. Complex arterial or venous reconstruction may increase the likelihood of thrombosis, as may the postoperative use of vasopressors. Loss of arterial inflow, if not causing early graft infarction and sepsis, leads eventually to ischemic cholangitis, biliary leak, and strictures, and usually precipitates re-transplantation. If urgent re-transplantation is needed, immunosuppression is reduced and antibacterial and antifungal agents given.

Hemorrhage

Hemorrhage requiring re-exploration is now unusual, but even patients closed with a dry surgical field may bleed in the immediate postoperative period. Recognition and timely intervention are essential. Bleeding may not be revealed by abdominal drainage and should be suspected in the setting of a rising heart rate, falling blood pressure, reduced skin temperature, and oliguria. A falling hemoglobin concentration should confirm the diagnosis. Although an abnormal PT is not routinely corrected post-transplant, because it is useful as a marker of improving synthetic function, signs of active bleeding should prompt volume resuscitation and administration of fresh-frozen plasma, platelets, and red blood cells as soon as possible. If the patient fails to stabilize after initial resuscitation in the ICU, then he/she should be returned to the operating room immediately. Failure to do so may compromise the newly implanted liver.

Although early biliary leak is uncommon, it will be readily detected by careful inspection of drain fluid for volume and especially color. The diagnosis is confirmed by measuring the concentration of bilirubin: if greater than that in the patient's serum, surgical exploration is usually required. Typically, the standard duct-to-duct anastomosis is converted to a Roux loop.

Post-ICU care

Management of the patients on the ward (initially in a high-dependency area) is best undertaken by a multi-disciplinary team that includes hepatologists, transplant surgeons, dietitians, and physiotherapists. Progress is highly variable between patients, but the dominant concerns and their management are outlined below.

Immunosuppression in our institution is usually tacrolimus (TAC)-based, with dosing adjusted to obtain serum trough levels of 10–15 ng/l. TAC is well-absorbed in the upper GI tract and the intravenous preparation is rarely used, even in the immediate postoperative period. The TAC level must be adjusted to take albumin binding into account, since hypoalbuminemia is common in the immediate postoperative period, and target values based on whole-blood measurements may be nephro- or neurotoxic.

Patients who are intolerant of TAC are given cyclosporine. In some patients, sirolimus may be more suitable because of nephro-protective and anti-neoplastic effects, but it is not used in the immediate postoperative period because of its inhibitory effect on wound healing. The use of prednisolone and azathioprine (AZA) is variable. Most patients are also given prednisolone, but those who undergo transplantation for hepatitis C virus are, if possible, maintained on a steroid-free regimen. It is our practice also to commence AZA once lymphocyte counts are greater than 0.5×10^9 /l. See Chapter 3 for more details.

Deterioration of graft function after initial stabilization is common, indicated by rising alanine aminotransferase and bilirubin. The most likely causes in the early postoperative period are vascular or biliary complications, sepsis, and rejection. Imaging of the transplanted organ is the first step, initially by ultrasound. Absence of arterial flow requires confirmation by direct or CT angiography and can occur with little or no biochemical change. It usually results in the need for re-transplantation. Once confirmed, appropriate anti-fungal and antibiotic therapy should be commenced and immunosuppression reduced. At re-transplantation, a conduit of donor iliac artery is anastomosed to the aorta, since the recipient celiac axis is often no longer usable.

Ultrasound should be followed by triple-phase CT if a biliary leak (usually heralded by a collection of fluid at the hilum) or infected collection is suspected, remembering that liver recipients may not complain of abdominal pain in the presence of biliary peritonitis. Tesla magnetic resonance imaging can be helpful, but interpretation in the immediate postoperative period is difficult. If there is graft dysfunction, any collection should be percutaneously sampled or drained and the fluid sent for bilirubin and culture. If a percutaneous approach is not possible, endoscopic ultrasound or laparotomy may be needed.

If a biliary leak is confirmed, the treatment of choice is formal reconstruction with a Roux-en-Y loop of jejunum. In most cases the leak is from the biliary anastomosis, but it may be from accessory ducts or even biopsy sites. Complete evacuation of the bile collection is essential as the hepatic artery typically traverses it and is often found to be in spasm.

Sepsis is common after transplant, especially after 5–7 days, and is frequently associated with liver dysfunction. The usual sites of postsurgical infection must be assessed (chest, wound, urinary tract, cannulation sites) and cannulae, catheters, and drains removed if possible. Intra-abdominal collections require drainage, either radiologically guided or surgical. Antimicrobial therapy must be initiated early and discussed with the microbiology team. Unusual causes of infection should also be considered, including organisms potentially transmitted with the donor organ. Many organs are retrieved from donors who themselves have had sepsis. Culture results from the donor and targeted antimicrobial treatment should be considered in recipients with unusual presentations of sepsis.

Acute cellular rejection

This usually first presents in the first week after transplant, signaled by rising bilirubin and hepatic enzyme levels, sometimes accompanied by eosinophilia, an unexplained rise in C-reactive protein, or pyrexia. Percutaneous liver biopsy is performed to confirm the diagnosis. When persistent ascites, thrombocytopenia, or other coagulopathy make this difficult or hazardous, a transjugular approach may be used, although this may be challenging if cavocavoplasty was used to implant the liver. Biopsy-proven acute cellular rejection is treated with pulsed intravenous methylprednisolone. This is usually very effective, although an attenuated response, or steroid-resistant rejection, is occasionally encountered and is often diagnosed only after multiple pulses. It may then be necessary to use anti-thymocyte globulin. This involves a 2-week course with doses adjusted against lymphocyte count.

Antibody-mediated rejection in liver recipients is very unusual but should be considered in cases of persistent rejection with vascular changes on histology and rising levels of donor-specific antibody. Treatment regimes vary but usually involve plasmapheresis and anti-lymphocyte agents.

Ongoing ascitic losses occur in patients who have had large volumes of ascites before transplant. This is usually self-limiting but may persist for several weeks. However, new-onset ascites should prompt investigation of portal venous and caval anastomoses. In particular, narrowing of the top caval anastomosis is associated with ascites, peripheral edema, and renal dysfunction. Imaging to confirm caval stenosis usually involves cavography with pressure studies and portal venous wedge pressure measurements. Treatment is difficult and in the early postoperative period may be best achieved with surgical revision. Later presentations are surgically hazardous and may be more safely managed by percutaneous stenting or dilatation.

Further reading

Fonouni H, Mehrabi A, Soleimani A, Müller SA, Büchler MW, Schmidt J. The need for venovenous bypass in liver transplantation. *HPB (Oxford)* 2008; **10**: 196–203.

Ramos E, Dalmau A, Sabate A, *et al.* Intraoperative red blood cell transfusion in liver transplantation: Influence on patient outcome, prediction of requirements, and measures to reduce them. *Liver Transpl* 2003; **9**: 1320–7.

Safadi A, Homsi M, Maskoun, *et al.* Perioperative risk predictors of cardiac outcomes in patients undergoing liver transplantation surgery. *Circulation* 2009; **120**: 1189–94.

Steadman R. Anesthesia for liver transplant surgery. *Anesthesiol Clin North Am* 2004; **22**: 687–711.

Chapter 25

Long-term management and outcomes

William Gelson and Graeme J.M. Alexander

Key points

- The most common causes of death after the first year following transplantation are recurrent and de novo malignancy, return of the original liver disease in the graft, sepsis, cardiovascular disease, and chronic rejection.
- Immune suppression should be tailored according to the disease causing the primary liver disorder, with varied doses or different agents.
- The most common cause of renal impairment after liver transplantation is calcineurin-inhibitor nephrotoxicity; substitution with mycophenolate mofetil or sirolimus may be required.

Early patient and graft survival, defined as the immediate postoperative period and the first year after liver transplantation, have both improved substantially since the procedure became adopted widely in the 1980s. In contrast however, survival for those patients who are alive after the first year has not improved in the longer term. This has been demonstrated in large cohorts from both the United Kingdom and the United States. Survival curves from the European Transplant Registry (Figure 25.1) show a similar pattern from year 3 onwards, where patients undergoing liver transplantation have a comparable survival when the operation was performed between 1968 and 1988 to those undertaken after 1988.

The comparison of long-term survival during each era is not "like for like," since the indications for transplantation and the underlying causes of liver injury have changed substantially with time, but the absence of a demonstrable improvement in long-term survival remains a cause for concern.

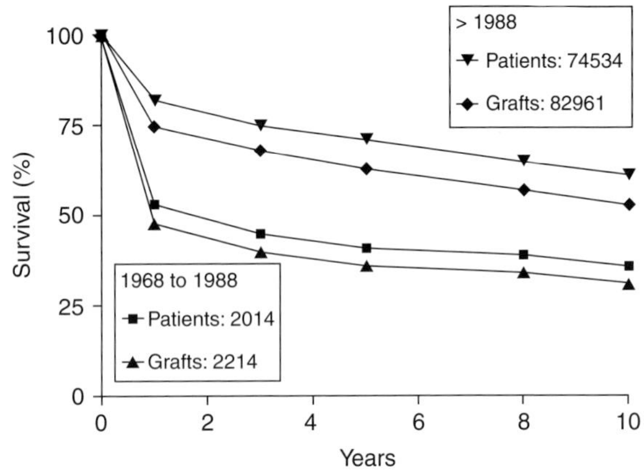

Figure 25.1 Patient and graft survival following liver transplantation in Europe. Engraftment was between May 1968 and December 2008. Graft and patient survival curves are shown for transplants before and after 1988. The curves demonstrate that short-term survival has markedly improved, whereas long-term survival has not. Data are taken from the European Liver Transplant Registry (www.eltr.org).

There are clear and consistent causes of late mortality (Table 25.1) that are common to all transplant programs and to each era, and one explanation for the lack of improvement in long-term survival is suboptimal management at an earlier stage for those conditions that lead to late deaths.

Late graft failure is much less common now than before, a change that can be attributed to technical improvements, experience, and a much lower likelihood of chronic rejection, so that recurrence of the original disease now represents the greatest challenge. It is not an inconsiderable challenge, since it is hard to think of many adult liver disorders that have not been reported to recur after liver transplantation.

Few studies examine those factors that predict late mortality. A preliminary analysis of the UK Transplant database using Cox regression analysis with

Organ Transplantation: A Clinical Guide, ed. A.A. Klein, C.J. Lewis, and J.C. Madsen. Published by Cambridge University Press.

Table 25.1 Causes of death after liver transplantation beyond year-1 in Europe

Hepatocellular carcinoma	22%
De novo malignancy	16%
Return of the original liver disease in the graft	14%
Sepsis	8%
Cardiovascular disease	7%
Chronic rejection	5%

death after year-1 as the outcome variable found that certain underlying liver disorders at the time of transplant carried an increased risk (these included alcohol-related, autoimmune hepatitis, cryptogenic or hepatitis C virus [HCV] related, and the presence of hepatocellular carcinoma [HCC] at the time of transplantation) and further that the choice of immune suppression was also influential, whereby prednisolone use at last follow-up was associated with an increased risk of death. The latter, of course, may be cause or consequence and requires further evaluation in prospective studies.

The etiological associations with survival after liver transplantation were corroborated by a recent study that examined "life years lost" after transplantation. When the UK liver transplant cohort survival was standardized and compared with that of the UK population at large, the etiologies of alcohol, autoimmune, HCV, and HCC were associated with loss of 14 years, 5 years, 17 years, and 24 years, respectively. Conversely, the etiologies of cryptogenic and primary biliary cirrhosis were associated with a gain in life years at 5 and 7 respectively. The cause of life years gained remains a matter of debate and may be in part due to the selection process of candidates for liver transplantation. Whatever the risk factors for patient loss, optimizing management and prevention of late complications is central to improving long-term outcome.

Immunosuppression

In common with other organ transplants, immune suppression in long-term survivors of liver transplantation involves a balance between effective control of rejection and complications related to therapy (discussed further in Chapter 3). Complications of immune suppression may be related to the original etiology (e.g., accelerated disease progression in viral hepatitis) or unrelated and similar to other organs (e.g., nephrotoxicity, infection, cardiovascular disease, or cancer).

Long-term corticosteroid use should be limited to those patients with a history of rejection that has been difficult to manage and dosing minimized by concomitant use of other forms of immune suppression. The biopsy appearances of late acute rejection may resemble "autoimmune hepatitis," and patients with this picture may respond to corticosteroids readily but relapse after withdrawal or dose reduction. The use of budesonide to minimize systemic side effects in this context is supported by anecdote and experience but not yet by randomized controlled trials (RCTs).

Azathioprine (AZA) or mycophenolate mofetil (MMF) are often used as long-term maintenance immunosuppression. There are no large head-to-head trials of these two agents in liver transplantation, and choice is center-specific. A minority of patients are intolerant of AZA, whereas a small number develop centrilobular injury that resolves after withdrawal. Calcineurin inhibitors (CNIs) are often the core therapy for immune suppression, again with no RCT evidence of benefit of a single regime.

The use of sirolimus (SRL) after liver transplantation is controversial. It is not endorsed by the US Food and Drug Administration because of two studies that demonstrated adverse outcome. The first showed an association of SRL with early hepatic artery thrombosis. The second revealed an excess mortality after switching from CNI to SRL in a group of patients with established grafts. The excess mortality did not reach statistical significance, and subsequent studies from the US Transplant Registry have demonstrated a survival benefit.

Management of the complications of immunosuppression

Common complications seen in long-term survivors of liver transplantation that are unrelated to the graft are shown in Table 25.2.

Metabolic syndrome

Up to 45% of liver transplant recipients have *metabolic syndrome*, defined as three or more of excessive weight gain, hypertension, diabetes, and hyperlipidemia.

Table 25.2 Common complications in long-term survivors of liver transplantation

Complication	Risk
Cardiovascular disease	
Cardiac event	RR approximately 3
Heart disease	Prevalence up to 18%
Metabolic syndrome	
Hypercholesterolemia	Prevalence 15–62%
Hyperlipidemia	Prevalence up to 33%
Hypertension	Prevalence 19–82%
Type 2 DM	SPR approximately 3
Obesity	Prevalence 7–30%
	SPR approximately 6
	Prevalence 29–47%
Malignancy	
Solid organ	SIR approximately 2.5 to 4
Lymphoma	SIR approximately 30
Other	
Osteoporosis	Prevalence 26%
Fractures in women	SIR approximately 2
Renal impairment	Prevalence 35–83%

SIR: standardized incidence ratio; SPR: standardized prevalence ratio; RR: relative risk.

Hypertension

The diagnosis of hypertension relies on a combination of clinic measurements, home measurements, and 24-hour ambulatory blood pressure monitoring. Given current anti-hypertensive guidelines, the target blood pressure should be 140/90 mmHg and lower (130/80 mmHg) in those with renal disease and/or diabetes mellitus. In the presence of diabetes mellitus or proteinuria, a reasonable first-line anti-hypertensive is an angiotensin-converting enzyme (ACE) inhibitor, with a calcium channel blocker as second line. In the absence of proteinuria, the converse applies with a calcium channel blocker as first-line therapy and combination with an ACE inhibitor as second line. Beta-blockade is less effective in liver transplant recipients treated with CNIs and may paradoxically increase central blood pressure.

Diabetes

Risk factors for type 2 diabetes include ethnicity, a positive family history, age greater than 45 years, glucose intolerance pretransplant, use of prednisolone and/or TAC, and the etiologies of HCV infection and cryptogenic (which probably reflects previous non-alcohol-related fatty liver disease in this setting). Effective management of diabetes is important, as it is associated with impaired long-term graft and patient survival. In one study, those who developed sustained post-transplant diabetes mellitus had a 10-year graft survival rate of 59% compared with 73% in non-diabetics and patient survival of 69% versus 78%. Diabetes is also a major risk factor for coronary heart disease, cerebrovascular disease, and peripheral vascular disease in liver transplant recipients.

Patients should be screened at each clinic visit with a random glucose, and hemoglobin A1c should be measured at least annually. Suspected diabetes mellitus should be confirmed with a fasting glucose and, where indicated, a formal glucose tolerance test. Management involves a combination of lifestyle advice, oral hypoglycemic agents, insulin, and reduction or discontinuation of corticosteroid therapy. Switching from CNI has not proved beneficial.

Hyperlipidemia

A fasting lipid profile should be measured annually and patients treated according to current guidelines with a statin in the first instance and a fibrate as second line. Dietary changes alone are ineffective. Simvastatin, atorvastatin, or pravastatin are appropriate first-line agents. The Framingham Cardiac Risk Score has not been validated for liver transplant recipients, who have an additional risk that in our view merits a lower threshold for treatment.

Obesity

Obesity is a risk factor for hypertension, type 2 diabetes, hyperlipidemia, and cardiovascular disease as well as surgical complications and graft dysfunction. It is common, with a rising incidence. CNIs and corticosteroids undoubtedly exacerbate the problem. Dietary advice and exercise may not be as effective as in clinical practice outside the transplant field. Therapeutic manipulation of immunosuppression (particularly corticosteroid avoidance) may be important, and pharmacological therapies such as Orlistat should be considered; in some cases, surgical referral should be considered.

Renal impairment

Renal failure has a significant impact on survival post-transplant and may double mortality 13 years after transplantation. It is also an additional, major risk factor for cardiovascular disease. The most common cause is CNI nephrotoxicity; other causes include diabetic nephropathy, hypertensive nephropathy, and HCV-associated glomerulonephritis.

In the case of CNI nephrotoxicity, successful approaches have included substitution with MMF or SRL. It is critical to recognize renal impairment at an early stage and take appropriate action before the changes become irreversible. In our view, any deterioration in renal function at any stage merits immediate review of pharmacotherapy. Dose of CNI may need to be reduced and plasma levels carefully monitored.

Osteoporosis

Bone mineral density is often low pretransplant despite prophylaxis and therapy, and falls further, often substantially, in the first 3 months following liver transplantation, rising to pretransplant or even healthy/normal age-matched values within 2 years. During this time fracture risk is highest.

Treatment with calcium, vitamin D, and bisphosphonates should be considered. Vitamin D deficiency is common before and after liver transplantation and often overlooked. Long-acting bisphosphonates are now available, which may have better compliance. CNIs are a probable risk factor for osteoporosis, but there is insufficient evidence to advise withdrawal in the presence of osteoporosis.

Neoplasia

Liver transplant recipients have an increased incidence of both cancers that are related to chronic viral infection and cancers related to the underlying disease. Examples of virus-related cancer include basal cell carcinoma; squamous cell carcinoma of the skin, cervix, and oropharynx; and lymphoma. Examples of etiology-related cancers include carcinoma of the colon in patients with primary sclerosing cholangitis (PSC) and esophageal carcinoma in alcohol-related liver disease.

Like other organ transplants, cancer is one of the most important causes of death in liver transplant recipients (discussed further in Chapter 4A). Skin cancers and lymphoma have an incidence of more than 10 times that of the background population, whereas for solid organ cancers, the risk is increased approximately four-fold. Most but not all solid organ malignancies are more common. Notably, the incidence of prostate and breast cancer does not appear to be increased. Preventative strategies include smoking avoidance, protection from sun exposure, and minimizing immune suppression so as not to suppress the anti-viral and anti-tumor effects of the host immune response.

Graft-related complications

Allograft rejection

Late acute cellular rejection (ACR) is similar both histologically and biochemically to early ACR, but may be difficult to distinguish from autoimmune (or perhaps more correctly alloimmune) hepatitis. A variety of clinical signs and symptoms may be observed, including fever, malaise, abdominal pain, hepatomegaly, and increasing ascites. Laboratory abnormalities include abnormal liver biochemistry, elevated inflammatory markers, and an eosinophilia. ACR is a pathological diagnosis with three major histological hallmarks: a mixed portal inflammatory infiltrate, non-suppurative cholangitis, and endothelialitis. Endothelialitis later can affect any transplanted vessel, including those inaccessible to biopsy, such as the cava.

The incidence of late ACR is between 7% and 23% and may coincide with a period of suboptimal immune suppression. Despite being a risk factor for chronic ductopenic rejection, late ACR usually responds either to therapeutic manipulation of immune suppression or a short course of high-dose intravenous methylprednisolone. Rarely, anti-thymocyte globulin will be required. In our center, patients with late ACR are maintained on at least dual-agent immune-suppressive therapy long-term.

Chronic ductopenic rejection (CDR) usually occurs in the first 2 years after transplantation. Its incidence is decreasing, probably as a consequence of improved immune suppression regimens and perhaps the introduction of more effective therapy for cytomegalovirus (CMV). The clinical onset is more insidious than ACR, with cholestasis being a prominent feature. Histology shows progressive ductopenia with inflammation, whereas features of a superimposed ACR may also be present. CDR may reverse with optimization of immunosuppression, but more often necessitates consideration of re-transplantation ultimately. The presence of bile ducts within more than 50% of portal triads is a good prognostic sign in terms of treatment response. Risk factors for CDR include recurrent episodes of ACR, late-onset ACR, CDR in a previous graft, untreated CMV infection, inadequate immune suppression, and primary biliary cirrhosis or primary sclerosing cholangitis as the underlying disease etiology.

Disease recurrence

Hepatitis B virus

Hepatitis B virus (HBV) graft infection led to death from liver failure in the majority of patients prior to the introduction of effective antiviral agents in the 1990s and remains a risk in (1) recipients positive for HBsAg pretransplant whether or not they are HBV DNA positive in serum, although the risk of graft infection is greater with a higher titre of HBV DNA; (2) HBV-naive recipients of grafts from anti-HBc positive donors; (3) recipients with suboptimal HBV prophylaxis post-transplant (either the lack of prophylaxis, a poor prophylactic regime allowing HBV mutants to arise, or poor patient compliance).

Prophylaxis with a combination of HBV immune globulin and at least two antiviral agents from lamivudine, adefovir, tenofovir, and entecavir is effective for those positive for HBsAg pretransplant, whereas a combination of two of these agents is effective usually for naive recipients of an anti-HBc positive donor. The choice of regime differs, often markedly, between centers, and the use of HBV immunoglobulin (Ig) may be determined by cost, but certain principles are common. Thus pretransplant therapy for HBV may select treatment-resistant mutants, so resistance profiling pretransplant is helpful in those with HBV DNA in serum at the time of liver transplant assessment. Some patients will have been treated before, sometimes without the knowledge or support of transplant physicians, which should inform post-transplant management. The frequency of administration and the dose of HBV Ig (if used) must be sufficient to maintain antibody levels above 100 IU/L at all times. Detection of HBsAg or HBV DNA post-transplant must be investigated urgently. The optimum duration of prophylaxis after transplantation (or perhaps more accurately, preventative therapy) is uncertain, and breakthrough after withdrawal of treatment as late as 5 years after transplantation has been reported. It is certainly possible to reduce the number of agents used after a period of 3–5 years of effective prophylaxis/therapy, but our view is that some form of treatment is essential in the absence of detectable immunity. The role of vaccination against HBV post-transplantation remains to be resolved, but there is insufficient evidence at present to support its use. Vaccination pretransplant for those naive to HBV is essential but not always effective.

Hepatitis C virus

Graft infection with HCV is almost invariable and probably occurs within hours of implantation. Chronic inflammation is inevitable and fibrosis progression more rapid, probably as a side effect of immunosuppression.

Between 10% and 30% of recipients with hepatitis C develop cirrhosis by year 5. This number increases to more than 40% by year-10. A rapidly progressive fibrosing cholestatic hepatitis affects a minority (2–5%). Protocol biopsies help to characterize disease progression. In the early post-transplant period, it may be difficult to distinguish between acute rejection and graft infection with HCV on histological grounds alone, but the clinical scenario is often informative; hepatitis in the first 28 days is most often rejection and that beyond 28 days is most likely to be HCV-related. Some centers employ additional histological assessment; the presence of Mcm-2 in the portal infiltrate is indicative of ACR, whereas the absence of lymphocyte Mcm-2 expression suggests HCV-related graft injury.

Advanced donor age is the most important risk factor for rapid progression of HCV-related fibrosis, but other factors include high levels of corticosteroid use or rapid withdrawal of immunosuppression. Therapy with pegylated interferon-α and ribavirin may be effective, with sustained virological response (viral clearance) achieved in approximately 20%. However, treatment side effects may be significant, and rates of acute rejection of up to 45% are reported. Although a recent Cochrane review found no mortality benefit with treatment (duration of follow-up was limited), many hepatologists are more confident now with antiviral therapy in the transplant setting than previously.

Autoimmune diseases

These carry an increased risk of ACR in the early stages and late ACR if immune suppression is decreased. In addition, all three conditions can be manifest on the grafted liver.

Primary biliary cirrhosis

At 10 years from transplantation, biochemical and histological changes characteristic of primary biliary cirrhosis are found in 60% of those recipients whose original disease was primary biliary cirrhosis. Initial immune suppression with cyclosporine rather than TAC may be beneficial in preventing the onset of these changes in the grafted liver but appears to have no benefit if used after these changes are established. Treatment with ursodeoxycholic acid may also be of benefit for established disease. Some patients with recurrent disease progress rapidly to cirrhosis with portal hypertension. Diagnosis relies on liver biopsy, as anti-mitochondrial antibody status is not informative. Graft failure secondary to recurrent primary biliary cirrhosis necessitates consideration of re-transplantation, but recurrent disease *per se* does not seem to affect graft or patient survival.

Autoimmune hepatitis

The risk of recurrent disease is such that long-term immunosuppression with two agents is recommended. Recurrent or de novo autoimmune hepatitis occurs in approximately 25% of grafts during the first 5 years after transplantation and more than 50% after 10 years of follow-up. Diagnosis is made by a combination of abnormal liver biochemistry, elevated serum IgG, and histological features.

Primary sclerosing cholangitis

PSC carries an increased risk of hepatic artery thrombosis and thus graft loss. Recurrence of PSC occurs in about 30% of allografts after 5 years and appears more aggressive in post-primary grafts, with rapid progression to liver failure in many cases. There are no strategies to prevent disease recurrence. Diagnosis involves a combination of cholangiography and liver biopsy. Treatment is of disease complications such as biliary stricture and re-transplantation in the face of graft failure.

Metabolic diseases

Iron overload may occur in patients who undergo transplantation for hemochromatosis and is prevented by maintaining iron stores at physiological levels with recurrent venesection. It is known that recidivism in those who undergo transplantation for alcohol-related liver disease is associated with a reduced survival.

Structural complications

Biliary stricture and incisional hernia are the most common late surgical complications after liver transplantation. Incisional hernias are managed by a combination of weight loss, supports, and surgical intervention. Anastomotic problems may present with a combination of abnormal liver tests, cholangitis, and jaundice. Management varies from antibiotic therapy and observation, through stenting to biliary reconstruction by means of a Roux-en-Y anastomosis. Non-anastomotic strictures are usually the result of ischemia, recurrent PSC, or cholangitis. If strictures are isolated, they may be managed by stenting and/or biliary reconstruction. If, as is often the case, strictures are multiple, management is with antibiotics and ursodeoxycholic acid. Progressive biliary disease or the development of secondary biliary cirrhosis should prompt consideration of re-transplantation.

Late hepatic artery thrombosis usually presents with liver abscess or biliary complications. It may, however, be an incidental finding at ultrasound, and liver function tests may be normal. Attempts at stenting and reconstruction are usually futile, and a further transplant may be required.

Portal vein thrombosis and stenosis are rare late complications. They may present with features of portal hypertension or be an incidental finding. Treatment of portal hypertension (beta-blockade or band ligation) and anti-coagulation is often required; alternatively, surgical or radiological portosystemic shunt should be considered.

Long-term follow-up of liver transplant recipients

Review frequency varies between centers and depends partly on patient morbidity. The aim of follow-up is to screen for graft dysfunction and the late complications of liver transplantation outlined previously in this chapter. Biannual review is a reasonable minimum requirement, with a consultation, blood pressure measurement, skin examination, urinalysis, and blood tests (full blood count, liver biochemistry, renal function tests, fasting glucose, HBA1c measurement, lipid profile, and trough immune suppression level for patients on CNI or SRL). Patients should undergo population-based screening (mammography, colon cancer surveillance, dermatology review, and cervical smear testing) as per local protocol. Dual-

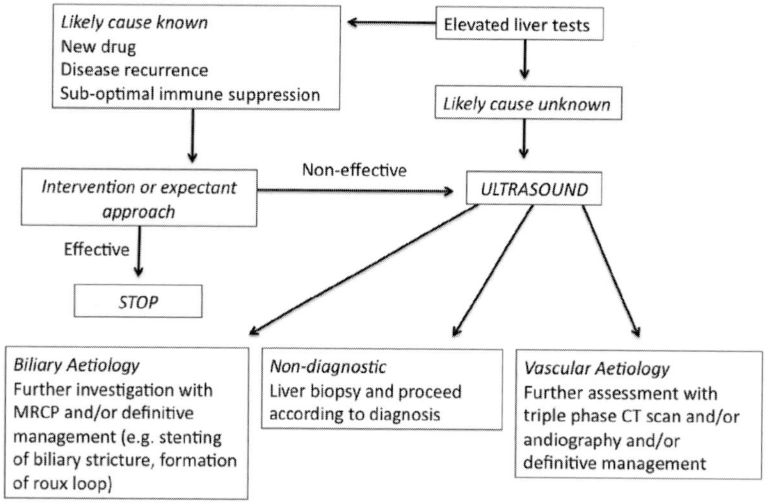

Figure 25.2 An approach to the management of abnormal liver tests in late survivors of liver transplantation. MRCP: magnetic resonance cholangiopancreatography.

energy x-ray absorptiometry (DEXA) scanning to screen for osteoporosis should be performed 2 years after transplantation and at least every 5 years thereafter.

Certain patient groups require additional investigations. These include 6-monthly ultrasound and α-fetoprotein surveillance for patients who undergo transplantation following HCC, endoscopy following primary sclerosing cholangitis, and protocol liver biopsies to identify disease progression following HCV infection.

Abnormal liver biochemistry is found in approximately 60% of patients, and minor abnormalities are usually managed expectantly. Significant elevations should prompt intervention and/or investigation. A management scheme for deranged liver tests late after liver transplantation is given in Figure 25.2.

Re-transplantation

Survival after liver re-transplantation is worse than after primary transplantation and decreases progressively with each new graft. In a period of donor shortage, second and subsequent liver transplants may be difficult to justify. Primary liver graft survival in Europe is presently 70% at 3 years, 65% at 5 years, and 55% at 10 years. The corresponding values for a second graft are 50%, 46%, and 37% and for a third 43%, 39%, and 30%, respectively. In the United Kingdom, one of the listing standards for liver transplantation is that projected 5-year mortality be greater than 50%. These data for post-primary grafts fall short of this and reflect the fact that the selection process for re-transplantation needs to improve.

Although selection for re-transplantation is currently center-dependent, there is evidence that nationally applied scoring systems may be informative. In the United States, the Model for End-Stage Liver Disease (MELD) score is used to select patients for primary grafts. With a score of greater than 25 immediately prior to transplantation, survival at 1 year is less than 60% for post-primary grafts, compared with less than 80% for first grafts. MELD score also predicts mortality in recipients with graft failure, with a score of 25 equating to a survival of 50% at 1 year, compared with 60% in patients with cirrhosis and liver failure before primary engraftment, i.e., patients with liver graft failure are more likely to die than patients with failure of their native liver.

Quality of life after liver transplantation

One of the major aims of liver transplantation is to improve quality of life. During the first 6 months after transplantation, physical and mental quality-of-life scores improve. Unfortunately, this trend is not sustained, and after year 1, emotional and mental health–related quality-of-life scores begin to decrease.

Employment is often used as a surrogate marker for quality of life. Approximately 50% of liver transplant recipients are employed, and studies have confirmed that those in work have a better quality of life than those out of work. Sexual dysfunction improves after liver transplantation. Although 30% of men report sexual inactivity before transplantation, only 15% report this afterwards. Fewer women seem to experience sexual dysfunction before transplantation (35%). This increases modestly to 40% after transplantation. Overall, few publications exist in the field of quality of life after liver transplantation. Given that quality of life is a major post-transplantation end point, further studies are required. In the mean time, psychosocial health should be considered as an important facet in the long-term management of liver transplant recipients.

Conception and pregnancy

The first successful pregnancy after liver transplantation was reported in 1978. As of December 2009 and since 1991, there have been 266 successful births in 152 liver transplant recipients recorded by the National Transplant Pregnancy Registry in the United States.

Liver-related complications are thought to include an increased risk of acute cellular rejection during pregnancy, affecting approximately 6%. This may be due to altered pharmacokinetics, which leads to lower trough levels of immunosuppressant, necessitating an increased frequency of monitoring and often increased dosing. Liver biopsy should be avoided whenever possible.

Maternal complications include increased risk of hypertension (34%), pre-eclampsia (25%), and diabetes (7%). Fetal complications include increased risk of low birth weight (35%), prematurity (40%), and fetal loss (26%). Pregnancies should be regarded as high risk and be managed in a center where support is available from a liver transplant team.

There is no definitive evidence that liver transplant immunosuppression is teratogenic. Prednisolone is safe, CNIs are probably safe, and the effects of SRL are unknown (but given the anti-proliferative effects of SRL, it should be avoided). There are a few case reports of teratogenicity in association with AZA without transplantation and a similar number of reports of teratogenicity in association with MMF use in renal transplant recipients. Overall they are probably both safe.

After pregnancy, care should be taken with dosing to prevent drug toxicity, as trough levels may increase. Breast feeding is usually discouraged due to theoretical toxicity in breast milk.

Potential future strategies

The "holy grail" of solid organ transplantation is often regarded as achieving immunological tolerance. Although this may be achieved in the future with new immunosuppressive strategies, it is apparent that some liver transplant recipients are already "operationally tolerant" in that they do not require long-term immunosuppression.

A handful of studies (the largest with 93 patients) have examined the withdrawal of immunosuppression from patients with established grafts. Approximately 20% of recipients seem to tolerate this in the medium term (maintain normal liver biochemistry) and 10% in the long term. Twenty percent develop clinically significant rejection, but graft loss is rare.

Studies of peripheral lymphocyte phenotypes and liver biopsy characteristics appear to be the most likely avenue in which rejection risk will be quantified. Biological agents that target peripheral lymphocytes destined for the liver appear to be the most likely candidates to provide targeted, liver-specific immune suppression.

More focus is required on late complications so that long-term outcomes improve. For every re-transplantation due to graft failure, a patient dies on the waiting list. Thus long-term graft preservation is not only pertinent to current recipients, but to future recipients also.

Further reading

Bacon BR, O'Grady JG, di Bisceglie AM, Lake JR. *Comprehensive Clinical Hepatology*. Philadelphia, PA: Elsevier, 2005.

Benten D, Staufer K, Sterneck M. Orthotopic liver transplantation and what to do during follow-up: recommendations for the practitioner. *Nat Clin Pract Gastroenterol Hepatol* 2009; **6**: 23–36.

ILTS/AASLD Transplant Course: Long-Term Outcomes of Adult and Pediatric Liver Transplantation. *Liver Transpl* 2009; **15** (S2), 1–94.

Chapter 26

Pediatric liver transplantation

Hector Vilca-Melendez and Giorgina Mieli-Vergani

Key points

- Liver transplantation is the accepted treatment for a wide variety of liver diseases in children.
- Over the past 10 years, a number of innovative surgical techniques have been developed to overcome the shortage of size-matched donors, particularly in children younger than 5 years of age.
- Graft and patient survival at 1 year has continued to improve, being currently greater than 85%.
- Complications are relatively common, but provided graft function is satisfactory, long-term survival is expected.
- Causes of early mortality include graft dysfunction and sepsis. Late mortality is most often due to sepsis, post-transplant lymphoproliferative disease, and non-adherence to immunosuppressive medication.

As more and more children have undergone liver transplantation (LT), the shortage of size-matched donors has become more of a concern and has led to the development of new surgical techniques based on the segmental anatomy of the liver. The use of reduced liver, as originally described by Bismuth and colleagues, provides a suitable size graft for a child, but wastes the rest of the liver mass. The so called "split" LT then evolved to provide two viable partial grafts that could be shared between a child and an adult. Living related LT has also played an important role in reducing the waiting time for a cadaveric organ and has now become a routine procedure in pediatric LT (discussed further in Chapter 22).

New and more varied immunosuppressive agents, better organ preservation, and improvement in peri- and postoperative care have greatly contributed to the success of LT. Currently, the 1-year survival in pediatric LT is approaching 95% for low-risk elective cases and is close to 80% even for acute liver failure.

Long-term management of post-transplant children entering into "normal" adulthood has become the new challenge for the transplant community. Factors intrinsic to this patient population, such as adherence to immunosuppression, drug therapy complications, psychosocial development and education, transition to adulthood, employment, and future parenthood, are now assuming great importance.

Indications for liver transplantation

LT should be considered for any child with end-stage liver disease with a predicted survival of less than 1 year or with a severe impact on quality of life. The pretransplant assessment and peri-operative management of children with liver disease require input from a large and experienced multi-disciplinary team. The decision on when to list for transplant is critical in order to minimize the risk of dying while on the waiting list and to ensure that the child is in optimal condition to survive transplantation. There are a number of factors that influence the timing of transplantation, including age, etiology of the underlying liver disease, past medical and surgical history, and quality of life.

At Kings College Hospital, two thirds of children are less than 5 years of age at the time of LT. Young age does not play a significant role in outcome, except for children less than 3 months of age, who tend to do less well.

Organ Transplantation: A Clinical Guide, ed. A.A. Klein, C.J. Lewis, and J.C. Madsen. Published by Cambridge University Press.

Clinical indications for LT include:

- Chronic liver disease with progressive liver failure and impaired synthetic function (prolonged international normalized ratio [INR] and low serum albumin)
- Severe jaundice with loss of muscle mass, failure to thrive, and severe osteoporosis
- Portal hypertension manifested by variceal bleeding and intractable ascites
- Encephalopathy, profound lethargy
- Spontaneous bacterial peritonitis, recurrent cholangitis
- Intractable debilitating pruritus

Some children develop hepatorenal or hepatopulmonary syndrome, which often reverses after LT. Pulmonary hypertension may be present in children with long-standing chronic liver disease: if unrecognized and severe (systolic >50 mmHg), this may increase the risk of death intra-operatively or in the early postoperative period. Developmental and/or growth retardation are common in children with chronic liver disease and should be addressed before and after LT.

Quality-of-life issues must be considered when deciding the timing of transplantation as they can have a profound effect on the child's future. These issues include the psychosocial aspects of living with chronic liver disease and educational prospects.

Chronic liver disease

Etiologies causing chronic liver disease in children and potentially leading to LT are summarized in Table 26.1. Some of the most important are described below.

Biliary atresia

This is a progressive obliterative cholangiopathy of unknown etiology that accounts for nearly 50% of children referred for LT. Kasai portoenterostomy is the best first treatment option if performed within 2 months of life, leading to clearance of jaundice in 80% of the cases. This success has been also linked to the experience of the surgical center performing the procedure. If complete correction of serum bilirubin is achieved, 50% of these children will keep their native livers up to their teenage years, but eventually 70–80% will require LT. Progressive cholestasis, recurrent episodes of cholangitis, cirrhosis with synthetic function failure, severe portal hypertension, and hepatic artery resistance index (HARI) ≥ 1.0 on Doppler ultrasound are all indications of progressive liver disease and of the need for LT. The differentiation between isolated biliary atresia (90% of cases) and biliary atresia splenic malformation (BASM) syndrome (10% of cases) is very important for surgical planning before LT, owing to the anatomical variations commonly found in BASM, including cardiovascular defects, polysplenia, situs inversus, absence of inferior vena cava (IVC), and preduodenal portal vein.

α_1-antitrypsin deficiency

This is one of the most frequent metabolic liver disorders that results in cirrhosis and requires LT in children. Clinical indications for LT are the same as for other cirrhotic disorders, but progression of disease is particularly rapid after the first signs of decompensation requiring early listing.

Non-cirrhotic metabolic liver disorders

Non-cirrhotic metabolic liver disorders that cause no structural damage to the liver but have deleterious systemic effects because of toxic metabolites or enzyme deficiencies should be considered for LT (Table 26.1). In these conditions, the purpose of LT is to improve the quality of life by correcting the metabolic defect, rather than being a life-saving procedure. Two other alternative strategies can be used to achieve this: hepatocyte transplantation and auxiliary partial orthotopic LT (APOLT). In both procedures, the aim is to provide the defective metabolite or enzyme preserving the whole or part of the native liver, thus providing a "safety net" in case of graft failure. The overall patient survival for LT for metabolic disorders is excellent, without significant difference in survival for cirrhotic and non-cirrhotic variants.

Alagille syndrome

This is an autosomal-dominant disorder that affects liver (intrahepatic bile duct paucity), heart (peripheral pulmonary stenosis, tetralogy of Fallot), eyes (posterior embryotoxon), and skeleton (butterfly vertebra, short stature) with characteristic dysmorphic facial features. A third of the patients with this condition require LT, and a thorough multi-organ assessment is necessary before LT, as cardiac problems may contraindicate the procedure. Renal tubular acidosis can

Table 26.1 Chronic liver diseases in children that may require treatment with liver transplantation

- Extrahepatic biliary atresia
  - Isolated biliary atresia
  - Biliary atresia splenic malformation (BASM) syndrome
- Metabolic liver disease
  - Cirrhotic
    - α_1-antitrypsin deficiency
    - Wilson's disease
    - Tyrosinemia type 1
    - Cystic fibrosis
    - Respiratory chain disorders
    - Glycogen storage disease type IV
    - Bile acid synthetic defect
  - Non-cirrhotic
    - Crigler-Najjar syndrome type 1
    - Glycogen storage disease type Ia and Ib
    - Propionic acidemia
    - Urea cycle deficiency
      - Ornithine transcarbamylase (OTC) deficiency
      - Arginosuccinate lyase (ALS) deficiency
      - Carbamoylphosphate synthetase (CPS1) deficiency
      - Citrullinemia
    - Primary hyperoxaluria
    - Familial hypercholesterolemia
    - Factor VII deficiency
    - Protein C deficiency
- Intrahepatic cholestasis
  - Syndromic
    - Alagille syndrome
  - Non-syndromic
    - Progressive familial intrahepatic cholestasis (PFIC)
      - Normal gamma glutamyl transferase (GGT)
        - PFIC-1 (Byler disease)
        - PFIC-2 (Bile salt export pump [BSEP] deficiency)
      - Elevated GGT
        - MDR3 deficiency
    - Idiopathic neonatal hepatitis
    - Parenteral nutrition related
- Chronic hepatitis
  - Autoimmune
    - Autoimmune hepatitis (AIH)
      - AIH type 1 (smooth muscle and/or antinuclear antibodies)
      - AIH type 2 (anti liver kidney microsome type 1 antibodies)
    - Autoimmune sclerosing cholangitis
  - Infectious origin
    - Postviral hepatitis (B, C, others)
- Liver tumors
  - Benign
    - Hemangioendothelioma (if large and non-resectable)
  - Malignant
    - Hepatoblastoma (if non-resectable)
    - Hepatocellular carcinoma (if small with no metastasis)
    - Fibrolamellar carcinoma (if small with no metastasis)
- Others
  - Polycystic liver disease
  - Budd-Chiari syndrome
  - Cryptogenic cirrhosis

cause renal impairment, whereas intracranial bleeding might be associated with a generalized vasculopathy caused by the disease. In our experience, dynamic cardiac testing with cardiac catheterization and dobutamine stress resulting in an increase in cardiac output greater than 40% indicates that the candidates may safely undergo LT. Profound cholestasis and intractable pruritus are common indications for transplantation in these patients; cirrhotic decompensation and development of HCC accelerate the need. Despite satisfactory 1-year survival rates after transplantation, the benefit seen in this systemic disease is limited, and catch-up growth is generally not satisfactory.

Autoimmune hepatitis

There are two types of autoimmune hepatitis (AIH) in childhood: type 1, characterized by smooth muscle antibody (SMA) and antinuclear antibodies, and type 2, characterized by anti-liver kidney microsomal type 1 antibody. Children with AIH frequently present acutely, particularly those with type 2, who can even develop fulminant hepatic failure, whereas a third have an insidious onset, often with flares and remissions, compatible with chronic liver disease and cirrhosis, particularly in type 1 AIH. Associated autoimmune disorders include inflammatory bowel disease, thyroiditis, nephrotic syndrome, and diabetes. Immunosuppressive therapy is the cornerstone of treatment for AIH, with initial high doses of prednisolone (with or without AZA) followed by progressive tapering over a period of 4–8 weeks. Second-line therapy for difficult-to-treat patients includes mycophenolate mofetil (MMF) and at times tacrolimus (TAC) or cyclosporine (CyA). Normalization of serum transaminases is seen after 6–9 months in 75–90%, but relapse occurs in up to 40% of patients and long-term treatment is usually necessary. LT is eventually required, usually several years after diagnosis in 10–20% of patients. A high incidence of chronic graft hepatitis is seen after LT, suggesting disease recurrence (10–35% of cases between 15–30 months post-transplant). In patients who undergo transplantation for AIH, it is prudent to continue with steroid-based immunosuppression after LT to prevent recurrence.

Hepatoblastoma

This is the most common malignant liver tumor in children. Its prognosis has been drastically altered by effective chemotherapy. Treatment schedules of the International Childhood Liver Tumour Strategy Group of the International Society of Pediatric Oncology (SIOPEL) have led to excellent response to chemotherapy, allowing previously unresectable tumors to be downsized to the point of resectability in more than 60% of cases, with very good survival rates. Those tumors that remain unresectable can be treated by LT (with grafts from cadaveric or living donors). Tumor recurrence is still the most common cause of death (20–25%) and in general is related to the presence of previous lung metastases. One or two courses of post-LT chemotherapy may be given, but this remains controversial.

Acute liver failure

Acute liver failure (ALF) is rare in children, but is associated with significant mortality (up to 70% without LT). The presence of encephalopathy is a clear indication for LT in adults with ALF, but in children it is more difficult to identify. Severe impairment of liver function requiring transplantation is defined by an INR >4, severe metabolic acidosis, cardiovascular instability, rapidly shrinking liver on ultrasound, and the presence of renal failure. Cerebral edema, with raised intracranial pressure and potential brainstem herniation, is the most serious complication, and multidisciplinary medical management is necessary to support the patient until a suitable organ is found, as this is the only effective treatment option. Contraindications for LT in ALF include:

- Irreversible neurological damage (persistent fixed and dilated pupils)
- Severe respiratory failure
- Active uncontrolled sepsis
- Underlying systemic disease not correctable by transplantation (e.g., mitochondrial cytopathies, hemophagocytic lymphohistiocytosis)

Causes of pediatric ALF treatable by LT are summarized in Table 26.2, and some of the most important etiologies are described below.

Table 26.2 Causes of acute liver failure in children that may require treatment with liver transplantation

Viral
Viral hepatitis, A to E
Seronegative hepatitis (non A–E)
Adenovirus, parvovirus, herpes simplex
Metabolic
Neonatal hemochromatosis
Tyrosinemia type 1
Wilson's disease
Fatty acid oxidation defects
Galactosemia
Drug- or toxin-induced
Acetaminophen overdose
Mushroom poisoning
Autoimmune
Autoimmune hepatitis (type 2 and type 1)
Giant cell hepatitis with Coombs-positive hemolytic anemia (it may recur post LT)

Attempts to support liver function until transplantation by using liver assist devices and hepatocyte transplantation are still in the experimental phase. The use of APOLT for ALF in children has produced patient survival rates (85%) comparable to those of whole liver replacement, with the added advantage of withdrawal of immunosuppression if the native liver regenerates. Hepatic regeneration, however, is slower in patients with seronegative hepatitis when compared with other etiologies.

Acute viral hepatitis

Acute viral hepatitis is the most common cause of ALF in children. It is predominantly seronegative in the United States and Europe, being characterized by severe impairment of liver synthetic function and bone marrow failure in 10% of cases. Hepatitis A and E are the most frequent cause of ALF in Asia.

Neonatal hemochromatosis

Neonatal hemochromatosis is a rare disorder associated with massive intrahepatic and extrahepatic iron deposition, and it is the most common cause of hepatic failure in the neonatal period. There is a high recurrence rate within families, but the pattern of inheritance is still unknown. It presents with severe liver failure at birth or immediately after, and the diagnosis is made when associated with at least two of the following findings: positive family history, elevated serum ferritin levels, confirmed extrahepatic iron deposition (salivary gland punch biopsy), and iron overload detected by magnetic resonance imaging. Initial medical treatment is attempted with anti-oxidant and iron-chelating agents; however, their efficacy has been questioned, and LT is recommended early, usually when severe coagulopathy or encephalopathy is present. The small size of these newborns represents a challenge in obtaining a size-match organ; therefore, while waiting for transplantation, exchange transfusions are recommended if INR is >5. Extensive neurological assessment must be performed before the surgical procedure. Despite all these precautions, patient survival rates after LT range from 50–60%; however, survivors have a good long-term outcome.

Wilson's disease

Wilson's disease is an autosomal-recessive disorder of copper metabolism that affects children after 3 years of age and may present as decompensated chronic liver disease or as acute liver failure. Diagnosis is made when the liver disease is associated with two of the following criteria: positive family history, low serum ceruloplasmin, high liver copper, presence of Kayser-Fleischer rings on eye examination, elevated 24-hour urinary copper excretion (before and/or after penicillamine challenge), and Coombs negative hemolytic anemia. The insidious chronic presentation can be successfully treated with long-term chelating agents, including penicillamine (or trientine) alone or in combination with zinc acetate or sulphate, but acute presentation with encephalopathy is generally fatal, and LT is the only effective option. For those cases with ALF but no encephalopathy, a prognostic scoring system has been devised to predict mortality and the need for LT based on readily available blood tests, including bilirubin, INR, aspartate aminotransferase, albumin, and white blood cell count. In our experience, children with a score of greater than 11 die without transplantation, but larger studies are necessary to validate this scoring system.

Surgical issues

Donor liver grafts

Donor liver grafts for children are most commonly obtained from donation after brain death (DBD) donors. Both donor and recipient should be ABO blood group compatible, but preferably an identical ABO-matched graft is used; however, under the age of 1 year, grafts from incompatible blood group donors can be used safely.

Pediatric donors who could provide size-matched organs are not common, and surgical techniques that allow the use of partial liver grafts for children from adult donors (reduced or split or living donor LT) have had a great impact on reducing the number of children dying on the waiting list. There is no upper age limit for liver donation, but livers from donors over 40 years of age tend to be used less commonly in children. Although there is no lower age donor limit, the use of livers from donors less than 6 months of age has been associated with a higher incidence of hepatic artery thrombosis.

Another increasingly important source of liver grafts is from donation after cardiac death (DCD) donors. It is possible to use liver grafts from DCD donors for pediatric recipients with satisfactory medium-term outcome. Only the best DCD donors, which fulfill strict quality criteria, should be selected for reduced or split LT for children.

Liver transplant procedure

The transplant procedure in a child commences with a bilateral subcostal incision, careful mobilization of the anatomical structures around the liver, particularly when the recipient has had previous operations resulting in dense adhesions (e.g., Kasai portoenterostomy), and excision of the diseased liver with or without the retro-hepatic vena cava. The implantation technique will depend on the type of graft used.

Whole liver graft

Orthotopic liver replacement using a whole-size pediatric graft is accomplished by anastomosing the vena cava, portal vein, and hepatic artery to the corresponding structures of the recipient and allowing blood reperfusion. Biliary reconstruction is generally achieved by end-to-end common bile duct anastomosis or hepatico-jejunostomy.

Reduced size liver grafts

Adult donor livers can be cut down to provide smaller grafts, based on the segmental anatomy of the liver. The graft can be reduced to a left lateral segment (segments II and III), the use of which can overcome a donor to recipient size discrepancy of 10:1. Use of the left or right lobe overcomes lesser degrees of size discrepancy. Further reduction of the left lateral segment is possible in order to provide a single segment graft (monosegment) to implant in very small babies. In our center, the part of the liver not used for the recipient after graft reduction is not discarded but rather is used for hepatocyte transplantation.

Split liver grafts

Split LT provides two grafts from a single donor, the left lateral segment for a child and the right lobe for an adult. Excellent patient and graft 1-year survival rates

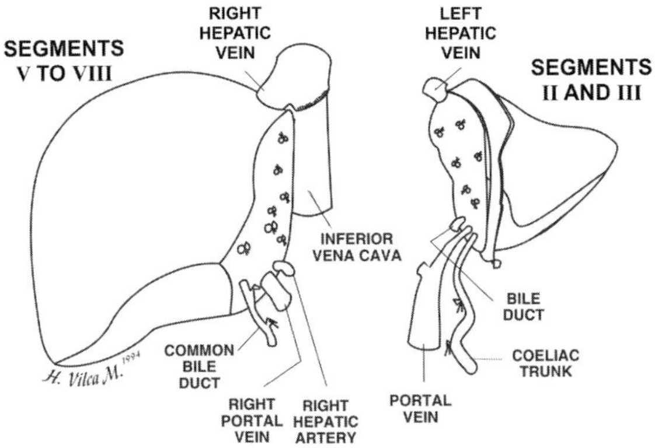

Figure 26.1 Split liver grafts. The splitting technique allows two patients to receive transplants from a single donor. The left lateral segment usually goes to a child and the right lobe to an adult.

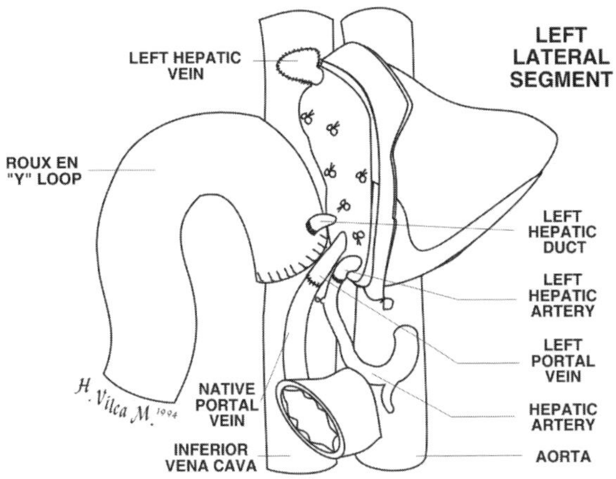

Figure 26.2 Living-related liver transplant. The left lateral segment from a living donor is generally used in pediatric liver transplantation.

have been achieved (90% and 87%, respectively; Figure 26.1). The liver is divided just to the right of the falciform ligament providing a left lateral segment for a child and an extended right lobe (segments IV–VIII) for an adult. The left hepatic artery and left portal vein are allocated to the pediatric graft if they are of a suitable size for a safe anastomosis. In most cases, the division at the hilum will result in one bile duct for the left lateral segment; but rarely, it might be necessary to perform two hepatico-jejuno anastomoses for biliary reconstruction.

Live donor grafts (see Chapter 22)

This surgical technique utilizes the left lateral segment from a living related donor (Figure 26.2). It was first performed in Brazil, but successful cases were subsequently carried out in Australia and the United States. Although it is performed worldwide with remarkable success, the actual donor morbidity/mortality remains unknown due to the lack of accurate reporting. In our center, live donation for children has become a routine operation, but a strict protocol to select the donors is essential. The advantages of this surgical modality include reduction of the time on the waiting list; scheduled, planned procedure; and shorter cold preservation times. Recipient survival is over 90% at 1 year, and for countries lacking cadaveric donation, living donation LT represents the only source of grafts for the pediatric population.

Auxiliary liver graft

Some pediatric patients with ALF or with liver-based metabolic disorders can be treated by APOLT. This technique includes the partial resection of the native liver (generally the left lateral segment) followed by the implantation of a size-matched partial graft. In ALF, this operation is technically more demanding than replacing the whole native liver, but allows withdrawal of immunosuppression when the native liver has recovered from the acute injury. In metabolic diseases, such as Crigler-Najjar syndrome, urea cycle defects and propionic acidemia, and in coagulation factor deficiencies, auxiliary grafting provides enough hepatocyte mass to correct the enzymatic/synthetic defect and at the same time preserves otherwise normal native liver to serve as a "safety net" in case of graft failure.

Immunosuppression

TAC is now the preferred agent for maintenance immunosuppression in pediatric LT. In the first 3 months, immunosuppression generally requires the use of steroids, which are rapidly weaned or withdrawn in the majority of children. In our center, steroids are rapidly weaned to a very low long-term maintenance dose (1–2.5 mg/day) together with low TAC levels (~5 mg/l) starting from 3 months after surgery. With the introduction of calcineurin inhibitors (CNIs), the rate of acute cellular rejection (ACR) has steadily decreased, but the better long-term outcome has led to an increase in CNI-related adverse effects. CNI-induced renal impairment can be as high as 60% in the pediatric transplant population, eventually leading to end-stage renal disease requiring renal transplantation. CNI-sparing regimes have been advocated involving either reduction in drug exposure and/or introduction of other immunosuppressive drugs. Dose reduction of CNIs can be achieved early by using induction with interleukin-2 receptor antibodies or anti-thymocyte globulin (ATG), or early after LT (around 3 months) with the addition of adjuvant drugs such as MMF, sirolimus (SRL), or everolimus. In cases of serious CNI-related side effects, it is possible to replace the CNI with MMF, but corticosteroid dose should be increased.

Post-transplant complications

The majority of complications and deaths occur within the first 3 months after LT. Hence early recognition and correction of these complications is essential to improve graft and patient survival.

Primary graft dysfunction

Primary graft dysfunction (PGD) is relatively rare (2–5%), and risk factors include donor characteristics, organ preservation, and technical or immunological complications in the recipient. Signs of poor graft function include hemodynamic instability, the need for inotrope support, metabolic acidosis, and coagulopathy. Urgent re-transplantation is the only real therapeutic option, but it carries significantly increased risk compared with primary LT.

Postoperative bleeding

Risk factors for post-transplant bleeding include poor graft function, renal failure, hemodialysis, and large intra-operative blood loss. Bleeding from the cut surface of a partial graft may reflect venous outflow obstruction. Exploratory laparotomy and surgical hemostasis is needed if the correction of a low platelet count or low fibrinogen does not achieve hemostasis. However, in up to 50% of cases, it is not possible to identify an active bleeding site during surgery.

Hepatic artery thrombosis

Hepatic artery thrombosis (HAT) is one of the most serious complications, which often leads to graft loss. The incidence in children varies from 5–8% and is less common in partial than full size liver grafts. Early HAT is generally linked to surgical risk factors including poor surgical technique, kinking of the artery, and previous endothelial injury (caused during organ retrieval). However, medical factors can also contribute to this complication, such as underlying prothrombotic disorders (anticardiolipin antibody), high hematocrit and raised blood viscosity, poor fluid management and arterial hypotension, and severe ACR causing liver swelling and increased resistance to arterial flow. Early recognition (scheduled Doppler ultrasound and urgent CT angiography) and immediate surgical revascularization may salvage the graft in up to one third of patients.

Late HAT (several years after transplantation) can occur, and the intrahepatic arterial supply invariably is revascularized by collateral vessels. Presentation is often subtle and the complications include mild liver dysfunction, late biliary stricture, recurrent low-grade cholangitis, intraparenchymal abscesses, and bacteremia. If hepatic collateralization is adequate, management is mainly conservative, but if the hepatic injury is severe, re-transplantation is required.

Portal vein thrombosis or stenosis

Portal vein thrombosis (PVT) occurs in approximately 2–15% of liver transplants, particularly in small children with a hypoplastic portal vein that is mainly associated with extrahepatic biliary atresia (EHBA). Surgical technical problems (e.g., a portal vein too short causing stretching or too long causing kinking) and previous PVT are recognized risk factors. Early PVT presents with graft dysfunction or gastrointestinal bleeding, and the diagnosis is confirmed by Doppler ultrasound and aortoportography. Sequential measurement of the spleen size is often a good guide regarding the continuing presence or development of portal hypertension, which is generally associated with a low platelet count and slight prolongation of the INR. Early surgical intervention to restore portal venous flow will usually rescue the graft.

Late portal vein complications present with signs of portal hypertension such as variceal hemorrhage or splenomegaly. The underlying cause may be technical, but on occasions remodeling of a partial liver graft causes stretching of the portal vein and possible thrombosis.

Venous outflow obstruction

This is uncommon and represents technical failure in the anastomosis of the graft to the hepatic veins or IVC. It may cause serious difficulty in controlling bleeding from the cut surface of the graft or in the longer term a clinical picture similar to Budd-Chiari syndrome. Suprahepatic caval stenosis is also rare and usually due to technical shortcomings. It presents with bilateral leg and lower trunk edema, renal impairment, and at times ascites. Doppler ultrasound, cavography, and pressure measurements will confirm the presence of a significant gradient across the stenosis. Dilatation using interventional radiological techniques may solve the problem.

Biliary complications

In children, biliary drainage at LT is re-established by bile duct–to–bile duct anastomosis (if the graft is size-matched) or more commonly by hepatico-jejunostomy (if a partial graft from an adult). Biliary leaks are the most common technical complications, occurring in 5–30% of children, and they might arise from the biliary anastomosis, the cut surface of partial liver grafts, the T-tube insertion site (if used), and unrecognized segmental bile duct left opened (generally, segment IV bile duct). Diagnosis can easily be made when bile appears in the abdominal drains, but it can present insidiously with fever or mild graft dysfunction, and only ultrasound-guided drainage of a collection will confirm the problem. Endoscopic or percutaneous cholangiography and stenting of the common bile duct will usually lead to resolution. Anastomotic biliary strictures occur in 10–35% of cases and generally within the first year after transplantation. They might be related to a previous bile leak episode and present with cholestasis, cholangitis, or features of biliary obstruction on liver function tests (mainly elevated gamma glutamyl transferase) or histology. Dilatation of the biliary tree may be seen on liver ultrasound. Endoscopic or percutaneous transhepatic balloon dilatation and, if indicated, placement of a biliary stent leads to the resolution of the majority of early strictures. Surgical reconstruction (e.g., hepatico-jejunostomy) is necessary if the stricture does not resolve with repeated dilatations.

Intrahepatic diffuse cholangiopathy is less frequent and tends to present late (often >12 months after transplantation) and is associated with hepatic artery thrombosis, preservation injury, and use of ABO-incompatible grafts. Very few patients can be managed conservatively, and the majority require re-transplantation.

Other surgical complications

Perforation of the small or large bowel is uncommon (6%) except in children with EHBA who have undergone previous surgery, in whom the incidence is over 10%. A low threshold for emergency laparotomy is needed to correct this complication and avoid a serious septic episode. Re-perforation is also a common event.

Immunological complications

ACR occurs in 40–60% of children within the first month, usually between 5 and 15 days after LT. ACR is suspected when there is a rise in the serum transaminase levels, but the diagnosis is only confirmed by liver biopsy. The typical histological features are of a dense periportal cellular lymphocytic and eosinophilic infiltration with endotheliitis and bile duct damage. The treatment of ACR is based on increasing immunosuppression, generally with daily boluses of methylprednisolone (10 mg/kg/day for 3 consecutive days). Steroid-resistant rejection occurs in approximately 6–30% of these patients, and rescue therapy with MMF seems to be effective in achieving good long-term graft function. The use of ATG or muromonab-CD3 for ACR carries numerous adverse effects, including a significant risk of over-immunosuppression. Grafts that do not respond to rescue therapy have a high chance of progressing to chronic rejection.

Late cellular rejection (LCR) can happen at 6 months or more post-transplantation, and it is not uncommon in children (8% of cases). It seems to be related to inadequate immunosuppression due to necessary dose reductions to avoid for example sepsis or post-transplant lymphoproliferative disorder (PTLD), but also to abnormal intestinal absorption or patients' poor adherence to medication. LCR can progress to chronic rejection and can also be complicated by the onset of de novo AIH.

Chronic rejection used to be a significant cause of graft loss, but its incidence is decreasing (5–10%). It generally happens within the first year post-transplant, with jaundice, pruritus, and elevated cholestatic liver function tests (alkaline phosphatase and gamma glutamyl transferase), with only mild to moderate elevation of the serum transaminases and preserved hepatic synthetic function. The diagnosis is histological and characterized by loss of bile ducts and arteriopathy. The treatment is to increase immunosuppression with TAC and/or SRL. This may reverse the changes in some children, but the majority progress to re-transplantation.

Infection

Bacterial, viral, or fungal infections are frequent in the postoperative recovery period. Risk factors pretransplantation include younger age (increased susceptibility to pathogens like coagulase–negative staphylococci or respiratory syncytial virus [RSV]), etiology (transplant for CF, biliary atresia and cholangitis, chronic liver diseases with spontaneous bacterial peritonitis), and donor infections (cytomegalovirus [CMV] and Epstein-Barr virus [EBV]). Post-transplant risk factors include poor graft function, graft ischemia (e.g., HAT), prolonged ICU stay, ventilator dependence, indwelling catheters, gut perforation, over-immunosuppression, and re-transplantation. Bacterial and fungal infections are a common early problem after LT (within the first month), whereas viral infection is more frequent later (CMV, EBV). Gram-negative septicemia and systemic fungal infection have a high mortality risk.

Bacterial pneumonia and IV line infections occur early after LT, and they should be treated aggressively. Gram-negative sepsis is often associated with a biliary leak, ascending cholangitis, bowel perforation, or graft ischemia (HAT). It is important to note that immunosuppressive therapy may minimize the clinical signs of sepsis. Prophylactic anti-microbial therapy is used for 5–7 days and is adjusted or stopped after the results of perioperative cultures. Most established infections can be successfully treated; however, colonization with multiple antibiotic-resistant bacteria is becoming a serious problem that requires the implementation of strict infection control measures.

The risk of fungal infections seems to be associated with pre-transplant fungal colonization and pyrexia and also with post-transplant immunosuppression, bacterial infections, and EBV infection. Fungal sepsis after LT is more common in patients with previous acute liver failure, liver re-transplantation, graft dysfunction, HAT, and bowel perforation. It should be suspected in any post-transplant patient with fever and high white blood count while receiving broad-spectrum antibiotics. *Candida* species are the most common pathogens; these generally respond well to fluconazole, caspofungin, and micafungin. Infections with *Aspergillus*, *Cryptococcus*, and mucormycosis and coccidioidomycosis, although less common, may carry a high mortality risk. Because of nephrotoxicity associated with the use of conventional amphotericin B, the liposomal form of the drug is preferred. Other options such as itraconazole or voriconazole require careful monitoring of graft function and immunosuppressive drug levels.

Herpes viruses are the most important viral pathogens post-transplant. CMV infection generally presents between 1 and 3 months after LT in children, and it can be caused by primary infection (e.g., from donor graft or blood products), reactivation of latent infection, or superinfection with different CMV strain. Prophylaxis with ganciclovir has decreased the rate and severity of CMV infection and should be used in high-risk cases (CMV-seropositive donor/seronegative recipient); however, prophylaxis may simply delay the onset of CMV disease. Monitoring of antigenemia (pp65 assay or CMV DNA polymerase chain reaction [PCR]) has had a significant impact on recipient management. Treatment continues until the CMV viral load is non-detectable.

Young children who are EBV negative before LT are particularly at risk of developing EBV-related PTLD (incidence of 4%). Determination of the EBV load by PCR predicts the risk of PTLD, but diagnosis must be confirmed histologically in enlarged lymph nodes or other affected tissues. Management of PTLD includes the withdrawal of immunosuppression alone or in combination with antiviral agents, with a success rate of 67%. Failure to respond or recurrence should be treated with monoclonal antibodies against CD-20 B cells (rituximab) or chemotherapy, depending on severity.

Other herpes viruses, such as herpes simplex virus and varicella zoster virus, potentially reactivate after transplantation, but treatment with acyclovir is generally highly effective.

The incidence of adenovirus infection after LT has decreased to 4% since the use of TAC-based immunosuppression. However, when present, it may cause fulminant hepatitis or necrotizing pneumonitis, often due to over-immunosuppression. Other common viral pathogens associated with upper and lower respiratory tract infections are influenza and RSV. Vaccination and/or antiviral treatment, when available, may help avoid significant and potentially life-threatening complications.

Re-transplantation

The incidence of re-transplantation for LT in children ranges from 9–29%. Common causes for re-transplantation are HAT (72%), PGD (19%), chronic rejection (15%), and biliary complications (10%). One-year patient survival rates of 67% have been reported in a multi-center study (including cases from 1996–2004); however, in other studies there was no survival difference between re-transplantation (91%) and primary LT (92%). Emergency re-transplantation (within 1 month after LT) appears to have a poorer prognosis. Allocation of a second liver because of failure of the first graft may be controversial if outcome is perceived as inferior, but re-transplantation is the only ethical option for the survival of those children needing this procedure.

Outcome and quality of life

Short-term survival after LT in children is excellent (1-year patient and graft survival >90% for elective cases) with no difference according to age, indicating the significant impact of improved surgical techniques and innovations in care for smaller recipients. LT for ALF in children still produces inferior outcomes (1-year survival of 75%), with early death related to multi-organ failure, sepsis, and neurological complications. Children who survive 1 year after LT generally continue to do well, with 5-, 10-, and 20-year patient survival rates of 86%, 82%, and 66%, respectively. Causes of late deaths include recurrence of malignancy, PTLD, and steroid-resistant rejection.

The initial obstacles to survival, particularly organ preservation, surgical technique, and immunosuppression, have been addressed, but the problems following successful transplantation are only now beginning to be recognized. Major interest has now turned towards the quality of life of long-term survivors. Twenty-year LT survivors will be seen more frequently over the next decade, and we should be attempting to address their needs now.

Health-related quality of life (HRQOL) assesses markers of overall well-being and functional outcomes, including physical, psychological, and social functions. However, HRQOL assessment is very difficult in the pediatric population due to intrinsic factors such as the age of patients (children or adolescents), neuro-developmental considerations, and source of reporting (parent or self-reporting), and family-related variables may cause significant bias in the results.

There is a strong correlation between quality of life, graft function, and complications requiring repeated hospital admission. After LT, the liver function tests normalize in the majority of patients, physical symptoms of end-stage liver disease improve or disappear (ascites, jaundice, pruritus, and fatigue), metabolic bone disease recovers, and those who were not able to walk before LT because of rickets or hypertrophic pulmonary osteoarthropathy are able to do so within a year. In general, transplant patients feel they have a normal level of physical function; however, HRQOL scores for physical function in this group of patients are lower than those in healthy children.

Psychosocial functioning also appears lower than in healthy children, especially in the area of education. The most common reason for delay in educational progress is missed school days before and after LT, but it may be also a consequence of developmental delay or learning disabilities (8%). However, in a study assessing children who had survived 20 years after LT, 90% completed high school and 50% attended college, indicating that we can expect improvement in their cognitive function.

Family factors play an important role in HRQOL. After LT, parents tend to view themselves as more relaxed and able to apply disciplinary boundaries. However, many families have difficulties in adjusting to the new situation. They miss the need to nurse their child through deteriorating health and they have anxiety about the child's long-term future, as it is not possible to give an absolute assurance that the child will remain well. Parents often report that their child's behavior is not entirely normal, and behavioral immaturity often persists in the form of acts of defiance or aggression, particularly in adolescents.

Adolescent transplant recipients are at increased risk of medication non-adherence, with incidence ranging from 17–53%. For the adolescent patient, this is a difficult period, with significant physical and emotional changes taking place, interaction with peers, the desire for autonomy from the family, and the imminent transfer of their medical care from pediatric to adult services. Furthermore, the development of secondary chronic illness due to immunosuppressive medication (e.g., renal dysfunction, weight gain, hypertension) carries a negative impact on their HRQOL. Other factors increasing the risk of non-adherence include inadequate knowledge of the medication regime, depression and anxiety, substance abuse, life stress, and inadequate relationship with the medical team. Transitional care programs for pediatric LT patients have been advocated to deal with these problems and to help in the gradual shifting of management skills from the medical team and parents to the adolescents themselves.

As the life expectancy of children undergoing transplantation continues to increase, we must be prepared for their future needs. These needs cannot be measured just as clinical outcomes after LT, but they should also consider improvement in quality of life. It is essential to ensure that important socioeconomic milestones are achieved by these patients: completing education, being in employment, and having their own families. It is likely that in the future, these factors will influence the timing of transplantation.

Further reading

Bartlett A, Rela M. Progress in surgical techniques in pediatric liver transplantation. *Pediatr Transplant* 2010; **14**: 33–40.

Bucuvalas J. Long-term outcomes in pediatric liver transplantation. *Liver Transpl* 2009; **15**: S6–11.

Dhawan A. Etiology and prognosis of acute liver failure in children. *Liver Transpl* 2008; **14**: S80–4.

Duffy J, Kao K, Ko C, *et al.* Long-term patient outcome and quality of life after liver transplantation: analysis of 20-year survivors. *Ann Surg* 2010; **252**: 652–61.

Hartley J, Davenport M, Kelly D. Biliary atresia. *Lancet* 2009; **374**: 1704–13.

Mieli-Vergani G, Vergani D. Autoimmune paediatric liver disease. *World J Gastroenterol* 2008; **14**: 3360–7.

Muiesan P, Vergani D, Mieli-Vergani G. Liver transplantation in children. *J Hepatol* 2007; **46**: 340–8.

Chapter 27

Recipient selection

Ernest I. Mandel and Nina E. Tolkoff-Rubin

Key points

- Thorough pretransplant evaluation is essential for maximization of both patient and graft survival.
- Cardiovascular evaluation and screening should be performed in nearly all patients.
- Screening for other chronic conditions, including infections and malignancy, should be performed, and they should be managed appropriately prior to transplantation.
- Morbidity and mortality, as well as quality-of-life considerations, should be taken into account when considering older candidates.
- A multi-disciplinary approach considering cognitive and other psychosocial factors is necessary to ensure successful transplantation.

Kidney transplantation is the renal replacement therapy of choice for suitable patients with advanced chronic kidney disease (CKD) or end-stage renal disease (ESRD), conferring both survival advantages and quality-of-life improvements over peritoneal dialysis and hemodialysis. With more than 80 000 patients currently awaiting transplantation in the United States, optimizing the selection of candidates is essential to ensuring the equitable allocation of this scarce resource. In addition, for those awaiting deceased donor transplantation, or for those fortunate to identify a potential living donor, a thorough pretransplant evaluation is needed to maximize both graft and patient survival.

Timing of referral

Observational studies suggest that survival after transplant is worse the longer a patient is on dialysis. Furthermore, patient and graft survival are improved in patients transplanted preemptively, that is, prior to the initiation of dialysis. Except for a zero antigen mismatch (for which patients can be eligible at an estimated glomerular filtration rate [eGFR] less than 20 ml/min/1.73 m^2), patients in the United States cannot undergo transplantation with a deceased donor kidney preemptively. Nonetheless, patients can be listed once their eGFR is below 20 ml/min/1.73 m^2, and, if they can identify a donor, preemptive living donor kidney transplantation should be pursued. Furthermore, the pretransplant evaluation and testing can take several months to complete, potentially delaying addition to the waiting list, and, therefore, especially in diabetics and others likely to progress to ESRD quickly, early referral is essential. For all these reasons, referral to a transplant center should likely be made once eGFR is found to be less than 30 ml/min/1.73 m^2.

The pretransplant evaluation

The preoperative evaluation of transplant candidates is a multi-disciplinary process that involves transplant surgeons, nephrologists, mental health professionals, social workers, dieticians, financial coordinators, and transplant coordinators. The goal of the evaluation is to identify any contraindications to transplantation, to determine immunologic factors impacting donor kidney options, to screen for comorbid conditions that need to be identified and managed prior to transplantation, and to assess psychosocial factors that could affect the success of the transplant. In the pages that follow, each of these components of the pretransplantation evaluation will be addressed.

Organ Transplantation: A Clinical Guide, ed. A.A. Klein, C.J. Lewis, and J.C. Madsen. Published by Cambridge University Press.

Table 27.1 Contraindications to transplantation

Active malignancy
Untreated infection
Severe comorbid conditions: cardiac, pulmonary, or vascular disease
Unable to manage: uncontrolled psychiatric illness or psychotic behavior, persistent substance abuse, or significant history of medical non-compliance
Primary oxalosis
Irreversibly limited potential for rehabilitation

Contraindications to transplantation

There are several absolute and relative contraindications to transplantation (Table 27.1). The greatest morbidity and mortality from transplantation occurs in the first year after transplant and consists of both cardiovascular and infectious complications. As such, patients with unmanaged cardiovascular disease and untreated or indolent infections should not undergo transplantation until these are addressed. In addition, to maximize the benefit of transplantation and the allocation thereof, patients with high near-term ($\leq$2 years) mortality, such as those with advanced or uncontrolled malignancy or severe non-renal disease, should likely not undergo transplantation. Patients with histories of medication non-adherence or psychiatric illness or social circumstances, including recreational drug abuse, that may limit their ability to adhere to post-transplantation care need to properly address these concerns prior to transplantation. Finally, the candidacy of patients with primary oxalosis should be considered carefully, with simultaneous liver and kidney transplantation being the option of choice. Several of these contraindications can be modified or intervened on prior to transplantation, as will be discussed. Identification of these absolute contraindications or modifiable, relative contraindications is the purpose of the pretransplantation evaluation.

Immunology

Tissue typing and histocompatibility

Immunologic evaluation begins with a thorough history of potential antigen exposure, including prior transplantation of any kind, blood product transfusion, and, in female candidates, prior pregnancy. Histocompatibility testing, including blood typing (ABO) and human leukocyte antigen (HLA) typing (A, B, DR, and at some centers, DQ), is performed to help identify both potential matches and to preclude recipient-donor pairings that would have poor outcomes. Additionally, patients with advanced kidney disease but not yet requiring dialysis can be listed preemptively for a zero antigen mismatch kidney, highlighting the importance of timely referral.

Recipient serum is also tested against a panel of cells representing a range of antigens in a local population. Known as the panel-reactive antibody (PRA), it is expressed as a percentage and is understood as the percentage of potential donor antigens against which the recipient's serum may react. Higher PRA suggests more difficulty finding a match, and as such, patients in the United States with PRA greater than 80% receive priority in organ allocation. The panel can vary from center to center and within center between different time periods. Because of this variation by location and time, the peak, or highest, PRA is used in determining priority in organ allocation when a donor organ is identified. Single-antigen bead technology has allowed the exact determination of HLA sensitization, so for many patients, *virtual cross-matching* confirms suitability of a particular donor organ (discussed further in Chapter 28).

ABO incompatibility and desensitization protocols

Advances in immunobiology have led to the development of desensitization protocols to allow for transplantation between ABO-incompatible or sensitized individuals. These protocols include some combination of plasmapheresis, intravenous immunoglobulin G, and preoperative immunosuppressants along with appropriate antibiotics for cytomegalovirus (CMV) and *Pneumocystis* prophylaxis in a now immunosuppressed host. Some protocols also include rituximab. At the pretransplantation visit, emphasis should be placed on identifying all potential living donors so that the latest protocols can be employed when possible.

Paired exchange and kidney list donation

In recent years, severe organ shortage has led to innovative solutions. One such solution is paired organ exchange, whereby recipients who have identified a willing donor who is otherwise not able to donate to them due to immunologic factors are paired with a similarly situated individual when the potential donors match each others' intended recipients. An alternative when a suitable living donor exchange is not possible involves pairing a recipient and their willing but incompatible donor with a recipient on the waiting list. The recipient at the top of the waiting list in the donor's blood group receives the living donor kidney, while the donor's recipient is given priority for a deceased donor kidney. These exchanges can be fraught with anxiety and disappointment, such that the setting of realistic expectations is essential at the first, and at subsequent, pretransplant visits.

Cardiovascular disease

Cardiovascular disease is the leading cause of death, and therefore graft loss, in the first year post-transplant. As such, preoperative assessment of cardiovascular disease is essential to improving patient and graft survival.

Ischemic heart disease

All patients presenting for transplantation evaluation are at increased risk for ischemic heart disease by virtue of their chronic kidney disease. For many, the underlying cause of kidney disease, particularly diabetes and hypertension, is also associated with increased risk. The preoperative history must focus on risk factors for and manifestations of ischemic heart disease, including Framingham risk factors, prior history of ischemic heart disease, and current signs and symptoms of ischemic heart disease, including assessment of exercise tolerance. Physical exam should include a thorough cardiovascular exam, and an electrocardiogram should be obtained. Nearly all patients should undergo non-invasive testing, with many centers choosing dobutamine stress echocardiography or nuclear sestamibi (Thallium stress test, myocardial perfusion scintigraphy). At least one study of pre-transplantation elective revascularization in diabetics has been shown to confer a survival advantage. Results of non-invasive testing that are suggestive of ischemic heart disease should therefore be followed up with cardiac catheterization and intervention where appropriate.

Structural heart disease

Systolic and diastolic heart failure, as well as significant valvular disease that can lead to heart failure, may impact transplant outcome. Moreover, severe heart failure and severe valvular disease may impact candidacy for transplantation surgery. Calcification associated with CKD places these patients at particular risk for developing valvular disease and subsequent consequences. As such, it is reasonable to assess function and valvular disease prior to transplantation via transthoracic echocardiography.

Peripheral vascular disease

Peripheral vascular disease is important both as a risk factor for ischemic heart disease as well as an important consideration in operative planning. Signs and symptoms of peripheral vascular disease, such as claudication; rest pain; past vascular insufficiency, including history of ulcerations, infections, or amputations; and in male patients, erectile dysfunction, should be elicited. Physical examination should include a thorough assessment of peripheral arterial pulses and lower extremities for signs of vascular insufficiency such as hair loss or ulcers. Symptoms or signs of peripheral arterial disease should be followed up with non-invasive vascular studies, and further evaluation and management initiated based on these results. Finally, in consultation with local transplant surgeons, CT of the iliac vessels without contrast may be indicated for assessment of vascular calcification and operative planning.

Tobacco use

Because of its strong association with cardiovascular disease in general, active tobacco use should be explored and cessation encouraged prior to transplantation. This should be re-addressed at each subsequent visit and medical management initiated or referral made to available cessation resources where applicable.

Hypercoagulable states

Patients with thrombophilic states are at risk for early graft loss. Many patients on hemodialysis via fistulae or grafts have experienced access clotting. Patients with systemic lupus erythematosus are at risk for anti-phospholipid antibody syndrome. Patients with a history of thrombotic events, whether classic venous thromboembolism, access clots, or more subtle suggestions such as recurrent miscarriages in women, should be screened for hypercoagulable states including factor V Leiden, prothrombin gene mutation, protein C and S deficiencies, anti-thrombin III deficiency, hyperhomocysteinemia, and antiphospholipid antibody syndrome (anti-cardiolipin and lupus anti-coagulant). If a thrombophilic state is identified, anti-coagulant therapy should be initiated and continued as indicated.

Infection

Pretransplant assessment of known infections and screening for other as yet unknown ones is necessary, both to ensure the safety of planned immunosuppression, as well as to determine, and possibly expand, the pool of donor candidates from which the potential recipient can draw.

Hepatitis B virus

Screening for hepatitis B virus (HBV) should be performed pretransplant, including both surface and core antibody testing. Viral load should be tested in all surface antigen–positive patients, as well as in surface antigen–negative patients who are core antibody positive to rule out acute infection. HBV e antigen testing should be performed in screen-positive patients as well. Patients with HBV should be referred for possible liver biopsy to assess the extent of liver disease, which would inform both transplant candidacy and the possible need for simultaneous liver transplant. In considering transplantation for patients with HBV, patients who are HBV surface antibody positive may receive a kidney transplant from an HBV core antibody–positive donor. Finally, post-transplant prophylactic lamivudine may be indicated for HBV suppression.

Hepatitis C virus

As in the case of HBV, screening for hepatitis C virus (HCV) should be performed prior to transplantation. All antibody-positive patients should have viral load checked to rule out false positives. Patients with HCV should be referred for liver biopsy and consideration of antiviral therapy for the same reasons mentioned above. If antiviral therapy is indicated, it should be administered pretransplant, as interferon and ribavirin can precipitate acute rejection. In considering transplantation for patients with HCV, patients with HCV genotype 1 may be considered for deceased donor kidneys from donors with known HCV of a less virulent genotype, although this remains an area of controversy. At the very least, knowledge of the genotype would be important in making this decision, and so the potential recipient's genotyping should be determined as part of the pretransplant evaluation. Finally, as yet, there is no available post-transplant prophylaxis against HCV.

Human immunodeficiency virus

Successful management of human immunodeficiency virus (HIV) with anti-retroviral therapy has made it possible to offer transplantation to HIV-infected patients while minimizing their infection risk in the setting of postoperative immunosuppression. Patients with HIV may therefore be viable transplant candidates, although many units would still consider HIV a contraindication. Preoperative infectious disease evaluation should be obtained to ensure optimal disease management, including achieving an undetectable viral load, and to review antiretroviral therapy for possible interactions with post-transplant immunosuppressive agents.

Tuberculosis

All transplant candidates, particularly those who are from or have traveled to endemic countries, or have other risk factors for mycobacterial exposure or disease, should have a tuberculin skin test as part of the transplant evaluation. Alternatively, blood antigen testing for tuberculosis (TB) can be performed, especially in patients at high risk for exposure or those likely to be anergic (lack of immunologic reaction to foreign substances), yielding a false-negative skin test. A positive test of either type, in the absence of a history of past treatment, should trigger further imaging and evaluation and would necessitate therapy for latent TB before transplantation due to the risk of reactivation of latent disease with immunosuppression. Once treated, post-transplant prophylaxis for treated latent TB is not indicated.

Other infections

Chronic bacterial infections, such as cellulitis, osteomyelitis, or upper or lower urinary tract infections, should be treated and clearance documented prior to transplantation. Such patients may benefit from consultation with an infectious disease specialist, especially one focusing on transplant infectious disease where available. Lesions at risk for becoming infected, such as active diabetic foot ulcers, should be assessed and managed prior to transplantation. Finally, all patients should be seen by a dentist to rule out any occult oral infections.

CMV antibody should be obtained to guide post-transplant prophylaxis needs coupled with donor characteristics. Screening for Epstein-Barr virus, herpes simplex virus, syphilis (rapid plasma reagin and fluorescent treponemal antibody), and human T-lymphotrophic virus-1 is recommended as well.

Screening for chronic infections not already discussed previously, such as schistosomiasis, strongyloides, histoplasmosis, coccidiomycosis, and Chagas disease, should be performed on a case-by-case basis for those from endemic areas and treatment initiated pretransplant as indicated. Prophylactic treatment may be needed long term after transplant as well.

Prophylactic vaccination

Vaccination history should be obtained and any needed vaccines administered in advance of any planned living donor transplant or as soon as possible for those awaiting a deceased donor. Relevant vaccines include *Haemophilus influenzae b*; hepatitis A virus and HBV; human papillomavirus; measles, mumps, and rubella (MMR); tetanus, diphtheria-acellular, and pertussis; polio; meningococcus; *Streptococcus pneumoniae*; varicella zoster virus (VZV); and influenza. Immune status should be confirmed for VZV, MMR, and HBV, and vaccine administered as indicated. Finally, potential transplant recipients should be given seasonal influenza, and any other relevant influenza vaccines, on an annual basis.

Malignancy

By general expert consensus, a prior history of malignancy precludes transplantation until a durable remission has been achieved. This is suggested to maximize both patient survival, given the risk of disease acceleration or recurrence on immunosuppressants, as well as graft survival, given the increased risk of host death with untreated or uncontrolled malignancy. Depending on the malignancy, a disease-free period of between 2 and 5 years is generally accepted as adequate. All transplant candidates should undergo age-appropriate cancer screening prior to transplantation for these same reasons. At the very least, this should include cervical smear and mammogram for female candidates, and colonoscopy for all candidates over age 50 years. Candidates with HBV or HCV should undergo appropriate screening for hepatocellular carcinoma, including serum α-fetoprotein and imaging. Despite the controversial nature of prostate cancer screening, given the importance of an intact lower urinary tract for the success of the transplant and the risk of outlet obstruction and allograft obstructive uropathy, as well as recipient mortality from aggressive prostate cancer, screening with prostate-specific antigen is advisable. Finally, especially with the risk of acquired cystic disease and possibly increased prevalence of renal cell carcinoma in ESRD patients, screening ultrasonography of the kidneys should be performed as part of the transplant work-up. Patients with suspicious lesions should undergo further evaluation. If the cancerous lesion is less than 3 cm, the patient can proceed with transplantation after undergoing nephrectomy without a waiting period. For lesions greater than 3 cm, transplantation should be deferred for the requisite 2- to 5-year period to ensure remission prior to transplantation.

Urologic disease

Because the transplanted kidney usually drains into the native lower urinary tract, underlying urologic disease can affect the transplant outcome. Although there is no evidence to suggest that routine screening for urologic disease improves graft or patient survival, those with known urologic disease, including history of congenital obstructive uropathy, bladder dysfunction, bladder or prostate cancer, nephrolithiasis with episodes of obstruction, or recurrent urinary tract infections, or those with symptoms suggestive of any of the above, should be evaluated by a urologist prior to transplantation. Results of such an evaluation should guide decision making regarding the need for preoperative medical management of any urologic condition, as well as the need for alternative allograft drainage (e.g., bladder augmentation or urinary diversion), or in the case of recurrent infection or retained nidus, the need for pretransplant native nephrectomy. Finally, it is reasonable to perform urinalysis and culture on all patients immediately prior to transplantation to ensure a sterile urinary tract.

Primary renal disease and risk of recurrent disease in the allograft

Risk of recurrent disease in the allograft varies by the etiology of the primary renal disease, as does the risk of graft failure from recurrent disease. For example, histologically, nearly all diabetics will manifest recurrent disease in the allograft, though allograft dysfunction from recurrent disease is unlikely. On the other hand, a small minority of patients with idiopathic focal segmental glomerulosclerosis (FSGS) or membranous nephropathy and a slightly higher percentage of those with atypical or familial hemolytic-uremic syndrome will manifest recurrent disease that will lead to graft failure. However, even these cases are confounded by the possible emergence of de novo disease (e.g., membranous nephropathy or thrombotic microangiopathy associated with certain immunosuppressants). Because the rate of recurrence as well as the clinical significance of recurrence (i.e., the rate of allograft dysfunction resulting from recurrent disease) is varied, the etiology of the primary renal disease in general should not affect the candidacy for transplantation. However, once recurrent disease has necessitated repeat transplantation, as can be the case in recurrent idiopathic FSGS, candidacy for further transplantation should be considered carefully. Given recent development of protocols for treating recurrent FSGS in the allograft, pretransplantation protein excretion should be assessed, especially when preemptive transplantation is being performed, preferably with a 24-hour urine collection or at least a spot protein/creatinine ratio. This will permit post-transplant screening for recurrent disease.

Diabetes mellitus

Patients with diabetes, whether or not diabetes is the primary cause of renal disease, comprise a large minority of kidney transplant candidates. Because diabetes confers increased risk for cardiovascular morbidity and mortality as well as infectious complications, management of diabetes should be optimized prior to transplantation, from glycemic and other metabolic control to podiatric care. Although, as mentioned above, allograft failure from recurrent diabetic disease is rare, because diabetics are at high risk for cardiovascular disease and infectious complications, type I, or juvenile onset, diabetics should be considered for simultaneous kidney and pancreas transplant to minimize future complications. Even when considering such options, a living donor kidney without pancreas transplantation would be preferred due to graft survival, which can then be followed by deceased donor pancreas transplant. If a living donor cannot be identified, then simultaneous deceased donor pancreas and kidney transplant would be the best option. In the future, diabetes management via islet cell transplantation, coupled with kidney transplantation, may be considered.

Obesity

Studies have shown that obesity, defined as body mass index (BMI) over 30 kg/m^2, confers a small but statistically significant increased risk of both graft failure and patient death. Obese patients also have higher perioperative risk, including risk of cardiovascular events and postoperative wound healing deficiencies leading to increased wound dehiscence and wound infection. Moreover, the long-term survival benefit of kidney transplantation over dialysis has been shown to diminish in patients with BMI greater than 40. As such, obese kidney transplant candidates should be strongly encouraged to lose weight either on their own or, in the case of those with BMI greater than 40, possibly in conjunction with weight loss surgery. Population-based studies suggest that obese patients can lose up to 10% of their body weight in a 6-month period with maximal effort, and in most cases this a reasonable goal to target. The actual cutoff for BMI above which weight loss should be considered mandatory prior to transplantation remains a center-by-center decision, although it would be reasonable to defer patients with BMI greater than 40 until significant weight loss has been achieved.

Age

At a minimum, patients considered for transplantation must have completed the immunizations described above and responded appropriately. As such, although there is no absolute minimum, candidates for transplantation are usually at least 1 year of age. On the other end of the spectrum, with the rapid growth of the ESRD population over 65 years of age, older patients account for an increasingly greater percentage of transplant candidates. Morbidity and mortality outcomes in older patients undergoing transplantation are

Table 27.2 Extended criteria kidney donor definition

Age >60 or 50–59 years and two of the following:
CVA as cause of death
Hypertension
Terminal creatinine >1.5 mg/dl

CVA: cerebrovascular accident.

favorable, including peri-operative morbidity and mortality as well as long-term patient and graft survival. However, the rate of infectious complications is markedly higher with advanced age. Therefore, the expected survival benefit from transplantation, considering the patient's life expectancy with and without transplantation, as well as quality of life after transplantation as compared with dialysis, must be taken into account when deciding about the candidacy of older patients. Furthermore, because older patients may not survive to transplantation due to long wait times, extended criteria donor (ECD; Table 27.2) kidneys should be considered for older transplant candidates as a means of shortening waiting list time.

Psychiatric, cognitive, and psychosocial evaluation

Neither psychiatric illness nor cognitive impairment should be considered a contraindication to transplantation. However, complicated postoperative medication regimes and the need for strict medication adherence means that a thorough assessment of the transplant candidate's psychiatric health and cognitive ability should be performed by an appropriate professional. A history of non-compliance may mean that candidates should be given an opportunity to prove ability to adhere to therapy, possibly by insisting on a time-limited trial whereby the patient can demonstrate ability and intention to comply. A history of substance abuse, including alcohol or illicit drugs, insofar as it increases risk of non-compliance with therapy and therefore graft loss, should prompt an evaluation and referral for counseling or treatment as appropriate prior to transplantation. Finally, assessment of candidates' social situation including social support structure should be conducted.

Managing the list

Following pre-transplantation evaluation and satisfactory completion of any needed testing, patients are added to the evaluating center's waiting list. Frequent re-evaluation of candidates should be performed to ensure ongoing suitability for transplantation, although how frequently is unclear. Immunological status should be automatically reassessed frequently with repeat tissue typing and antibody testing via updated PRA status. As for other factors, at the very least, regular reassessment of cardiovascular and infectious disease status is advisable, possibly as often as every 2 years.

To ensure ability to accept organ offers in a timely fashion, in addition to regular reassessment of candidacy, some centers maintain a second or parallel lists of candidates, such as those eligible for or willing to consider ECD kidneys.

Further reading

Bunnapradist S, Danovitch GM. Evaluation of adult kidney transplant candidates. *Am J Kidney Dis* 2007; **50**: 890–8.

Kasiske BL, Cangro CB, Hariharan S, *et al.* The evaluation of renal transplant candidates. *Clinical practice guidelines. Am J Transplant* 2001; **2(Suppl 1)**, 3–95.

Kasiske BL, Snyder JJ, Matas AJ, Ellison MD, Gill JS, Kausz AT. Preemptive kidney transplantation: The advantage and the advantaged. *J Am Soc Nephrol* 2002; **13**: 1358–64.

Montgomery RA, Zachary AA, Ratner LE, *et al.* Clinical results from transplanting incompatible live kidney donor/recipient pairs using kidney paired donation. *JAMA* 2005; **294**: 1655–63.

Pilmore H. Cardiac assessment for renal transplantation. *Am J Transplant* 2006; **6**: 659–65.

Chapter 28

Sensitization of kidney transplant recipients

Nick Pritchard

Key points

- The most important alloantibodies are directed against human leukocyte antigen (HLA) and are formed in response to exposure to foreign HLA molecules, usually at the time of blood product administration, previous transplant, or during pregnancy.
- The role played by non-HLA antibodies in graft injury is increasingly recognized.
- *Virtual cross-matching* is the process of predicting the likelihood of a significant antibody-mediated immune event between recipient and graft; it may be used in pretransplant risk assessment and can also assist with the process of organ allocation.
- Desensitization may allow transplantation of presensitized patients with donor-reactive HLA or ABO antibodies by reducing antibody levels to such a degree to make transplantation safe.

For many years, the importance of HLA antibody–antigen interactions to transplant outcome has been appreciated. Matching donor and recipient HLA antigens has led to better transplant outcomes, and there is good evidence showing that responses to mismatched HLA antigens are the principal element determining immunological outcomes after solid organ transplantation. This chapter considers the importance of recipient sensitization with particular reference to renal transplantation. It considers the clinical relevance of both HLA and non-HLA antibodies in graft outcomes. As part of this, it discusses strategies for antibody testing and application of those tests to clinical practice and the assessment of immunological risk. Finally, it looks at the strategies to improve the likelihood of transplantation in a highly sensitized population and outcomes in this particular group.

Sensitization

Definitions of sensitization

Sensitization is defined as the presence of preformed alloantibody in the serum of prospective transplant recipients. The most important alloantibodies are directed against HLA. They are formed in response to exposure to foreign HLA molecules, usually at the time of blood product administration, previous transplant, or during pregnancy. More recently non-HLA antibodies directed against endothelial cell targets have been shown to be associated with antibody mediated rejection (AMR) and poor long-term graft outcomes.

Quantization of sensitization

Anti-HLA antibodies are also called panel-reactive antibodies (PRA) because they have historically been quantified by testing the potential recipient's serum against a "panel" of lymphocytes harvested from a number of individuals with a wide range of HLA types. Using a complement-dependent cytotoxicity cross-match (CDC) to detect the presence of antibodies in the recipient serum against lymphocyte surface antigens, the extent of sensitization is determined by calculating the percentage of donors in the panel where cell lysis occurs. To define levels of sensitization, patients with a PRA of 0–10% are considered to be non-sensitized, whereas highly sensitized patients are considered to be those patients with a PRA of greater than 85%. These criteria are arbitrarily determined to define subgroups of patients, but the level of sensitization

Organ Transplantation: A Clinical Guide, ed. A.A. Klein, C.J. Lewis, and J.C. Madsen. Published by Cambridge University Press.

appears to have a graded effect on outcomes: the higher the PRA, the poorer the outcome.

Measurement of PRA by CDC has been largely replaced by more sensitive and less cumbersome solid-phase assays, which report a calculated PRA or population-reactive antibodies. The antibody specificities of all HLA antibodies present in the recipient serum are determined. Then from knowledge of the HLA antigen frequency in the donor population, the proportion of donors against which the serum will react can be calculated. The calculated PRA for any individual will be higher than the CDC-PRA because of the increased assay sensitivity, but it does provide a more reliable and standardized measure of sensitization.

Causes of sensitization

Sensitization occurs through the development of long-lived B-cell memory responses in response to exposure to foreign antigen and most importantly HLA molecules. The three primary sources of such exposure are pregnancy, blood transfusion, and previous transplants. These sensitizing events have an additive and interacting effect on the PRA. Beyond these three clear causes for sensitization, there may be other factors that contribute to sensitization, including, for example, infection. Interestingly, a significant minority of patients (approximately 10% of males and 20% of nulliparous women) receiving their first transplant with no previous history of blood transfusion appear to be sensitized (PRA > 10%). The cause for this is as yet unidentified. This may be due to failure to identify previous transfusions and unrecognized pregnancy in women, but there may be some cross-reactivity or heterologous immunity from other previous immune interactions.

Clinical relevance of HLA and non-HLA antibodies

De novo development of HLA antibody post-transplant

The majority of patients receiving a first renal transplant have no detectable HLA antibody at the time of transplant. Following transplant, approximately 25% of recipients will develop de novo HLA antibody, and most will develop this within the first year. The HLA antibodies that develop are donor-specific in only 50% of patients and non-donor HLA in the other 50%. Development of de novo donor-specific antibody (DSA) does not necessarily induce acute AMR, which occurs in less than 5% of renal transplants. Despite the absence of acute AMR, the risk of graft loss is three times higher following the development of HLA antibody, and outcomes are equally poor regardless of whether or not this is donor-specific. However, DSA is associated with the development of chronic AMR and transplant glomerulopathy.

Pre-formed HLA antibody present at the time of transplant

The presence of HLA antibody at the time of transplant implies previous exposure to and subsequent development of persistent B-cell memory responses to the relevant HLA antigen. Depending on the level of antibody present, hyperacute rejection (HAR) or accelerated AMR may occur at the time of transplantation. The level of antibody present is defined by laboratory testing, and this provides an assessment of immunological risk.

In addition to this humoral or B-cell sensitization, it is increasingly being realized that a component of preformed allo-specific T-cell memory may also be present in potential recipients. A number of studies have shown a high frequency of donor-reactive memory T cells. These can occur independently of the presence of high levels of alloantibody and B-cell sensitization; T-cell sensitization is less clearly related to alloantigen exposure because cross-reactivity within the T-cell repertoire is common, and it is possible for recipient T cells to recognize peptide associated with donor major histocompatibility complex molecules. The presence of such a memory T-cell response increases the risk of T-cell–mediated rejection (TCMR). However, as yet it is not routine in most centers to screen for T-cell sensitization, and there is no clear evidence that high levels of T-cell sensitization has significant impact on long-term graft and patient survival.

Non-HLA antigens

With better identification and understanding of the interaction between the presence of HLA alloreactivity and cross-match results, the role played by non-HLA antibodies in graft injury is increasingly recognized. The origin of non-HLA antibodies is less clear

Table 28.1 Common molecular targets for non-HLA antibody responses in solid organ transplants

Specificity	Allograft type	Type of rejection
MICA	Kidney, heart, pancreas	HAR, AR, CR
Vimentin	Heart	AR, CR
AT_1R	Kidney	AR
HMA-1 & -2	Kidney	HAR, AR
ICAM-1	Heart	Uncertain

MICA: major histocompatibility complex Class I-related chain A; AT_1R: angiotensin II type 1 receptor; HMA-1 & -2: hepatic membrane associated antibodies-1 & -2; ICAM-1: intracellular adhesion molecule-1; HAR: hyper-acute rejection; AR: acute rejection; CR: chronic rejection.

than HLA alloreactive antibodies. Non-HLA antibodies that have been identified as having a deleterious effect in transplantation are heterogeneous, with a wide range of different specificities. Relevant antibodies have been identified with reactivity against epithelial cells, endothelial cells, and monocytes. They can occur through alloimmunization through the same mechanisms as HLA sensitization, and the presence of non-HLA antibodies is strongly associated with HLA pre-sensitization. However, autoreactive non-HLA antibody may occur without sensitizing events and are found in patients with autoimmune disease.

It is estimated that 10% of C4d-positive acute rejection episodes in renal transplants are due to non-HLA antibodies. In HLA-identical renal grafts, non-HLA antibodies may be responsible for up to 80% of irreversible rejection episodes. Non-HLA immune responses contribute substantially to kidney failure, with transplants from HLA-identical siblings failing more frequently in recipients with higher PRAs. Of the different factors contributing to graft loss, 38% of graft failures are due to non-HLA antibody, 18% are due to HLA antibody, and 43% are due to non-immunological causes.

The full range of clinically relevant specificities that non-HLA antibodies may interact with is still not elucidated. However, there are an increasing number of antibodies against a wider range of non-HLA specificities that have been identified. These have been implicated in mediating a wide range of clinically relevant immune injuries. A discussion of the details of these different antibodies is beyond the scope of this chapter, but they are summarized in Table 28.1.

Defining the role of non-HLA antibody–antigen interactions in transplant outcome is still in its infancy. Clarification of the pathogenetic mechanisms by which non-HLA antibodies arise, how they contribute to graft injury, and the impact they have on long-term outcomes is crucial and to date remains uncertain. The importance of non-HLA immune responses is increasingly being recognized, and they are likely to become more important as problems related to HLA response are better understood and managed.

Pretransplant risk assessment based on cross-match and antibody screening results

In most UK centers, a CDC and flow cytometry cross-match (FCXM) against T and B cells is routine practice prior to transplantation, with interpretation in the context of up-to-date solid-phase antibody screening results. A schema incorporating results from all of these assays is shown in Table 28.2. Alongside the laboratory data defining the presence and level of any DSA, the past sensitization history must be taken into consideration. Relevant factors that increase the risk of immune-related problems are shown in Table 28.3, and this further refines the immunological risk of the donor–recipient pair.

In general terms, the vast majority of transplants undertaken would be from the low-risk category, with most centers preferring to avoid higher risk procedures. However, the availability of polyclonal antibodies such as anti-thymocyte globulin and monoclonal agents against CD25, CD20, and CD52 for use in induction protocols to reduce the risk of rejection or as treatment for refractory AMR allows successful transplantation of higher risk patients. In this way, although some categories of antigen may be absolute barriers to transplantation, some higher risk donor–recipient combinations may, in certain situations, be seen as carrying acceptable levels of risk. Factors relating to donor, recipient, and locally available resources will play a role in the final decision regarding what constitutes an acceptable level of risk and how it is managed.

Virtual cross-matching

With the introduction of solid-phase assays for detection of anti-HLA antibody, it has become possible to determine the presence of HLA-DSA "virtually" by

Table 28.2 Immunological pretransplant risk assessment based on donor cross-match and antibody screening

Cross-match method						
CDC-XM		FCXM				
T cell	B cell	T cell	B cell	Current or historical	Antibody screening results	Interpretation
+	+	+	+	Current	IgG HLA Class I DSA	Very high risk[a]. Probable HAR.
–	+	–	+	Current	IgG HLA Class II DSA	Very high risk[a]. HAR unlikely (reported only in high titre HLA-DR) but accelerated/refractory AMR and poor long-term prognosis.
–	+	–	+	Current	Weak IgG HLA Class I DSA	High risk[b]. B cells express higher levels of HLA Class I than T cells, thus B+/T– XM may indicate low levels of HLA Class I DSA.
–	–	+	+	Current	IgG HLA Class I DSA	High risk[b]. Lower titre DSA detected by more sensitive FCXM. HAR unlikely but high risk of severe accelerated AMR.
–	–	–	+	Current	IgG HLA Class II DSA	Intermediate risk[c]. Significant risk of acute and chronic AMR[d].
+	+	+	+	Historical	IgG HLA Class I DSA	High risk[e]. Risk of anamnestic 2° T & B cell.
–	+	–	+	Historical	IgG HLA Class II DSA	High risk[e]. Risk of anamnestic 2° T & B cell.
–	+	–	+	Historical	Weak IgG HLA Class I DSA	Intermediate risk[c].
–	–	+	+	Historical	IgG HLA Class I DSA	Intermediate risk[c].
–	–	–	+	Historical	IgG HLA Class II DSA	Intermediate risk[c].
–	–	–	–	C or H	IgG HLA Class I or II DSA	Low risk. DSA detected by solid-phase assay alone. Significance remains unclear.
+	+	+	+	C or H	Negative	Low risk. Autoreactive IgM/IgG non-HLA Ab.
–	–	+	+	C or H	Positive not donor HLA specific	Low risk.

[a] Absolute veto to transplantation.

[b] HAR unlikely but risk of severe early AMR and considered a contraindication to transplant in most centers.

[c] Intermediate-risk transplants should be avoided if reasonably possible (i.e., short waiting time, easy to avoid unacceptable mismatches) but may be undertaken with appropriate clinical caution; consideration for enhanced immunosuppression and antibody removal and close post-transplant antibody monitoring.

[d] In the past +B cell FCXM even in the presence of DSA was considered low risk. Retrospective analysis of B+/T– XM transplants has subsequently shown the presence of HLA Class II DSA to be a risk for acute and chronic AMR.

[e] Risk of anamnestic secondary T- and/or B-cell response; need to consider high-risk immunosuppression strategy, the duration, titre, and priming source of antibody and repeat mismatches (pregnancy or re-graft). Historical positive cross-matches caused by cross-reactive alloantibodies (avoiding the main specificity and priming stimulus) constitute intermediate immunological risk and are less likely to be associated with refractory T- or B-cell response.

Table 28.3 Factors increasing immunological risk for transplant.

DSA titres	Persistently high DSA titres Rising DSA titres Past positive, current negative titres
High PRA	Broad sensitization (even if non–donor-specific) Presence of > 1 DSA (esp. If Class I and Class II)
Transplant history	History of previous early rejection and graft loss Number of previous transplants
HLA match	Increased number of mismatches Type of mismatch (e.g., DR mismatch) Repeat mismatch
Recipient–donor relationship	Husband → wife or child → mother risk previous exposure
Sensitizing events	Number of previous pregnancies or blood transfusions

comparing recipient HLA antibody specificities with HLA typing of the donor. *Virtual cross-matching* is the process of predicting the likelihood of a significant antibody-mediated immune event between recipient and graft. Virtual cross-match has applications in pretransplant risk assessment and can also assist with the process of organ allocation.

Uses of virtual cross-matching

The virtual cross-match is at least as sensitive as FCXM for the detection of HLA-DSA but gets around the problems of non-specific binding of irrelevant antibodies, which produce a false-positive result. A negative virtual cross-match in a non-sensitized patient, provided a full sensitization history is available, and knowledge of previous screening may allow a cross-match to be omitted pretransplant. This reduces cold ischemic time and improves graft outcome. Unfortunately, in sensitized patients, the error rate for the virtual cross-match is too high (15%) to allow for omission of the cross-match. To clarify differences in terminology between UK and US readers, this specific use of solid-phase assays to avoid a pretransplant cross-match is in the United Kingdom what is recognized as a virtual cross-match; in the United States, a wider definition incorporating all the elements discussed in this section is considered as virtual cross-matching.

The converse position of a positive virtual cross-match can eliminate unnecessary work and expedite deceased organ allocation by predicting the presence of unacceptable antigens without the need for formal cross-match testing. A positive virtual cross-match forms the basis for identifying patients who would be suitable for augmented immunosuppression or desensitization. The ability to accurately predict positive cross-matches is used in identifying compatible donor-recipient pairs in paired-donor exchange programs.

Correlation of virtual cross-matching with cell-based assays

The key factors when considering the utility of virtual cross-matching are how well it correlates with the results from CDC and FCXM testing and ultimately how the virtual cross-match predicts clinical outcomes. The correlation of the virtual cross-match with CDC has been shown to be low, but this probably reflects the significantly higher sensitivity of the solid-phase assays to detect HLA antibody. The correlation, as might be expected, was much higher compared with FCXM and was greater than 85% in most studies but is slightly lower in highly sensitized individuals. The predictive value of a negative virtual cross-match in a clinical setting is good; it is associated with a very low risk for early AMR. This has been shown in a number of studies in which the risk of early rejection has been as low as 4% and allograft survival is good even among sensitized patients.

The predictive value of a positive virtual cross-match depends very much on the immunosuppressive regimen that is utilized. It is increasingly clear that transplanting in the presence of DSA is possible with little impact on short-term outcomes as plasmapheresis and antibody therapies become more widely used. In the absence of these treatments, when the cross-match assay is negative and the presence of a DSA is detectable by solid-phase assay alone, then the presence of antibody does predict poorer outcomes. In CDC negative transplants with DSA detected by solid-phase assay, the incidence of AMR is higher, and graft survival is also lower in recipients in whom DSAs are present compared with those in whom they are not. When FCXM is negative and HLA-DSA is detected by solid-phase assay, there is an increased risk of AMR, but short-term outcomes appear good and the impact on long-term outcomes is less certain. Thus the presence of HLA-DSA detectable only by solid-phase assay does represent a significant risk for AMR and possible

Table 28.4 Causes for inaccuracies in virtual cross-matches

Possible causes for false-negative virtual cross-match	
AMR caused by non-HLA antibody	Non-HLA antibodies that will not be detected as the virtual cross-match is HLA restricted. The incidence of early AMR related to non-HLA antibody is very low, and these events prove problematic to detect with currently available assays.
Incomplete donor HLA typing	Current solid-phase assays cover the most frequent allelic variants of HLA-A, -B, -Cw, -DRb1, -DRb3–5, -DQb, and –DP loci. Unfortunately, donor HLA typing often does not include HLA-Cw and -DP and does not have allelic resolution. DSA against these antigens has been shown to lead to AMR, but the exact relevance of preformed Cw- and DP-DSA is not fully understood. However, until full HLA typing of donors is undertaken, the virtual cross-match will not identify all potential DSAs.
Failure to detect relevant HLA antibody	DSA directed against an epitope that is not represented in the assay panel or the presence of interfering substance preventing detection of relevant antibodies are rare but recognized problems.
Possible causes for a false-positive virtual cross-match	
In vitro artefact	HLA molecules used for testing may be denatured by the production process, producing novel epitopes or exposing epitopes that are not accessible in vivo, allowing antibody binding which in the clinical setting is not relevant.
Variable pathogenicity of the DSA	DSA may bind to donor HLA but does not induce graft injury. To date, no routinely available characteristic of HLA-DSAs (e.g., HLA Class, sensitizing event, DSA level) has been found to be unequivocally predictive of clinical significance. A number of other putative pathogenic factors that may affect the clinical impact of HLA-DSA have been proposed, but as yet these remain unproven.

worse long-term outcomes but not is not in most centers a contraindication to transplantation.

Problems with virtual cross-matching

There is good correlation between virtual cross-matches, FCXM, and clinical outcomes, but the results are not perfect. Some of these differences can be explained by the differences in sensitivity of cell-based and solid-phase assays, but there are technical and procedural problems that may also contribute. Common causes for false-positive and false-negative virtual cross-matches are outlined in Table 28.4. It is clear that there are a number of aspects of virtual cross-matches that require improvement. On the technical side, expansion of the solid-phase assay panels to include more potential epitopes and exact and complete donor HLA typing will improve accuracy. In addition, the improvement of the assay itself to eliminate technical false positives is required. From an immunological viewpoint, a better understanding of the important factors that contribute to pathogenicity of antibodies in a transplant setting are required to improve the final risk assessment. However, the virtual cross-match can be seen as a useful tool in many areas of transplantation, and the addition of solid-phase assays to the immunological assessment pretransplant does improve understanding of the overall risk (see Table 28.2).

Transplantation options for highly sensitized individuals

There are multiple problems faced by patients who are sensitized, and these form a considerable part of those waiting for transplantation. Approximately one third of patients on the UK transplant register have detectable HLA antibody, and more than half of these are highly sensitized (PRA $>$ 85%). Although these highly sensitized individuals are prioritized for well-matched deceased donor kidneys, they may well wait for many years before receiving a transplant. This in itself is a very significant problem, as time waiting for a transplant is the most important modifiable risk factor that determines long-term patient and graft survival. However, as the accuracy of immunological risk assessment has improved, the options available for the successful transplantation of highly sensitized recipients has increased.

The options include paired-donation programs, acceptable mismatch programs, and desensitization. The first two options do require relatively large organ exchange organizations in order to be effective but are increasingly being introduced. Desensitization is not reliant on large donor pools, but the outcomes seen are still currently not well defined. In order for optimal treatment to be offered to highly sensitized patients, all three in combination probably provide the optimal solution.

Paired-kidney donation

Paired-donor schemes involve the recruitment of living donor–recipient pairs who are unable to progress to transplantation because of ABO blood group or HLA incompatibility. Full ABO and HLA details are then collated, and the pool of donors and recipients are entered into a computer algorithm to produce the maximum number of acceptable donor and recipient pairs. Those pairs identified are then subsequently cross-matched to confirm the results of the positive cross-match before proceeding to transplant. The details of the algorithms used differ to some degree between different programs but are optimized to allow for the maximum utilization of available live donor organs. Unfortunately, a large proportion of the recipients within paired donor matching schemes are sensitized, and only a small percentage of patients who are highly sensitized receive transplants through this route; in the UK paired donor scheme, only 18% of patients with PRAs of 85–94% and 2% of patients with PRAs greater than 95% have received a transplant. However, for those who are successful in getting a transplant, the outcomes from within these programs are excellent and comparable to those of standard live donor transplantation.

Acceptable mismatch programs

Acceptable mismatch programs have developed as a means to increase the probability that highly sensitized patients receive a suitable cross-match negative organ from a deceased donor. The organ allocation algorithm of most centers and organizations includes the HLA specificities against which the patient is sensitized. This then avoids the allocation of unacceptable mismatches, which would lead to a positive cross-match. For highly sensitized patients, identifying all HLA antibody specificities is extremely difficult. Therefore, these programs identify specificities against which the recipient has never developed antibodies to generate a number of acceptable mismatches, which, alongside the patient's HLA phenotype, is used for allocation. Antibodies against HLA-A, -B, -C, -DR, and -DQ are identified by solid-phase assay and confirmed using cell-based techniques. Organs are then allocated at the highest priority on the basis of blood group compatibility. These programs have provided a number of advantages over the standard practice of prioritizing highly sensitized patients through the allocation of additional points in the allocation algorithm. First, the rate of transplantation is increased, with approximately 60% of highly sensitized patients undergoing transplantation within 2 years (compared with 20% using the standard allocation program). The second benefit is that in contrast to sensitized patients receiving a graft through the standard program, both short-term and long-term graft survival appears to be identical to that of non-sensitized patients. Although this offers a huge benefit for highly sensitized patients, it is not an answer for all. About 40% of patients will not find an acceptable donor from the donor population, and for these patients, desensitization remains the only option.

Desensitization

Desensitization is the process that allows transplantation of presensitized patients with donor-reactive HLA or ABO antibodies. Complete removal of antibody is impossible, so the purpose of these protocols is to reduce antibody levels to such a degree to make transplantation safe.

ABO incompatible transplantation

Transplantation across ABO incompatibility carries a high risk for HAR, and so all living donor transplants are performed with ABO compatibility. Unfortunately, up to 35% of potential living donor transplants are ABO incompatible (ABOi). More than 1000 ABOi transplants have been preformed worldwide between all possible combinations of ABO incompatibility. ABO antibody testing does provide some difficulties. There is very wide variation in ABO titers between individuals, but in general, levels are higher in blood group O individuals. Measurement of ABO immunoglobulin (Ig) G and IgM antibody titers is performed by agglutination assay using either tube dilution or solid-phase card techniques with antibody titers assayed against reference red blood cells (RBCs) and in some cases donor RBCs. Recipient serum is serially diluted, and the last dilution where positive agglutination occurs determines the antibody titer. Unfortunately, these assays are subject to wide inter- and intra-institutional variability related to differences in protocols and observer reporting. This has lead to differences in reported starting titers that can be desensitized (1:256–1:1024) and safe antibody titer for transplant (1:4–1:16) between different centers. The ABO antibody titer at assessment also informs decisions over the number of antibody treatments that are

Table 28.5 Comparison of different antibody removal techniques

	Plasma exchange	DFPP	Immunoabsorption
Plasma volume treated	1	2–3	3
Coagulopathy	++++	++	+/–
Use of clotting products	+++	+	–
Hypocalcemia	++++	++	+
Length of treatment	2 hours	3–4 hours	6–8 hours
Cost	+	++	++++

DFPP: double-filtration plasmapheresis.

likely to be required and also the likelihood of AMR, which is higher in those with titers greater than 1:128 before antibody removal.

HLA incompatible transplantation

Assessment for HLA incompatible (HLAi) transplant should include analysis of the CDC, FCXM, and solid-phase assay plus a detailed review of the sensitization history. As previously discussed (see earlier note and Table 28.3), the antibody specificity, Ig isotype, antibody strength, and variation over time (current versus historical) should be determined. Antibody strength is determined by serial dilution of recipient serum in CDC and FCXM. As with ABOi, the strength of antibody is defined by the dilution at which the cross-match becomes negative. Antibody strength may also be assessed by fluorescence intensity in FCXM. Although cell-based assays remain the mainstay of this process, solid-phase assays, which have increased sensitivity and specificity and the capability of partial or full automation, are increasingly used. Some centers have correlated solid-phase assay results with cross-match results to establish acceptable DSA levels for desensitization and transplantation. As with ABOi assays, it is important to note that these correlations are center-specific due to variations in laboratory protocols and equipment. Consideration of a number of factors in the sensitization history of any recipient must be taken into account in decisions about whether or not to proceed to desensitization (See Table 28.3). These in conjunction with the laboratory data define acceptable levels of DSA that could successfully be desensitized, the amount of plasma removal treatment that may be required, and a target level acceptable for transplantation. These thresholds vary between centers; some centers would insist on a negative CDC before progressing, whereas others accept some level of positive CDC when additional treatment post-transplant is possible.

Desensitization treatment protocols

The immunosuppressive protocols that have been developed have three elements: DSA (either HLA or ABO) is eliminated or reduced to safe levels, new antibody production is inhibited, and augmented immunosuppressive regimes to prevent cellular rejection are generally employed.

Antibody removal

Antibody removal is performed by either plasma exchange, double-filtration plasmapheresis, or immunoabsorption. There are pros and cons to each of these methods (Table 28.5), but all are capable of adequate antibody removal for desensitization. Following antibody removal by whatever method, a rebound increase in plasma Ig levels is seen. This is partly through redistribution of Ig from the extravascular space and partly through re-synthesis, and the precise contribution of these two factors is unclear. Redistribution is overcome by further antibody removal to deplete total-body Ig levels.

Reduction in antibody production

A number of agents have been employed to reduce antibody production. Splenectomy was widely used in the past, particularly in Japan. However, it has been largely replaced by rituximab, which appears equally effective. Splenectomy is now almost exclusively reserved for the treatment of AMR unresponsive to standard treatment in certain centers. Intravenous Ig has pleiotropic immunosuppressive effects on both humoral and cellular immune responses but is thought to inhibit antibody production through

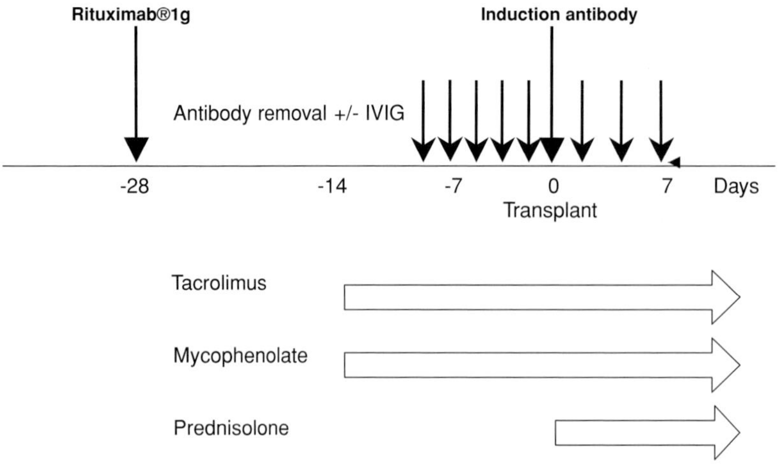

Figure 28.1 Treatment protocol for desensitization. IVIG: intravenous immunoglobulin.

binding inhibitory Fc receptors on plasma cells and through induction of apoptosis in both plasma cells and B cells. It has been employed in three different ways in desensitization. It has been used after each antibody removal treatment at low dose (100 mg/kg) to inhibit antibody re-synthesis. In some protocols it is given at intermediate dose (500 mg/kg) immediately before transplantation to reduce antibody production. High-dose intravenous Ig (2 g/kg) has been used for both live donor and deceased donor transplantation administered as four doses 1 month apart prior to transplantation. This protocol does not employ antibody removal but appears to produce similar results. Rituximab is probably the most widely employed method for inhibition of antibody production. Most centers employ a single-dose regimen (1000 mg or 375 mg/m^2), which has been shown to eliminate all circulating B cells.

Augmented immunosuppressive regimens

In most situations, augmented immunosuppression employing tacrolimus, mycophenolate mofetil (MMF), and steroid are employed. This is principally employed to inhibit cell-mediated responses, but in addition, MMF may have an impact on antibody production. These are usually commenced 7–14 days before transplant. The use of induction antibody treatment is universal. In ABOi transplants, anti-CD25 antibodies have been employed. However, because of the significantly higher risk of TCMR in HLAi transplants, it is usual to employ T-cell depleting antibodies such as Thymoglobulin or Alemtuzumab. A number of different protocols have been developed world-wide incorporating these elements, but most follow a similar outline, which is described in Figure 28.1.

Postoperative protocols

Following ABOi and HLAi transplant, antibody removal protocols vary between centers; most use three to five elective antibody removal treatments, but some centers adjust treatment according to antibody titers (Table 28.5). ABO antibody titers are measured daily for the first 2 weeks and then two to three times per week for a further 2–4 weeks. A rapidly rising titer is seen in approximately 10% and most centers would treat this with further antibody removal, as it may predict AMR. Subsequent antibody monitoring is infrequent, and later rises in antibody titer are not uncommon but in the absence of graft dysfunction do not appear to be significant for long-term outcomes. At any stage that graft dysfunction is detected, ABO antibody titers should be checked in case of AMR. However, it should be noted that C4d deposition is seen in 75% of ABOi transplants and is not significant in the absence of other features of AMR.

In HLAi transplants, DSA levels are monitored using solid-phase assays. This is partly through the difficulties of access to donor blood samples and partly because of the technical complications provided by the use of rituximab and Alemtuzumab interfering with cell-based assays. Antibody screening is similar to ABOi transplantation with monitoring daily or on alternate days for the first 2 weeks and then two to three times per week for a further 2–4 weeks, with most episodes of rejection occurring within this period.

Ongoing infrequent monitoring of DSA levels beyond this period is usually performed. Rapidly rising DSA levels or graft dysfunction requires transplant biopsy to exclude AMR, which is common. The significance of rising DSA levels in the absence of rejection and the finding of C4d deposition on biopsy without other evidence of rejection is unclear. If these occur in the first 4–6 weeks after transplant, many centers would treat with further antibody removal. Beyond that period, management is usually expectant with increased monitoring for the development of graft dysfunction.

Outcome following desensitization

The incidence of TCMR in ABOi transplantation is similar to that in ABO-compatible transplants (10–20%), as might be expected. The incidence of AMR is approximately 10% and is more common in those patients with higher initial antibody titers (>1:128) and those with early and rapid return of ABO antibodies after transplant. World-wide data suggest that both short-term (1 year) and long-term (>5 years) outcomes are excellent, with both patient and graft survival comparable to that of ABO-compatible transplants.

Unlike ABOi transplant, HLAi transplants have inferior outcomes to those in HLA-compatible live donor transplants. There is an increased incidence of DGF. The incidence of TCMR is significantly higher than seen in HLA-compatible transplants, with a 20–60% risk of severe rejection. The risk of AMR is also significantly higher compared with ABOi transplant, with an incidence of between 30–40%. One-year graft survival is approximately 85% (c.f. 95% for HLA-compatible transplants), which is similar to that seen for deceased donor transplants. Longer term data are insufficient to draw clear conclusions on patient and graft survival compared with HLA-compatible transplantation. However, some reports have shown early graft loss due to arteriopathy and glomerulopathy, particularly in those with HLA Class II DSA. Additional concerns remain over the likely increased rates of opportunistic infections and malignancy that may occur given the significantly elevated immunosuppressive load that these patients receive.

Further reading

BSHI/BTS Joint Guidelines for the Detection and Characterisation of Clinically Relevant Antibodies in Allotransplantation. Available at www.bts.org.uk and www.bshi.org.uk, May 2010.

Doxiadis II, Claas FH. Transplantation of highly sensitized patients via the acceptable mismatch program or desensitization? We need both. *Curr Opin Organ Transplant* 2009; **14**: 410–3.

Fuggle SV, Martin S. Tools for human leukocyte antigen antibody detection and their application to transplanting sensitized patients. *Transplantation* 2008; **86**: 384–90.

Jordan SC, Peng A, Vo AA. Therapeutic strategies in management of the highly HLA-sensitized and ABO-incompatible transplant recipients. *Contrib Nephrol* 2009; **162**: 13–26.

Tambur AR, Ramon DS, Kaufman DB, *et al.* Perception versus reality? Virtual crossmatch – how to overcome some of the technical and logistic limitations. *Am J Transplant* 2009; **9**: 1886–93.

Chapter 29

Live donor kidney donation

Arthur J. Matas and Hassan N. Ibrahim

Key points

- For a patient with end-stage renal disease, the best option is a living (related or unrelated) donor transplant.
- A transplant before initiation of dialysis (preemptive transplant) is associated with better post-transplant outcomes than a transplant after initiation of dialysis.
- Mortality associated with donor nephrectomy is about 0.03%, and major morbidity is less than 1%.
- Long-term outcome (survival and quality of life) after donor nephrectomy is similar to that of the age-matched population.

Patients with chronic kidney disease (CKD) need to make two important decisions, with each requiring careful consideration. The first is whether to proceed with transplantation or dialysis as primary therapy. Ideally, this decision should be made early in the course of CKD. Patients need to understand the risks and benefits of each treatment modality. The second is whether to proceed with living donation or to go on the waiting list for a deceased donor transplant.

When compared with maintenance dialysis, a successful transplant is associated with significantly longer life and significantly better quality of life. However, a transplant is associated with the risks of surgery and of immunosuppression-related complications. Whereas in practice, patients transition from dialysis to transplant (e.g., after being on the waiting list) or from transplant to dialysis (e.g., after graft failure), a decision early in the course of CKD that transplantation is to be the primary therapy may facilitate early transplantation. Transplant results are significantly better for recipients who undergo transplant before initiating dialysis (preemptive transplant) or after a short course of dialysis versus recipients who undergo transplant after a more prolonged dialysis course. This was clearly shown in a study of "paired-kidney" deceased donor transplants, in which one kidney from the donor was transplanted to a recipient who had been on dialysis less than 6 months and the other kidney (from the same donor) was transplanted to a recipient who had been on dialysis more than 24 months (Figure 29.1). At 60 months post-transplant, recipients with less than 6 months of pretransplant dialysis had 20% better graft survival.

With regard to choosing between living donation or deceased donor transplantation, there is no doubt that a living donor transplant is the best option. For the recipient, the surgery for living and deceased donor transplants are almost identical, and the immunosuppression is similar. Yet, patient and graft survival are significantly better after a living donor transplant. In addition, having a living donor transplant is far more likely to permit preemptive transplantation. Importantly, when considering living donor transplants, the results of related (human leukocyte antigen [HLA] non-identical) and unrelated transplants are identical. Figure 29.2 shows the 5-year graft survival outcome for first transplants by donor source. HLA-identical living donor transplants have the best outcome, and all subgroups of living donor transplants do better than deceased donor transplants. Note, however, that living unrelated transplants have the same outcome as non-identical living related transplants. The fact that unrelated donor kidney transplants are associated with excellent long-term results has allowed marked expansion of the donor pool and permitted development of non-directed donation and paired exchanges.

Organ Transplantation: A Clinical Guide, ed. A.A. Klein, C.J. Lewis, and J.C. Madsen. Published by Cambridge University Press.

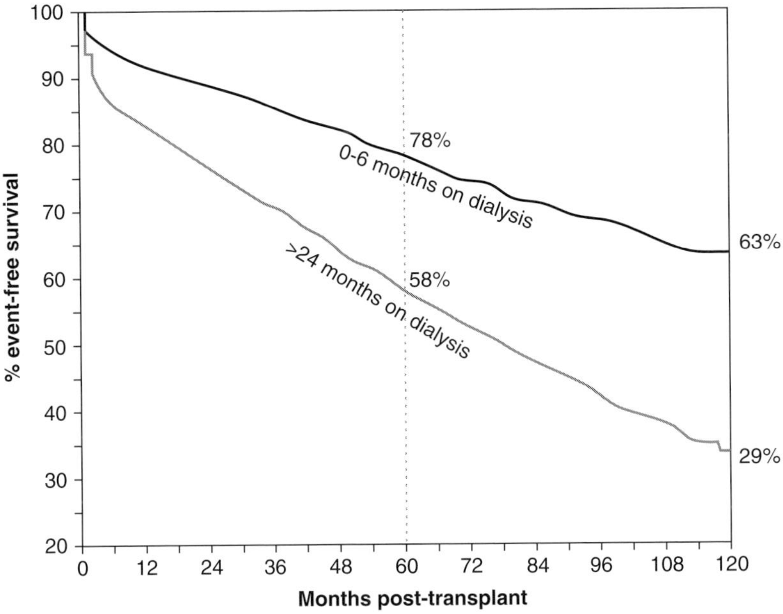

Figure 29.1 Unadjusted graft survival in 2405 recipients of paired kidneys with short compared with long end-stage renal disease time. From Meier-Kriesche HU, Kaplan B, Waiting time on dialysis as the strongest modifiable risk factor for renal transplant outcomes: A paired donor kidney analysis, *Transplantation* 2002; **74**:1377–81, with permission from Wolters Kluwer Health.

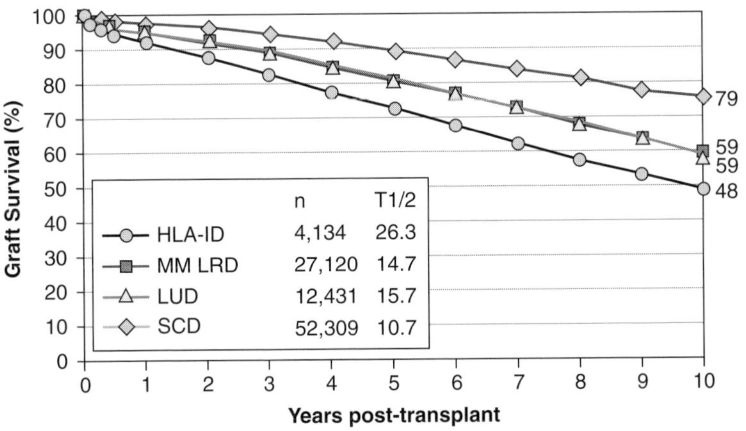

Figure 29.2 Actuarial graft survival and half life (t ½): first transplant by donor source. Based on = Organ Procurement and Transplantation Network/United Network for Organ Sharing data as of July 2009. First transplants of kidney only, done between January 1996–December 2005. Patient death was considered a graft loss. MM: mismatched; LRD: living related donor; LUD: living unrelated donor; SCD: standard criteria deceased donor. Mike Cecka, personal communication.

The major concern about living donor transplantation is the risk to the donor. The donor operation is a major procedure that is associated with morbidity, mortality, and the potential for adverse long-term consequences, secondary to living with a single kidney. A major concern regarding the use of living donors has been whether unilateral nephrectomy predisposes to the development of kidney disease and/or premature death. A transplant program considering living donation should have well-defined protocols to fully inform donor candidates about the potential risks of the procedure and to make sure that consent is voluntary. Our protocol includes a screening interview at the time of initial contact by a potential donor, followed by sending the donor candidate a package containing both written information and a video about donor risk. If the donor contacts us again after reviewing the material, a clinic visit for evaluation is scheduled. At that time, the candidate meets with the surgeon, nephrologist, coordinator, and social worker/advocate. The goal of the evaluation is to determine that the prospective donor is healthy and will tolerate the operation, has two normally functioning kidneys, and has no diseases that would affect renal function or could be transmitted with the kidney graft. A critical aspect is making sure that the candidate has complete information on the risks and benefits of donation so as to be able to make an informed decision. As they decide whether or not to proceed with their evaluation and donation, prospective donors must be informed of the risks. They must also recognize that time will be lost from work and family. Although the cost of the donor's evaluation and surgery is paid for by the recipient's insurance (in the United States), the donor is away from work for several weeks, often without compensation for lost wages or traveling expenses. Recipient surgery and immunosuppression are discussed in Chapters 30 and 3, respectively. In the following sections, we review data on donor risks and outcomes.

Donor surgical risks

Laparoscopic donor nephrectomy has been associated with less pain and a faster recovery for the donor than conventional open nephrectomy; as a result, in the last decade, laparoscopic nephrectomy has become the procedure of choice at many transplant centers. Importantly, the surgical risks for laparoscopic and open nephrectomy are similar. Peri-operative mortality has been reported in a number of studies to be 0.3–0.4%. The most common causes of death have been pulmonary embolism, bleeding, and infection. Major morbidity has occurred in less than 1% of donor nephrectomies, and minor complications in less than 10%. There are minimal differences between open and laparoscopic nephrectomy. Given that laparoscopic nephrectomy is an intra-abdominal procedure, one long-term concern is the potential for bowel obstruction.

Long-term donor outcome

A major concern is whether donor uninephrectomy leads to adverse long-term outcomes. This concern has been driven by both clinical and experimental studies. Donor uninephrectomy leads to the immediate loss of about 50% of renal function. Compensatory changes take place in the remaining kidney, and within 6 weeks, measured renal function is about 75–80% of pre-nephrectomy. Studies in the general population (and a number of subgroups) have noted that mild decreases in renal function correlate with increased long-term mortality and increased cardiovascular risk. One such subgroup is kidney transplant recipients: mild renal dysfunction after kidney transplantation is associated with increased risk for cardiovascular disease, cardiac death, and major cardiac events.

Experimental data have suggested that renal ablation is associated with compensatory changes that lead to subsequent progressive renal dysfunction. Of note, most of these studies have been in the rat model. In this model, renal dysfunction is preceded by increasing proteinuria. Thus it has been a concern that some living donors have developed proteinuria shortly after donation. In spite of these concerns, every study of long-term donor follow-up, to date, has shown donor survival to be similar to or better than that of the age-matched general population. Similar observations have been made after uninephrectomy (when there is a normal contralateral kidney) in the non-donor population. There have been no data to suggest increased cardiovascular disease after donor nephrectomy. Perhaps donor nephrectomy is not associated with sufficient renal dysfunction to increase the risk for cardiovascular disease; alternatively, we may not have followed donors long enough to be able to discern any increase in the risk. Additional long-term studies are needed to resolve this issue.

Stability of long-term renal function of donors is also of concern after kidney donation. As described above, in the rat model, renal ablation has led to subsequent progressive renal dysfunction, and the damage is proportional to the amount of renal tissue removed. The importance of this experimental observation is that humans have an age-related loss of renal function. A possibility is that the remaining kidney will slowly lose functional mass (with aging) and that this will reach a critical threshold where progressive renal disease is inevitable. However, the injury seen in the rat model appears to be species-specific; similar progression to renal failure has not been seen in other animal models. In humans who are not kidney donors, evidence that a reduction in renal mass may lead to progressive renal failure comes from studies of children born with abnormal kidneys and from reports of progressive damage developing in patients born with only one kidney. In such situations, it has not always been clear that the patient had one normal kidney. In contrast, other long-term (>40 years) follow-up studies of non-donors who underwent nephrectomy for unilateral disease have not shown progressive deterioration in renal function.

Prospective living donors are screened to determine that they have two normal kidneys at the time of nephrectomy. To date, numerous studies have examined renal function, proteinuria, and hypertension. Isolated cases of renal failure after donor nephrectomy have been reported, and the United Network for Organ Sharing (UNOS) database has noted that 172 former donors have been listed themselves for a deceased donor kidney. Of these, some had donated one kidney before the establishment of the UNOS database, making it difficult to determine a denominator and calculate the incidence of end-stage renal disease (ESRD). However, no large, single-, or multi-center series (with numerator and denominator well-defined) has demonstrated any evidence of progressive deterioration of renal function in a significant proportion of living donors. In recognition of this benign course, most insurance companies do not increase premiums for kidney donors. A limiting factor in most of these studies is that the average follow-up time has been less than 20 years. Given that most living donors have a life expectancy of more than 20 years, longer follow-up is necessary.

In the largest study to date, we have recently reviewed long-term outcome in our donor population. Between 1963 and 2007, 3698 patients underwent donor uninephrectomy at our institution. We were able to collect follow-up information on 99%. Donors were matched with the general population for age, sex, and race or ethnic group and outcome compared. We found that the long-term survival of donors was similar to the matched controls. ESRD developed in 11 donors, a rate of 180 cases per million persons per year, as compared with a rate of 268 per million per year in the general population.

In addition, in our study, a subset of donors returned to our institution for detailed studies: measurement of the glomerular filtration rate (GFR) and urinary albumin excretion and assessment including the prevalence of hypertension, general health status, and quality of life. Of the subgroup of donors having detailed studies (12.2 ± 9.2 years after donation), 85.5% had a GFR of 60 ml/min/1.73m^2 or higher, 32.1% had hypertension, and 12.7% had albuminuria. The risk of proteinuria, contrary to other studies, was similar to age, sex, ethnicity, and body mass index (BMI) matched controls; a finding that clearly challenges commonly held beliefs regarding donor risk. Older age and higher BMI, but not a longer time since donation, were associated with both a GFR that was lower than 60 ml/min/1.73m^2 and hypertension. A longer time since donation, however, was independently associated with albuminuria. Most donors had quality-of-life scores that were better than population norms, and the prevalence of coexisting conditions was similar to that among controls from the National Health and Nutrition Examination Survey who were matched for age, sex, race or ethnic group, and BMI. When donors with more than 20 years of follow-up were compared with matched controls, again there were no differences.

Donor quality of life

Numerous studies, using a variety of standardized instruments (most commonly the SF-36, a short-form 36-question survey) have studied living donor quality of life. In general, living donors report a similar or better quality of life, as compared with the general population. When concerns were raised, they were related to possible negative effects on recovery and future health, the amount of time to return to routine daily activities and commitment, the financial consequences and implications, and the potential penalization by life or health insurance companies. In addition, many living donors report feeling abandoned after surgery by the transplant program and are disappointed by the lack of any follow-up after their hospital discharge. These concerns need to be taken into consideration by every living donor program. In general, the hospital culture is centered on "the sick." Because donors are not viewed as being "sick," they may not get the attention they deserve.

Risk factors for less positive quality of life after donation have also been identified, including poor donor or recipient physical outcome, a negative personal donor–recipient relationship, and financial hardship. In addition, most studies are of living related donors. It needs to be determined whether unrelated donors have similar outcomes, since their relationship dynamic and motivation to donate is complex. Most of the aforementioned studies were done in donors who underwent open nephrectomy. It will be important to learn whether the same issues develop after laparoscopic nephrectomy. Such information can help transplant programs design protocols to increase living donor satisfaction.

Pregnancy after donation

Historically, some centers would not accept women of child-bearing age as donors because of concern that there would be increased risk of pre-eclampsia, eclampsia, and renal damage in the context of pregnancy after uninephrectomy. As the shortage of organs has become more severe, and wait times for a deceased donor kidney have increased, most centers now accept women of child-bearing age as donors. Although the numbers are limited, studies to date have not shown increased maternal or fetal risks for pregnancies after donation when compared with the general population. However, and albeit with small numbers, there is a suggestion that post-donation pregnancies may be associated with increased risk of pre-eclampsia.

Future concerns

Population studies have shown that smoking, obesity, hypertension, and elevated blood glucose levels are associated with an increased risk of proteinuria and kidney disease. In the United States today there is an epidemic of type 2 diabetes and of hypertension; the rate of both diseases increases as the population ages. Therefore, many donors may end up with one or both of these diseases. Both are well-described causes of ESRD. In addition, many centers currently accept obese donor candidates. Studies are necessary to determine whether there is increased long-term risk for such donors.

A critical question is whether living donors who subsequently develop any form of kidney disease, even years after nephrectomy, will have an accelerated course to renal failure. We have recently studied the outcome of living donors who develop type 2 diabetes after donation. In our entire experience (n = 3777), 154 donors developed type 2 diabetes at a mean of 17.7 ± 9.0 years after donation. Mean follow-up after development of diabetes has been 7 years. To date, estimated GFR is no different between donors with diabetes and those without during similar follow-up duration after donation; diabetic donors, however, were more likely to be hypertensive and proteinuric.

Limitations of current data

Numerous questions remain regarding the surgical and peri-operative risks, long-term outcome, and quality of life for living kidney donors:

1. What is the very long-term outcome of donor nephrectomy? Most published studies have a mean follow-up of less than 15 years. Those with longer follow-up have not demonstrated any increased risk. However, larger numbers and longer follow-up are necessary. Many donors are in their 20s and 30s at the time of donation. We need 50–60-year follow-up after donation to be able to inform future candidates about the true long-term risk.
2. To date, reports of long-term follow-up (>20 years) are limited to "ideal" donors selected over 2 decades ago. Due to the tremendous organ shortage, there has been loosening of the criteria for acceptance for donors. As discussed above, some centers now accept donors with single-drug hypertension and/or obesity. It behooves those centers using "expanded criteria living donors" to define the short- and long-term outcome for such donors. If risks are increased (versus "ideal" donors), then future candidates need to be informed.
3. Is proteinuria or mild renal dysfunction (seen in some living donors) associated with an increased risk of cardiovascular disease or mortality?
4. If living donors develop native kidney disease or another disease that might affect their remaining kidney (particularly type 2 diabetes), will they suffer an accelerated course to renal failure?

Acknowledgments

We thank Stephanie Daily for her help in the preparation of the manuscript of this chapter.

Further reading

Abecassis M, Bartlett ST, Collins AJ, *et al.* Kidney transplantation as primary therapy for end-stage renal disease: a National Kidney Foundation/Kidney Disease Outcomes Quality Initiative (NKF/KDOQITM) Conference. *Clin J Am Soc Nephrol* 2008; **3**: 471–80.

The Authors for the Live Organ Donor Consensus Group. Consensus statement on the live organ donor. *JAMA* 2006; **284**: 2919–26.

Evans RW, Manninen DL, Garrison LP, Jr, *et al.* The quality of life of patients with end-stage renal disease. *N Engl J Med* 1985; **312**: 53–9.

Ibrahim HN, Foley R, Tan L, *et al.* Long-term consequences of kidney donation. *N Engl J Med* 2009; **360**: 459–69.

Meier-Kriesche HU, Kaplan B. Waiting time on dialysis as the strongest modifiable risk factor for renal transplant outcomes: a paired donor kidney analysis. *Transplantation* 2002; **74**: 1377–81.

Wolfe RA, Ashby VB, Milford EL, *et al.* Comparison of mortality in all patients on dialysis, patients on dialysis awaiting transplantation, and recipients of a first cadaveric transplant. *N Engl J Med* 1999; **341**: 1725–30.

Chapter 30

Surgical procedure

Paul Gibbs

Key points

- Each hour of cold ischemia will affect the long-term outcome of the kidney transplant, and cold ischemic times should be kept to a minimum.
- Identification of the bladder during surgery may be improved by filling the bladder through the catheter with a dilute methylene blue solution.
- If there is significant atherosclerosis, with calcification resulting in non-compressible, solid arteries that cannot be clamped, it may be necessary to use the common iliac artery or even on occasion the aorta to perform the arterial anastomosis.
- If the transplanted kidney fails and transplant nephrectomy is performed within a short time, mobilization and removal of the kidney is usually straightforward.
- If using older donor kidneys, reduced renal function may necessitate transplantation of both kidneys to a single recipient; these can usually be placed together into the same iliac fossa.

When discussing renal transplantation with prospective recipients, the procedure is usually described as a moderate-sized operation, and although this is true in most cases, it is not one to be taken lightly. A first transplant in a "virgin" iliac fossa is indeed relatively straightforward, but it is also true that the operation can be very technically challenging. A previous transplant, severe atherosclerosis as is the case in many renal failure patients, or limited access due to either patient size (both the depth of the iliac fossa and adiposity of the patient) or the size of the kidney can lead to considerable surgical difficulties.

Cadaveric donor nephrectomy

The most common surgical approach used for cadaveric donor nephrectomy is the en bloc technique through a large abdominal incision. This technique permits rapid removal of the kidneys, therefore reducing the risk of renal vascular spasm and irreversible anoxic injury due to prolonged warm ischemia. The heart and liver teams often begin the dissection simultaneously. The kidneys can be dissected free and easily removed after in situ flushing with preservation solution of the graft and the liver and pancreas have been removed. If the heart is not harvested, the descending aorta can be cross-clamped in the left pleural cavity without prior dissection. An aortic cannula is placed below the renal artery and fixed. The supraceliac aorta is clamped, and cold perfusate is instilled into the kidneys through the aortic cannula, using, for example, University of Wisconsin (UW) solution. A vent in the inferior vena cava (IVC) prevents venous engorgement and drains the perfusate. After the hepatectomy and pancreatectomy are complete, dissection is carried out in a bloodless field. The right colon and duodenum are mobilized and reflected up into the left upper abdomen. The lesser splanchnic nerves and left mesocolon are divided to expose the left kidney. Deep dissection mobilizes both kidneys medially with Gerota's fascia. Both ureters are identified and transected close to the bladder and dissected up to the level of the lower renal pole. The IVC and aorta are divided just below the level of the aortic cannula. The en bloc dissection is completed by incising the prevertebral fascia while the aorta and IVC are retracted upward, together with the kidneys and ureters. The kidneys are separated on

Organ Transplantation: A Clinical Guide, ed. A.A. Klein, C.J. Lewis, and J.C. Madsen. Published by Cambridge University Press.

ice following removal from the donor: the left renal vein is divided to include a cuff of IVC, whereas the IVC remains with the right kidney. From the posterior aspect, the aorta is opened and the renal arteries identified, and then the kidneys are separated. A total of 250–300 ml of cold perfusate is flushed through each kidney using a cannula in each renal artery. The kidneys are bagged in perfusate solution and stored on ice for transportation to the recipient hospital. All remaining back table preparation is left for the recipient surgeon.

Cold ischemia

Transplantation using organs from cadaveric donors is always performed with the overriding need to minimize the cold ischemic time of the organ. The length of time acceptable to store an organ is variable and for kidneys can be extended out to 48 hours. However, it is now well established that each hour of cold ischemia will affect the long-term outcome of the kidney transplant, and cold ischemic times should be kept to a minimum and certainly below 24 hours.

The standard cadaveric transplant

Technique

Prior to the patient being anesthetized, the kidney should be inspected and back table dissection performed to ensure that it is not damaged. The renal artery and vein are freed from any retroperitoneal fat, and any polar arteries are identified and if necessary reconstructed by anastomosis to the main artery if they have not been included on the aortic patch. Where there are multiple veins, smaller ones may be tied, although it may be prudent to anastomose both veins where they are of equal size. Care must be taken to avoid denuding the ureter of its peri-ureteric tissue, as this may render it ischemic.

Following induction of anesthesia, the patient is catheterized and the operative site prepared and draped. A curvilinear incision is made in the iliac fossa, extending from the midline supra pubic area to the level of the anterior superior iliac crest, although in patients with access problems, this can be extended further. The oblique muscles are divided, but in most cases it is possible to leave the rectus abdominis intact. The peritoneum is mobilized medially to expose the iliac vessels; during this mobilization, the round ligament is usually divided in females and the spermatic cord mobilized and retracted medially in males. The inferior epigastric vessels are also usually divided, although very occasionally, if there is any doubt about the blood supply of the lower abdominal wall they can be preserved. The external iliac artery and vein are dissected free, taking care not to damage lymphatics unnecessarily. The renal vessels are anastomosed end to side to the external iliac vessels using standard vascular clamps to control the iliac vessels and usually 5/0 monofilament suture such as Prolene. Individual surgical preference dictates which is anastomosed first, although most commonly the vein precedes the artery.

Once each anastomosis is complete, the renal vessel is clamped and blood flow restored to the leg. This allows the anastomosis to be tested and even on occasion revised without compromising the kidney's circulation by further interruption after reperfusion. Once both anastomoses are satisfactory, the kidney is reperfused with blood.

There are a number of techniques for anastomosing the ureter to the bladder. These include the Leadbetter–Politano or a direct vesico-ureteric anastomosis. In the latter technique, a small anterior cystostomy is made, dividing the muscle layers of the bladder and making a small opening in the mucosa of the bladder. Direct mucosa to mucosa anastomosis is performed using interrupted absorbable sutures. The bladder muscle layer is then closed over the distal end of the ureter as an anti-reflux measure. A short double J stent can be used to protect this anastomosis; this is usually removed at 6 weeks. It is important to trim the ureter back as far as possible to ensure an adequate blood supply to the ureteric side of the anastomosis and minimize either anastomotic leaks or stenosis.

Identification of the bladder can be surprisingly difficult, especially in patients on long-term peritoneal dialysis in whom the peritoneum has thickened or with a small shrunken bladder due to many years of anuria. Identification may be improved by filling the bladder through the catheter with a dilute methylene blue solution.

An alternative to using the patients' bladder is to perform a direct anastomosis with the recipients' native ureter, spatulating both ureteric ends. The native ureter is usually divided, and even if there is residual renal function in the native kidneys, this rarely results in troublesome hydronephrosis. This uretero-ureterostomy is usually protected with a double J stent, although passing the stent antegrade down the native ureter is often not possible and a small cystostomy may need to be made to allow retrograde passage of the stent.

The Leadbetter–Politano procedure involves the creation of a submucosal tunnel along which the ureter is tunneled before being brought through the mucosal layer into the bladder. The distal ureter is spatulated, everted, and secured to the bladder mucosa, creating a ureteric nipple. The technique requires an anterior cystostomy. Finally, in patients with bladder dysfunction or absence, it is sometimes necessary to drain the urine into an ileal conduit. This is an isolated segment of vascularized small bowel, which is widely used by urologists as a replacement bladder following total cystectomy. Ideally it should be created prior to the patient being placed on the waiting list. In this instance, the ureter is anastomosed end to side to the bowel wall, ensuring mucosa-to-mucosa apposition. The anastomosis can be stented in the same way as the standard technique and brought out through the stoma on the skin surface.

There are a number of variations to this standard technique, which can be utilized depending on circumstances. If healthy, the internal iliac artery can be divided and swung up to allow end-to-end anastomosis with the renal artery. This is useful in cases where there is no aortic patch on the renal artery and is therefore widely used in live donor transplants. The internal iliac vein can be divided to allow better access to the external vein where the right kidney is being transplanted. This is to make the venous anastomosis more accessible, as the right renal vein is short. Various techniques for lengthening the vein have also been described, usually utilizing a segment of the donor vena cava. In the majority of cases, this is not required.

Many patients with renal failure have significant atherosclerosis, with calcification resulting in noncompressible solid arteries that cannot be clamped. In these cases and also in re-transplants into the same iliac fossa, it may be necessary to use the common iliac artery or even on occasion the aorta to perform the arterial anastomosis. Careful preoperative assessment by computed tomography scanning should allow identification of calcified arteries before listing for transplantation.

Peri-operative care

General anesthesia is the norm for kidney transplant recipients. Most will be fasted prior to surgery; however, tracheal intubation and muscle relaxation are generally employed to allow optimum surgical access. Central venous access is generally obtained (often using ultrasound guidance as multiple lines may have been placed in the past), but invasive arterial monitoring is not often required. The patient should be catheterized, usually once anesthetized. Immediately prior to reperfusion of the donor kidney, most centers administer a cocktail of drugs comprising methyl prednisolone as immunosuppressant, mannitol, and sometimes frusemide. Adequate intravascular filling is required to maximize organ perfusion; some clinicians target a central venous pressure (right atrial pressure) of at least 10 mmHg at this point. It is also important to maintain blood pressure, especially as the donor may have had significant hypertension.

After waking (at the end of the procedure), the patient is usually looked after in a high-dependency area or step-down unit. Hourly urine measurements and careful fluid balance is imperative. A Doppler ultrasound may be performed within a few hours of the operation to achieve a baseline reading of renal arterial flow, even when there is good immediate function. In patients with no function, this is obviously crucial to ensure that the vessels are patent.

Living donor renal transplant (see Chapter 29)

A live patient donating a kidney is a challenging situation in which any complication must be strenuously prevented. The preferred donor procedure is a laparoscopic nephrectomy, with mobilization of the kidney assisted by the use of a hand port, usually through a small infra-umbilical midline incision through which the kidney is removed. Choice of which kidney is removed is dependent mainly on the arterial anatomy, avoiding if possible the need for multiple renal artery anastomoses in the recipient, although often the left kidney may be a less challenging procedure. The split in function between the kidneys should also be taken into account.

Recipient procedure

This is essentially the same as for a cadaveric renal transplant, with the main difference being the arterial anastomosis. Because there will not be an aortic patch, use of the internal iliac artery (when disease-free) for the arterial anastomosis is common, although the external iliac artery may need to be used in cases where there is significant disease. The other technical challenge is that both the vein and artery are often shorter in a live donor kidney, making performance of the anastomosis more technically challenging. There is also a high incidence of two renal arteries due to early bifurcation of the main renal artery and the length of artery lost due to the stapling required in laparoscopic retrieval. One method of dealing with multiple renal arteries is to excise a length of the internal iliac artery including its first branch. This can then be used as a Y graft and anastomosed to the two renal arteries on the back table, eliminating the need to perform difficult arterial anastomoses at depth in the iliac fossa. End-to-end reconstruction of the internal iliac is then performed, allowing an easier, safer anastomosis.

Pediatric transplantation (see Chapter 33)

The number of children who become donors is thankfully very small, which means that the many children requiring renal transplantation will receive an adult organ, whether from a cadaveric or live donor. This has implications with regard to the size match of kidney to recipient, and it is often necessary in smaller children to place the kidney within the peritoneal cavity and anastomose the renal vessels to the aorta and the vena cava. The initial incision needs to be longer then in adults, extending as far as the tip of the 12th rib. The kidney is usually placed retroperitoneally behind the cecum, ensuring access to enable percutaneous biopsies to be performed in the postoperative period. Otherwise the procedure is essentially the same as for an adult transplant.

En bloc renal transplantation

In very small child donors (age $<$ 2 years), the risk of thrombosis of the kidney if used as a single organ is very high; these kidneys are therefore often transplanted as a pair, en bloc, still attached to the aorta and vena cava into both children and adults. This allows the aorta and cava to be used to perform the vascular anastomoses, considerably reducing the risk of thrombosis. The proximal end of both great vessels is oversewn and the distal end anastomosed end to side in the usual manner. Alternatively, the aorta and cava can be anastomosed as interposition grafts into transected iliac vessels. The disadvantage of the latter technique is that if graft nephrectomy is required in the early postoperative period, the donor vessels will also need to be removed, resulting in the need to reconstruct the iliac vessels.

Donation after cardiac death cadaveric donors

The number of kidney transplants from donation after cardiac death (DCD) donors has increased substantially over the last 10 years. These donors may be quite elderly (age $>$ 70 years) and as a consequence have a higher incidence of pre-existing renal disease. It is prudent to biopsy kidneys from elderly donors or those with significant past medical history including diabetes or hypertension, and recent practice has seen the successful transplantation of both kidneys into one patient where the biopsy has revealed significant glomerulosclerosis. Both kidneys unless very large can be transplanted into the same iliac fossa, with the proximal kidney being anastomosed onto the common iliac artery and vena cava. It is important to remember to implant the proximal kidney first so that it can be reperfused while the second kidney is implanted. Although DCD kidneys have a lower immediate function rate compared with donor kidneys after brain death, the medium- and long-term outcome seems to be comparable, and they are a valuable extra source of kidneys for transplantation.

Complications

Early vascular complications include both bleeding and thrombosis. Hemorrhage sometimes occurs up to a week later if there is ongoing wound infection. It can be arterial or venous, and the subsequent hematoma can be large enough to obstruct urine flow and cause hydronephrosis. All significant hematomas should be evacuated, even if there is no ureteric obstruction to reduce the risk of ongoing infection.

Arterial thrombosis is uncommon and is usually a technical issue. When identified, it requires immediate re-exploration if there is a chance of saving the kidney. Unfortunately, the kidney has often already infarcted and has to be removed. Renal vein thrombosis is more common (around 6% in some series) although still unusual and can result in the sudden loss of the kidney within the first week after transplantation. Its cause is usually not technical; all patients should have a thrombophilia screen performed, although an abnormality is rarely found. Immunological factors may also play a role, although the exact mechanism remains uncertain.

Ureteric complications are the commonest specific complication. The incidence is in the region of 10–15%. The majority of cases are due to ischemia and usually require revision surgery to re-implant the ureter into the bladder. This can be a difficult operation, especially if there is a long-standing infection resulting in dense fibrosis. Options include direct re-implantation into the bladder of the ureter if there is enough length, the formation of a Boari flap from the bladder wall where the ureter is short, or use of the native ureter, which can be anastomosed directly to the renal pelvis if necessary. Ureteric complications are often serious due to the ongoing infection and result in the loss of a kidney.

Late vascular complications are usually stenosis of the arterial anastomosis or a stricture in the renal artery. There is a possibility that this may be related to clamping the artery during implantation. Radiological stenting may sometimes be possible; however, surgical bypass of the stenosis is otherwise performed using a saphenous vein graft.

Transplant nephrectomy

Unfortunately, a transplant nephrectomy is sometimes required. If performed within a short time after transplant, mobilization of the kidney is usually straightforward, as is its removal. It is usually prudent to remove the donor vessels, as if left in situ with ongoing rejection, they have been known to rupture, causing life-threatening hemorrhage. The defect in the iliac vein and artery usually requires a small vein patch to allow closure without stenosing the vessel. The long saphenous vein is the usual source for this.

Late nephrectomy of failed grafts is not routinely performed. It is indicated for a number of clinical reasons, including persistent bleeding from a failed kidney due to ongoing rejection following withdrawal of immunosuppression, chronic infection, or the need to create space for another transplant if both iliac fossae have previously been used for transplantation. This needs to be done prior to re-listing. The kidney is usually densely adherent to the surrounding tissue, and mobilization can be slow and needs to be intracapsular. It is important for dissection to remain close to the kidney because damage to the iliac vessels is easy at this stage as they are often lying close to the kidney as a result of fibrosis. The kidney is resected, dividing all vessels high in the hilum, leaving the donor vessel anastomoses to the iliac vessels intact. At this stage after a transplant, rupture and bleeding is not a significant concern.

Further reading

Mangus RS, Haag BW. Stented versus nonstented extravesical ureteroneocystostomy in renal transplantation: a meta-analysis. *Am J Transplant* 2004; **4**: 1889–96.

Odland MD. Surgical technique/post-transplant surgical complications. *Surg Clin North Am* 1998; **78**: 55–60.

Steffens J, Stark E, Haben B, Treiyer A. Politano-Leadbetter ureteric reimplantation. *BJU Int* 2006; **98**: 695–712.

Wilson CH, Bhatti AA, Rix DA, Manas DM. Routine intraoperative ureteric stenting for kidney transplant recipients. *Cochrane Database Syst Rev* 2005; **4**: CD004925.

Chapter 31 Peri-operative care and early complications

Lorna Marson and John Forsythe

Key points

- Careful assessment and preoperative preparation of the renal transplant recipient is essential, paying particular attention to hydration status, cytomegalovirus prophylaxis, and immunosuppressive regime.
- Dialysis immediately before transplant surgery is associated with delayed graft function.
- Close postoperative monitoring is required, especially of urine output and fluid balance.
- A high level of suspicion must be maintained for postoperative hemorrhage, as this may compress the transplanted kidney, causing vascular thrombosis and permanent damage.
- Complications following renal transplantation include delayed graft function, hemorrhage, acute rejection and unwanted effects of immunosuppressive therapy.

This chapter aims to describe the management of the renal transplant recipient from the time of their admission to hospital to discharge, including immediate preoperative preparation, postoperative management, and early post-transplant complications. Surgical aspects of the transplant procedure are covered in Chapter 30.

Preoperative evaluation

All patients undergoing renal transplantation will have been assessed prior to listing for transplantation, but they still require a thorough review on admission for transplant, as some time may have elapsed since their assessment visit.

History

Any change in the patient's condition since the time of transplant assessment should be sought. In particular, history of recent infection will be important in the decision of whether or not the transplant should proceed. Review of any urinary problems is useful at this stage. Other salient points to note in the history include details of dialysis, including time of last treatment and any access or other related problems. Volume of urine output (if any) per day should be determined and a history of past or present urinary tract problems documented. Evidence of recent or current infection should be sought, including access site (vascular or abdominal wall, including peritonitis). Other important factors include previous surgery and evidence of ischemic heart disease and peripheral vascular disease. Recipient blood group, tissue typing, and virology (cytomegalovirus [CMV], Epstein-Barr virus, human immunodeficiency virus [HIV], hepatitis B virus [HBV], and hepatitis C virus [HCV]) must be recorded in the notes.

Donor details should also be included in recipient clerking, including age, cause of death, blood group, and tissue typing. All donor details in the notes should be made anonymous. In many centers across the world, the recipient has access to their own clinical notes, and therefore significant donor details recorded in the notes would threaten donor anonymity. Important clinical factors that may have some relevance to graft outcome should be recorded.

Examination

A full physical examination of the patient should be performed, including observation of fluid status, peripheral pulses, and abdominal scars/hernias. In addition, it is essential to examine for signs of active

Organ Transplantation: A Clinical Guide, ed. A.A. Klein, C.J. Lewis, and J.C. Madsen. Published by Cambridge University Press.

infection. Careful fluid replacement may be required prior to the transplant operation.

Investigations

Essential investigations prior to surgery include full blood count, blood urea nitrogen, creatinine and electrolytes, baseline calcium/liver function tests, blood glucose, clotting screen/INR (if on warfarin), and blood group and save. Viral serology status should also be checked, in particular, CMV, HIV, HBV, and HCV.

A negative donor–recipient human leukocyte antigen (HLA) cross-match is required in order to proceed with transplantation. This subject is covered in detail in Chapter 28.

Preoperative management

Dialysis

Hemodialysis is indicated before transplantation if serum potassium is greater than 5.5 mmol/l or significant fluid overload is present. It is worth noting that preoperative hemodialysis is associated with an increased risk of delayed graft function, probably due to hypovolemia. The majority of patients will require only 2–3 hours of dialysis. This should be performed with minimal anticoagulation and with the aim of leaving the patient at 1–2 kg above their dry weight.

Patients may be "nil by mouth" for some time prior to surgery. In these circumstances, fasting has the effect of increasing the risk of hyperkalemia, and an intravenous (IV) infusion of glucose-containing solution will help control the rise in potassium.

Drug therapy

Antihypertensive medications

These should all be reviewed during the preoperative evaluation. In general, beta-blockers should be continued; however, angiotensin-converting enzyme inhibitors and related drugs should be stopped peri-operatively. Other anti-hypertensive medication should be withheld in the early postoperative period and kept under regular review.

Anti-platelet and anti-coagulation therapy

Aspirin therapy can be continued peri-operatively, as it has not been shown to increase the risk of postoperative hemorrhage. A combination of aspirin and clopidogrel is used in patients who are at high risk of a vascular event or who have had a drug-eluting coronary stent placed – usually for a defined period such as 12 months. Some centers may suspend such patients from the transplant waiting list until completion of dual therapy when they can be reactivated on aspirin alone.

Pretransplant management of oral anti-coagulants

In living donor transplant recipients, warfarin should be discontinued 5 days prior to the transplant, and the international normalized ratio (INR) should be monitored. An INR less than 1.5 is acceptable for the transplant to take place. If preoperative anti-coagulation is required, this can be administered via IV unfractionated heparin once the INR is subtherapeutic. This should be stopped 6 hours before transplant. Alternatively, subcutaneous low-molecular-weight heparin may be used, but its effect is unpredictable in patients with chronic kidney disease and so should be used with caution.

In deceased donor transplant recipients, the INR should be checked urgently on admission. If the INR is greater than 1.4, reversal of warfarin should be considered using either prothrombin complex concentrate or 1–2 mg of vitamin K. The disadvantage of vitamin K is a relative lag time until the reversal of anticoagulation and a very variable impact on coagulation thereafter. Fresh-frozen plasma may also be administered (to replace clotting factors) when there is no availability or no experience in using prothrombin complex concentrate.

Immunosuppressive therapy

Most centers use induction therapy with two doses of an anti-CD25 monoclonal antibody such as basiliximab at induction of anesthesia and on postoperative day 4.

Prophylaxis

Deep venous thrombosis prophylaxis

Although the risk of deep venous thrombosis (DVT) post-transplant is relatively low (in the region of 2%), the use of DVT prophylaxis is recommended, with compression stockings and administration of subcutaneous heparin (5000 units) at anesthetic induction and daily thereafter until the patient is mobile.

Table 31.1 Donor and recipient CMV status and risk of disease

Donor (D)/recipient (R) status	Risk of CMV disease
D+/R+	10–30%
D+/R–	50–80%
D–/R+	0–30%
D–/R–	0%

Antibiotic prophylaxis

A single dose of prophylactic antibiotic at the time of surgery is indicated. The choice of drug will vary according to the individual unit's protocol.

CMV prophylaxis

The risk of developing CMV disease postoperatively varies depending on the donor and recipient CMV status (Table 31.1). Undoubtedly there is a role for prophylaxis: to reduce the risk of CMV disease during the early months following transplantation when the patients are most heavily immunosuppressed, although it may just delay the onset of CMV disease.

Different prophylaxis strategies may be adopted, including universal prophylaxis given to all patients for whom the donor is CMV positive. The length of prophylaxis is currently under debate, but a recent study in renal transplantation has demonstrated better control of disease when prophylaxis is given for 200 days, rather than 100 days. Some centers do not administer prophylaxis at all, but rather regularly monitor CMV levels by polymerase chain reaction assay for the first 6 months following transplantation. Treatment with valganciclovir is then commenced when a threshold number of viral copies have been reached.

Prophylaxis against pneumocystis

Trimethoprim-sulfamethoxazole is usually prescribed for a period of 3–12 months post-transplant as prophylaxis against pneumocystis.

Consent

In most cases a patient information booklet will have been given to the patient well in advance. This allows the patient to take in the necessary details of the operation and the balance of risk between transplantation and remaining on dialysis. Ideally, consent should be taken well in advance of the day of surgery.

Once the results of all the investigations are obtained and a decision has been made to proceed with the transplant, informed consent should be obtained, particularly if there are factors making the kidney higher risk. A brief description of the procedure should be given, including the length of time for the operation, the presence of drains, and a urinary catheter postoperatively. In addition, it is wise to mention the presence of a ureteric stent and the need to remove this sometime after the transplant. It is also important to warn the patient that the kidney may not work straight away after transplantation. This is particularly important if the donor history makes this more likely, e.g., donation after circulatory death (DCD) donor. In situations in which there is an increased risk of complication postoperatively, e.g., transmission of infection or malignancy, this should also be discussed with the patient. This should include the balance of risk between accepting such an organ and remaining on the waiting list for future transplant.

The early postoperative phase

The presence or absence of primary function in the early postoperative phase is very important. Primary function is expected in all living donor transplants and most deceased donor procedures, particularly if the donor was donation after brain death (DBD) with a short cold ischemic time. Prolonged cold ischemic time is associated with an increased risk of delayed graft function, which in turn affects acute rejection rates and long-term outcome.

Fluid management

Urine output may vary between none and several liters over 24 hours. The patient must therefore be closely monitored postoperatively. Fluid balance assessment should be made using vital signs, central venous pressure, urine output, and daily weights. Early observation of trends in vital signs and urine output allows the rapid diagnosis of problems such as hemorrhage, or more rarely, thrombosis.

Administration of IV fluids is required to replace fluid losses and to maintain circulating volume. Fluid loss after transplant comprises urine output, insensible losses (approximately 500 ml/24 hours), and loss from surgical drains. This fluid should be replaced with crystalloid at a rate of approximately urine output (for the last hour) plus 40 ml/hr for maintaining fluid status. This should be carefully monitored on an hourly basis for the first 24 hours following transplant.

It is noted above that different combinations of donor/recipient will give rise to differing risk of delayed graft function. This should be borne in mind when assessing the patient in the first hours following transplant. For instance, in a live donor transplant (which has been completely uncomplicated), the absence of urine or the presence of very small urine output should be a serious finding demanding urgent investigation and action (see next section).

Evaluation of the oliguric/anuric patient

If an early postoperative check reveals that the patient is passing little urine, a thorough clinical assessment must be undertaken. The patency of the urinary catheter should be first checked. Hematuria may contribute with the formation of small clots, and gentle bladder washouts are required. Fluid status should be determined, and if hypovolemia is suspected, careful fluid challenges (such as a 250-ml saline bolus) should be tried and the response noted. There is a significant incidence of vascular complications after renal transplant (approximately 2%). If other causes of low urine output have been excluded, then a Doppler ultrasound scan should be performed, which should detect a vascular abnormality.

Postoperative analgesia

Most patients will be managed with patient-controlled analgesia (PCA), with intravenous morphine or fentanyl. In addition, they should be prescribed regular paracetamol. Following removal of the PCA, regular oral opioids will be required, but care should be taken to avoid unwanted side effects, including nausea, vomiting, itching, and decreased consciousness, since these agents are metabolized partly through renal handling.

Early postoperative complications

Delayed graft function

If the patient is euvolemic, with a well-draining urinary catheter and a normal Doppler ultrasound scan, the likely cause of a low urine output is delayed graft function (DGF) secondary to acute tubular necrosis. DGF is defined as the need for dialysis within the first week following transplant. DGF is unusual in living donor transplants (2–5%). It complicates 10–30% of all deceased donor grafts and is most common in DCD kidneys (50–80%). Renal function recovers in the majority of patients, often within the first few days, but it may take several weeks.

Risk factors for the development of DGF include donor factors such as donor age older than 60 years, hypertension, retrieval factors such as requirement of inotropic support, increased warm ischemic time (e.g., in DCD), prolonged cold ischemia, and recipient factors such as obesity, HLA sensitization, hemodialysis within 24 hours prior to surgery, and long second warm ischemic time. Long-term consequences of DGF include increased acute rejection risk, higher serum creatinine at 1 year, and, if DGF is combined with acute rejection, reduced long-term graft survival.

DGF is managed by careful attention to fluid balance and avoidance of drug toxicity. The patient should undergo a protocol biopsy on day 5 to ensure that there is no concomitant rejection process. If DGF persists, the biopsy should be repeated every 7–10 days, until the onset of graft function. Reduction of calcineurin inhibitor (CNI) levels is also appropriate once the biopsy has demonstrated the absence of rejection, with a target trough level for tacrolimus (TAC) of approximately 5 ng/ml, using other agents to augment overall immunosuppression.

Technical complications

Wound

Risk factors for wound complications following renal transplantation are obesity, long duration of dialysis, elderly patients, high doses of immunosuppressive drugs such as prednisolone or sirolimus, and diabetes. Wound infection may be superficial or deep. If superficial, thorough cleaning and consideration of antibiotic therapy is required. Deep wound infections, involving fascial or muscular layers, may require surgical drainage and laying open. Antibiotic treatment is indicated if there are systemic signs of sepsis. A less common complication is wound dehiscence, which also may be superficial or deep, requiring primary or secondary closure as appropriate.

Postoperative hemorrhage

Usually occurring within the first 24 hours following transplantation, this should be identified rapidly through careful monitoring of the patient's fluid status, and persistent signs of hypovolemia, even if they are subtle, should be assumed to be due to bleeding until proven otherwise. Other signs of bleeding are excessive amounts of drain fluid and increased analgesia requirement. If the patient is stable, a Doppler ultrasound scan may be useful, as it may reveal a peri-nephric hematoma, but this may also just delay definitive management. There should be a high level of suspicion and the patient should return to the operating theater if there is any doubt. Ongoing bleeding into a relatively small anatomical space will cause pressure on the renal vessels and may lead to vascular thrombosis. When the patient returns to surgery, the most common site of hemorrhage is around the renal hilum, not the anastomosis.

Graft thrombosis

This predominantly occurs within the first week post-transplant. Venous thrombosis is more common, occurring in between 2–4%. Renal artery thrombosis is rare, with an incidence of around 1%. Risk factors for graft thrombosis include retrieval injury to donor vessels, atherosclerosis of donor or recipient vessels, technical error with the anastomoses, angulation of the vessels, or external compression from a hematoma or lymphocele. In addition, persistent postoperative hypotension may lead to thrombosis as a result of the low flow state. Graft thrombosis should be excluded in cases where there is acute graft dysfunction, particularly if there was initial function and abrupt anuria or oliguria ensues, despite adequate fluid management. In addition, in a situation where the kidney would be expected to have primary function, such as a living donor transplant, and the patient is oliguric or anuric, this should be excluded as a matter of urgency. Venous thrombosis will cause severe pain as the graft becomes swollen. Urgent Doppler ultrasound will confirm the diagnosis, with absent venous flow and reversed arterial diastolic flow. The patient should be returned to surgery urgently if there is to be any chance of salvaging the graft. Graft nephrectomy is by far the most likely outcome, and the patient must be warned of this prior to return to the operating theater.

Urological complications

Ureteric leak or obstruction may occur due to a surgical problem, distal ureteric ischemia, or immunological damage to the ureter. Ureteric leak tends to occur in the early postoperative phase and presents with increased wound pain and/or increasing fluid discharge from the wound or drain, commonly occurring following removal of the urethral catheter. Ultrasound may detect fluid around the kidney, which, if aspirated, should be sent for biochemistry. A urine leak is confirmed if the fluid contains high levels of creatinine and potassium.

Management includes replacement of the urethral catheter. If a stent is in place, it is likely that the patient will require surgical treatment. If, however, there is no stent in place at the time that the leak is detected, some time may be bought by placing a percutaneous nephrostomy and performing a nephrostogram, which will help delineate the site of the leak. Some centers will attempt to treat the problem by antegrade placement of a stent across the site of the leak. However, the best treatment is usually surgical re-exploration and repair, often by performing a new ureteric to bladder anastomosis. Ureteric obstruction is usually a late complication following renal transplantation and can be largely avoided in the early postoperative phase by the routine use of a ureteric stent.

Lymphocele formation

This complication commonly occurs between 2 weeks and months following transplantation and is due to leakage from recipient lymphatics dissected at the time of surgery. The fluid can build up to a large quantity and exert significant compression on the transplanted kidney, giving rise to ureteric obstruction. In some situations the lymphocele may press on the iliac veins, with increased swelling and discomfort in the leg on the side of the transplant. Aspiration may be required as a matter of urgency to reduce the pressure. Definitive treatment is surgical, with fenestration of the peritoneum overlying the lymphocele, allowing drainage of the lymphatics into the peritoneal cavity. This can usually be performed laparoscopically and be aided by the use of laparoscopic ultrasound to ensure no damage to surrounding structures.

Early immunological complications

Acute rejection

Acute rejection occurs in 10–25% of renal transplants and is most common during the first 3 months following transplantation. Risk factors for the development of acute rejection include sensitization (through previous transplant, pregnancy, and blood transfusion), HLA mismatches, and DGF. In addition, the immunosuppressive regimen adopted will have an impact; induction therapy with anti-CD25 antibodies reduces acute rejection rates, mycophenolate mofetil (MMF) is a more effective agent than azathioprine (AZA), and TAC is probably associated with lower rates of acute rejection than cyclosporine in renal transplantation.

Patients present with acute graft dysfunction, with increasing serum creatinine and oliguria. This is usually detected by medical staff as the patient is often asymptomatic. Doppler ultrasound scan is required to exclude other causes of renal dysfunction, such as ureteric obstruction or vascular complications, usually followed by renal biopsy. In addition, serum should be sent for antibody screening, particularly if antibody-mediated rejection (AMR) is suspected.

Treatment should be commenced prior to biopsy results if there is a high index of suspicion, in the form of pulsed IV methylprednisolone (250–500 mg). Immunosuppression should be optimized, with careful monitoring of CNI levels. The majority of rejection episodes are treated effectively with pulsed steroids, but when the response is poor or there is a rapid return of rejection following treatment, alternative therapies can be used, such as polyclonal antibodies, e.g., anti-thymocyte globulin (ATG).

Early antibody-mediated rejection

Acute AMR accounts for approximately 10% of rejection episodes in the early post-transplant period. The diagnosis can be difficult to make and is based on biopsy findings of acute tissue injury, with endothelial cells staining positive for C4d (discussed further in Chapter 2). In addition, AMR is associated with the presence of anti-donor HLA donor-specific antibodies (DSAs) on serological testing. AMR is caused by the binding of DSAs to graft endothelial cells, which leads to complement activation and endothelial cell injury.

The aim of treatment of AMR is to remove DSAs, which may reduce the likelihood of further injury, and to reduce vascular inflammation. Daily plasma exchange removes circulating DSAs, and pulsed doses of methylprednisolone reduce vascular inflammation, with the added benefit of treatment of any associated T-cell–mediated rejection.

T-cell–mediated rejection

This accounts for the majority of rejection episodes and is characterized by lymphocytic infiltration of the interstitium, tubules, and vessels. Such rejection is classified according to the Banff 1997 working classification, as outlined on Table 31.2. The majority of rejection episodes are confined to the tubulointerstitium, with vascular involvement associated with worse response to therapy and reduced graft survival.

Table 31.2 Banff 1997 classification of T-cell–mediated rejection (TCMR)

Borderline changes
Suspicious for TCMR
No arteritis
Tubulitis without significant interstitial inflammation or
Interstitial inflammation without significant tubulitis
Acute TCMR
Acute tubulo-interstitial rejection
1A: Significant interstitial inflammation and moderate tubulitis 1B: Significant interstitial inflammation and severe tubulitis
Acute vascular rejection
2A: mild or moderate arteritis with or without interstitial inflammation or tubulitis
2B: Severe arteritis with or without interstitial inflammation or tubulitis
3: Transmural arteritis ± fibrinoid necrosis

Early complications of immunosuppressive therapy

CNIs

Monitoring of levels is essential to ensure adequate drug exposure while minimizing exposure to toxic side effects such as nephrotoxicity. Initially, trough levels should be taken regularly and the treatment dose should be amended accordingly. Optimal levels will depend on various factors such as HLA mismatch, whether the kidney is DCD or DBD, and the presence of previous sensitizing events. Patients with deteriorating renal function in the context of high TAC levels can be managed with dose reduction in the first instance, progressing to biopsy if this does not result in improved function. Histologically, TAC toxicity is associated with arteriopathy, with vascular hyaline deposits.

Another less common but devastating side effect of CNIs is the development of thrombotic microangiopathy, with deterioration in renal function in association with biopsy findings of endothelial cell swelling and capillary thrombi with fibrinoid necrosis in arterioles. It may or may not be associated with hematological abnormalities, such as falling platelets and microangiopathic hemolytic anemia. CNIs should be stopped and daily plasma exchange may be required until a response is seen, continuing treatment on alternate days thereafter for 2–4 weeks. This strategy can be accompanied by treatment with ATG to cover the CNI-free period before considering options for long-term immunosuppression.

Anti-proliferative agents

Early complications include myelosuppression, with a fall in hemoglobin, white blood cells, and platelet count, requiring cessation of therapy if severe. MMF is commonly associated with diarrhea, which can be managed by altering the dosing regimen from 1 g twice daily to 500 mg four times a day. An alternative preparation, Myfortic, is available, which, in some patients, has fewer gastrointestinal side effects, and so this could be tried, or the patient could be switched to AZA if the diarrhea is severe.

Steroids

The majority of side effects of steroids occur in the later period following transplantation. However, poor glycemic control may be an early side effect, in both diabetic and non-diabetic patients.

Further reading

Luan FL, Stuckey LJ, Park JM, Kaul D, Cibrik D, Ojo A. Six-month prophylaxis is cost effective in transplant patients at high risk for cytomegalovirus infection. *J Am Soc Nephrol* 2009; **20**: 2449–58.

Racusen LC, Colvin RB, Solez K, *et al.* Antibody-mediated rejection criteria – an addition to the Banff 97 classification of renal allograft rejection. *Am J Transplant* 2003; **3**: 708–14.

Racusen LC, Solez K, Colvin RB, *et al.* The Banff 97 working classification of renal allograft pathology. *Kidney Int* 1999; **55**: 713–23.

Taylor CJ, Kosmoliaptsis V, Sharples LD, *et al.* Ten-year experience of selective omission of the pretransplant crossmatch test in deceased donor kidney transplantation. *Transplantation* 2010; **89**: 185–93.

Yarlagadda SG, Coca SG, Formica RN Jr, Poggio ED, Parikh CR. Association between delayed graft function and allograft and patient survival: a systematic review and meta-analysis. *Nephrol Dial Transplant* 2009; **24**: 1039–47.

Chapter 32 Long-term management and outcomes

Sharon Mulroy and John D. Firth

Key points

- Advanced donor age is the strongest predictor of poor long-term graft survival.
- Transplant glomerulopathy is an alloimmune-mediated lesion that is strongly linked to anti–human leukocyte antigen (HLA) class II antibodies.
- Proteinuria is common after renal transplantation (45% of cases at 1 year) and is an important marker of graft injury.
- Renal transplant recipients are at a 3–5-fold higher risk of cancer than the general population.
- Urinary tract infection is the most common infection in kidney transplant recipients and usually occurs in the first year following transplantation.
- Chronic allograft nephropathy (CAN) remains the most common cause of chronic graft dysfunction, where the mainstay of treatment is calcineurin inhibitor reduction or withdrawal.

Kidney transplantation is a common and routine treatment. Over the last 20–30 years, there have been great improvements in short-term graft survival. This is explained by a number of factors, including advances in human leukocyte antigen (HLA) typing and cross-match techniques, newer immunosuppressive agents, and better methods for the prevention and treatment of early infection. Very good short-term results now mean that management emphasis is increasingly on medium- to long-term outcomes. However, the rate of attrition of "established" grafts (*graft half-life*) has not improved substantially over many years, with approximately 4% of grafts continuing to fail each year. Chronic graft dysfunction, the progressive loss of glomerular filtration rate (GFR) occurring months and years after transplantation such that most patients eventually lose their grafts, remains a major challenge for transplant clinicians. This chapter concentrates on issues that arise from 6 months after transplant onwards and considers issues in the early post-transplant period only insofar as they affect long-term management and outcome.

Graft and patient survival

The Organ Procurement and Transplantation Network/US Scientific Registry of Transplant Recipients report shows an increasing number of renal transplants performed in the United States between 1998 and 2007, with deceased donors increasing from 7898 to 10 083 and live donors increasing from 4409 to 6033. One-year graft survival has also increased during the same time from 88.8 to 91.4% for patients receiving grafts from deceased donors and 94.6 to 96.5% for those receiving grafts from live donors. One-year patient survival is also excellent at 95.9% for recipients of deceased donor kidneys and 98.7% for recipients of live donor kidneys in 2007. Long-term survival is also good, with 10-year graft survival of 43.3% and 59.3% for recipients of deceased and live donor grafts, respectively, and patient survival of 61.2% and 77.1%, respectively. Extended criteria donor graft survival is inferior, with 80.6% 1-year and 27% 10-year survival in 1998, the first year for which 10 year data is available. The largest report looking at the difference between donation after cardiac death (DCD) and donation after brain death (DBD) donors (1998–2004) showed that approximately 3% of kidneys were from DCD donors but that there was no difference in 5-year patient (81%) and graft (67%) survival rates. However, there was a difference in the

Organ Transplantation: A Clinical Guide, ed. A.A. Klein, C.J. Lewis, and J.C. Madsen. Published by Cambridge University Press.

Table 32.1 Risk factors associated with poor graft survival

Donor factors	Advanced age Hypertension Vascular disease Type (living better than cadaveric)
Peri-transplant factors	Type of cadaveric donor (cardiac death less good than brain death) Long cold ischemia time
Immune factors	High panel-reactive antibody titres Many HLA mismatches Acute rejection (some types)
Non-immune factors	Donor/recipient size/gender mismatch Recipient hypertension Poor drug compliance Drug toxicity Recurrent disease Infection – CMV, BKV

incidence of delayed graft function: 41% and 24% for DCD and DBD, respectively.

Causes of graft loss

A number of factors are correlated with poor graft outcome (Table 32.1 and Figure 32.1). With the advent of more powerful immunosuppressive medications and the expansion of the donor pool to include older donors with cardiovascular comorbidity, the impact of HLA matching on outcomes in deceased donor transplantation has diminished considerably. Advanced donor age is now the strongest predictor of poor long-term graft survival.

Death with a functioning graft

Although patient survival after transplantation is superior to that of patients who remain on dialysis, it is still inferior to that of the general population. Indeed, death with a functioning graft is the single most important cause of graft loss, accounting for up to 50% of all graft failures occurring after the first year after transplant. The most common causes of death in renal transplant recipients are premature cardiovascular disease, infection, and malignancy, all of which are exacerbated by or caused by immunosuppression.

Chronic graft dysfunction

Chronic graft dysfunction is the progressive loss of GFR beginning months or years after transplantation. It is extremely common and in most patients ultimately leads to graft failure (also see Chapter 4B). Specific causes of graft injury are listed in Table 32.2 and are discussed in detail next, but it is important to recognize that graft injury is often multi-factorial.

Injury begins prior to transplantation. The peri-transplant process results in variable acute injury dependant on the mode of patient death and degree of ischemia–reperfusion injury, which occurs on a variable background of pre-existing donor kidney disease (age, hypertension, vascular disease). The importance of such injury is emphasized by studies of living spousal donor kidneys that reveal enhanced survival compared with cadaveric transplants, despite poor HLA matching.

Graft injury continues after transplant in response to both immune and non-immune-mediated mechanisms and leads to chronic graft dysfunction, the terminology of which is confused. The most common cause is *chronic allograft nephropathy* (CAN), a term that should be applied to grafts with damage characterized by interstitial fibrous and tubular atrophy (IF/TA) identified on biopsy. The term "chronic

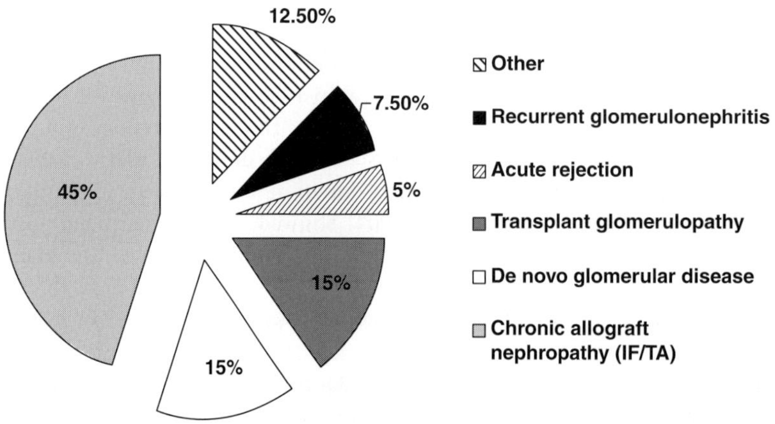

Figure 32.1 Causes of graft loss (censored for mortality).

Table 32.2 Causes of graft injury

Pretransplant factors	
Acute peri-transplant injury	Ischemia–reperfusion injury Brain death
Pre-existing donor disease	Cold ischaemia time Age-related GFR loss Hypertension Atheromatous vascular disease
Post-transplant factors	
Immune-dependent	Acute T-cell or antibody-mediated rejection Subclinical acute cellular rejection Chronic antibody-mediated rejection Transplant glomerulopathy Recurrent glomerulonephritis
Immune-independent	Recipient factors Hypertension Diabetes mellitus Renovascular disease Transplant artery stenosis Atheromatous disease Calcineurin inhibitor toxicity Urinary obstruction Urinary sepsis CMV (associated with "over-immunosuppression") BKV (associated with "over-immunosuppression")

rejection" has often been used incorrectly in this context but should be reserved for the situation in which biopsy has shown an immune-mediated cause (cell or antibody mediated) of graft injury. To further dissuade from imprecise usage of the term CAN to describe any form of chronic graft dysfunction, the 2007 Banff classification recommended that it be replaced in description of renal transplant biopsy findings with the phrase "interstitial fibrosis and tubular atrophy without evidence of specific aetiology" (IF/TA), with an emphasis on differential diagnosis from specific causes of graft injury.

Chronic allograft nephropathy

Chronic allograft nephropathy (IF/TA without evidence of specific etiology) is not a diagnosis but describes a non-specific response to graft injury that is the most common reported cause of death-censored renal allograft loss (Figure 32.1). Moderate to severe CAN (IF/TA) is present in 25% of renal transplants at 1 year and 90% by 10 years. Clinically it is characterized by progressive renal dysfunction, hypertension, and variable proteinuria. Its onset is unpredictable and the clinical course variable, reflecting the fact that CAN (IF/TA) is the common end point of many different causes of graft injury. The most important risk factors for CAN (IF/TA) are acute rejection, donor age, pre-existing donor disease, and exposure to calcineurin inhibitors (CNIs).

Transplant glomerulopathy

Transplant glomerulopathy is a specific histological lesion characterized by thickened glomerular capillary walls that have double contours, with reduplication or lamination of the glomerular basement membrane on electron microscopy. The condition can be subclinical as an isolated histological lesion, but over time is associated with progressive worsening of histopathological change and the development of CAN (IF/TA) and chronic vasculopathy. Incidence increases with time, beginning in the first year after transplant (4% of all biopsies at 1 year, increasing to 20% at 5 years). Clinical presentation is with proteinuria (often nephrotic range), hypertension, and allograft dysfunction.

There is strong evidence from animal models and clinical studies that transplant glomerulopathy is an alloimmune-mediated lesion that is strongly linked to anti-HLA class II antibodies. Donor-specific antibodies (DSAs; most commonly class II) are present in up to 75% of cases, and staining with C4d is usually (but not always) positive. Risk factors include prior sensitization, the presence of HLA antibodies (class II > class I) prior to transplantation, and acute rejection. There is a high incidence in patients undergoing desensitization protocols (see Chapter 28).

Even in the absence of significant proteinuria or graft dysfunction at diagnosis, transplant glomerulopathy is a progressive condition associated with poor outcome. In one study of patients undergoing protocol biopsy at 1 year, more than 50% of those with the condition reached a combined end point of graft loss or loss of greater than 50% GFR over the next 36 months.

Chronic antibody-mediated rejection

Chronic antibody-mediated rejection is diagnosed based on the triad of presence of circulating DSAs, positive C4d staining, and morphologic evidence of chronic tissue injury on allograft biopsy including transplant glomerulopathy (glomerular double contours), peritubular capillary basement membrane multi-layering, IF/TA, and arteriolar fibrous intimal thickening. The condition is present in 10–30% of biopsies done to evaluate chronic graft dysfunction and is associated with poor graft outcome. Risk factors include prior sensitization, DSAs (class II > class I), and the degree of HLA mismatch. The contribution of non-HLA antibodies is poorly understood.

Recurrent glomerulonephritis

Recurrent glomerulonephritis is common but does not always lead to allograft loss, with recurrent disease often following an indolent course. Overall, 10-year graft survival is similar in patients with biopsy-proven glomerulonephritis as their primary renal diagnosis as for those with other causes of renal failure, and hence glomerulonephritis is not a contraindication to transplantation in most cases. Biopsy-proven glomerulonephritis is the primary cause of graft loss in around 20% of kidney transplant recipients, with the 10-year incidence of allograft loss due to recurrent glomerulonephritis being 8.4% in one large series. Recurrence rates vary between the different types of glomerulonephritis, with primary focal segmental glomerulosclerosis (FSGS), immunoglobulin A (IgA) nephropathy, and atypical hemolytic uremic syndrome (HUS) being most likely to recur.

Focal segmental glomerulosclerosis

Primary FSGS recurs in 30–40% of renal transplants, perhaps more commonly in grafts from living donors. Recurrence usually (>80%) occurs within the first year and may happen within hours of transplantation. Risk factors include rapid progression of the primary disease to end-stage renal failure (<3 years), pediatric recipients, and recurrence in a previous renal allograft. Indeed, recurrence in a second graft is almost inevitable (>80%) in the event that a first renal allograft is lost to recurrent FSGS. Several studies have reported a variable response to plasmapheresis (up to 50%), but relapse occurs in more than half of these patients when the treatment is stopped. Others have reported success with rituximab or cyclophosphamide, but this is anecdotal (case reports and small series).

IgA nephropathy

IgA nephropathy recurs in approximately 30% of patients by 10 years after transplant, with graft loss resulting in up to 10%. The risk of recurrence is higher with a transplant from a living related donor, but this is not a strong contraindication as outcomes still compare favorably with those of cadaveric grafts. Aggressive recurrence is rare, and as with native IgA disease, there is no proven treatment, although corticosteroids and cyclophosphamide have been tried.

Atypical hemolytic uremic syndrome

Recurrence in patients who develop end-stage renal disease following diarrheal associated (D+) HUS is very uncommon. Atypical (no diarrhea; D–) HUS (aHUS) is a rare disorder caused by dysregulation of complement pathways that results in the development of thrombotic microangiopathy within the kidney. Recurrence occurs after transplantation in approximately 50% of patients with aHUS, and no intervention has been shown to be effective, with graft loss almost inevitable.

Renovascular disease

Transplant renal artery stenosis (RAS) usually presents between 3 months and 2 years after transplant, but can occur at any time. It is a relatively common and potentially curable cause of refractory hypertension and graft dysfunction, usually presenting with an asymptomatic rise in creatinine (possibly in relation to commencing an angiotensin-converting enzyme [ACE] inhibitor or an angiotensin receptor blocker [ARB]), hypertension that is difficult to treat, and/or fluid overload. The presence of a bruit is neither sensitive nor specific.

RAS usually arises close to the surgical anastomosis, but may occur more distally. It is the result of intimal scarring and hyperplasia in response to injury to the donor or recipient vessels during harvesting or transplantation. Stenoses may also occur several years after transplant as a result of development of atheromatous disease in the renal transplant artery or more proximally in the iliac vessels.

Polyomavirus associated nephropathy

Polyomaviruses (BK virus [BKV], JC virus [JCV], and SV40) are small, non-enveloped dsDNA viruses that can infect, and remain latent in, a large number of target tissues, including urothelium, becoming reactivated during states of immunosuppression. In more than 95% of cases, polyomavirus-associated nephropathy is caused by BKV, which is an emerging problem in renal transplantation, with reported incidence varying from 1–10%.

There are no known clinical risk factors that clearly identify the kidney transplant recipient who will develop BKV nephropathy. Pretransplantation seroprevalence for BKV varies from 60–80%. BKV nephropathy is more frequent in seronegative recipients of a seropositive donor kidney (BKV D+/R–), but it is not confined to this group, and BKV reactivation may come from the donor or recipient. A high overall burden of immunosuppression is a risk factor for BKV nephropathy, but there is no compelling evidence that any particular immunosuppressive agent is worse (or better) than any other.

BKV reactivation is common after renal transplantation, with viruria detected in up to 30% of patients. BKV infection can be detected by polymerase chain reaction (PCR) for BKV DNA in plasma or urine and by examination of the urine cytologically for BKV inclusion-bearing epithelial cells (decoy cells) or by electron microscopy for viral particles. These tests are sensitive for detecting active viral replication but are not specific for nephropathy. A negative BKV urine or plasma PCR excludes the diagnosis of BKV nephropathy. Quantitative PCR for BKV in plasma may be predictive for BKV nephropathy, with a threshold value (≥10 000 copies/ml) having been suggested, below which the condition is unlikely.

Biopsy remains the gold standard for diagnosis of BKV nephropathy, which causes interstitial inflammation and tubular cytopathic changes, often with visible viral inclusions. However, these changes may be patchy and isolated to the medulla and may be missed in up to one third of patients if a single core is taken; hence at least two cores should be examined. Diagnosis should be confirmed by immunohistochemical staining specific for BKV or cross-reacting SV40 large T antigen. The histological differentiation of BKV nephropathy from acute cellular rejection can be difficult, but the absence of definitive features of acute cellular rejection such as endothelialitis is helpful.

Late diagnosis of BKV nephropathy, or misdiagnosis (and treatment) as acute rejection, results in rapid loss of graft function in more than 50% of patients. Early diagnosis and timely reduction in immunosuppression has improved outcomes significantly.

Strategies to improve graft function

The multiple mechanisms of graft injury that are associated with or lead to long-term attrition (Table 32.2) mean that no single intervention is, or is likely to be, effective in preserving graft function. Most patients with progressive loss of GFR are asymptomatic and present with a rise in serum creatinine, by which time significant graft damage (IF/TA) may already have occurred. Some centers therefore advocate protocol biopsy to facilitate the early detection of IF/TA and its specific causes, but biopsy is not without hazard, and there is no evidence that this approach results in improved long-term graft outcomes. Serial measurement of GFR may make earlier detection of graft dysfunction possible.

Table 32.3 Clinical history and investigation of graft dysfunction

Clinical history – points of particular relevance
Original diagnosis and clinical course of primary renal disease
Number and severity of previous rejection episodes
Urological symptoms
Compliance with medication
Drugs Nephrotoxic agents, e.g., NSAIDs, ACE inhibitors/ARBs Drugs that raise plasma creatinine but not by reducing GFR, e.g., trimethoprim
Investigations
HLA antibody screen to look for de novo donor-specific antibody (DSA)
Current and historical calcineurin inhibitor levels
BK virus screening
Urine Microscopy Culture Urinary protein quantification Cytology
Ultrasound renal transplant
Colour Doppler renal transplant artery
Assess bladder emptying
+/– Imaging native kidneys

Any deterioration in graft function requires a thorough clinical history, examination, and investigation to exclude potentially reversible causes such as dehydration, obstruction, urinary tract infection, transplant renal artery stenosis, or BKV nephropathy (Table 32.3). If initial investigations do not reveal a cause for the loss of GFR, then renal transplant biopsy is necessary in most patients to make an accurate diagnosis, with it being particularly important to distinguish between (1) ongoing immune-mediated graft injury, which will usually require enhancement of immunosuppression; (2) CAN (IF/TA), for which the mainstay of treatment is CNI reduction or withdrawal; and (3) BKV nephropathy, for which reduction in overall immunosuppressive burden is generally required.

Management of chronic allograft nephropathy (IF/TA)

There is no consensus regarding the best management of CAN (IF/TA). The differential diagnosis between CNI-related nephrotoxicity and other causes of renal graft injury remains very difficult. Histological lesions considered relatively specific for CNI toxicity (see above) can occur through other processes, and there is considerable inter- and intra-observer variability in the histological scoring of renal transplant biopsies. Despite these difficulties, in the absence of any evidence of ongoing immune-mediated graft injury, CNI toxicity remains the major modifiable factor for progressive CAN (IF/TA).

Immunosuppressive regimens that avoid CNI use completely are generally regarded as being associated with an unacceptable risk of acute rejection. Recent efforts have therefore focused on devising regimens that minimize CNI exposure, either by substitution with a mammalian target of rapamycin (mTOR) inhibitor or maintenance on prednisolone and an anti-metabolite alone (usually mycophenolate mofetil [MMF] if tolerated at a therapeutic dose). Although there are many uncontrolled studies in this area, there are few randomized controlled trials, and none have focused on longer-term graft outcomes. Some data suggest that tacrolimus (TAC) may be less nephrotoxic than cyclophosphamide (CyA), but long-term outcome data are lacking.

CNI reduction and withdrawal

The main risk of CNI withdrawal is acute rejection. A meta-analysis of 13 studies of CNI withdrawal and subsequent maintenance on an anti-metabolite and prednisolone showed that the excess risk of acute rejection is around 10% when CyA is withdrawn from an azathioprine (AZA)-based regimen. This caused great concern, but subsequent long-term data revealed a trend toward improved graft survival in patients weaned from CyA (relative risk [RR] for graft failure = 0.92). Nevertheless, concern regarding acute rejection has meant that maintenance therapy with AZA and steroids is not routine practice, although it may be a good option in some cases of CAN (IF/TA).

Box 32.1 Recommendations for CNI withdrawal

Patient > 6–12 months post-transplant
No evidence of current immune-mediated acute or chronic graft injury on renal transplant biopsy
Able to tolerate a therapeutic dose of anti-metabolite
- Mycophenolate mofetil 2 g daily or mycophenolate sodium 1440 mg daily
- Azathioprine (1.5–2 mg/kg per day)

Start prednisolone 10 mg once daily if not on corticosteroids
Reduce cyclosporine dose by 30–50% every 2–4 weeks
Increased graft surveillance until CNI withdrawal is complete

MMF has replaced AZA in routine protocols in many centers over the last decade. However, despite the widely held prejudice that it is a more effective immunosuppressant than AZA, CyA withdrawal in patients receiving CyA, MMF, and corticosteroids is also associated with an increase in acute rejection, up to 10% of cases in some studies. This is balanced by stabilization of, or improvement in, short-term graft function and a trend toward a sustained improvement in graft function at 5 years. There are little data on TAC withdrawal, but similar principals probably apply. Due to these concerns regarding the safety of CNI-free immunosuppression, recent studies have looked at minimizing CNI exposure in combination with interleukin-2 (IL-2) antibody induction, MMF, and steroids. This strategy seems safe and effective in the short term, but long-term outcome data are needed.

Practical details of how to withdraw CNIs are given in Box 32.1. Such withdrawal has an additional benefit in that it may also reduce hypertension and dyslipidemia.

Several early studies reported that replacement of CNI with sirolimus (SRL) in patients with CAN resulted in short-term improvement or stabilization of graft function in most cases, although many could not tolerate the new drug, and discontinuation rates were high. However, it is now clear that SRL is not the hoped for panacea. In many studies it has been shown that switching to SRL produces poor outcomes in patients with significant proteinuria. Recent data from a large randomized controlled trial (the CONVERT Trial) did not show a significant improvement in GFR after SRL conversion. A subset of patients with well-preserved

Box 32.2 Recommendations for CNI conversion to an mTOR inhibitor

No evidence of current immune-mediated acute or chronic graft injury on renal transplant biopsy
No significant proteinuria
Malignancy
Start prednisolone 10 mg once daily if not on corticosteroids

graft function (GFR > 40 ml/min) and normal urinary protein excretion did show a modest benefit, but patients with GFR less than 40 ml/min tolerated conversion to SRL poorly, with an unacceptable number of treatment-related adverse events. There is now consensus that waiting until there is advanced permanent graft damage is associated with poor outcomes after conversion to SRL, but it seems reasonable to consider conversion in patients with early CAN (IF/TA) and without significant proteinuria (Box 32.2). The occurrence of post-transplant malignancy provides a further rationale for switching.

Use of novel immunosuppressive agents

It is hoped that novel non-nephrotoxic immunosuppressive agents may offer better options for CNI-free induction and maintenance regimens in the future, but many initially promising possibilities have not delivered. Recent studies using costimulatory blockade with belatacept in combination with MMF showed results that have encouraged some, but a significant excess of post-transplant lymphoproliferative disorder (PTLD) indicates that a substantial note of caution is in order.

Management of chronic antibody-mediated rejection and/or transplant glomerulopathy

There are no data from randomized controlled trials (RCTs) that any specific therapy improves long-term outcome when renal transplant biopsy shows chronic antibody mediated rejection and/or transplant glomerulopathy. Some studies have reported success with conversion to TAC- and MMF-based regimens. Other strategies involve antibody removal (plasmapheresis), intravenous immunoglobulin, and rituximab.

Screening for and management of polyoma virus–associated nephropathy

Many centers now advocate screening, by urine cytology or BKV PCR (plasma or urine), for the first 2 years after transplantation. This allows the early identification of patients with BKV reactivation who are at risk of developing BKV nephropathy and timely intervention by preemptive reduction in immunosuppression before irreversible parenchymal damage (IF/TA) occurs. Various strategies have been employed, with one approach being to withdraw the anti-metabolite and to minimize steroid dose in recipients on a standard CNI-based triple therapy regimen.

There are observational data that cidofovir and the fluoroquinolones may improve viral clearance, and both have been shown to have anti-BKV activity in vitro, but there is no strong evidence that they offer any advantage above reduction in immunosuppression alone. Intravenous IgG has also been used to treat BKV nephropathy. Given its immunomodulatory effects, as well as anti-BKV properties, this might offer benefit in patients with concurrent acute rejection, but because of its cost and unproven efficacy, intravenous IgG should not be used routinely.

The main risk of reducing immunosuppression is acute rejection, but failure to clear virus leads to poor graft function and outcome. Close monitoring of viral titers and graft function is essential. It may take several weeks for BK-virus specific immunity to recover, during which time viremia persists and renal injury may continue to accumulate. Following reduction in immunosuppression, if BKV titres do not fall, further reduction in immunosuppression may be required, and further biopsy is indicated to exclude rejection (or other pathology) if graft function worsens. Repeat imaging to exclude obstruction is also sensible in this context because BKV has been associated with the development of ureteric stricture.

Other long-term issues

Adherence to treatment

Non-adherence is common and is often overlooked in the busy transplant clinic. Studies have estimated up to 50% of transplant patients may be non-adherent at some time; the spectrum of behaviors ranges from the occasional missed dose to consistently missing

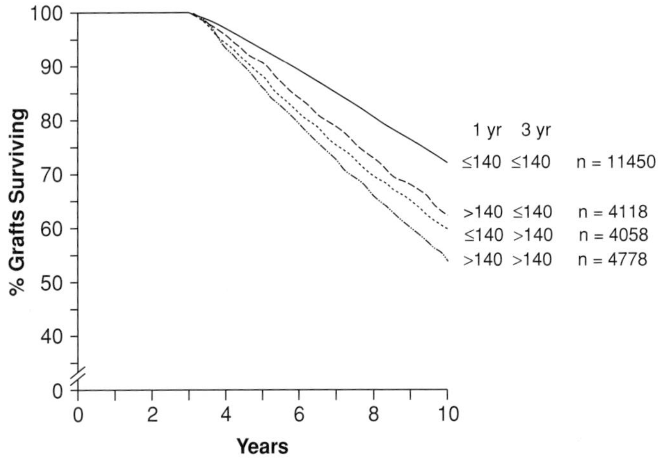

Figure 32.2 Kidney transplant survival from 3–10 years in relation to systolic blood pressure at 1 and 3 years post-transplant. The respective 1- and 3-year pressures are indicated to the right of each curve, together with the number of patients (n) studied.

all medication doses. Decreased adherence is associated with acute rejection and a seven-fold overall risk of allograft loss and is thought to precede up to one third of allograft failures, particularly late allograft losses. Non-adherence is often non-intentional. Common barriers include simple forgetfulness, the complexity of immunosuppressive regimens, problems with filling prescriptions (including cost in many countries), and lifestyle factors. Improved communication and a clear understanding of the patient's perspective are important in identifying a solution. Intentional non-adherence, where the patient does not want to take their medication, is more difficult to address. Again, it is very important to gain the patient's perspective. Drug-related side effects, the patient's own beliefs regarding their medications, and peer pressure (particularly among adolescents) are all important factors.

Anti-proteinuric measures

Proteinuria is common after renal transplantation (45% of cases at 1 year) and is typically low grade ($\leq$500 mg/d in two thirds of cases). It is an important marker of graft injury: there is a strong association between proteinuria and reduced graft survival, with the level of proteinuria further stratifying this risk – 3.9% of recipients with proteinuria less than 150 mg/d 1 year post-transplant will have lost their graft by 5 years, compared with 41.2% with proteinuria greater than 3000 mg/d. Given this, it seems reasonable that anti-proteinuric measures are applied rigorously. These include the use of the maximum tolerable dose of an ACE inhibitor and/or ARB, but it must be admitted that there are no firm data to say that such treatment alters allograft survival.

Prevention of cardiovascular morbidity and mortality

The incidence of cardiovascular disease is very high after kidney transplantation, with the annual rate of fatal or non-fatal cardiovascular events being 3.5–5.0%, much higher than that of the general population. Strategies to reduce cardiovascular risk focus on minimizing time on dialysis, prevention and aggressive treatment of traditional cardiovascular risk factors (hypertension, diabetes mellitus, dyslipidemia, discouragement of smoking), and preservation of graft function.

Management of hypertension

Hypertension is extremely common in renal transplant recipients, with prevalence 50–90% in various studies. It remains an independent risk factor for cardiovascular events after transplantation and is associated with reduced graft survival (Figure 32.2). However, there have been no RCTs in renal transplant recipients to determine whether blood pressure lowering improves graft survival, and if so, what blood pressure should be targeted. Nevertheless, in view of the potential benefits to both patient and graft survival, the general consensus is that hypertension should be treated aggressively, and most transplant physicians target a blood pressure of less than 130/80 mmHg as recommended for other populations of high-risk patients.

Table 32.4 Causes of post-transplant hypertension

Drugs – CNI, corticosteroids
Kidney allograft dysfunction
Renovascular Transplant renal artery stenosis Atheromatous arterial disease proximal to the allograft artery anastomosis
Factors relating to native kidneys

There are many reasons why renal transplant recipients have hypertension (Table 32.4). When the blood pressure is difficult to control, and particularly when it is associated with unexplained graft dysfunction, or there is more than 20% decline in renal function after introduction of an ACE inhibitor or ARB, patients should be screened for transplant RAS.

Color Doppler ultrasonography is a non-invasive method of diagnosing transplant RAS (87–94% sensitivity, 86–100% specificity), but is very dependent on the skill and experience of the operator. Magnetic resonance angiography is non-invasive and very sensitive, but gadolinium cannot be used in the many patients with a GFR less than 30 ml/min because of the risk of nephrogenic sclerosing fibrosis. Angiography remains the gold standard, but is invasive and should be reserved for patients with positive screening investigations or in whom there is a strong clinical suspicion despite negative ultrasound Doppler. Local complications include groin hematoma and pseudo aneurysm formation. There is a risk of contrast-induced nephrotoxicity, and cholesterol embolic disease has been reported.

Percutaneous transluminal angioplasty is the treatment of choice for most patients with a hemodynamically significant transplant RAS. Re-stenosis is common (30%) and may be treated by repeat angioplasty with or without stenting. Drug-eluting stents may offer an advantage in the prevention of re-stenosis, but their use in peripheral vascular disease has been disappointing, and there are very little data on their use in the treatment of transplant RAS. Surgery may be required for patients with stenoses who are unsuitable for angioplasty, or in whom angioplasty has been unsuccessful.

Aside from the specific matter of transplant RAS, all patients should be given advice on lifestyle modifications (relating to low-salt diet, exercise, alcohol intake, and weight loss), which can produce small but beneficial effects on blood pressure. With regard to antihypertensive drugs, there is insufficient evidence to strongly recommend any particular class of anti–hypertensive. Our practice is to follow guidelines for the general adult population (e.g., British Hypertension Society Guidelines), taking into account post-transplant complications and relevant comorbid factors (Table 32.5).

Table 32.5 Use of common anti-hypertensive agents in kidney transplant recipients

Agent/class	Advantages/indications common in kidney transplant recipients	Disadvantages/contraindications common in kidney transplant recipients
Angiotensin-converting enzyme inhibitors (ACEi)/angiotensin receptor blockers (ARBs)	Proteinuria Heart failure with systolic dysfunction Post-myocardial infarction Transplant erythrocytosis	Hyperkalemia Anaemia Transplant renal artery stenosis
Calcium channel blockers	Chronic stable angina Increased CNI levels (allow reduction in dose/cost)	Edema Gum hypertrophy (some agents) Increase CNI levels (if not anticipated)
Thiazide diuretics	Heart failure with systolic dysfunction Hyperkalemia Edema	Hyperuricemia – gout Dyslipidemia Impaired glucose tolerance Hyponatremia
Beta-blockers	Heart failure with systolic dysfunction* Chronic stable angina Post myocardial infarction	Hyperkalemia Dyslipidemia Impaired glucose tolerance
Alpha-blockers	Bladder outflow obstruction	Edema Postural hypotension

CNI, calcineurin inhibitor (e.g. cyclosporine, tacrolimus)
*Carvedilol, bisoprolol, metoprolol.

Table 32.6 Risk factors for the development of new-onset diabetes after transplantation (NODAT)

Pretransplant
Obesity
Ethnicity (African American or Hispanic)
Age (>60 years)
Family history of type 2 diabetes
Hepatitis C virus and CMV disease
Impaired fasting glucose
Post-transplant
Immunosuppression (in order of diabetic potential) Corticosteroids Tacrolimus Cyclosporine Sirolimus
Post-transplant weight gain

CMV: cytomegalovirus.

Pretransplant diabetes

Even though the survival benefits seen after transplantation are greater among patients with diabetes than those without, both patient and graft survival are worse in diabetic than non-diabetic renal transplant recipients (5-year post-transplant patient survival of approximately 70% versus 90–95%). This is a major issue given that diabetes is the cause of end-stage renal disease in 15% of renal transplant recipients and that type 2 diabetes is increasingly present as a comorbid condition as the average age of patients on the transplant waiting list rises. The excess mortality in diabetic patients is almost entirely as a result of cardiovascular deaths, although infective causes are also more common.

New-onset diabetes after transplantation

New onset diabetes after transplantation (NODAT) is common, with incidence in the first year after transplant reported in the range 5–20% and US registry data recently declaring a prevalence of 41% at 3 years post-transplantation. This is an important matter because, despite its short duration, NODAT is associated with reduced long-term graft survival (RR graft failure = 1.63) and increased cardiovascular mortality (RR death = 1.87).

NODAT is caused by insufficient insulin release in response to an increase in insulin resistance. Risk factors are listed in Table 32.6. Lifestyle modification aimed at increasing exercise and avoiding post-transplant weight gain can be helpful, but immunosuppression is the major and obviously modifiable issue. It has been hard to quantify the relative risks of different immunosuppressants on the development of NODAT; RCTs have used varying definitions of the condition, with widely different immunosuppressive regimens and doses of particular immunosuppressants.

One strategy to reduce the incidence of NODAT is to transplant patients without using steroids. However, as discussed previously in the context of management of CNI toxicity and BKV nephropathy, the clear risk of reducing overall immunosuppression is acute rejection. Some (but not all) studies of early (within 3 months) or late steroid withdrawal from CyA-based regimens have reported an unacceptable risk of this condition. By contrast, steroid-free immunosuppression (or early steroid withdrawal) in conjunction with TAC, MMF, and antibody induction (both IL-2 blocking and T-cell depleting) seems safe in low immunological risk recipients. If NODAT is diagnosed, then in the absence of rejection, it may be reasonable to modify immunosuppression. The strategy most often used is rapid steroid reduction and conversion from TAC to CyA.

Regarding targets for glycemic control, standard practice is to aim for the same as in the non-transplant population (HbA1C <7%) using a standard approach. All of the standard dietary, oral hypoglycemic, and insulin treatments can be employed, excepting that as for other patients with chronic kidney disease, metformin (or other biguanides) should not be given to renal transplant recipients with estimated GFR (eGFR)less than 30 ml/min.

Management of dyslipidemia

Many renal transplant recipients have dyslipidemia, often caused or exacerbated by impairment of renal function and immunosuppressive medications. Based on the fact that such patients are at very high cardiovascular risk, it is generally accepted that modifiable risk factors such as dyslipidaemia should be treated aggressively, although there is no RCT evidence of benefit in hard clinical end points in the renal transplant population. Aside from dietary intervention and lifestyle modifications, the drugs most commonly employed (as in other patient groups) for elevated low-density lipoprotein cholesterol levels (>2.6 mmol/l) are the statins, but there is concern

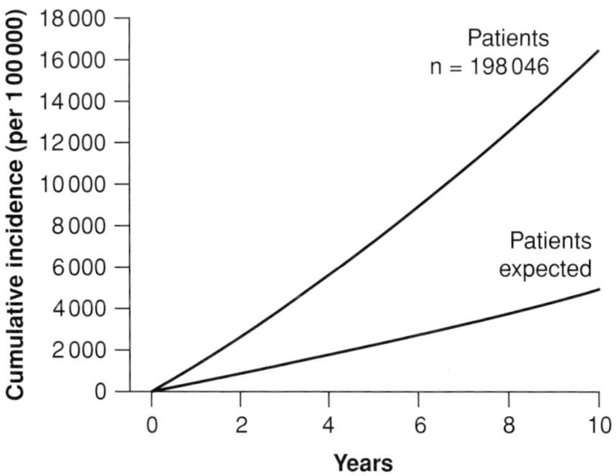

Figure 32.3 Incidence of all types of malignant tumors in cadaveric renal transplant recipients compared with the expected incidence in the general population.

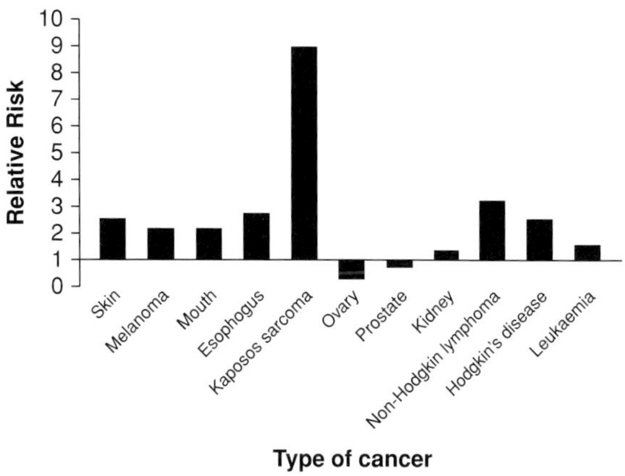

Figure 32.4 Relative risk of cancer in renal transplant recipients compared with patients on the waiting list.

regarding the high incidence of clinically significant myopathy when these are used concurrently with CyA, which increases the blood levels of all statins regardless of their pathway of metabolism.

Significant elevation of serum triglycerides (> 5.65 mmol/l) that persists despite lifestyle modifications and treatment of secondary causes is usually treated with ezetimibe. Nicotinic acid can be used as an alternative, but fibrates are generally avoided due to risk of myositis/rhabdomyolysis.

Malignancies (see also Chapter 4A)

Renal transplant recipients are at 3–5 fold higher risk of cancer than the general population (Figure 32.3), and the cancers that they develop are often more aggressive, with poor survival. However, the situation varies greatly for different types of cancer: some common cancers (including breast and prostate) do not occur more frequently; non-melanoma skin cancer and PTLD are particularly common (Figure 32.4).

Women with renal transplants should be offered and encouraged to accept regular breast and cervical screening. All renal transplant recipients will have urinalysis performed as part of regular clinic monitoring: the development of new hematuria should trigger investigation of the urinary tract because of the increased risk of renal cell cancer in the native kidneys (often with acquired cystic disease) and of bladder cancer. Screening for skin malignancy is also required.

The cumulative risk of non-melanoma skin cancer after renal transplantation is 2.3% at 1 year and 7.4% at 3 years, with very high rates (> 50%) reported after long-term follow-up of patients in sunny parts of the world. Treatment is by local excision.

PTLD

PTLD is driven by Epstein-Barr virus present in latent form in B lymphocytes. It occurs in 1–2% of renal transplant recipients, most often presenting with lymphadenopathy, graft infiltration, and central nervous system or gut involvement. The usual initial management is by step-wise reduction of immunosuppression, which requires close monitoring but is effective in more than 50% of cases, with standard chemotherapy (often combined with rituximab) used if this does not lead to the desired response. See Chapter 4A for further details.

Management of immunosuppression in the patient with malignancy

Malignancy arising in a renal transplant recipient should generally be treated in the same manner as it would be in any other patient with comparable renal function. However, given that therapeutic (regarding the transplant) immunosuppression may have played some role in inducing the malignancy, the issue of whether or not the patient's transplant immunosuppressive regimen should be altered should be considered. There is a difficult balance to be struck here: from the point of view of treating the malignancy, complete withdrawal of immunosuppression would be best, yet this would inevitably lead to rejection and loss of the renal transplant, which is something that few patients would wish to consider in any circumstances. Data on which to base rational decisions is sparse. Most patients and most transplant physicians will attempt to find a compromise where immunosuppression is reduced but not withdrawn, with close monitoring of transplant function. In tumors that are clearly caused or exacerbated by immunosuppressive drugs, there is a very strong rationale for doing this, and as previously discussed, this strategy is well established for the management of post-transplant lymphoproliferative disorder. For solid organ tumours without a clear viral aetiology, the rationale is less clear and any changes need to balance the risks of the tumor versus the risk of graft loss and quality of life on dialysis.

Aside from simply reducing immunosuppression, there are theoretical grounds for thinking that switching to an mTORi (e.g., sirolimus, as discussed in the management of CAN) may be helpful in a patient with malignancy because these agents have both antiproliferative and immunosuppressive properties. Data from registries and randomized trials has shown the incidence of *de novo* post-transplantation malignancy is lower in sirolimus treated patients, but their role when malignancy has occurred is less clear. Data from small trials and case reports suggests that early conversion to mTORi is beneficial in non-melanoma skin cancer, Kaposi's sarcoma, and renal cell carcinoma, but the difficulty of switching to a drug that many patients find difficult to tolerate because of side effects should not be underestimated.

Infectious diseases

Urinary tract infection

Urinary tract infection (UTI) is the most common infection in kidney transplant recipients. Most occur in the first year following transplantation. Analysis of the US Renal Data System database has shown that late UTI (>6 months after transplantation) is associated with poor renal allograft survival and increased mortality.

Escherichia coli is the most common uropathogen in renal transplant patients; *Enterococcus* species, *Pseudomonas*, coagulase-negative staphylococci, *Enterobacter*, and other organisms (group B streptococci and *Gardnerella vaginalis*) also occur. Antibiotics should be given for 7–14 days, and an anatomical cause (vesico-ureteral reflux, neurogenic bladder, bladder outflow obstruction) should be excluded in any patient with relapsing (recurrent) UTI. Asymptomatic bacteriuria is common, but there is no consensus regarding whether this should be treated, and in one study, treatment did not prevent symptomatic UTI.

Other infections

Acute surgical issues have resolved by 6 months after transplant. Most patients are well and have returned to normal activities, and their immunosuppression has been minimized to that required for long-term maintenance. Most infections occurring beyond this point are typical community-acquired infections and, aside from UTIs, include upper and lower respiratory tract infection (viral or bacterial) and gastroenteritis (usually viral). However, atypical or opportunistic infections are more common than in the general population and should be sought if the clinical picture is not obvious and/or initial treatment is unsuccessful. These are discussed in Chapter 4C.

Transplant bone disease

Bone disease in renal transplant patients is complex: many patients have pre-existing chronic kidney disease–mineral bone disease (CKD-MBD; which may persist after transplantation), osteoporosis, or previous parathyroidectomy. Renal transplant patients are at high risk of fracture, but it is not proven that low bone mineral density (BMD) or a loss of BMD predicts this as it does in the general population; indeed, it is known it does not predict fracture risk in patients with stage 4–5 CKD. Unfortunately, there are no good data looking at the effect of bone-specific therapy on patient-level outcomes (mortality or fracture risk) in renal transplant patients.

In patients with relatively good renal function (eGFR > 30 ml/min), it is reasonable to check BMD regularly and offer appropriate treatment to those in whom this is low. This might be with vitamin D, active analogues of vitamin D, and/or a bisphosphonate depending on the presence of CKD-MBD as indicated by levels of parathyroid hormone, calcium, phosphate, alkaline phosphatase, and vitamin D.

Specific side effects of particular immunosuppressants

Aside from the notable general side effects of immunosuppression, most importantly including susceptibility to some malignancies and some infections (as discussed above), long-term transplant recipients frequently suffer side effects specific to particular immunosuppressants.

Steroids are especially problematic: most of their complications arise and become clinically apparent within the first 6 months, but those that commonly declare themselves clinically later than this include osteoporosis, avascular necrosis of bone, tendon ruptures, and cataracts.

Aside from nephrotoxicity and diabetes (as discussed above), complications of CNIs that often arise or progress after 6 months include hyperuricemia/gout, distal limb pain, neurotoxicity, and (with CyA) coarsening of facial features, gum hypertrophy, and hypertrichosis. Longer term side effects of AZA and MMF include marrow suppression, and (with AZA) alopecia.

Chronic kidney disease

Most renal transplant recipients have stage 3 CKD, meaning an eGFR of between 30 and 60 ml/min, and most, for reasons discussed above, can expect this to decline to stage 4 CKD (eGFR 15–30 ml/min) and stage 5 CKD (eGFR < 15 ml/min) over years. They will therefore require diagnosis and management of the complications of CKD, in particular of renal mineral and bone disorder and of renal anemia. Discussion of these is outside the scope of this chapter, and the reader seeking information should consult a general nephrology resource.

Pregnancy

Women with advanced chronic renal failure and/or receiving dialysis are rarely able to conceive and produce a live birth, hence for many such women a significant reason for wanting a transplant is the desire to have children. The risks of pregnancy and childbirth to both mother and child are higher in renal transplant recipients than in women without medical problems, but pregnancy is usually successful in women with stable, satisfactory renal transplant function, and considerations of pregnancy are a routine part of long-term management.

Factors affecting pregnancy outcome

Standard advice is that women wishing to conceive should have stable and satisfactory renal function and wait at least 1 year after transplantation before attempting to conceive, which takes them beyond the period of greatest risk of acute rejection and viral infection. Regarding women with CKD of any sort, the chances of a successful outcome to pregnancy reduce with increasing impairment of renal function. The transplant kidney is not affected by nor is it a contraindication to a vaginal delivery. Deliveries are more likely to be by Cesarean section, but this is due to medical indications.

Medical management before and during pregnancy

Aside from general measures appropriate to all pregnant women (e.g., encouragement to stop smoking, folic acid supplementation), the most important requirement is for careful review of the patient's medications. Prednisolone (<15 mg/d), AZA, CyA, and TAC are thought to be safe in pregnancy, but MMF (early pregnancy loss; severe structural abnormalities including hydrocephaly, cleft lip and palate, microtia, and absence of external auditory canals) and SRL (teratogenic in animal studies; very little clinical experience) are not.

Further reading

Augustine JJ, Hricik DE. Steroid sparing in kidney transplantation: changing paradigms, improving outcomes, and remaining questions. *Clin J Am Soc Nephrol* 2006; **1**: 1080–9.

El-Amm JM, Haririan A, Crook ED. The effects of blood pressure and lipid control on kidney allograft outcome. *Am J Cardiovasc Drugs* 2006; **6**: 1–7.

Golshayan D, Pascual M. Minimization of calcineurin inhibitors to improve long-term outcomes in kidney transplantation. *Transpl Immunol* 2008; **20**: 21–8.

Yarlagadda SG, Klein CL, Jani A. Long-term renal outcomes after delayed graft function. *Adv Chronic Kidney Dis* 2008; **15**: 248–56.

Zachariah MS, Tornatore KM, Venuto RC. Kidney transplantation and pregnancy. *Curr Opin Organ Transplant* 2009; **14**: 386–9.

Chapter 33

Pediatric kidney transplantation

Khashayar Vakili and Heung Bae Kim

Key points

- Kidney transplantation has become the treatment of choice for pediatric patients with end-stage renal disease.
- Transplantation has been shown to provide improved long-term survival compared with dialysis as well as improved growth and development in children.
- Advances in immunosuppression medications, surgical technique, and postoperative care continue to improve graft and patient survival rates.
- Disease recurrence, chronic allograft nephropathy, and complications of immunosuppression remain significant causes of morbidity and mortality in children following renal transplantation.

Pediatric end-stage renal disease (ESRD) requires renal replacement therapy by either dialysis or kidney transplantation. Most patients will transition between these two modalities at least once during their lifetimes. The decision to institute renal replacement therapy is based on the presence of complications that include fluid overload, electrolyte disturbances, symptomatic uremia, failure to thrive, metabolic bone disease, and psychomotor developmental delay. In the majority of instances, the initiation of hemodialysis or peritoneal dialysis precedes renal transplantation. However, in the absence of contraindications, kidney transplantation is the treatment of choice for children with ESRD, as it provides numerous benefits when compared with long-term dialysis. These benefits include decreased morbidity and mortality, improvements in quality of life, and improvements in growth and development.

Pediatric kidney transplantation requires a dedicated team of specialists including pediatric nephrologists, transplant surgeons, pediatric urologists, transplant coordinators, dialysis personnel, nutritionists, pharmacists, social workers, psychologists, infectious disease specialists, and others. This multi-disciplinary approach to the care of these patients is critical in achieving long-term graft and patient survival. Although there are some similarities between adult and pediatric kidney transplantation, there are many aspects of the medical and surgical care of the pediatric transplant patients that are somewhat unique and are the focus of this chapter.

Much of the data presented in this chapter are based on the North American Pediatric Renal Trials and Collaborative Studies (NAPRTCS), which has collected data since 1987 on about 17 000 children with ESRD and about 10 000 children with renal transplants.

Indications and contraindications for renal transplantation

Chronic kidney disease (CKD) is defined as kidney damage based on pathological abnormalities or markers of dysfunction in urine or blood and is the same as adult staging of CKD. Renal replacement therapy is indicated for patients who progress to stage 5 CKD.

Diseases leading to ESRD in children differ significantly from those in adults. The primary diagnoses and demographics for pediatric patients undergoing renal transplantation in 2008 are shown in Table 33.1. The majority of ESRD cases in infants and young children are a result of congenital or inherited disorders, whereas acquired renal disease is more prevalent in older children and young adults. The etiology of ESRD has an important impact on the preparation

Organ Transplantation: A Clinical Guide, ed. A.A. Klein, C.J. Lewis, and J.C. Madsen. Published by Cambridge University Press.

Table 33.1 Diagnoses and demographics of pediatric patients undergoing renal transplantation

Primary diagnosis	%
Aplasia/hypoplasia/dysplasia	15.9
Obstructive uropathy	15.6
Focal segmental glomerulosclerosis	11.7
Reflux nephropathy	5.2
Chronic glomerulonephritis	3.3
Polycystic disease	2.9
Medullary cystic disease	2.8
Hemolytic uremic syndrome	2.6
Prune belly	2.6
Congenital nephrotic syndrome	2.6
Familial nephritis	2.3
Cystinosis	2.0
Pyelo/interstitial nephritis	1.8
Membranoproliferative glomerulonephritis type I	1.7
Idiopathic crescentic glomerulonephritis	1.7
Systemic lupus erythematosus nephritis	1.5
Renal infarct	1.4
Berger's (IgA) nephritis	1.3
Henoch-Schönlein nephritis	1.1
Membranoproliferative glomerulonephritis type II	0.8
Wegener's granulomatosis	0.6
Wilms' tumor	0.5
Drash syndrome	0.5
Oxalosis	0.5
Membranous nephropathy	0.4
Other systemic immunologic disease	0.3
Sickle cell nephropathy	0.2
Diabetic glomerulonephritis	0.1
Other	9.8
Unknown	6.2
Gender	
Male	59.4
Female	40.6
Race	
White	59.8
Black	16.9
Hispanic	16.7
Other	6.6

Based on data from North American Pediatric Renal Trials and Collaborative Studies (NAPRTCS).

of the patient for transplantation, postoperative management, and overall graft survival. For example, patients with obstructive uropathy may require pretransplant bladder reconstruction to allow for adequate graft drainage following transplant. Failure to adequately prepare the bladder can result in early graft loss. Diagnoses with a significant recurrence rate such as focal segmental glomerulosclerosis (FSGS) or atypical hemolytic uremic syndrome (HUS) may require special protocols to decrease the risk of disease recurrence. In extreme cases such as type 1 primary hyperoxaluria, simultaneous liver transplantation may be required to prevent recurrence of the primary disease.

Some contraindications to transplantation include presence of metastatic malignancy, active infection with hepatitis B, severe multi-organ failure, positive direct cross-match, or irreversible debilitating brain injury. In approaching a patient following complete resection for malignancy, the long-term probability of tumor-free survival is the main determining factor in proceeding with kidney transplantation. For example, many centers allow for a 1-year recurrence-free period following resection of a bilateral Wilms' tumor before planning kidney transplantation. Relative contraindications include ABO incompatibility, previous positive direct cross-match, active autoimmune disease (lupus erythematosus, anti-glomerular basement membrane), human immunodeficiency virus (HIV) infection, psychomotor or psychiatric illness necessitating custodial care, chronic hepatitis C virus (HCV) infection, significant history of non-compliance, or lack of family support or adequate home supervision.

Preoperative management and evaluation

Kidney transplantation should be performed after a thorough work-up and preparation of the patient as well as the family. Allowing adequate time for correction of nutritional deficits and metabolic derangements are vital to minimizing post-transplant complications. In addition, because the majority of pediatric patients receive adult-size kidneys, the size of the child has to be suitable to accept an adult-size kidney. This generally is of concern in infants weighing less than 6.5 kg or with a length of less than 65 cm. As a result, renal transplantation in infants less than 1 year of age is not common. Whenever possible, infants should be supported with dialysis until they grow to an appropriate size for transplantation.

In the majority of cases, pediatric kidney transplantation is performed once a patient has developed ESRD and is on maintenance dialysis. However, about 25% of children undergo preemptive transplantation, with the highest rate in the 6–12-year-old age group. Preemptive transplantation is thought to have many potential benefits, including avoidance of dialysis and improvement in growth and development.

A thorough multi-disciplinary evaluation is necessary prior to renal transplantation. The recipient is generally evaluated by a nephrologist, transplant surgeon, urologist, transplant nurse coordinator, social worker, psychologist, dietician, and pharmacist. A history and physical examination should be performed, with special emphasis on identification of associated anomalies for children with congenital renal anomalies. The size and shape of the recipient's abdomen and prior abdominal operations are used as a guide to select the most suitable position for the kidney allograft. From a surgical standpoint, particular attention should be paid to the quality of the femoral pulses. A history of femoral venous catheters, abnormalities on examination, or pelvic malformations should prompt a radiographic evaluation (ultrasound, computed tomography [CT] or magnetic resonance imaging [MRI]) of the abdominal arterial and venous vasculature. Standard laboratory tests include complete blood count, electrolytes, urea, creatinine, coagulation parameters, liver function tests, and panel reactive antibodies. Urine should be analyzed and cultured. Cardiac and pulmonary evaluation should include chest X-ray, electrocardiogram, pulmonary function tests, and echocardiogram when indicated. Serologic tests should be performed, including cytomegalovirus (CMV); Epstein-Barr virus (EBV); HIV; toxoplasmosis; hepatitis B virus (HBV); HCV; measles, mumps, rubella (MMR); varicella zoster virus (VZV); and herpes simplex virus (HSV). Patients should have up-to-date vaccinations, including HBV, tetanus, hemophilus influenza type b, polio, MMR, VCV, pneumococcal vaccine, influenza, and hepatitis A virus prior to transplantation if at all possible. The use of immunosuppression medications after transplantation may blunt the appropriate response to killed vaccines and preclude the use of live-virus vaccines. Any live-virus vaccines should be given at least 4 weeks prior to transplantation.

In contrast to the adult population, lower urinary tract anomalies in children with renal failure are quite common. Common diagnoses associated with lower urinary tract anomalies include vesicoureteral reflux, posterior urethral valves, neurogenic bladder, Prune belly syndrome, and bladder or cloacal exstrophy. Based on the NAPRTCS report, about 25% of pediatric kidney transplant recipients have lower urinary tract anomalies. The goal of the pre-transplant urologic evaluation is to ensure the establishment of a suitable urinary conduit with the aim of minimizing the future risk of injury to the kidney allograft. Pretransplant work-up may include determination of urinary flow rate, post-void residual volume, cystoscopy, urodynamics, or voiding cystourethrogram.

Bladder pressures over 40 cmH_2O have been shown to result in allograft damage following kidney transplantation. Pretransplant strategies to decrease bladder pressure may include the use of anticholinergics and intermittent catheterization, which may be used in patients with high post-void residuals. These strategies will also need to be continued after transplantation. In some cases, the bladder cannot be adequately assessed due to oliguria or diversion. Reconstruction of the urinary tract in patients with functional kidneys prior to transplantation will allow cycling of the bladder. If the urinary tract is not in continuity with the bladder, intermittent catheterization may be used for bladder cycling. Despite the above strategies, sometimes the bladder will continue to be inadequate in size and function and the patient will therefore require urinary reconstruction. Patients with inadequate bladder capacity will benefit from augmentation with small intestine, colon, or stomach. Gastric remnants can result in loss of acid in urine and result in metabolic alkalosis. In most cases, the bladder reconstruction is performed prior to transplantation.

Overall, about 60% of the kidney grafts are from living donors with the parents comprising the majority (81%) of the living donors. The remainder of children receive kidneys from either donation after brain death (DBD) or donation after cardiac death (DCD) donors. DBD donors yield higher quality grafts and therefore constitute the majority of pediatric deceased kidney donors. The use of DCD donors for pediatric patients has become more controversial given the recent changes in the allocation system, which allow for pediatric patients to be preferentially allocated kidneys from younger deceased donors (under age 35).

Grafts from living donors tend to have shorter ischemic times and a higher 5-year graft survival (85%) compared with deceased donor grafts (80%). One obvious disadvantage of living donors is the risk to the

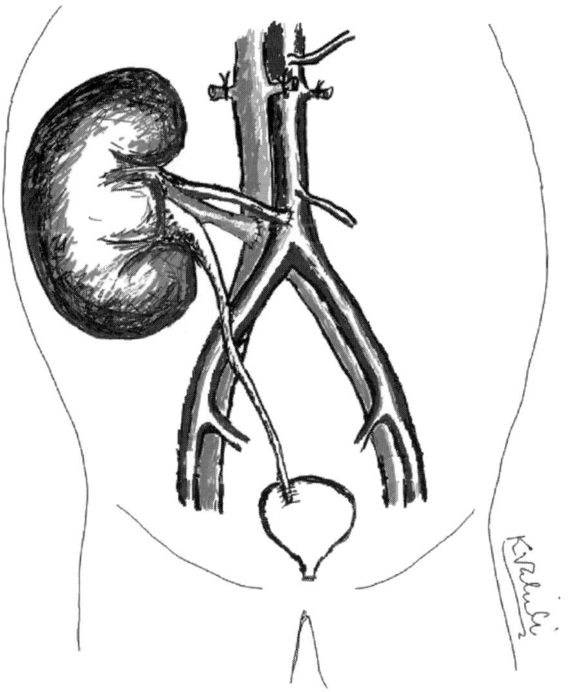

Figure 33.1 Intraabdominal kidney transplant with anastomoses to the distal aorta and vena cava following bilateral native nephrectomies.

donor. Therefore, potential donors undergo a rigorous work-up prior to being selected as a donor. Grafts from living donors that will be at high risk of early failure secondary to recipient immune status or recurrent disease should generally be avoided.

Surgical technique

In the pediatric population, the size of the patient dictates the position of the renal allograft (discussed further in Chapter 30). The preferred location for the placement of the renal allograft is in either the right or left iliac fossa via a retroperitoneal approach with vascular anastomoses to the iliac vessels. In children weighing less than 20 kg, an adult-sized allograft usually requires an intra-abdominal approach, which provides more space for the kidney (Figure 33.1). In this case, the distal aorta and vena cava are used for inflow and outflow, respectively, due to the small size of the iliac vessels. The intra-abdominal approach also allows for native nephrectomies at the time of transplantation when indicated. Indications for native nephrectomy include hypertension, recurrent urinary tract infections, significant proteinuria, or high urine output. Excess proteinuria may result in hypoimmunoglobulinemia as well as increased risk of thrombosis due to loss of coagulation inhibitors. In order to minimize the risk of thrombosis after transplantation, native nephrectomies are performed prior to transplantation in patients with severe proteinuria such as infants with congenital nephrotic syndrome. However, in most other cases, native nephrectomy can be performed at the time of transplant. If the kidney graft is to be placed via a retroperitoneal approach into the iliac fossa, then native nephrectomies can be performed laparoscopically prior to transplantation.

In certain congenital malformations, vascular anatomic aberrations can be encountered, such as left-sided vena cava, intraperitoneal aorta, or predominant abdominal azygous system. However, with careful preoperative vascular mapping (CT or MRI) and planning, these anatomic variations should not necessarily preclude renal transplantation.

Postoperative management

Maintenance of adequate circulating volume and perfusion pressures are important during and following renal transplantation. Excessive volume overload in the operating room or in the early postoperative period, especially in small recipients, can result in pulmonary edema and the requirement for prolonged ventilatory support. IV dopamine infusion can be used in the early postoperative period to maintain adequate perfusion pressures (mean arterial pressure > 60–65 mmHg). In addition to replacement of insensible losses, urine output should be replaced in a 1:1 ratio in the first few days following transplantation to prevent hypovolemia. Output is generally replaced with 1/2 normal saline, with adjustments made to electrolyte balance based on urine and blood studies. Glucose should be included in the baseline insensible fluid rate until the patient is able to tolerate enteral fluids. Particular attention should be paid to the patient requiring significant fluid replacement due to early renal allograft diuresis, as these patients can develop significant electrolyte abnormalities. Hyperphosphatemia may be observed until normal graft function is achieved, requiring treatment with phosphate binders. However, once the graft starts functioning well, hypophosphatemia and hypomagnesemia may result, necessitating initiation of oral supplements. Increase in blood creatinine concentration may be secondary to acute tubular necrosis, hypovolemia, vascular compromise, ureteral obstruction, or rejection. Based on the overall clinical scenario, appropriate diagnostic work-up should be carried out.

Most centers perform a baseline imaging study (ultrasound or mercaptoacetyltriglycine [MAG3] scan) within the first 24 hours following transplantation. Further imaging is usually dictated by the subsequent clinical course. If vascular compromise is suspected postoperatively due to a decrease in urine output or increasing creatinine, a Doppler ultrasound should be used to evaluate blood flow through the renal artery and vein. A nuclear medicine scan (MAG3) can be used to assess perfusion, excretory function, or the presence of urine leak. The radioisotope is concentrated in the urine, and a slow rate of excretion can be seen in acute tubular necrosis and rejection. Visualization of radioisotope outside the urinary tract is suggestive of a urine leak.

The urine reservoir (bladder or a urinary conduit) is decompressed with an indwelling catheter for the first 5–6 days following surgery to allow for adequate healing of the ureteral anastomosis. A surgical drain placed at the time of surgery is monitored for quality and quantity of output. If a urine leak is suspected, testing the creatinine concentration in the drain fluid can aid in diagnosis.

Hypotension and severe hypertension should be avoided in the early postoperative period. Low blood pressure may lead to hypoperfusion in an adult-size kidney in a pediatric recipient, which may in turn lead to a delay in function. Adequate circulating volume should be ascertained and vasoconstrictors should generally be avoided due to the increased risk of renal vasoconstriction. Hypertension can be treated with calcium channel blockers (nifedipine and amlodipine), hydralazine, beta-blockers, and alpha-blockers. Angiotensin-converting enyzme inhibitors and angiotensin receptor blockers are avoided in the first several weeks after transplant due to the risk of inducing renal insufficiency.

Immunosuppression

Based on the NAPRTCS 2008 annual report, interleukin-2 antibodies are the most commonly used agents for induction therapy for both living donor (51%) and deceased donor (50%) pediatric renal transplants. Antibody induction therapy, defined by administration of antibody at transplant or on day 1 post-transplant, was initiated in about 54% of recipients in 2007.

Steroid dose reduction is of particular interest in the pediatric population since steroids can have many profound negative effects, including growth retardation, glucose intolerance, hypertension, aseptic bone necrosis, and impaired wound healing. Currently the maintenance regimen of prednisone, tacrolimus (TAC), and mycophenolate mofetil (MMF) is used for the majority (about 30%) of transplants. With the introduction of MMF and TAC, the use of azathioprine and cyclosporine has declined significantly over the past 10 years. In addition, the use of prednisone has decreased from 95% in 1996 to 61% in 2007 per the NAPRTCS 2008 report. Many centers have developed strategies to wean the patient off steroids within the first 1–2 years following transplantation.

Postoperative complications

Delayed graft function

Generally, a well-functioning kidney graft will have excellent function within the first 1–3 days, resulting in normalization of serum creatinine concentration. However, in some cases, reaching normal renal graft function takes longer than expected. In most cases, acute tubular necrosis (ATN) is the main cause of this delayed function. Based on NAPRTCS data, delayed graft function can be seen in 5% of living donor and about 16% of deceased donor transplants. Risk factors for ATN in the living donor transplants include greater than five prior blood transfusions, history of prior transplants, age less than 24 months, black race, native nephrectomy, and prior dialysis. Risk factors for ATN following deceased donor transplant include more than five blood transfusions, prior transplant, cold ischemia time greater than 24 hours, native nephrectomy, black race, donor age less than 2 years or greater than 50 years, and prior dialysis. Grafts with early ATN have a lower 5-year survival rate (65%) compared with grafts without ATN (85%).

Graft thrombosis

Vascular thrombosis of the renal graft is a devastating event seen in about 2–3% of pediatric renal transplants and is a major cause of graft failure in the first year following transplant. Vascular thrombosis usually occurs within the first several days following surgery; however, it can also occur after several weeks. The clinician should be alerted to the possibility of vascular compromise if there is a sudden decrease in renal function that results in oliguria or anuria. The diagnosis can be established by obtaining a Doppler ultrasound of the graft to evaluate blood flow into the kidney. In addition, an MAG3 radionuclide scan can be used to establish the diagnosis. In nearly all cases, vascular thrombosis results in the loss of the graft, requiring removal of the graft. The only chance at salvaging the graft is if re-operation and thrombectomy is carried out within the first few hours following thrombosis.

NAPRTCS has demonstrated increased risk of graft thrombosis in living donor recipients with prior transplantation. Cold ischemia time longer than 24 hours has been associated with increased risk of thrombosis. Donors older than 5 years of age and the use of antibody induction therapy are associated with decreased risk of thrombosis.

Hemorrhage

Postoperative hemorrhage may result in the development of a hematoma around the graft, thereby causing compression of the renal parenchyma and renal vasculature. A compartment syndrome may develop, which will place the graft at risk of ischemia, infarction, and eventual failure. This is particularly true in the case of grafts placed in the retroperitoneal space. Clinically significant bleeding will require return to the operating room for control of bleeding and evacuation of hematoma. Prompt recognition of clinically significant postoperative bleeding is important in order to minimize the risk of injury to the graft and the patient.

Urologic complications

Urologic complications following transplantation occur in about 5–10% of cases. The most common urologic complications following transplantation include ureteral leak, stricture, kinking, extrinsic compression, and clinically significant vesicoureteral reflux. Obstruction of the urinary flow results in decreased urine output and hydronephrosis. Obstruction may be secondary to edema at the ureterovesical anastomosis, kinking of the ureter, or extrinsic compression from a lymphocele. An ultrasound or MAG3 scan can be used for definitive diagnosis. Depending on the cause of obstruction, insertion of a ureteral stent or percutaneous drainage of the lymphocele may resolve the obstruction. In rare instances, revision of the ureteral anastomosis may be necessary. Pre-existing bladder or ureteral pathology may increase the chance of post-transplant urologic complications. Prior urologic surgery, pretransplant obstructive uropathy, or vesicoureteral reflux may increase the risk of urologic complications following transplantation. The effect of urologic complications on long-term graft survival is not very clear. In the case of ureteral obstruction, prompt relief of obstruction will likely not have long-term detrimental effects on the graft. Some studies have shown that vesicoureteral reflux may result in higher rates of graft dysfunction and failure. This is likely secondary to recurrent urinary tract infections, which have been correlated with increased risk of long-term graft failure.

Recipients with previous bladder augmentation procedures are at higher risk of developing UTIs as well as metabolic acidosis. The intestinal segment absorbs urinary ammonia and ammonium chloride, which along with secretion of bicarbonate leads to metabolic acidosis.

Due to the high incidence of lower urinary tract dysfunction in the pediatric population with ESRD undergoing renal transplantation, careful preoperative planning and meticulous operative technique are necessary to minimize the risk of post-transplant urologic complications. The involvement of a pediatric urologist is crucial in obtaining optimum outcome in patients with complex urologic problems.

Graft rejection

Graft rejection occurs at least once in about 40–50% of kidney grafts. Over the past 25 years, the probability of rejection within the first year following transplant has decreased significantly, owing to improvements in immunosuppressive regimens. Based on NAPRTCS data, the probability of first rejection within 12 months after living donor and deceased donor transplants is 8.7% and 17.7%, respectively. In the late 1980s, the probability of rejection within the first year was more than 50%. Some of the risk factors for rejection following deceased donor transplantation include black race, two HLA-DR mismatches compared with no mismatches, and no induction therapy. In living donor transplantation, recipient age, HLA-DR mismatches, and ATN are risk factors for rejection.

Definitive diagnosis of graft rejection requires a graft biopsy for histologic and immunohistochemical evaluation in addition to other appropriate investigations to exclude other causes of rise in serum creatinine. Biopsy is generally performed percutaneously and under ultrasound guidance.

Chronic allograft nephropathy and chronic rejection

Chronic allograft nephropathy (CAN) is the most common cause of eventual graft failure in the pediatric transplant population, comprising about 35% of all causes of graft failure. It is clinically manifested by a gradual decline in renal function over a course of months to years. CAN has replaced what was previously referred to as chronic rejection. The exact pathophysiology of CAN has not been elucidated; however, immunological as well as non-immunological mechanisms have been proposed. Some studies have demonstrated a correlation between acute rejection and eventual development of CAN. Non-immunological risk factors such as hyperfiltration secondary to relatively low nephron mass, large recipient size, African-American race, older or female donors, and long ischemic times have also been suggested.

Unfortunately, there is no treatment for CAN, and once it is diagnosed, renal function usually continues to decline. Medical therapy should be focused on reducing associated problems including hypertension and proteinuria. Because there appears to be an association between acute rejection episodes and the development of CAN, aggressive and adequate treatment of acute rejection is crucial. Prevention of CAN is especially important in the pediatric population as poor renal function has a significant effect on growth. Recently, avoidance of calcineurin inhibitors is being evaluated as a potential strategy to decrease the incidence of CAN following renal transplantation.

Disease recurrence after renal transplantation

The original disease process leading to renal failure may recur in the transplanted kidney. Some disease processes and their recurrence rates include FSGS, 14–50%; atypical HUS, 20–80%; typical HUS, 0–1%; membranoproliferative glomerulosclerosis type 1, 30–77%; membranoproliferative glomerulosclerosis type 2, 66–100%; systemic lupus erythematosus, 0–30%; immunoglobulin A (IgA) nephritis, 35–60%; Henoch-Schönlein nephritis, 31–100%; and primary hyperoxaluria type 1, 90–100%.

The presentation of disease recurrence can vary widely, ranging from subclinical elements of the original disease to full disease recurrence and eventual renal failure. Based on NAPRTCS 2008 data, recurrent disease leads to graft failure in 6.8% of cases, which makes it one of the top four causes of graft failure. FSGS is one of the most common causes of ESRD in children. FSGS recurrence in the allograft leads to graft loss in 50% of patients. Recurrence may occur immediately after transplantation, resulting in severe proteinuria, ATN, and small vessel thrombosis. There is no established treatment or prevention regimen for FSGS recurrence; however, plasmapheresis and rituximab have been used with some success.

The most common cause of typical HUS in children is enteropathic bacteria, and this does not usually result in ESRD or recurrence in the kidney graft. However, atypical HUS or "non–Shiga toxin-associated" HUS can lead to ESRD as well as recurrence after transplantation. Atypical HUS may occur in the setting of deficient von Willebrand factor–cleaving protease (ADAMTS-13), metabolic disorders, or dysfunction in complement regulation. Complement dysfunction may result from factor H, I, B, or C3 mutations or the presence of anti-factor H antibodies. Due to a high rate of recurrence and graft failure, factor H and I mutations are considered by some to be contraindications to renal transplantation. However, treatment with plasmapheresis and fresh-frozen plasma has produced some positive results. Because factor H is produced in the liver, some advocate combined liver–kidney transplantation in this setting.

Primary hyperoxaluria type 1 is an autosomal-recessive disease caused by deficiency in peroxisomal alanine-glyoxylate aminotransferase (AGT), which leads to an overproduction of oxalate. High levels of oxalate lead to urolithiasis, nephrocalcinosis, and eventually chronic kidney disease. Because the enzyme AGT is produced in the liver, liver transplantation is necessary to restore normal enzyme function. The chance of disease recurrence in the transplanted kidney without a liver transplant is 90–100%; therefore, most patients undergo a combined liver and kidney transplant. Dialysis is used in the pretransplant setting to maintain normal serum oxalate levels and is continued in the post-transplant setting to prevent early oxalate deposition and damage to the graft. Oxalate is deposited and stored in a wide variety of tissues, and therefore it is slowly released into the blood following transplantation. Native nephrectomies are required since the kidneys are a major site of oxalate deposition.

Autoimmune diseases such as IgA nephropathy, Henoch-Schönlein purpura, lupus nephritis, and anti-neutrophil cytoplasmic antibodies (ANCA)-associated vasculitis may recur after transplantation but do not lead to graft loss in the majority of cases.

Patient and graft survival

Based on the NAPRTCS 2008 report, the 1- and 5-year graft survival rates for pediatric living donor kidney transplantation are about 95% and 85%, respectively. Graft survival rates following deceased donor kidney transplantation are 93% and 75%, respectively. Some of the leading causes of graft failure in decreasing order of frequency are chronic rejection (or CAN), acute rejection, vascular thrombosis, death with functioning graft, recurrence of original kidney disease, and patient discontinuation of medication.

Patient survival rates at 1 and 5 years following transplantation are 98% and 95%, respectively. Infants younger than 24 months of age receiving a deceased donor organ have had lower survival rates in the past, but this has improved over the past 20 years. The leading causes of death (percent of all causes) are cardiopulmonary (15.4%), bacterial infection (12.6%), malignancy (10.6%), viral infection (8.1%), and non-specified infection (7.9%). The overall rate of malignancy is about 2.4% and about 80% of malignancies are related to post-transplant lymphoproliferative disorder. Risk factors associated with mortality include young recipient age, ATN within 30 days post-transplant, and specific underlying renal diseases including congenital nephrotic syndrome, oxalosis, and Drash syndrome.

Further reading

Cochat P, Fargue S, Mestrallet G, *et al.* Disease recurrence in paediatric renal transplantation. *Pediatr Nephrol* 2009; **24**: 2097–108.

Fine RN, Martz K, Stablein D. What have 20 years of data from the North American Pediatric Renal Transplant Cooperative Study taught us about growth following renal transplantation in infants, children, and adolescents with end-stage renal disease? *Pediatr Nephrol* 2010; **25**: 739–46.

Harmon WE. Pediatric kidney transplantation. In Avner ED, Harmon WE, Niaudet P, Yoshikawa N (eds). *Pediatric Nephrology*, 6th ed. Berlin: Springer, 2009.

Humar A, Matas AJ. Kidney transplantation. In Humar A, Matas AJ, Payne WD (eds). *Atlas of Organ Transplantation*. Berlin: Springer, 2009.

North American Pediatric Renal Trials and Collaborative Studies (NAPRTCS) Annual Report (2008). Available at: https://web.emmes.com/study/ped/annlrept/annlrept.html (accessed March 1, 2010).

Sheldon C, Shumyle A. Urological issues in pediatric renal transplantation. *Curr Opin Urol* 2008; **18**: 413–8.

Chapter 34

Pancreatic transplantation

Dixon B. Kaufman

Key points

- The results for all types of pancreas transplantation have improved over the past decade, in large part due to advances in immunosuppression.
- A successful pancreas transplant produces a normoglycemic and insulin-independent state virtually immediately after revascularization.
- The benefits of adding a pancreas transplant to ameliorate diabetes are profound – it saves lives.
- As with other organ transplants, episodes of acute rejection appear to predispose to late allograft loss.
- Surgical complications are more common after pancreas transplantation compared with kidney transplantation and occur in 5–10% of cases. These are usually seen within 6 months and are an important etiology of pancreas graft loss.

Rationale of pancreas transplantation for patients with diabetes mellitus

There are nearly 3 million people in the United States with type 1 diabetes mellitus (DM1) and 35 000 new cases diagnosed each year that result from autoimmune destruction of the insulin-producing cells in the pancreas. $CD4^+$ and $CD8^+$ T cells and macrophages infiltrate the islets, but clinical symptoms may not appear until as much as 80% of the beta cells are destroyed. Antibodies directed against glutamic acid decarboxylase (GAD 65), a protein tyrosine phosphatase-like molecule (IA-2), and insulin are seen, but not all patients with auto-antibodies go on to develop diabetes, and auto-antibodies sometimes disappear many years after the onset of diabetes. Increased susceptibility has been linked to particular human leukocyte antigen (HLA) combinations and immunoregulatory gene polymorphisms, as well as certain insulin gene alleles.

Exogenous insulin saves patients from rapid demise, but even the combination of newer formulations of insulin and sophisticated administration regimens does not prevent DM from being the leading cause of blindness and renal failure in adults and the seventh leading cause of death in the United States. Death is sometimes due to massive, acute hyperglycemia and ketoacidosis, but is more often due to secondary diseases (especially cerebral and coronary vasculopathy) arising from less severe hyperglycemia occurring over time. The development of secondary comorbidities is tightly linked to chronic glucose control, as measured by the percentage of non-enzymatically glycosylated hemoglobin (HbA1c). HbA1c levels in diabetics may be as high as 20%, whereas normal values range from 4–5.9%. Any decrease in HbA1c is considered beneficial, but efforts to achieve normal HbA1C by increasing doses of insulin are limited by the incidence of hypoglycemia.

Iatrogenic hypoglycemia causes 2–4% of deaths in people with DM1, with less severe episodes manifesting as behavior change, cognitive impairment, seizure, and coma as the glucose-dependent brain cells decline and then fail. The risk of death is highest in patients with asymptomatic hypoglycemia, in whom the early

Organ Transplantation: A Clinical Guide, ed. A.A. Klein, C.J. Lewis, and J.C. Madsen. Published by Cambridge University Press.

signs of hypoglycemia (sweating, hunger, anxiety, palpitations, and tremor) are absent because of autonomic failure, either as a result of diabetes-associated autonomic neuropathy or a blunted epinephrine response following repeated hypoglycemic episodes. Glucagon is the primary insulin counter-regulatory hormone, but the injected insulin cannot respond to hypoglycemia and continues to suppress the release of glucagon. Because the autonomic pathway normally serves as a back-up glucose-raising mechanism, these patients lack the trigger both to take in external sources of glucose and to mobilize internal glucose stores.

The only treatments that have been demonstrated to normalize HbA1c levels, influence the progression of secondary complications, and avoid hypoglycemia involve beta-cell replacement therapy with pancreas or islet transplantation. Pancreas transplantation is superior to islet transplantation with regard to the efficiency and durability of achieving glycemic control and its beneficial effects on diabetic secondary complications. A successful pancreas transplant produces a normoglycemic and insulin-independent state virtually immediately after revascularization. It reverses the diabetic changes in the native kidneys of patients with very early diabetic nephropathy, prevents recurrent diabetic nephropathy in patients undergoing a simultaneous pancreas–kidney transplant, reverses peripheral sensory neuropathy, stabilizes advanced diabetic retinopathy, and significantly improves the quality of life.

However, there are important considerations of pancreas transplantation that currently precludes it as therapy for all patients with DM1. First, it is unrealistic that all patients with DM could receive a pancreas transplant. There are too many patients with DM1 and too few organs for transplantation. Second, pancreas transplantation involves significant surgery. Third, lifelong immunosuppression is required to prevent graft rejection. Therefore, the indications for pancreas transplantation are very specific and narrow. There are three circumstances where consideration for pancreas transplantation is reasonable for patients with DM1: (1) select patients who are also excellent candidates for kidney transplantation; (2) patients with a well-functioning kidney transplant receiving immunosuppression; (3) select patients who are extremely brittle or have significant frequency and severity of hypoglycemic unawareness such that the risks of surgery and immunosuppression are less morbid than the current state of ill health.

Indications and contraindications to pancreas transplantation

Approximately 1300 pancreas transplants are performed annually in the United States. Two thirds involve a simultaneous pancreas and kidney transplant (SPK) for patients with diabetes and chronic or end-stage renal failure. There are approximately 2200 candidates registered on the United Network for Organ Sharing (UNOS) waiting list. Ninety percent of SPK transplants are in recipients with DM1, and only about 10% (<90 cases annually) are select recipients with DM type 2 (DM2). The benefits of adding a pancreas transplant to ameliorate DM are profound: it saves lives.

Approximately 1500 candidates are registered on the UNOS waiting list for solitary pancreas transplants. Solitary pancreas transplant falls into two categories. The first group are patients with DM who have received a previous kidney transplant from either a living or cadaveric donor. The pancreas-after-kidney (PAK) group accounts for approximately 20% of patients receiving pancreas transplants. The main consideration is that of surgical risk, since the risk of immunosuppression has already been assumed. Most PAK recipients have received a prior living donor kidney allograft. The second group are non-uremic, non-kidney transplant patients with DM1. In this situation, one assesses the risk of immunosuppression to be less than the current clinical condition with conventional exogenous insulin administration. These patients with DM have extremely labile disease, such that there is difficulty with day-to-day living, associated with frequent emergency room visits and hospitalizations for hypoglycemia or diabetic ketoacidosis. Other patients may have significant difficulty with hypoglycemic unawareness that results in unconsciousness without warning. This can be a devastating condition for these select patients, affecting their employment and their ability to drive, with concern about suffering lethal hypoglycemia while asleep. The indications for a pancreas transplant alone (PTA) are essentially identical to those patients being considered for an islet transplant. However, in the former situation, there are fewer contraindications with respect to body mass index and insulin requirements.

Evaluation of candidates for pancreas transplantation

There are significant pre-existing comorbidities of pancreas transplant candidates with advanced renal disease, and it should be assumed that coincident extra-renal disease is present. Advanced vascular disease (in particular, coronary artery disease) is the most important comorbidity to consider in patients with DM1 with diabetic nephropathy. It has been estimated that DM1 uremic patients carry a near 50-fold greater risk of cardiovascular events then the general population. Because of the neuropathy associated with diabetes, patients are often asymptomatic because ischemia-induced angina is not perceived. Virtually all DM1 uremic patients should undergo coronary angiography because non-invasive tests are relatively insensitive; however, care should be given to minimize contrast agents. This patient group also experiences an increased rate of stroke and transient ischemic attacks. Deaths related to cerebral vascular disease are approximately twice as common and occur at a younger age in patients with DM and end-stage renal disease. Peripheral vascular disease is significant, and DM1 uremic patients are at risk for lower limb amputation secondary to ulcers associated with advanced somatosensory neuropathy.

Diabetic retinopathy is nearly ubiquitous, and significant vision loss may have occurred. A patient with significant vision loss must have adequate support systems to ensure they are able to manage the post-transplant regime.

Autonomic neuropathy is prevalent, commonly underestimated, and may manifest as gastropathy, cystopathy, and orthostatic hypotension. Neurogenic bladder dysfunction is an important consideration in patients receiving a kidney transplant either simultaneously or prior to subsequent pancreas transplantation. Inability to sense bladder fullness and empty the bladder predisposes to urine reflux and high post-void residuals. This may adversely affect renal allograft function and increase the incidence of bladder infections and pyelonephritis. The combination of orthostatic hypotension and recumbent hypertension results from dysregulation of vascular tone. Therefore, careful re-assessment of post-transplant anti-hypertensive medication requirement is important. Patients with severe gastroparesis may have difficulty tolerating oral immunosuppressive medications and prophylactic agents. Motility agents such as metoclopramide, domperidone, or erythromycin may be useful.

Mental or emotional illnesses including neuroses and depression are common. Diagnosis and appropriate treatment of these illnesses is an important pre-transplant consideration, with important implications for ensuring a high degree of medical compliance.

Pancreas organ allocation

UNOS is now in the process of redesigning the pancreas allocation for pancreas transplantation to better address the needs of patients with DM with and without concurrent renal failure since currently, waiting time for SPK transplant varies widely across the United States and there is a lack of specific listing criteria. Under the new system, if a uremic DM1 candidate on the list for an SPK transplant is allocated a pancreas from a local deceased donor, then the kidney would also be offered from the same deceased donor. SPK and PTA candidates would also be combined onto a single list. Allocating the cadaveric pancreas (with kidney for SPK transplant) prior to procurement of the organs has distinct advantages: (1) the transplant center performing the pancreas transplant could also procure the pancreas; (2) the patient can be admitted to the hospital for re-evaluation simultaneously, rather than sequential to the procurement of the organ; (3) cold ischemia time will be shorter. Pancreas allografts do not tolerate cold ischemia as well as kidney and require revascularization within 24 hours from procurement.

Transplant surgery and surgical complications

Deceased donor pancreas selection

Identification of suitable cadaveric donors for pancreas transplantation is one of the most important determinants of outcome.

Several anatomical and physiological factors have been identified that affect the results of pancreas transplantation. In general, the criteria that determine an appropriate donor for pancreas transplantation are more stringent than for kidney or liver donors. Important considerations include weight, age, hyperglycemia, hyperamylasemia, adiposity, and vascular anomalies.

Obese donors weighing more than 100 kg are frequently not found to be suitable pancreas donors

Table 34.1 Contraindications of pancreas procurement for transplantation

1. History of type 1 diabetes mellitus
2. History of type 2 diabetes mellitus
3. History of previous pancreatic surgery
4. Intra-abdominal trauma to the pancreas
5. Donor age < 10 years and > 55 years (relative contraindication)
6. Donor weight < 30 kg and > 100 kg (taken in consideration with height)
7. Intraoperative assessment A. Vascular supply B. Severe edema, significant adipose infiltration, significant fibrosis or mass C. Pancreatic hemorrhage or trauma

because of DM2 or a high degree of adipose infiltration of the pancreas. Importantly, pancreata from relatively older donors (age 55–65 years) and obese organ donors are associated with very successful islet isolation recovery required for an islet transplant. Therefore, all deceased organ donors should be considered for procurement of pancreas and islets for transplantation.

Hyperglycemia and hyperamylasemia are very frequently observed in deceased organ donors. Hyperglycemia is not a contraindication to pancreas procurement for patients who are known not to have DM1 or 2. Deceased donor assessment may also include HbA1c levels. Hyperamylasemia is concerning, but reports have indicated that it has no meaningful influence on pancreas graft function post-transplant. Pancreatitis or pancreatic injury in the case of a donor with trauma should be ruled out at the time of procurement.

Perhaps the most important determinant of the suitability of the pancreas for transplantation is by direct examination of the organ during surgical procurement. The degree of fibrosis, adipose tissue, and specific vascular anomalies can be accurately assessed. Pancreata with heavy infiltration of adipose tissue are believed to be relatively intolerant of cold preservation and have the potential for a high degree of saponification due to reperfusion pancreatitis that follows revascularization. These organs may be more suitable for islet isolation.

The important vascular anomaly that must be evaluated during procurement is the occurrence of a replaced or accessory right hepatic artery originating from the superior mesenteric artery. Experienced procurement teams will be able to successfully separate the liver and the pancreas either in situ or on the backbench without sacrificing quality of either organ for transplantation.

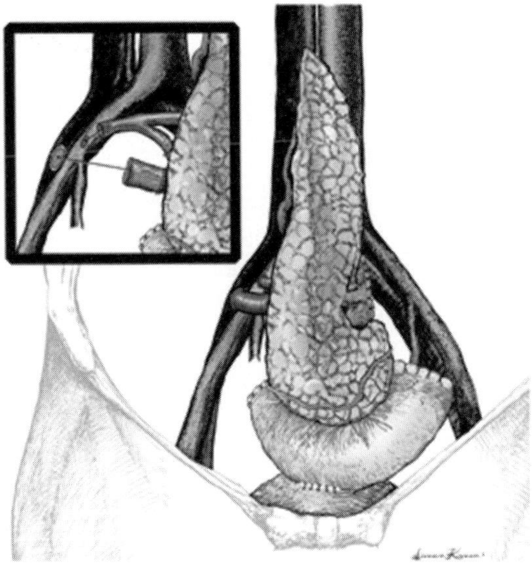

Figure 34.1 Pancreaticoduodenal allograft with exocrine bladder drainage and systemic venous drainage. Illustration by Simon Kimm.

The use of donation after cardiac death donors for pancreas transplantation has been reported, although with a higher rejection rate at the time of procurement. If the pancreas is deemed suitable, there is the added consideration of the effect of delayed kidney graft function in a uremic SPK candidate.

The use of living related and unrelated pancreas donors has also been described. A distal pancreatectomy is performed for a segmental pancreas transplant. Anecdotal cases of combined live donor partial pancreatectomy and nephrectomy have also been reported. These procedures are not widely performed and are confined to one or two pancreas transplant programs.

Pancreas transplant surgery

The surgical techniques for pancreas transplantation are diverse, and there is no standard methodology used by all programs.

The principles include providing adequate arterial blood flow to the pancreas and duodenal segment, adequate venous outflow of the pancreas via the portal vein, and management of the pancreatic exocrine secretions. The native pancreas is not

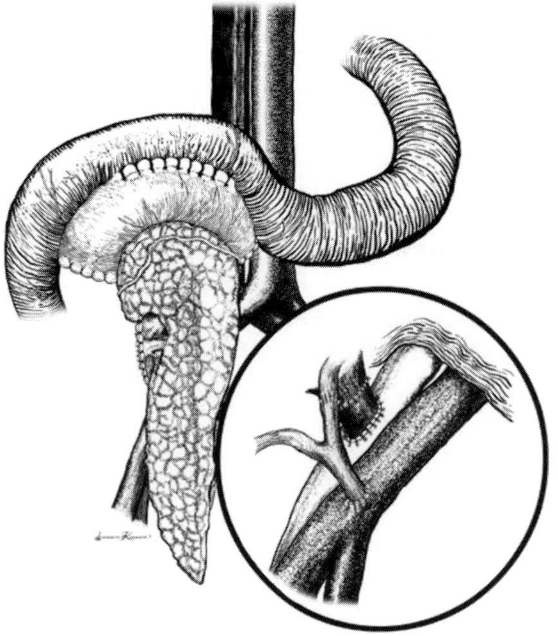

Figure 34.2 Pancreaticoduodenal allograft with exocrine enteric drainage and venous systemic drainage. Illustration by Simon Kimm.

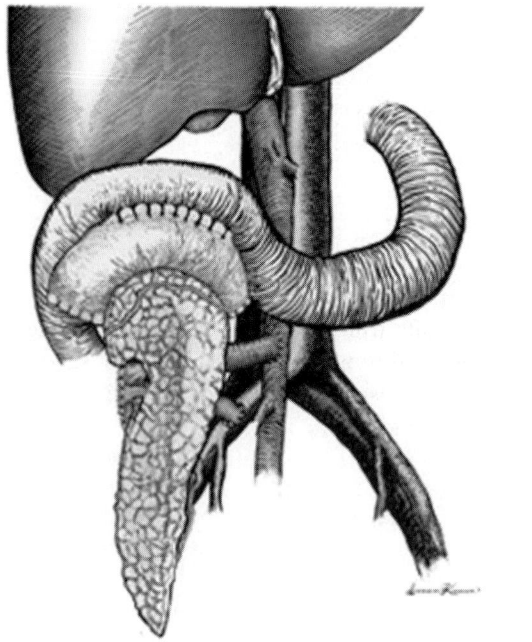

Figure 34.3 Pancreaticoduodenal allograft with exocrine enteric drainage and portal venous drainage. Illustration by Simon Kimm.

removed. Pancreas graft arterial revascularization is typically accomplished utilizing the recipient right common or external iliac artery. The Y-graft of the pancreas is anastomosed end to side. There are two choices for venous revascularization: systemic and portal. Systemic venous revascularization commonly involves the right common iliac vein or right external iliac vein. If portal venous drainage is utilized, it is necessary to dissect out the superior mesenteric vein (SMV) at the root of the mesentery. The pancreas portal vein is anastomosed end to side to a branch of the SMV. This may influence the methodology of arterial revascularization using a long Y-graft placed through a window in the mesentery to reach the right common iliac artery. Portal venous drainage of the pancreas is more physiological with respect to immediate delivery of insulin to the recipient liver. This results in diminished circulating insulin levels relative to that in systemic venous-drained pancreas grafts. There has not been documented any clinically relevant difference in glycemic control.

Handling the exocrine drainage of the pancreas is the most challenging aspect of the transplant procedure. Pancreatic exocrine drainage may be handled via anastomosis of the duodenal segment to the bladder or anastomosis to the small intestine. Enteric drainage of the pancreas allograft is physiological with respect to the delivery of pancreatic enzymes and bicarbonate into the intestines for reabsorption and can be constructed with or without a Roux-en-Y. The enteric anastomosis can be made side to side or end to side with the duodenal segment of the pancreas. The risk of intra-abdominal abscesses is extremely low, and the avoidance of the bladder-drained pancreas has significant implications with respect to the potential complications that include bladder infection and the frequent requirement for enteric conversion. Currently, more than 80% of pancreas transplants are performed with enteric drainage and the remainder with bladder drainage.

Complications of pancreas transplantation

Surgical complications are more common after pancreas transplantation compared with kidney transplantation. Non-immunological complications of pancreas transplantation account for graft losses in 5–10% of cases. These occur commonly within 6 months of transplant and are an important etiology of pancreas graft loss in SPK transplantation.

Thrombosis

Vascular thrombosis is a very early complication typically occurring within 48 hours. This is generally due to venous thrombosis of the pancreas portal vein. The etiology is not entirely defined but is believed to be associated with reperfusion pancreatitis and the relatively low-flow state of the pancreas graft. To minimize graft thrombosis, prudent selection of donor pancreas grafts, short cold ischemia times, and meticulous surgical technique are necessary. Approximately 5% of pancreas grafts will need to be removed because of portal venous thrombosis. Arterial thrombosis is less common and is usually associated with anastomosis to atherosclerotic vessels.

Acute venous thrombosis results in a sudden rise in serum glucose and is occasionally associated with pain directly over the pancreatic graft and occasionally ipsilateral lower extremity swelling from extension of the thrombus into the common iliac vein. Confirmatory non-invasive perfusion imaging of the graft is performed using technetium-99m hexamethyl propylene amine oxime. Ultrasonography can also be used to determine vascular flow in the allograft. Management requires urgent operative intervention, either thrombectomy with vascular revision or graft excision. The findings at surgery are an ischemic, dusky, non-viable pancreas and duodenal segment with fresh clot in the graft portal vein. Salvage of the thrombosed graft is not to be expected but has occasionally been described.

To reduce the incidence of pancreatic graft thrombosis, anti-coagulation is routinely used. Most centers employ a combination approach involving heparin and an anti-platelet agent early postoperatively, although this increases the risk of hemorrhage. The management of mild postoperative bleeding is more acceptable than the irreversible consequence of allograft thrombosis.

Hemorrhage

Bleeding from the vascular anastomotic site or cut surfaces of the pancreatic graft will result in an intra-abdominal hematoma. Clinical suspicion, the physical examination, serial blood counts, and attention to abdominal drain output suggest postoperative hemorrhage. Discontinuation of anti-coagulants/anti-platelet agents and correction of coagulation abnormalities using conventional therapies is usually effective. Aggressive resuscitative efforts and operative intervention are essential if hemodynamic instability develops. The hematoma should be removed, exploration performed to identify any source of bleeding, and the viability of the pancreas (and kidney) confirmed. Gastrointestinal bleeding may occur in enteric-drained pancreas transplant from a combination of peri-operative anticoagulation and bleeding from the suture line of the duodeno-enteric anastomosis. It may be recognized by a fall in hemoglobin, melena, or positive fecal occult blood. This is usually self-limiting; therefore, conservative management is usually sufficient. Occasionally, interventional radiological embolization of a bleeding vessel or re-operative exploration is required.

Transplant pancreatitis

Transplant pancreatitis occurs to some degree in all patients. A temporary elevation in serum amylase and lipase levels usually occurs for 48–96 hours after transplant. These episodes are transient and mild without significant clinical consequence.

Complications of the bladder-drained pancreas transplant

Bladder-drained pancreas transplantation is associated with many mild to moderately severe complications that arise because of the unusual physiology of pancreatic exocrine secretions draining into the bladder. The pancreas transplant will eliminate approximately 500 ml of bicarbonate-rich fluid with pancreatic enzymes into the bladder each day. Change in pH of the bladder accounts, in part, for a greater increase in urinary tract infections.

Sterile cystitis, urethritis, and balanitis may occur after bladder-drained pancreas transplantation. This is due to the effect of the pancreatic enzymes on the urinary tract mucosa. This is more commonly experienced in male recipients. Urethritis can progress to urethral perforation and perineal pain. Treatment options include conservative treatment or operative enteric conversion.

Careful monitoring of serum electrolytes and acid–base balance is necessary because metabolic acidosis routinely develops as a consequence of bladder bicarbonate excretion and often requires oral bicarbonate supplementation. Patients are also at risk of dehydration, orthostatic hypotension, and electrolyte disturbance due to large volume losses that may require fluid replacement.

Reflux pancreatitis can result in acute inflammation of the pancreas allograft, mimicking acute rejection with symptoms of pain with hyperamylasemia. It is believed to be secondary to reflux of urine through the ampulla into the pancreatic ducts and may occur even in the presence of mild prostatic hypertrophy. This frequently occurs in patients with neurogenic bladder dysfunction and necessitates investigation of the cause by pressure flow studies and cystourethrography. Recurrent graft pancreatitis requires enteric conversion.

Urine leak from breakdown of the duodenal segment is the most serious postoperative complication of the bladder-drained pancreas, and a high index of suspicion is required. It is usually encountered within the first 2–3 months post-transplant but can occur many years later. Typical presentation is abdominal pain with elevated serum amylase, which can mimic reflux pancreatitis or acute rejection. Supporting imaging studies with CT and cystography confirm the diagnosis. Operative intervention is usually required when the degree of leakage determines whether direct repair, enteric conversion or graft pancreatectomy is indicated.

Complications of the enteric-drained pancreas transplant

The most serious complication of the enteric-drained pancreas transplant is that of a leak and intra-abdominal abscess. Patients present with fever, abdominal discomfort and leukocytosis, commonly 1–6 months post-transplant. Computed tomography imaging and percutaneous drainage of intra-abdominal fluid for Gram stain and culture is essential. Bacteria and often fungi are commonly found, and broad-spectrum antimicrobial therapy is essential. Surgical exploration and repair of the enteric leak is necessary. A decision must be made regarding whether the infection can be eradicated without removing the pancreas allograft. Incomplete eradication of the infection will result in progression to sepsis and multi-organ failure. Peri-pancreatic infections can result in development of a mycotic aneurysm at the arterial anastomosis, which may rupture, and requires allograft pancreatectomy. A number of factors have contributed to the reduction in incidence of intra-abdominal abscess: greater recognition of the criteria for procuring suitable cadaveric pancreas allografts; improved peri-operative antibiotic prophylaxis, including anti-fungal agents; minimizing anti-rejection immunotherapy and reduction in acute rejection. There is no convincing evidence that a Roux-en-Y intestinal reconstruction decreases incidence.

Immunological aspects of pancreas transplantation

Immunosuppression for pancreas transplantation

The outcome of pancreas transplantation with respect to graft survival and rejection rates is dependent on the choice of immunosuppression agents used. The risk of pancreas allograft rejection is much greater than that observed with kidney transplantation. The precise reasons are not well defined but likely involve greater immunogenicity of the pancreaticoduodenal graft. The majority of pancreas transplant programs use lymphocyte-depleting induction therapy combined with tacrolimus, mycophenolate mofetil (MMF), or sirolimus and prednisolone. Induction therapy is used with greater frequency in pancreas transplant recipients than for any other solid-organ recipients. One reason is the relatively higher risk of rejection observed for pancreas transplant recipients as compared with other solid organ transplants. This combination has significantly improved graft survival rates. There are steroid avoidance protocols described for pancreas transplantation and reports of successful steroid withdrawal.

Pancreas allograft rejection

An understanding of the kinetics of the tissue injury during acute rejection is essential to making a timely diagnosis. Destruction of beta cells occurs relatively late following initial injury of the acinar tissue. Therefore, the diagnosis of pancreas graft rejection by hyperglycemia is a late and often irreversible situation. Detection of changes in acinar cell function is the basis for early suspicion of pancreas graft rejection. The graft is usually inflamed and patients may experience pain and discomfort around the graft due to peritoneal irritation. This, coupled with elevation in the serum amylase or lipase and, if bladder-drained, reduction in urinary amylase, may be the initial presentation of acute rejection.

The gold standard for confirming the diagnosis of pancreas graft rejection is pancreas graft biopsy. The biopsy may be performed by several methods, including percutaneous, transcystoscopic in a bladder-drained pancreas, or open surgical biopsy. The usefulness of pancreas graft biopsy to confirm the clinical suspicion of rejection is so important that the surgical procedure of pancreas transplantation should include consideration of the intra-abdominal location of the pancreas to make it accessible for percutaneous biopsy. This is especially important in PTA and PAK transplant procedures.

In SPK transplant, it is the kidney allograft that is the best indicator of a rejection episode and will manifest as a rise in serum creatinine. This will prompt ultrasound and biopsy of the kidney allograft. Concurrent pancreas graft rejection would be treated by the renal anti-rejection therapy. It is extremely uncommon for isolated pancreas allograft rejection to occur in SPK transplantation (1–2%), and the diagnosis requires both kidney and pancreas transplant biopsies. Treatment is guided by severity and may involve pulsed steroids or anti-lymphocyte immunotherapy with successful treatment in excess of 90%, if diagnosed promptly. The incidence of pancreas rejection has been reduced from approximately 80% to less than 20% in the modern era of transplant immunosuppression.

Results of pancreas transplantation

The results of pancreas transplantation are typically described in terms of both patient and pancreas graft survival. Pancreas graft loss is defined as patient death with a functioning graft or loss of insulin independence irrespective of whether the pancreas allograft is in place or removed. The most valuable and complete information on the results of pancreas transplantation comes from the UNOS Registry and the International Pancreas Transplant Registry (IPTR).

Outcomes of patient and graft survival

The results of SPK transplantation in terms of patient and graft survival have shown steady improvement over time. According to results from the UNOS Registry, SPK recipients who underwent transplantation in 2006 achieved 1-, 3-, and 5-year patient survival rates of 94.8%, 90.8%, and 86.6%, respectively. Pancreas graft functional survival rates for the same post-transplant time periods were 84%, 77%, and 73.2%, respectively. Kidney graft functional survival rates for the same post-transplant time periods were 91.8%, 84.4%, and 78.7%, respectively. Single-center reports from UNOS show wide variability of kidney and pancreas graft survival rates.

According to the IPTR, there was no clinically significant difference in pancreas graft outcome in bladder-drained pancreases versus the enteric-drained pancreas. There is also no clinically significant difference in outcome in systemic venous drainage versus portal drainage. The immunologic risk for graft loss for technically successful cases of SPK transplantation has decreased over time. The current rate of immunological loss is only 2% at 1 year. Relative risk factors for pancreas graft loss in SPK recipients have been determined and include increasing recipient age and prolonged preservation time (>24 hours), and positive effects were shown for the use of MMF.

Effect of pancreas transplantation on secondary complications of diabetes

Recipients of a successful pancreas transplant maintain normal plasma glucose levels without the need for exogenous insulin therapy. This results in normalization of HbA1c levels and a beneficial effect on many secondary complications of diabetes, including blood pressure, diabetic neuropathy, autonomic neuropathy-associated sudden death, and diabetic nephropathy. The durability of the transplanted endocrine pancreas has been established with the demonstration that normalization of HbA1c is maintained for as long as the allograft functions. The potential lifespan of the transplanted pancreas is not precisely known since there are surviving pancreas allografts greater than 20 years post-transplant still functioning.

The quality of life of pancreas transplant recipients has been studied widely. The functioning pancreas allograft leads to even better quality of life when compared with that of recipients of a kidney transplant alone. Virtually all patients of a successful pancreas transplant report that managing their life, including immunosuppression, is much easier than prior to transplantation. Successful pancreas transplantation will not elevate all patients with diabetes to the level of health and function of that of the general population, but transplant recipients consistently report a significantly better quality of life than do patients who remain diabetic.

Further reading

American Diabetes Association. Economic Costs of Diabetes in the U.S. in 2002. *Diabetes Care* 2003; **26**: 917.

Axelrod D, Sung R, Meyer KH, Wolfe RA, Kaufman DB. Systematic evaluation of pancreas allograft quality, outcomes, and geographic variation in utilization. *Am J Transplant* 2010; **10**: 837.

Ojo AO, Meier-Kriesche HU, Hanson JA, *et al.* Impact of simultaneous pancreas-kidney transplantation on long-term patient survival. *Transplantation* 2001; **71**: 82.

OPTN/UNOS Pancreas Transplantation Committee Report to the Board of Directors, Juen 21–22, 2010, Richmond, VA. Available at: http://optn.transplant.hrsa.gov/CommitteeReports/board_main_PancreasTransplantationCommittee_6_24_2010_9_59.pdf

Salvalaggio PR, Davies DB, Fernandez LA, Kaufman DB. Outcomes of pancreas transplantation in the United States using cardiac-death donors. *Am J Transplant* 2006; **6**: 1059.

Chapter 35

Pancreatic islet transplantation

Heidi Yeh and James F. Markmann

Key points

- Successful islet transplantation would result in larger numbers of insulin-independent recipients compared with whole organ pancreas transplantation, both because of a larger donor pool and a larger transplant candidate pool.
- Improving isolation techniques and novel immunosuppression are resulting in islet auto-transplantation outcomes approaching those of whole organ pancreas transplantation.
- Islet auto-transplantation is available as a method of avoiding diabetes in pancreatectomy patients.

Endogenous insulin production can be restored by beta (β) cell replacement, most commonly achieved through whole organ pancreas transplantation as described in Chapter 34. This involves a major vascular procedure, which may be difficult for long-standing diabetics who have developed severe peripheral vascular disease or are poor candidates for major procedures because of coronary artery disease. Although the presence of exocrine tissue is useful for early detection of inflammation in the transplanted organ, severe transplant pancreatitis due to ischemia or rejection can result in serious morbidity, and even mortality. For many patients, these short-term risks outweigh any survival advantage offered by improved glycemic control.

In contrast, the main risk associated with isolated islet transplantation is that of chronic immunosuppression. The exclusion of exocrine tissue removes the risk of post-transplant pancreatitis with its attendant problems, and the infusion of a cell preparation obviates the requirement for disrupting major blood vessels as would be required for whole organ implantation. Even in patients who could tolerate the invasive surgery required for the latter, recovery after islet transplantation would be much shorter and easier.

Furthermore, whole organ pancreas transplantation is limited by the insufficient number suitable for transplant: only 16% of deceased donors yield a transplantable pancreas. Good-quality islets, on the other hand, can be obtained in sufficient numbers from older and higher body mass index (BMI) donors with less stringent hemodynamic requirements than whole organ pancreata, so that potential islet donors from the current donor pool represent more than 1000 additional recipients a year who could achieve insulin independence.

Islet isolation does involve an additional 20 hours of processing time, USD 40 000 of expense (not including the cost of processing pancreata that yield islets of insufficient number or of setting up an islet processing facility), and as many as six staff members beyond that needed for whole organ transplantation. More importantly, islet transplantation is historically neither as efficient nor as durable as whole organ pancreas transplantation and is therefore not yet a satisfactory replacement for pancreas transplantation. However, emerging data suggest that newer protocols in islet transplantation may yield comparable results to those of pancreas transplantation, and if this trend continues, islet transplantation will no longer be considered an experimental procedure.

Organ Transplantation: A Clinical Guide, ed. A.A. Klein, C.J. Lewis, and J.C. Madsen. Published by Cambridge University Press.

Deceased donor allotransplant

Recipient selection

The aforementioned complications limit islet transplantation to patients with type 1 diabetes mellitus (DM1; confirmed by stimulated C-peptide < 0.3 ng/ml, in addition to clinical history) requiring insulin for at least 5 years and one of the following complications despite appropriate medical care and good compliance: hypoglycemic unawareness or metabolic lability characterized by either frequent episodes (two or more per year) of severe hypoglycemia in which the patient is unable to treat him- or herself or has had hospital admission for ketoacidosis. These complications represent a higher risk of mortality from diabetic disease, therefore increasing the benefit of immunosuppression over exogenous insulin treatment, even if insulin independence may not be permanent.

Poor quality of life because of diabetic retinopathy, autonomic neuropathy (gastroparesis, postural hypotension, neuropathic bowel or bladder), or persistent, severe neuropathic pain has been considered as an indication for improved glycemic control by islet transplantation. Although it is well-documented that progression of microvascular disease is slowed or halted by lowering HbA1c, it is not as clear that established disease can be reversed, so secondary comorbidities are not commonly used as justification for islet transplantation. However, DM1 patients with a well-functioning kidney transplant may be candidates for islet transplantation after kidney transplant (without one of the above complications) if they show evidence of poor glycemic control on insulin, e.g., HbA1c $\geq$ 7.5%, since they are already on immunosuppression. Islet transplant has not yet been associated with renal graft loss and in fact may prolong renal graft function and survival. There have also been reports that islets transplanted after successful kidney transplant show better function and survival than those transplanted alone.

Simultaneous islet and kidney transplantation is an option in DM1 patients who qualify for a kidney transplant, but have not yet received one. This has not yet been widely adopted in clinical trials because the immunosuppression regimen for kidney transplantation is well established and quite effective and includes components that had been thought to preclude successful islet transplantation. Although some islet after kidney candidates undergo trial weaning and replacement of the islet-toxic components of their immunosuppression prior to islet transplantation, many remain on their kidney immunosuppression and do equally well, so this may be less of a concern. Too few simultaneous islet and kidney transplants have been performed to ascertain the risk to a newly transplanted kidney done under islet transplant immunosuppression.

In addition to the usual screening done for solid organ transplant, weight and insulin requirement are important factors in considering candidacy for islet transplantation. Specific numbers vary by center and trial, but body weight greater than 75–90 kg make it unlikely that an adequate number of islets will be procured to achieve insulin independence, even with islets recovered from two or three donors. Patients with BMI greater than 26–30 kg/m^2 who require more than 50–60 IU/d of insulin are likely to have peripheral insulin resistance in addition to DM1 and are also unlikely to become insulin independent with islet transplantation.

Processing

In the 1970s, the first attempts to use islet transplantation clinically were stymied by the inability to extract and purify islets. It was not until 1986 that the development of automated islet-cell processing made it possible to collect sufficient numbers of islets to reverse diabetes, albeit only for a few days. Current technologies are all based on this method described by Camillo Ricordi.

Islet donors undergo the same screening as solid organ donors, although acceptable age and BMI for islets are much higher than for whole pancreas. Generally, the pancreas is harvested as if for whole organ transplant, then stored and transported, on ice, either in standard preservation solution or at the interface between a preservation solution and a second layer of oxygenated perfluorocarbon. If the latter method is used, the duodenum and spleen are usually removed prior to storage. This second layer is meant to provide enough oxygen to the organ by diffusion to support whatever low rate of metabolism continues during cold storage and prevent anoxic injury. It has shown promise in animal models, especially with prolonged storage times, but has not yet shown a clear advantage in clinical use where the cold storage time is kept to a minimum. The pancreas should accumulate less than 12 hours and preferably less than 8 hours of cold ischemia time.

Processing begins with dissecting the duodenum and spleen off, if not already done, and clamping off the main and accessory ducts before dividing the pancreas at the neck. Cannulas are inserted into the main pancreatic ducts of each piece at the cut surface. An enzyme blend containing collagenase is then infused through the ducts until the two halves are well distended. For about a decade, Liberase HI (manufactured by Roche), which contained both collagenase and a neutral protease, thermolysin, had been used as the standard reagent. Because production involved contact with material from bovine brain, there was concern about the risk of transmitting bovine spongiform encephalopathy with the islets, so this was discontinued in 2007. The standard switched to a collagenase only preparation (manufactured by Serva), which required addition of a protease. This switch was associated with reports of decreased islet yields, but this has improved with alterations in processing techniques, and formal studies have not affirmed such observations. Roche now makes a mammalian tissue-free version of Liberase HI, which otherwise appears, in initial studies, to produce acceptable islets. However, variability in the potency of enzyme blends from one lot to another continues to be an issue.

The pancreas is then cut into small pieces and placed into a digestion chamber, which is warmed, in order to activate the enzymes. The digestion chamber continuously shakes, adding mechanical disruption to enzymatic digestion. Continuous flow of fluid through the chamber removes the smallest fragments of tissue, which are sampled and visually inspected. When intact islets are visualized, the fragments are diluted with cold culture media or other physiological solution and kept cool to prevent further digestion. The fibrous network of ducts and vessels remains in the digestion chamber. Further purification can be done by density-gradient separation, as highly purified islets are less dense than islets still attached to exocrine tissue. The goal is greater than 30% purity and greater than 70% viability (as determined by fluorescent dye exclusion or inclusion), and it is more difficult to get high-purity islets from younger donors, although cell clusters from younger donors are speculated to contain pancreatic duct stem cells that may develop into insulin-producing cells post-transplant.

A sample of the fluid may be taken for long-term microbiological culture in order to identify any rare pathogens that may be infused into the patient, and antibiotics are added to the final tissue collection. For clinical use, the islets should be Gram stain and endotoxin negative. The latter is important not only for prevention of systemic inflammatory response syndrome (SIRS) in the recipient but also to prevent a local inflammatory response that will prevent subsequent engraftment or spur rejection. These islets may be cultured for up to 72 hours to "rest" the islets and allow them to recover from any ischemic or traumatic injury. This can also be helpful if extra time is needed to prepare the patient with pre-transplant immunosuppression.

Islets are quantified by packed tissue volume (5–10 ml per infusion) and by islet equivalent (IE). An IE is defined by both insulin content, generally determined with an insulin granule binding dye such as diphenylthiocarbazone and size, based on a spherical islet of mean diameter 150 μM. It is rare to get more than 600 000–700 000 islets per pancreas, with higher BMI donors tending to yield more islets, and the number is usually much lower. Only 30–60% of islet isolations result in material adequate for transplantation.

Infusion

The islets (Figure 35.1) are resuspended into 50–200 ml of solution supplemented with human serum albumin and heparin. More than 90% of islets are transplanted into the liver by infusion through the portal system. This can be done percutaneously or through a mini-laparotomy and are allowed to infuse under gravity. Percutaneous infusion requires only local anesthesia and is performed by interventional radiology via transhepatic catheterization of the portal venous system. Portal vein pressure is recorded before, during, and after the infusion; if pressures exceed 22 mmHg, the infusion is temporarily halted to allow pressure to drop back below 18 mmHg. Careful monitoring of portal pressures and cessation of infusion as necessary have largely eradicated complications such as portal hypertension and splenic hemorrhage. Because there is no reversal of heparin, coils and gelatin-sponge pledgets are left in the puncture tract during catheter removal to decrease the risk of bleeding. This probably decreases the very low risk of biliary leakage and arteriovenous fistula as well. Alternatively, access to the portal vein can be gained by open placement of an infusion catheter into an appropriately sized omental vein. This is done under general anesthesia through a small abdominal incision in the operating room. The vein is ligated upon withdrawal of the

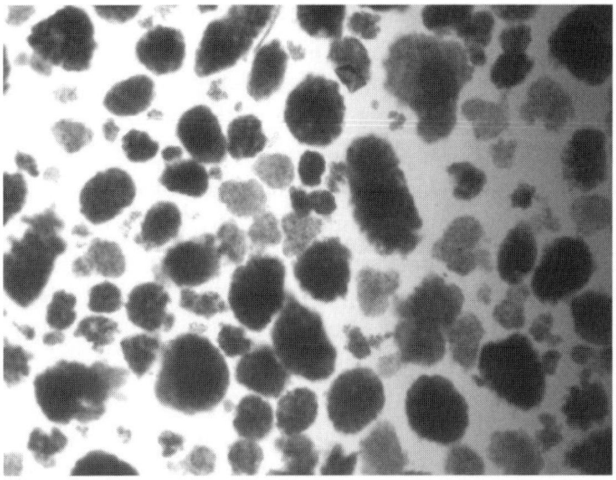

Figure 35.1 Islets isolated from deceased donor pancreas, ready for infusion. Photograph courtesy of J. Lei, MD, MBA, Massachusetts General Hospital.

infusion catheter. The incidence of branch portal vein thrombosis (no complete portal vein thrombosis has been reported) is similar with both procedures and has decreased with newer purification techniques, lower islet cell volumes, and the use of heparin, both 70 IU/kg of heparin in the infusate and a continuous infusion post-procedure. Hepatic macro-infarction has not been reported in humans, but mouse models show peri-islet areas of hepatic necrosis by reflected light confocal microscopy. This probably corresponds to the small and transient rise in serum aminotransferases seen after intraportal islet infusion. However, it does not appear to have any clinical sequelae.

An average of 8000–12 000 IE/kg recipient body weight is needed to achieve insulin independence, although insulin independence has been reported with less than 6000 IE/kg. Less than 5000 IE/kg body weight as an initial infusion is not generally considered worth exposing the patient to foreign material and immunosuppression, and two to four infusions may be required for insulin independence. Islets from multiple donors may be combined into a single infusion, if the donors are simultaneously available, or infusions may be given serially, either when the initial infusion results in decreased insulin requirements without complete insulin independence, or when an initially successful graft function decreases to the point of the recipient requiring insulin again.

The liver became the preferred site of transplantation because animal studies showed that fewer islets were required to reverse diabetes than in any other easily accessible sites. Intrahepatic placement of transplanted islets offers some physiological advantages, allowing insulin to be released through its usual route of delivery through the liver, exposing hepatocytes to "portal" concentrations of insulin that stimulate glucose storage, and permitting the liver to play its normal role in regulating systemic insulin levels. Portal circulation contains the highest concentrations of immunosuppression, which is advantageous in an islet alone patient, but this may prove toxic in a patient with a coexisting kidney allograft, which requires maintenance of adequate immunosuppressive levels in the systemic circulation.

There are additional reasons that intraportal infusion may be deleterious to islets. Although the liver has an arterial as well as portal venous blood supply, parenchymal oxygen levels are lower than in the pancreas, probably particularly so for islets lodged in the small vessels of the portal system. Islets in the liver have greater exposure to any ingested toxins or those released by gut bacteria, and the high glucose and lipid levels in post-prandial mesenteric blood may stress β cells as well. Scattered throughout the liver, it is difficult to biopsy islet allografts for monitoring purposes, and in the unlikely chance that the islets were contaminated by microbes or malignant cells, they could not be removed without damaging or removing the liver. Auto-islets transplanted into the livers of pancreatectomized dogs eventually lost function in nearly 80% of animals within 15 months, suggesting that the liver does not support long-term survival of islets, even in the absence of auto- and allo-immunity.

Furthermore, placement of islets in a vascular space exposes them to immediate blood-mediated inflammatory reaction (IBMIR). IBMIR occurs when proinflammatory factors such as tissue factor and monocyte chemoattractant protein 1 are upregulated by islet cells during brain death and organ procurement. These engage the coagulation and complement systems, platelets, and polymorphonuclear neutrophils (PMNs) when transplanted islets come in contact with blood in the portal vein. In addition, collagen and other extra-cellular matrix proteins present in islet clusters are prothrombotic and trigger inflammation. Some speculate that as much as 75% of the transplanted islet mass is lost to IBMIR, compounded by inflammation induced locally by hypoxic hepatocytes surrounding islet emboli in the portal vessels.

Many other sites have been used in the laboratory, including the spleen, pancreas, peritoneum, stomach wall, bone marrow, testis, brain, and systemic venous circulation (lodging in the lung), but only a few have been used clinically. Placement of islets under the kidney capsule is frequently used in mice, but was used only briefly in the early days of clinical islet transplantation; surgical access to the kidney capsule is highly invasive and the space has lower oxygen tension than the liver parenchyma. Intramuscular islet transplantation has been done in humans (at subtherapeutic doses) and is of special interest because of easy accessibility for biopsy, but in animals, it has required coadministration of a growth factor or a prevascularized device to achieve metabolic function and seems to induce vigorous leukocyte infiltrates. One patient who received autologous islets into the brachioradialis muscle continued to require insulin after pancreatectomy for hereditary pancreatitis, but was C-peptide positive for at least 2 years. One attempt was made at a combined intrathymic and intraportal transplantation, but the patient failed to become insulin independent in spite of receiving pooled islets from seven donors, and nothing is known of the contribution that thymic injection made to long-term C-peptide positivity. Pilot studies have been done and larger trials are underway for subcutaneous placement of both allo- and xeno-islets in macrocapsules or within vascularized prostheses, but few data are available now.

Engraftment and function

Many strategies are used to promote better engraftment. Heparin is given at the time of infusion to prevent portal vein branch thrombosis, but heparin also has important anti-inflammatory activities. In addition to its anti-platelet and anti-thrombin properties, heparin inhibits complement activation and impairs leukocyte function by disrupting leukocyte adhesion molecules' interaction with their ligands and inhibiting PMN elastases and proteases. Low-molecular-weight dextran sulfate can also be given with islet infusion. It is associated with a lower risk of bleeding than heparin, and in addition to its anti-coagulant properties, it also inhibits complement activation. Other drugs are primarily anti-inflammatory agents, but do carry some increased risk of bleeding. Etanercept is a fusion protein consisting of the extracellular binding portion of human tumor necrosis factor receptor linked to the Fc portion of human immunoglobulin (Ig) G1. It binds and deactivates tumor necrosis factor alpha (TNFα), which is directly toxic to β cells, as well as participating in IBMIR. Its use at induction improves marginal mass allograft outcomes in rodents and has been associated with better likelihood of insulin independence in marginal mass studies in humans.

One simple method of decreasing β-cell toxicity has been to maintain patients on gradually decreasing amounts of insulin during and after islet transplantation. This allows the islets to recover and engraft before exposing them to hyperglycemia and increasing their metabolic demands. Insulin dosing obviously needs to be carefully monitored to avoid hypoglycemia, and glucose may need to be administered.

Agents such as exenatide/Byetta aim to improve the function of existing islets. Exenatide is a synthetic version of a hormone first isolated from Gila monster saliva, which enhances glucose-dependent insulin secretion and suppresses glucagon secretion. It is in clinical use to improve glycemic control in type 2 diabetes mellitus in conjunction with oral hypoglycemics and also appears to increase the likelihood of achieving insulin independence and prolong insulin independence in uncontrolled studies.

Immunosuppression (also see Chapter 3)

Classically, glucocorticoids have played a major role in post-transplant immunosuppression. However, steroids are known to inhibit insulin secretion by β cells and may exert a direct toxic effect on them, as well. At the same time, steroids increase the demand for insulin by simultaneously stimulating liver gluconeogenesis and inhibiting peripheral uptake of glucose. It was not until 1990 that a steroid-free immunosuppression regimen including tacrolimus was reported to result in long-term insulin independence of one patient. In that series, however, patients did not have autoimmune diabetes and had become diabetic as a result of upper abdominal exenteration (requiring liver transplant at the same time). Furthermore, only five of nine patients were insulin-free 6 months after transplant. Real enthusiasm for islet transplantation as treatment for DM1 arose from initial reports of the results of the "Edmonton protocol," which combined steroid-free immunosuppression with infusions from one to four donors, as necessary to achieve insulin independence. Seven of seven patients in a single-center study became insulin independent and remained insulin independent 5.5–15 months later at the time of publication.

The international trial of the Edmonton protocol included 36 patients at nine international sites who received induction with daclizumab and maintenance with sirolimus (SRL) and tacrolimus (TAC). Fifty-eight percent were insulin independent at any point during the study, 44% were insulin independent 1 year after the final transplant, and only 14% were still insulin independent 2 years after transplant. An additional 28% required insulin but no longer had hypoglycemic episodes at 1 year, and a total of 70% were still C-peptide positive at 2 years. There was a great deal of center variability, with some centers achieving 1-year insulin independence in 100% of their patients, whereas other centers had no patients who were insulin independent at 1 year. A 5-year follow-up from Edmonton, as a single-center study, reported 10% who were insulin independent and 80% who were C-peptide positive.

Part of the issue may be that TAC (perhaps a generalized calcineurin inhibitor [CNI] effect) can cause deficiencies in insulin secretion, reducing insulin mRNA and protein production, as well as decreasing β-cell proliferation. Animal studies suggest that CNIs also reduce peripheral tissue sensitivity to insulin. SRL has also been shown to prevent β-cell division, inhibiting replacement of β cells lost to attrition. The effects of TAC and SRL on β-cell proliferation are additive.

Some new immunosuppression protocols attempt to address this problem by minimizing exposure to TAC and/or SRL. Clinical trials with daclizumab or basiliximab induction and maintenance with belatacept and mycophenolate mofetil (MMF) are underway, with early, unpublished results of five of five patients insulin independent after a single infusion for 70–305 days.

Another TAC-free protocol used anti-thymocyte globulin for induction and efalizumab together with either SRL or MMF for maintenance. Efalizumab is of particular interest in transplant for DM1 because it has the potential to inhibit T cells that do not require costimulation for activation and proliferation (especially in the setting of lymphopenia inducing immunosuppression), such as memory T cells that would be present in autoimmune diseases such as DM1. There are unpublished reports that four of five patients remain insulin independent 150–240 days after withdrawl of efalizumab for safety reasons (some patients remain on single-agent maintenance with SRL or MMF only) and have increased number of regulatory T cells (Tregs) and reduced allospecific T-cell activity.

Other protocols still using TAC and/or SRL have also been promising. Teplizumab is a humanized mouse anti-CD3 antibody that is also in clinical trials for newly diagnosed DM1 as an attempt to preserve the remaining β cells. In an islet transplantation pilot study using teplizumab for induction with SRL and low-dose TAC maintenance, four of six patients were insulin independent at 1 year and three of six were still insulin independent at 3 years. At this time, there are still ongoing trials with teplizumab.

Some current islet transplantation trials use alemtuzumab induction and TAC/MMF maintenance. A pilot study reports 90% insulin independence at 2 years. An unpublished study has 10 of 12 insulin independent patients with maximum follow-up of 4 years (the remaining two patients stopped immunosuppression because of meningitis and a brain abscess, both of which have resolved with treatment and immunosuppression withdrawal). These are small numbers of patients, but these results parallel long-term outcomes with whole organ pancreas transplantation. Alemtuzumab has also been used in China for simultaneous islet and kidney transplants with promising results at 1-year follow-up. The fact that CD52 is present on natural killer cells, monocytes, and macrophages raised the possibility that alemtuzumab might reduce IBMIR, and quantitative function tests at 3 months do suggest improved engraftment. There is also evidence that islet transplant patients on alemtuzumab have donor-specific Tregs that produce interleukin-10 and decreased allo- and islet-specific T-cell reactivity.

The 2009 annual report of the Collaborative Islet Transplant Registry suggests that T-cell–depleting induction is associated with a 0.3–0.8-fold lower hazard ratio of losing insulin independence than interleukin-2 receptor blockade induction. Unpublished subanalysis of data collected by the Collaborative Islet Transplant Registry suggests that the use of T-cell–depleting induction is associated with higher rates of initial insulin independence and longer persistence, approaching that of whole organ transplantation.

Post-transplant monitoring

In the International Trial of the Edmonton Protocol, insulin independence was defined as HbA1 less than 6.5%, fasting glucose ≤ 140 mg/dl three or fewer times a week, and post-prandial glucose ≤ 180 mg/dl four or fewer times a week, in the absence of exogenous insulin. C-peptide, particularly valuable in monitoring graft function in patients who have developed an insulin requirement after being insulin independent, helps determine whether immunosuppression should be continued in order to maintain some level of endogenous insulin production.

Many patients who require supplemental insulin still experience freedom from hypoglycemic episodes and metabolic lability. It is likely that the residual islet mass is responsible for enough insulin production that if the islets stop releasing insulin in response to hypoglycemia, the exogenous insulin is not sufficient to completely inhibit glucagon release from α cells. α cells may also become more responsive because of the intervening avoidance of hypoglycemic episodes while the patient was insulin independent. Preventing severe hypoglycemic episodes and metabolic lability not only avoids hospital admissions and risk of death, but also provides a significant improvement in the patient's quality of life, even if insulin administration is required. Patients with partial graft function often have lower HbA1c levels when compared with pretransplant or to those with negative C-peptide, and this has been associated with fewer cardiovascular deaths and better atherosclerotic profiles. These benefits are generally thought to be worth the risk of continued immunosuppression.

Provocative testing such as measuring glucose and insulin responses to mixed meals and intravenous glucose can give more quantitative information regarding declining islet function before the development of insulin requirements, but the indications for treatment are not yet clear. Similarly, anti-islet antibodies are monitored with the rationale that re-appearance after transplant may signal impending rejection, but their significance is still ambiguous and not definitively worth the risks of increasing immunosuppression. Anti-HLA antibodies have been associated with rejection in solid organ transplants and declining islet function, as well. There has been one case report of an insulin-independent patient who developed anti-HLA antibodies 6 months prior to developing poor glycemic control eventually requiring treatment with insulin. A course of rituximab and intravenous IgG resulted in recovery of insulin independence and loss of anti-HLA antibody expression.

Standard surveillance for diabetic complications should continue as for usual clinical care of a diabetic patient and to document their progression or regression following islet transplantation. Although markers are being developed for visualization of intrahepatic islets by positron emission tomography and magnetic resonance imaging, there is not yet a standard imaging technique.

Auto-transplant and living donor allo-transplant

The remaining cases of insulin-deficient diabetes follow surgical removal of the pancreas for chronic pancreatitis or for pancreatic cancer and occasionally, non-specific inflammatory destruction of the endocrine tissue by chronic pancreatitis. There is a fairly large experience with islet auto-transplant for chronic pancreatitis, but because of the risk of malignant cells contaminating the islet preparation, there is only one report from Germany of islet auto-transplant done for pancreatic adenocarcinoma. The patient never achieved insulin independence and died 2.5 years later from tumor recurrence, although not in the liver.

Insulin independence occurs less often with islet auto-transplantation: 32% at 1 year in the University of Minnesota series of 173 patients, with the first transplanted in February 1977. However, it must be remembered that islet auto-transplants are all single-donor infusions, the donor has a diseased pancreas and may be non-ideal for other reasons, and that many transplants in the series were done before islet isolation techniques had been optimized (75% of the auto-transplant recipients received 5000 or fewer IE/kg). However, of those who do achieve insulin independence, 74% remained so at 2 years, 69% at 5 years, and 28% at 10 years. One of the patients continues to be insulin independent over 13 years later. In contrast, among islet allo-transplant patients who achieve insulin independence, only 45% remained so at 2 years and less than 10% at 5 years.

The experience in islet auto-transplant suggests that late attrition in allo-transplants is not due solely to using the liver as the site of transplant, as suggested by previously mentioned dog studies. There are a small number of autopsy specimens from islet allo-transplant patients who died from other causes, but who had increasing insulin requirements with partial graft function. Although those show loss of islet mass without evidence of immune damage or infiltration, the difference between autograft and allograft persistence suggests that much of the gradual loss of islet mass is likely immune-mediated. The fact that 32% of patients can achieve islet independence when only 25% received more than 5000 IE/kg supports the thought that poor engraftment involves factors peculiar to deceased donors, which are exacerbated by prolonged cold storage.

There has also been one report of successful living donor islet transplant in Japan. The recipient was diabetic because of pancreatitis and suffered from hypoglycemic unawareness. Her mother, the donor, donated her distal pancreas, which yielded more than 400 000 islets. The immunosuppression regimen followed the Edmonton protocol, supplemented with infliximab, an anti-TNFα monoclonal antibody. At the 2-month follow-up, both donor and recipient were insulin independent.

Future of islet transplantation

It is likely that islet allo-transplantation will soon be equivalent to whole organ pancreas transplantation in terms of graft function and survival, while retaining the advantage of being a much lower risk procedure. Recent trials suggest that as many as 80% of patients achieve insulin independence. Graft survival has also improved significantly. In the Edmonton international trial, insulin independence persistence rates were 24% at 2 years, but this had improved to approximately 40% at 3 years for transplants done between 1999–2004, and then to approximately 60% at 3 years for transplants done after 2004. For islet transplantation to become standard treatment for DM1, further improvements are needed in immunosuppression and in durability and effectiveness. Furthermore, more sources of islets are necessary. This last issue is being approached by efforts at developing animal sources of islets and engineering β cells in vitro, either from stem cells or re-programming differentiated cells. Once islet allo-transplant becomes more reliable, living donors may be considered.

Minimizing IBMIR, which may begin with donor management, is crucial to improving engraftment rates and the effectiveness of islet transplantation. The risk of bleeding limits the dosage and duration of heparin for the purposes of IBMIR, but alternate forms of heparin such as 2-O,3-O-desulfated heparin, which retain their anti-inflammatory properties and have much lower anticoagulation activity, may be an option. In the laboratory, one group has coated islets with heparin to hide the proinflammatory components from their receptors in the bloodstream, minimizing systemic exposure to anti-coagulation. Other agents with combined anti-coagulant and anti-inflammatory properties, such as activated protein C and CD39, are under investigation.

To prolong graft survival, more effective and safer forms of immunosuppression are constantly being sought. Besides developing new pharmaceuticals and bioagents, tolerance induction and encapsulation technology are also possible methods to protect allo-islets from the recipient immune system. Probably the most poorly defined factor in islet transplantation is the long-term, non–immune-related loss of islet mass that is observed in animals and humans. This will require a better understanding of β-cell homeostasis.

Further reading

Clinical Islet Transplantation Consortium. Available at: www.citisletstudy.org.

Collaborative Islet Transplant Registry. Available at: www.citregistry.org.

Fiorina P, Shapiro AMJ, Ricordi C, Secchi A. The clinical impact of islet transplantation. *Am J Transplant* 2008; **8**: 1990–7.

International Islet Transplant Registry. Available at: www.med.uni-giessen.de/itr.

Islet Cell Resource Center. Available at: icr.coh.org.

Nath DS, Hering BJ. Islet cell replacement therapy. *Clin Lab Med* 2005; **25**: 541–56.

Chapter 36

Intestinal transplantation

Stephen J. Middleton, Simon M. Gabe, Neville V. Jamieson, and Andrew J. Butler

Key points

- Parenteral nutrition remains the first-line treatment for irreversible intestinal failure.
- Intestinal transplantation now offers most patients an improvement in quality of life as compared with complicated parenteral nutrition.
- Survival is now better than that of lung and approaching that of liver transplantation, and systems are being developed to more accurately predict postoperative survival of individual patients.
- Intestinal transplantation is a cost-effective alternative to parenteral nutrition as the costs of the procedure equate to the combined costs of 2 years on parenteral nutrition, after which a cost saving is made.
- Acute rejection of a functioning graft is invariably associated with a change in its function; the stomal output is usually increased and more watery in consistency.

The technical ability to transplant the intestine was recorded over a century ago; however, many attempts at this procedure over the intervening years did not achieve even short-term graft or patient survivals. Success, in terms of medium-term survival with fully functioning grafts, was finally reported in the late 1980s. The key factor in the progression of the technique was the development of suitable immunosuppressive regimes.

The exponential increase in the use of the procedure in the 1990s has been superseded by a less dramatic rise over the last 10 years, which now has almost reached a plateau at about 200 procedures worldwide per year (Figure 36.1). This trend can be

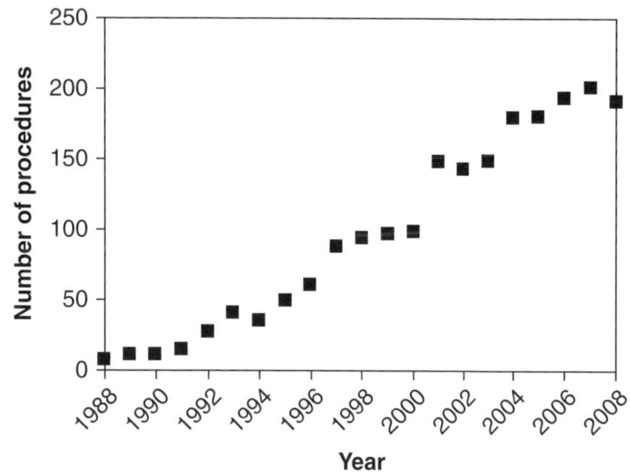

Figure 36.1 Intestinal transplantations undertaken per year (adults and children). Adapted from the International Registry, with permission: www.lhsc.on.ca/itr.

partly accounted for by the presence of an initial reservoir of patients who required the surgery leading to a rapid rise in its use and then by the steady increase in transplant centers offering the procedure and gradual broadening of indications which maintain the rate of use at the current level. As results improve, the technique is offered to patients earlier, and if this trend continues, it may be used as an alternative to parenteral nutrition (PN) over the next 5 to 10 years rather than being an option only when PN cannot continue due to complications.

Current survival chances are probably best represented by the data from the international registry. One-, 5-, and 10-year survivals are approximately 65%, 40%, and 30%, respectively, but if the last 10-year experience is considered, survival figures have improved to 75%, 50%, and 40%, respectively, and in adults 5-year survival is approaching 60%. There are slight differences in survival between types of procedures (isolated intestine, intestine and liver, or multivisceral)

Organ Transplantation: A Clinical Guide, ed. A.A. Klein, C.J. Lewis, and J.C. Madsen. Published by Cambridge University Press.

undertaken. These tend to fluctuate, and currently combined small intestine and liver grafts are associated with a better survival, at least if the comparison is made between those surviving the first postoperative year. The experience of the center is also an independent risk factor, with those centers with less volume having an inferior survival record. Interestingly, most of the improved survival has been seen in the first year, after which the survival curves have not changed over the last two decades. This suggests that the main focus of attention should now turn to outpatient care and follow-up and the understanding and prevention of chronic rejection.

Management of patients with irreversible intestinal failure

PN remains the primary treatment for patients with irreversible intestinal failure. This is currently associated with a better survival chance than intestinal transplantation, with 10-year survival in the literature of 43–71%, and when well tolerated can lead to excellent duration and quality of life. However, occasionally due to complications of PN or to progression of an underlying disease process, PN cannot be safely continued and transplantation is then considered (Table 36.1). Such transplantation candidates can be divided into three categories:

1. Patients with life-threatening complications of PN, such as (a) failing vascular access, (b) PN-related liver disease, or (c) severe recurrent line-associated sepsis.
2. Patients with indications for extensive evisceration of abdominal organs requiring concurrent transplantation.
3. Patients requiring transplantation of other abdominal organs.

A fourth category is emerging that considers patients with very poor quality of life on PN as potential candidates.

When caring for this group of patients it is essential to appreciate that they may benefit from a transplant in the future and should not be allowed to drift through a downward spiral of PN complication or disease progression without considering transplantation as an option. Certain subgroups of patients on PN have a worse prognosis and should be monitored more closely to allow timely referral. These include those with ultra-short bowel syndrome who tend to develop intestinal failure associated liver disease and visceral myopathy or neuropathy who develop liver disease and central venous catheter sepsis.

Timing of intestinal transplantation

Much of the improvement in postoperative survival is due to the realization that patients need to be in good physical and psychological condition to survive the procedure. There is evidence that survival is inversely associated with comorbidity, and clinical scoring systems that will semi-quantify this risk are being developed. Therefore, patients who have active reversible comorbidity are not usually offered transplantation. Those with sudden loss of intestine due to conditions such as volvulus or superior mesenteric artery thrombosis should be established on PN and all efforts made to improve and stabilize their physical and psychological condition. Many such patients will remain well and content on PN and currently would not be considered as candidates for transplantation.

Patients who cannot be established on stable PN are usually not candidates for transplantation as they are unlikely to survive the procedure. Those initially established on PN who subsequently develop complications or experience progression of an underlying disease process should be evaluated for their suitability for transplantation. Certain groups of patients on PN can be considered as high risk for PN complications and therefore potential candidates for earlier transplantation. The main PN-related indications in adults and children are loss of vascular access and PN-related liver disease (Table 36.1). Patients who lose two or more major venous access sites are candidates for assessment as it is important to evaluate them while venous access remains sufficient for transplantation. The risks associated with the transplantation procedure are increased when venous access falls below two or three major veins, depending on the extent of the planned surgery. Those who develop liver disease need careful evaluation as it may be possible to avoid liver transplantation if the small intestine is transplanted before progression to severe liver disease. This progression can often be insidious and is a leading cause of death on the transplantation waiting list.

Occasionally, patients find their quality of life considerably impaired by PN and explore the possibility of intestinal transplantation as a way of improving it. A cautious approach should be taken in these

Table 36.1 Summary of indications for intestinal transplantation

1. Life-threatening complications of PN
a) Progressive liver disease
• Severe liver disease or progressive disease despite all remedial actions
b) Recurrent septic episodes
• IF patients who have severe septic complications (i.e., life-threatening line infection needing admission to ITU, or recurrent fungal or yeast or candidal infections)
c) Lack of central venous access (including femoral veins)
• For isolated intestine: venous access limited to three major sites
• For intestine as part of a cluster graft: venous access limited to four major sites
2. Very poor quality of life thought to be correctable by transplantation.
3. Patients with indications for extensive surgery involving partial or complete evisceration:
Adults
a) Surgery to remove a large proportion of the abdominal viscera, which is considered untenable without associated multi-visceral transplantation (e.g., extensive desmoid disease, extensive severe mesenteric arterial disease requiring intervention)
b) Localized malignancy considered to be amenable to curative resection, which would necessitate extensive evisceration (e.g., localized neuroendocrine tumors and cholangiocarcinoma – particular caution should be exercised with this group)
Children
a) Surgery that will lead to:
• Terminal gastrostomy
• Terminal duodenostomy
• Ultra short bowel: In children <10 cm, with or without ileocecal valve
• Recurrent fluid and electrolyte management problems needing frequent hospital admission
4. Patients requiring transplantation of other abdominal organs
a) When the transplantation procedure is expected to preclude the possibility of future intestinal transplantation (loss of vulnerable and limited venous access, further HLA sensitization)
b) When the risk is increased by excluding the intestine from the graft (predictable problems related to administering immunosuppression [e.g., line sepsis], ongoing severe intestinal disease such as diabetic visceral neuropathy, or ultra short bowel syndrome, causing fluid, electrolyte, and acid–base balance problems [damage to renal graft]), and when the need for subsequent intestinal transplantation is considered likely

situations as there will likely be a trade-off between gain in quality of life and reduced longevity. This can be difficult for patients to appreciate, and all efforts must be made to ensure that they have full psychiatric and psychological evaluation and support. It is also important to appreciate that quality of life may not improve after transplantation and they will not return to a medication-free and morbidity-free life that they often seek. Most patients will be vulnerable to infections and drug side effects, although these factors are usually well tolerated. It is also very important for patients to appreciate that intestinal transplantation does not currently guarantee a life without a stoma. If an overriding reason for a patient to have a transplant is to remove their stoma, then it should be explained that they will have an ileostomy after the procedure. There may be the possibility of joining the transplanted small bowel onto the patients native colon (if still present) after a number of years, but this is currently an area of development.

The process and requirements for intestinal transplantation

The transplant team

The establishment of an effective and comprehensive team of health professionals is one of the key factors for the success of a program. Core members should include a lead gastroenterologist, a lead surgeon, and at least one additional named senior colleague in each of these disciplines with adequate experience and knowledge to provide support and cover. There should be an established team of transplant surgeons with sufficient numbers to prevent overcommitment of any individual during very active periods. Specialist nurse coordinators provide the platform of organization and nursing expertise. In addition to the core team, there must be many other interested parties who are invited as named opinions in their specialty. As the program expands, this list of allied professionals becomes wide-ranging.

Referral and assessment of adult patients

Patients thought to be candidates are usually assessed during a short programmed admission to the transplant center when a comprehensive evaluation of their gut function, anatomy, and comorbidity is undertaken. In the United Kingdom, all adult patients are then discussed at the National Forum for Adult Intestinal Transplantation, at which recommendations regarding the most appropriate management plan are made. In each case, this process is a prerequisite to receiving National Commissioning Group financial support to undertake the procedure.

It is important to involve external peer review before listing patients for transplantation. This encourages uniformity of practice and improves the selection process. A detailed preoperative assessment of patients allows their preoperative status to be semi-quantified and included when considering center performance statistics.

Particular attention should be given to those who are likely to fall through the window of opportunity. These patients often have progressive disease, which may advance to a point that contraindicates transplantation or results in death while on the waiting list. Examples of this include patients who are rapidly losing venous access points and those bleeding from portal hypertension. Special consideration should also be given to PN-dependent patients who require transplantation of other organs and may benefit from a cluster graft including intestine rather than receive a subsequent intestinal graft in the setting of an existing graft and consequent immunosuppression.

Selection of type of grafts

Intestinal transplantation is frequently undertaken as part of a composite graft containing other intra-abdominal organs. This is often required to resolve disease or restore function of vital organs and occasionally for technical reasons to reduce the risks associated with the surgery.

Where irreversible intestinal failure is the only significant dysfunction, "isolated" intestinal grafts are used. This has the theoretical advantage over other options as it is potentially reversible in the case of catastrophic rejection. Associated pancreatic disease such as in type 1 diabetes mellitus or gastroparesis as found in patients with visceral neuropathy or myopathy may warrant transplantation of stomach, duodenum, pancreas, and small intestine. This is often termed a "modified multi-visceral" graft because it excludes the liver. When undertaken in conjunction with the liver, it is termed multi-visceral". When disease is limited to the small intestine and liver, such as in intestinal failure related liver cirrhosis, a combined liver/intestine graft is offered to patients. The international registry report that isolated grafts are the commonest (59%), multivisceral account for 24%, and combined intestine/liver for the remaining 17%.

Listing and problems on the waiting list

In the United Kingdom, adult patients are considered by the National Forum for Adult Intestinal Transplantation for their suitability as candidates for transplantation and are also assessed locally for the feasibility of the transplant in each individual case. There may also be local concerns about comorbidity and complexity of peri- and postoperative care that must be considered. Once listed, the final preoperative preparations are made and they are registered with the central governing organization (UK Transplantation). At this stage it is important to inform all those involved in the current or future care of the patient, confirm that tissue typing have appropriate samples, a precise surgical plan has been made, and fully informed written consent for this plan and other possible outcomes obtained. The typical waiting time for a suitable donor in the United Kingdom is 9 months, and during this period patients are subject to deterioration. Patients on the waiting list need to be followed carefully to ensure that they are in a position to undergo transplantation if called. This usually involves reviewing them twice a month until transplantation.

Conditions leading to the need for intestinal transplantation

The majority of patients have irreversible intestinal failure and are not able to continue PN because of complications. Some have conditions that require extensive evisceration that cannot be undertaken without transplantation. A short bowel is the commonest underlying condition in both pediatric and adult patients. In the pediatric transplanted population, it accounts for 68% of patients and is predominantly the result of gastroschisis (24%), necrotizing enterocolitis (16%), volvulus (10%), and intestinal atresia (9%). In adult transplanted patients it accounts for 58% and is predominantly the result of volvulus (10%), Crohn's disease (8%), and trauma (7%).

Dysmotility including visceral myopathies and neuropathies represent another large group of patients (approxmately 14% overall). Adult patients with this condition tend to have a worse prognosis on PN and are consequently considered to be a high-risk group. They tend to get central venous catheter sepsis and lose venous access as well as develop liver disease and should therefore be watched more closely. Referral for consideration of transplantation should occur promptly if these complications occur.

The majority of patients with tumors (7% overall) have desmoids. These benign but locally invasive tumors also need very careful monitoring. Early referral may allow a less extensive transplant procedure. The growth of desmoids can suddenly accelerate, and this should trigger an immediate discussion with a transplant center. Patients transplanted because of other tumors have usually had a relatively localized neuroendocrine tumor or cholangiocarcinoma. The survival of some of these patients has been very good, extending over 5 years, although a detailed study of the outcome of this group has not been published.

Transplantation in pediatrics

Pediatric transplantation is not the specific subject of this chapter. However, the general principles of how and when to use intestinal transplantation for adults can also be applied in most cases to pediatrics. Perhaps the greatest difference from adults arises from the underlying primary diseases and the interaction with family members. Certain aspects of the postoperative social and psychological care also differ from those of adults. Schooling and adolescence are particularly challenging, whereas adults tend to find employment a major problem.

The immediate preoperative period

On admission for the transplantation procedure, baseline tests should be repeated, and it is important to check that written informed consent for the proposed surgery is in the notes and confirm that the patient is aware of the likely postoperative situation in the intensive treatment unit (ITU). The psychological status of the patient has a major effect on their postoperative recovery; it is important to make it clear to them that they will experience frequent setbacks postoperatively and that this is to be expected and should not be taken as an indication that the procedure is failing.

The surgery

The assessment summary and protocol should be available wherever the patient is being managed. It is common for the surgery to take 12–16 hours, after which patients often remain on ITU for 3–4 days, then high-dependency unit for 2–4 weeks before transfer to the ward for 4–6 weeks. This timeline is obviously subject to large variations. Peri-operative immunosuppression is summarized in Table 36.2.

Splenectomy

Many patients require a splenectomy. The need for this cannot always be predicted; therefore, it is our practice to prepare patients for this eventuality. Appropriate preoperative vaccinations are given and postoperative prophylaxis with penicillin V.

Other considerations

If renal transplantation is also undertaken, mannitol 20% 100 ml intravenously (IV) and furosemide 20 mg IV should be given before revascularization.

Postoperative care

Immunosuppression

Tacrolimus (TAC) should be started on the second postoperative day. It can be given orally, but its absorption should be confirmed by an absorption profile. Blood levels taken at intervals over 12 hours provide a guide to the efficiency of absorption. and 12 hour trough levels of 8–12 ng/ml are satisfactory

Table 36.2 Peri-operative immunosuppression

Agent	Dose	Start	Stop	Comments
Methylprednisolone	500 mg IV	1 hour before lymphocyte-depleting agent	Single dose	Important to cover possible cytokine release from lymphocyte depletion
Methylprednisolone	20 mg IV BID	Day 1	Day 7	Taper steroids depending on clinical picture
Methylprednisolone	10 mg IV BID	Day 7	Day 14	Stop if no signs of rejection
Chlorpheniramine	10 mg IV	1 hour before lymphocyte-depleting agent	Single dose	Important to cover possible cytokine release from lymphocyte depletion
Anti-lymphocyte antibody (Campath)	30 mg SC	Intraoperatively and day 1	Day 0 and 1 only	SC route minimizes effects from cytokine release
Tacrolimus	Aim for trough levels of 8–12 ng/ml	Day 2	Continue long term	Well absorbed from stomach; watch for renal impairment

Note: The choice of the agents used may vary between centers. BID: twice a day; IV: intravenously; SC: subcutaneously.

(Table 36.2). If the IV route is required, then an infusion delivering 0.05 mg/kg over 24 hours is commenced, aiming for levels at 24 hours of approximately 123–150 ng/ml. If the oral dose fails to achieve a satisfactory level, then IV TAC should be administered. When converting from IV to oral dosing, the dose ratio is usually considered to be 1:3. The target level should be reduced in the face of hypoalbuminemia. Steroids should be commenced on day 1, with IV methylprednisolone 20 mg administered twice a day (BID) for 7 days, then reduced to 10 mg BID for 7 days, and then stopped if no evidence of rejection. Mycophenolate mofetil (1g BD Po) can be used as an adjunct to tacrolimus when tolerated.

Antibiotics

These should be broad spectrum, and the patient's microbiological history should be considered. Virological monitoring should include cytomegalovirus (CMV) polymerase chain reaction/immunoglobulin M weekly or at each outpatient appointment from month 2–9 or at suggestion of CMV symptoms.

Prophylaxis against deep venous and graft venous thrombosis

Prophylaxis is given against deep venous thrombosis and graft venous thrombosis with low-molecular-weight heparin. In addition, aspirin is started on discharge or if platelet count rises above 500×10^9/L. Long-term anti-coagulation should be considered if thrombophilia is found or suspected.

Salt and water balance

Large shifts of fluid and electrolytes are often encountered postoperatively. The reasons for this have yet to be fully elucidated. In the first 2 weeks, sodium losses can occur by as much as 1 Mole per day, predominantly via the kidneys and also from high stomal output. The latter usually occurs after the third postoperative day and continues for 2–3 weeks. Occasionally this is protracted and requires large doses of loperamide. Codeine is less well tolerated and should be avoided if possible. In resistant cases it is worth a trial of separating dietary fluids from solids. Measuring fluid and electrolyte losses accurately is vital, and appropriate replacement is one of the most challenging aspects of the procedure.

Renal function

Special consideration must be given to renal function. Even in the absence of a renal graft, it is common to encounter renal impairment. This tends to occur in the second and third week, probably due to progressive TAC nephrotoxicity. Caution should be exercised as patients often have very low serum creatinine levels secondary to low lean body mass, and the relative change in creatinine should be noted.

Nutrition

It is common practice to commence PN, through a dedicated line when possible, 24–48 hours postoperatively. We find that a 24-hour period free from PN is useful to focus on regaining fluid and electrolyte balance after the operation. A Jejunal feeding tube should be placed at the time of surgery. As soon as there are signs of intestinal motility (usually after a few days), jejunal feeding is started and built up gradually over 10–14 days to full requirement if tolerated. This often takes longer, and the transition from PN to jejunal feeding must be tailored for each case. Likewise, the introduction of oral feeding varies widely; sips can be started as soon as nasogastric drainage tails off, but food is usually not commenced for 10–14 days to allow the anastomosis to heal. We often find that patients are slow to take oral food; some of this arises from the commonly encountered nausea, but it also seems to be related to their preoperative feeding state in that those who took very little or no food preoperatively have a tendency to find eating more difficult postoperatively. As oral feeding is established, the jejunal feeding can be tailed off. This usually takes 6–8 weeks, and there is often need for a small amount of residual jejunal feeding. On occasion, stopping jejunal feeding is required to stimulate patients to take their nutritional requirement orally. IV glutamine may be included in the postoperative regime in order to facilitate enterocyte recovery.

Physiotherapy

Early mobilization and chest physiotherapy are of key importance. Attention to the musculoskeletal system so that the complications associated with the prolonged surgery and ITU care can be minimized should be another focus.

Postoperative complications

Rejection of intestinal graft

Between 50% and 75% of patients experience rejection in the first few postoperative months. This figure varies widely partly because of the lack of consensus regarding the definition of acute rejection and also because of the heterogeneity of the anti-rejection regimes used, and this is commonest in the early postoperative period. The median time for the first episode of acute rejection to occur is about 2.5 weeks after surgery, and this underscores the need to take frequent biopsies to monitor rejection in the first month. Most acute rejection episodes occur in the first year, after which the level of monitoring can be considerably reduced and eventually stopped. It is our practice to take surveillance biopsies three times a week for the first month and twice a week during months 2 and 3, unless the patient is discharged, in which case once a week reducing to twice a month in months 2 and 3 is usually more realistic, but this should be tempered by the patient's ability to inform the center in the event of an alteration in stomal output or other sign of deterioration. From months 4–6 inclusive, once per month is usually appropriate and after this every 2 months for the first year and when appropriate according to clinical progress. Biopsies are taken from the distal small intestine via the stoma (at least 15 cm proximal to the stoma to avoid artefact, using small cup non-spiked forceps), and if present, regular colonic graft biopsies should be taken in addition. In situations when there is clinical suspicion of rejection but routine biopsies are normal, additional biopsies from the proximal intestine should be studied if access to this region is possible.

Diagnosis of intestinal graft rejection

Acute rejection of a functioning graft is invariably associated with a change in its function. The stomal output is usually increased and more watery in consistency. In addition, there are often signs of an inflammatory response with fever and elevated C-reactive protein, and serum albumin may fall. Immediate ileoscopy is required, and mucosal biopsies should be taken for urgent analysis by an experienced histopathologist. If there are ongoing signs despite a negative histological assessment for rejection, a clinical decision should be made, as it is possible for rejection to affect only a segment of small bowel. Other investigations can be helpful, such as white blood cell scintigraphy, positron emission tomography scanning, and capsule endoscopy. Nevertheless, it is not uncommon to encounter a situation where a clinical decision must be made on the basis of probability and risk–benefit assessment. In the majority of cases, a pulse of IV methylprednisolone 500 mg daily for 3 days will not cause harm and will often settle mild to moderate rejection. The clinical response to this can be evaluated and assists in formulating a view concerning the diagnosis of rejection. Escalation to anti-rejection agents with more adverse side effect profiles such as anti-thymocyte globulin (ATG) and alemtuzumab, however, should only be considered when the evidence for rejection is strong. Patients at high risk of CMV infection are likely to develop severe symptomatic disease if they receive antibody treatment for rejection. Pneumocystis carinii pneumonia prophylaxis should always be provided, and if patients are given ATG, they

Table 36.3 Common infections following intestinal transplantation in the United Kingdom

Infection	Stage	Location	Frequency	Likely pathogens	Clinical features	Diagnosis	Treatment
Bacterial	Immediate/ Early > mid > late	Central line–related, 29% Superficial surgical site, 17% Pneumonia, 14% Abdominal collection/peritonitis, 14%	Bacterial infections account for 69% of all infections, 60% of these are caused by gram positive organisms.	*Staphylococcus aureus* (including MRSA) *Escherichia coli* *Klebsiella* *Pseudomonas* Coagulase-negative staphylococci: IV line infections only	Brisk deterioration/septic shock/and organ-specific features (respiratory, urinary, intra-abdominal) Lower grade sepsis with coagulase-negative staphylococci	Blood cultures/ pneumococcal/ legionella urinary antigens/ Organ-specific: BAL; sputum; urine culture Intra-abdominal scans, radiologically guided percutaneous aspiration for accessible intra-abdominal collections	Initially broad-spectrum antibiotics, then adjust to include sensitivities of known organisms. Vancomycin if known MRSA-positive or if cross-infection occurring. (Use to cover possible MRSA if infection severe) Take special note of previous infections, particularly antibiotic-resistant organisms and current hospital-acquired pathogens. Remove infected IV lines; drain collections.
Fungal	Early < mid Median time to first fungal infection 181 days	Aspergillosis (30%) Wound, pulmonary, disseminated, cerebral	Fungal and candidal infections account for 14% of all infections.	*Aspergillus fumigatus*	Antibiotic-resistant pneumonia Aspergillosis serious, particularly disseminated, and intra-cerebral is usually fatal.	Chest CT can be diagnostic, respiratory samples other than BAL and trans-bronchial biopsy unlikely to be helpful. PCR investigation.	Aspergillosis with amphotericin B/AmBisome, voriconazole, or caspofungin
Candidal	Immediate/early	Candidiasis (>60%) oropharyngeal, genitourinary, wound-related, line infections		*Candida albicans*	Antibiotic-resistant sepsis	Blood and urine culture, line tip culture	AmBisome/Abelcet Caspofungin Fluconazole if mild/known to be sensitive Line removal if infected
Viral	Early < mid > late Median time to first viral infection 91 days Late episodes usually recurrence	CMV, look for colitis, hepatitis, and retinitis. EBV – PTLD late	Viral infections, 17% 60–85% of donor population are CMV positive. Activity in recipient usually implies reactivation.	Influenza, RSV, or CMV parainfluenza-3 CMV VZV HSV-1/2 EBV Human herpes virus 6 Adenovirus	Flu-like illness, pneumonia (Influenza, RSV, CMV, parainfluenza) Organ disease (CMV) Severe Chicken pox or zoster, pneumonitis (VZV) Systemic infection, organ disease (HSV-1/2) From glandular fever to PTLD (EBV) Systemic infection, fever (Human herpes virus 6) Systemic infection, organ disease (adenovirus)	Nose and throat swab, nasopharyngeal aspirate, BAL, PCR	Antivirals, depending on circulating strains (parainfluenza-3) Nebulized ribavirin (parainfluenza-3) Ganciclovir (CMV) Acyclovir (VZV, Herpes simplex 1/2) Discuss with virologist and hematologist (EBV) Discuss with duty virologist (Herpes virus-6) Cidofovir (discuss with duty virologist) (Adenovirus).

Immediate: first postoperative week; early: 2 weeks to 2 months postoperative; mid term: 2 months to 12 months postoperative; late: 12 months onwards. BAL: bronchoalveolar lavage; CMV: cytomegalovirus; CT: computed tomography; EBV: Epstein-Barr virus; HSV: herpes simplex virus; MRSA: methicillin-resistant Staphylococcus aureus; PCR: polymerase chain reaction; PTLD: post-transplant lymphoproliferative disorder.

should also receive full-dose intravenous ganciclovir for the duration of that treatment.

The histological changes of rejection are often subtle and can be misleading. Several particular histopathological features of acute rejection have been described in patients pretreated with lymphocyte-depleting antibodies, such as sparse neutrophil infiltration in the lamina propria leading to more prominent eosinophilic infiltration and sometimes eosinophilic cryptitis. The presence of apoptotic bodies in the crypt bases is perhaps the most specific feature but again must be semi-quantified and judged in the clinical context.

Acute vascular rejection is less common. When it occurs it can be rapid and overwhelming. It seems to occur independently from acute cellular rejection and is correlated with human leukocyte antigen (HLA) panel-reactive antibodies (PRAs) and positive T/B-cell cross-matches.

Tissue typing

HLA matching does not seem to reduce the incidence of acute rejection. The presence of donor-specific antibodies increases the risk of acute rejection, and PRA correlates with the incidence of acute rejection of the intestinal graft. Therefore, recipients are screened for PRAs in the preoperative assessment and during their time on the waiting list. It is also often useful to check PRAs in the postoperative period to assist in the diagnosis of rejection.

Treatment of systemic sepsis

Patients are heavily immunosuppressed such that onset of systemic sepsis is a medical emergency. This may be the first sign of rejection as a consequence of translocation of bacteria. Consultation with a microbiologist who is familiar with the clinical scenario is essential. Cultures should include blood, urine, and stomal effluent; swabs of throat, wounds, or IV sites; and drain fluid. Viral studies for Epstein-Barr virus, CMV, herpes simplex virus, and adenovirus should be undertaken and the advice of a virologist sought. A small intestinal biopsy should also be performed in cases of systemic sepsis of possible graft origin, such as concomitant increased ileostomy output, but there should be a low threshold for this in any case. Patients with chest signs should be considered for bronchoalveolar lavage. Organisms previously identified from patient specimens should be reviewed and

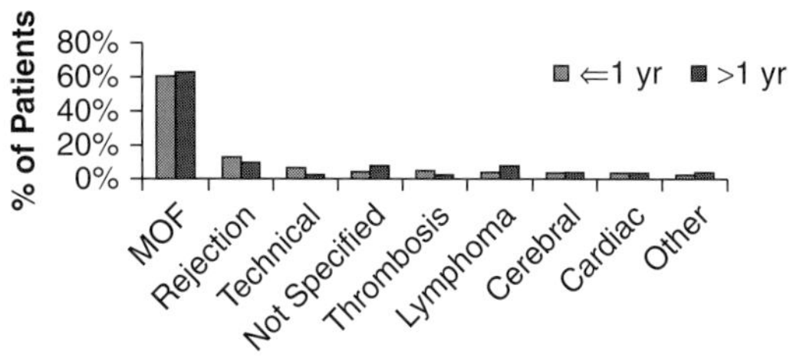

Figure 36.2 Causes of death following intestinal transplantation (adults and children). MOF: multi-organ failure. Adapted from the International Registry, with permission: www.lhsc.on.ca/itr.

taken into consideration. When IV lines appear clinically infected, they must be removed and catheter tips sent for culture. In the absence of an obvious source of infection, IV lines need to be removed when possible (Table 36.3). Broad spectrum antimicrobial agents should be commenced according to microbiologist advice and protocol.

The postoperative period following discharge from hospital

The postoperative mortality rate remains relatively steep for about 5 years and then begins to plateau. This emphasizes the importance of close monitoring of patients for at least 5 years and the need for rapid intervention for any deterioration in health while they remain in this relatively high-risk period. It has been our experience that patients continue to have problems after 5 years, requiring occasional hospitalization for short periods about once a year, usually for transient sepsis or dehydration. It is essential to have a well-organized follow-up schedule that allows detection of problems at an early stage. For patients who cannot get back to the center quickly, a shared care policy with local primary and secondary care providers is important. Psychological issues tend to come to the forefront as the physical problems occur less frequently.

Causes of postoperative death

In the early days of intestinal transplantation, the main cause of death was acute cellular rejection followed rapidly by sepsis and multi-organ failure (Figure 36.2). Since the advent of lymphocyte-depleting induction immunosuppression, this has largely been replaced by sepsis and multi-organ failure without acute cellular rejection as the initiating event. The use of single- or double-agent maintenance immunosuppression has reduced the incidence of severe postoperative sepsis, and this has partly accounted for the improvement seen in survival over the last 10 years.

Special considerations

Pregnancy

Younger patients frequently want to consider reproduction soon after the transplant procedure. There is some experience in the literature of intestinal and multi-visceral patients successfully conceiving and delivering healthy children. One of the main considerations is the potential teratogenicity of immunosuppression as discussed in Chapter 31. Mycophenolate mofetil and sirolimus (SRL) should probably be avoided. Again, it is important to involve a high-risk pregnancy service well in advance of this scenario so that preparations can be made to appropriately manage these patients who may have reproduction as their ultimate aim.

Travel

Patients who are vaccinated prior to transplantation have a better chance of remaining immune than those vaccinated after the procedure while on immunosuppression. In general it is wise to encourage patients not to travel to regions where the medical care is limited and/or risk of infection high. Intercurrent infection may provoke rejection, and differentiating between gastrointestinal infection and rejection can be difficult.

Intercurrent surgery

The main consideration here is the increased risk of infection because of immunosuppression. The further out from transplantation the better, given that the influences of lymphocyte depletion often last for a year or more. If patients are taking SRL, they may need conversion to TAC prior to the procedure and remain on this until healing is complete. It is also of critical importance to fully brief the surgeon and staff undertaking any intercurrent surgery and if possible have the patient regularly reviewed by a transplant clinician.

Employment

Quality of life following transplantation is of great importance. In addition to being a primary aim of the transplantation, we consider it to be a key factor in the long-term survival of patients. Many patients feel a lack of self-worth and purpose if they cannot gain employment. This is compounded by the tendency for employers to avoid them because of the perception that they are unreliable due to their health status.

Further reading

Grant D. Current results of intestinal transplantation. The International Intestinal Transplant Registry. *Lancet* 1996; **347**: 1801–3.

Lloyd DA, Vega R, Bassett P, Forbes A, Gabe SM. Survival and dependence on home parenteral nutrition: experience over a 25-year period in a UK referral centre. *Aliment Pharmacol Ther* 2006; **24**: 1231–40.

Middleton SJ, Nishida S, Tzakis A, *et al.* Cambridge-Miami score for intestinal transplantation preoperative risk assessment: initial development and validation. *Transplant Proc* 2010; **42**: 19–21.

Middleton SJ, Pollard S, Friend PJ, *et al.* Adult small intestinal transplantation in England and Wales. *Br J Surg* 2003; **90**: 723–7.

Todo S, Reyes J, Furukawa H, *et al.* Outcome analysis of 71 clinical intestinal transplantations. *Ann Surg* 1995; **222**: 270–80.

Chapter 37

Composite tissue allotransplantation

Face transplantation

Maria Siemionow and Can Ozturk

Key points

- In recent years, face transplantation has become a clinical reality and in the future may become a standard procedure.
- Face transplantation is still classified as "experimental" since there are not yet sufficient scientific data regarding long-term outcome.
- To date there are two scalp and 14 facial allograft cases reported.

The face and scalp are aesthetically and functionally very important parts of the human body. Burn injuries, gunshot wounds, animal attacks, and extensive tumor surgery are the primary causes of traumatic facial deformities. These deformities may present with single or composite tissue defects involving skin, muscle, and/or bone, as well as different functional and aesthetic units. The face consists of six major aesthetic units, comprised of forehead, eye/eyebrow, nose, lips, chin, and cheek. Primary closure, skin grafting, local flaps, tissue prelamination and prefabrication, distant flaps, tissue expansion, and free tissue transfers are traditional reconstructive choices for covering facial defects. There are currently few reports of total face reconstruction using a full-thickness skin grafting technique.

Conventional surgery

Skin grafting is not an ideal reconstruction method for extensive facial defects because of the relatively poor color and texture match, poor functional outcome, and secondary deformities such as ectropion and microstomia due to graft contraction. There are many different kinds of local flaps used in covering specialized parts of the face, such as nose, cheek, and lips. These flaps have an ideal color and texture match with the original missing tissue; however, their application applies to only small or moderate defects. Prelamination and prefabrication of flaps is used in reconstructing more complex facial tissue defects such as nasal lining and eye-socket defects. Expanded skin flaps are frequently used in facial reconstructive surgery to provide identical color and texture. Functional and aesthetic results are better when compared with those of other reconstructive options. They are ideal for covering moderate skin and soft tissue defects if the adjacent tissues are not compromised. Microsurgical free tissue transfers are the technique of choice not only for reconstruction of extensive composite tissue defects, but also for repairing small but technically challenging parts of the face such as oral and nasal lining. Walton showed successful results of functional restoration of nasal airway and nasal aesthetic units by using various artistic combinations of cartilage grafts, forehead flaps, and prefabricated radial forearm free flaps. The scapular/parascapular, serratus, latissimus dorsi, anterolateral thigh, rectus abdominis, and fibula flaps are the other free flap options commonly used in facial and scalp reconstruction. There are various cases of scalp and partial face replantation published in the literature. Replantation provides the best functional and aesthetic outcome because the defect is reconstructed with original missing tissue. However, this is only possible in selected cases.

Face transplantation

Face allotransplantation is an alternative option for complex facial defects that cannot be reconstructed with the above procedures. Composite tissue allotransplantation (CTA) is a new developing field of modern plastic and reconstructive surgery. The "composite tissue" is a combination of different types of tissues

Organ Transplantation: A Clinical Guide, ed. A.A. Klein, C.J. Lewis, and J.C. Madsen. Published by Cambridge University Press.

such as skin, fat, muscle, nerve, and bone that originate from ectoderm and mesoderm. The complexity of these grafts may challenge immune responses in the donor's body, making graft acceptance and tolerance more difficult to achieve when compared with solid organ transplants.

Experimental studies on CTA began with the rat hind-limb allograft models in the 1960s. Following development of successful solid organ transplantation in clinical practice, the first clinical CTA was a hand transplant, which was performed in Ecuador in 1964. Despite immunosuppressive therapy including steroids and azathioprine, the hand was amputated after 2 weeks due to rejection. In September 1998, Dubernard and colleagues performed the world's first successful hand allotransplant in Lyon, France. The immunosuppression protocol included anti-thymocyte globulin (ATG), tacrolimus (TAC), mycophenolate mofetil (MMF), and prednisolone. To date more than 50 forearm and hand transplants have been performed worldwide. In 2008, Machens and Höhnke in Munich, Germany, performed the first whole arm allograft transplant. Cavadas and colleagues in Valencia, Spain, have also proposed leg allograft transplantation, although to date only syngeneic transplantation has occurred. The successful results of hand and limb transplantation made face transplantation feasible.

Cadaver studies

A series of cadaver dissections were performed in preparation for face transplantation. The sequence of procedures in mock facial transplantation is described in Table 37.1.

Computer modeling and identity issues

Biomodeling has come into clinical use with the stereolithography apparatus, a computer-controlled technique that builds anatomically accurate skeletal models from radiological data. Using computer-based models, the face looks neither like the donor nor the recipient prior to injury, but carries more of the characteristics of the recipient skeleton than of the donor soft tissues. However, an unrealistic presentation of the final appearance of the face is the main disadvantage of these programs.

Table 37.1 Sequence of procedures in mock facial transplantation

1.	Transfer of the donor facial flap into the recipient's facial defect
2.	Coaptation of the supraorbital, infraorbital, and mental nerves
3.	Anchoring of the flap at the region of the mandibular and zygomatic ligaments
4.	Anchoring of the flap to the preauricular region, mastoid fascia, and temporal fascia
5.	Anchoring of the flap to the frontal bones
6.	Closure of the upper and lower gingivobuccal incisions
7.	Closure of the upper and lower conjunctival incisions
8.	Anastomoses of the external carotid arteries
9.	Anastomoses of the facial veins
10.	Coaptation of the great auricular nerves
11.	Anastomoses of the external jugular veins
12.	Closure of the skin incisions

Preparation for face transplantation

Patient selection process

The patient selection process must comply with the institutional review board–approved protocol. The optimal candidates for face transplantation should be patients between 18 and 60 years of age with minimal coexisting medical illness who agree to comply with lifelong immunosuppression therapy and show a strong desire to proceed with face transplantation.

Potential candidates should be evaluated by a multi-disciplinary face transplant team, which may include plastic surgeons; transplant surgeons;, ear, nose and throat (ENT) surgeons; immunologist; psychiatrist; infectious disease specialist; social worker; and bioethics specialist. Physical evaluation includes recording of facial tissue defects, current functional status of the facial muscles, and sensory deficits. Screening for epstein-barr virus, cytomegalovirus, human immunodeficiency virus, and hepatitis viruses is also performed. Tissue typing and detection of human leukocyte antigen (HLA) antibodies is determined as for solid organ transplantation.

Imaging is required to analyze the details of the facial defect and determine necessary structures for allotransplantation. This includes computed tomography (CT; head, neck, chest, and abdomen), magnetic resonance imaging (MRI; to determine the soft tissue defect and abnormalities) and CT angiography (vessel mapping) of the head and neck, carotid Doppler studies, electromyogram, and nerve conduction studies. After clinical review of the physical and psychological condition of potential candidates, patients who are accepted for transplant give informed consent. A thorough explanation of potential risks and possible outcomes of the procedure should be given, including potential complications of the surgery (i.e., graft failure, infection, death), lifelong immunosuppression and related complications, acute/chronic graft failure/rejection, graft-versus-host disease, possible further salvage or revision surgeries, and the importance of compliance and rehabilitation.

Clinical cases of face transplantation

To date there have been two scalp transplants and 14 facial allotransplantation cases reported in the literature and in media (Table 37.2). In 1982, Buncke and colleague performed the first scalp isotransplantation between identical twins (same blood group and HLA tissue type). The patient, who had lost 60% of her scalp tissue due to avulsion trauma, was treated with split-thickness skin grafts taken from her identical twin. Later, the patient was treated with two free scalp flaps from her identical twin. No immunosuppressive agent was given. The second scalp transplantation case in the literature was performed by Jiang and colleagues in 2005. This 72-year-old male patient had stage IIIC recurrent cutaneous malignant melanoma of the scalp vertex. After wide excision of the tumor, the defect was reconstructed with a CTA including cephalo-cervical skin flap and bilateral ears that were taken from a brain-dead male donor. The patient received the combination of MMF, prednisone, and daclizumab as immunosuppressive therapy. According to the authors, there were no signs of rejection and no tumor recurrence during a 4-month follow-up.

In November 2005, Dubernard and colleagues performed the first partial facial allotransplant in Amiens, France. The recipient was a 38-year-old woman with a myocutaneous defect of the central face area due to a dog bite. The donor was a 46-year-old with identical blood group and five of six HLA antigen matches with the recipient. A radial forearm flap from the donor was transferred with facial CTA to the left submammary fold of the recipient for monitoring of immunological response of the grafts, aiming to diminish damage to the facial allotransplant by skin biopsies.

A description follows of the fourth facial allotransplant in Cleveland, Ohio, in 2008. The patient was a 45-year-old woman who had a midface defect after a shotgun injury in 2004. Two months after the trauma, the patient was transferred to The Cleveland Clinic and had 23 autologous reconstructive operations prior to the facial allotransplantation procedure. None of these autologous reconstructions provided adequate functional or aesthetic results. Her facial defect included absence of a nose with underlying maxillary bone, loss of orbicularis oculi and orbicularis oris muscle function, scarred lower eyelids with ectropion, right-eye enucleation, and facial nerve deficit (Figure 37.1). She could not eat solid food or drink from a cup and her speech was slurred due to palatal damage. She required a tracheostomy for ventilation and a percutaneous gastrostomy tube for nutrition. The donor was a woman matching the patient in age, race, and skin complexion. There was mismatch of both blood group (donor group A, recipient group AB) and HLA tissue type (two of six matches). After identifying recipient vessels, the soft tissues, bones, and hardware from previous surgeries were removed. The template of the recipient's facial defect was outlined based on three-dimensional graft architecture. The CTA was included over 535 cm^2 (80% of donor face) of facial skin and included Le Fort III midfacial skeleton, infraorbital floor, bilateral zygoma, lower eyelids, nose, anterior maxilla with teeth, anterior hard palate, alveolus, upper lip, parotid glands, and intraoral mucosa. After fixation of bone components, microvascular end-to-end anastomosis of the bilateral facial arteries and veins was accomplished with an ischemic time of 2 hours and 40 minutes and total operation time of 22 hours. After 2 months she was discharged from hospital (Figure 37.2). She had revision surgery to remove excess tissue 18 months after transplant. Rehabilitation consisted of passive and active facial muscle exercises, speech therapy, sensory re-education, and facial acceptance re-education, which began 48 hours after transplantation. The sensory recovery of the graft was confirmed by presence of 7-mm two-point discrimination at 8 months; however, motor recovery improved over 1 year post-transplant. Finally, the patient gained missing facial functions such as nasal breathing, smelling, drinking, eating, and speaking intelligibly. She is satisfied with her facial

Table 37.2 Anatomical and surgical details of facial transplant patients reported to date

Patient	CTA design	Vessel and nerve repair	Sensory and functional recovery
Patient 1, 38 y, F – 2005 Amiens, France	Upper and lower lips, perioral muscles. Partial nose with alar and triangular cartilages, anterior septum. Cheek, partial oral, and nasal mucosa.	Bilateral facial a. and v. (end to end). Bilateral infraorbital and mental nerve. Left mandibular branch (end to end).	Light touch (10 weeks) Temperature (6 months) Eat and drink (1 week) Labial contact (6 months) Chin and nose pyramidal muscle motion (12 months) Smile (14–18 months)
Patient 2, 30 y, M – 2006 Xian, China	Upper lip, nose, the right anterior maxilla, sinus. Right zygoma with lateral orbital wall, right parotid gland, and partial masseter.	Right external maxillary a. and anterior facial v. (end to end). Right facial nerve not well coapted.	Light touch (3 months) Temperature (8 months) Unable to smile completely. Facial nerve not functional. Eat, drink, and talk normally.
Patient 3, 29 y, M – 2007 Paris, France	Lower two-thirds of face, including skin, soft tissue, lips, chin, cheeks, nose, bilateral parotid glands, parotid ducts, and intraoral mucosa.	Bilateral external carotid arteries and thyrolingofacial trunks (end to end). Bilateral facial and infraorbital nerves.	Light touch (3 months) Temperature (3 months) Eat and speak (10 days) Orbicularis oris and oculi voluntarily contract (6 months) Spontaneous mimicry (9 months) Trigeminal and facial motor function (12 months)
Patient 4, 45 y, F – 2008 Cleveland, OH	Le Fort III midfacial skeleton, total infraorbital floor, bilateral zygoma, lower eyelids, nose, anterior maxilla with teeth, anterior hard palate, alveolus, upper lip, parotid glands, and intaroral mucosa.	Bilateral common facial arteries, left external jugular, posterior facial, and right facial veins (end to end). Bilateral facial nerve repair interpositional nerve grafts.	Smell (2 days) Light touch (5 months) Temperature (5 months) Upper lip occlusion Facial mimicry Eats and drinks from a cup. Speaks more clearly.
Patient 5, 28 y, M – 2009 Paris, France	Cheek, nose, parotid glands, and ducts. Upper and lower lips. Premaxilla, chin and intraoral mucosa.	Bilateral external carotid a., external juguler vein and thyrolinguofacial trunk. Bilateral facial nerves.	None reported
Patient 6, 37 y, M – 2009 Paris, France	Upper two-thirds of face and entire scalp with bilateral ears, forehead, lower eyelids, nose, bilateral cheeks, bilateral parotid glands and parotid ducts, intraoral mucosa.	Bilateral external carotid arteries and thyrolinguofacial trunks (end to end). Bilateral facial, supraorbital, and infraorbital nerves.	None reported
Patient 7, 59 y, M – 2009 Boston, MA	Midfacial tissue including skin, soft tissue, nose, upper lip, bilateral cheek, bilateral parotid ducts, maxilla with teeth and palate.	Left external carotid, right facial a. (end to end), bilateral facial vein. Bilateral facial and infraorbital nerves.	None reported

CTA = composite tissue allotransplantation; F: female; M: male; y: years (age).

appearance, and has regained self-confidence and social reintegration.

Care after face transplantation

Monitoring

Inspection for facial allograft viability and observation for signs of rejection such as erythema, edema, and blistering should be done on a daily basis, in addition to Doppler monitoring and tissue oxygenation measurements. Standard blood tests for monitoring immunosuppression including renal function should also be performed.

Immunosuppression

Currently, there is no standard immunosuppressive protocol. A number of different induction and maintenance therapy protocols and different viral and

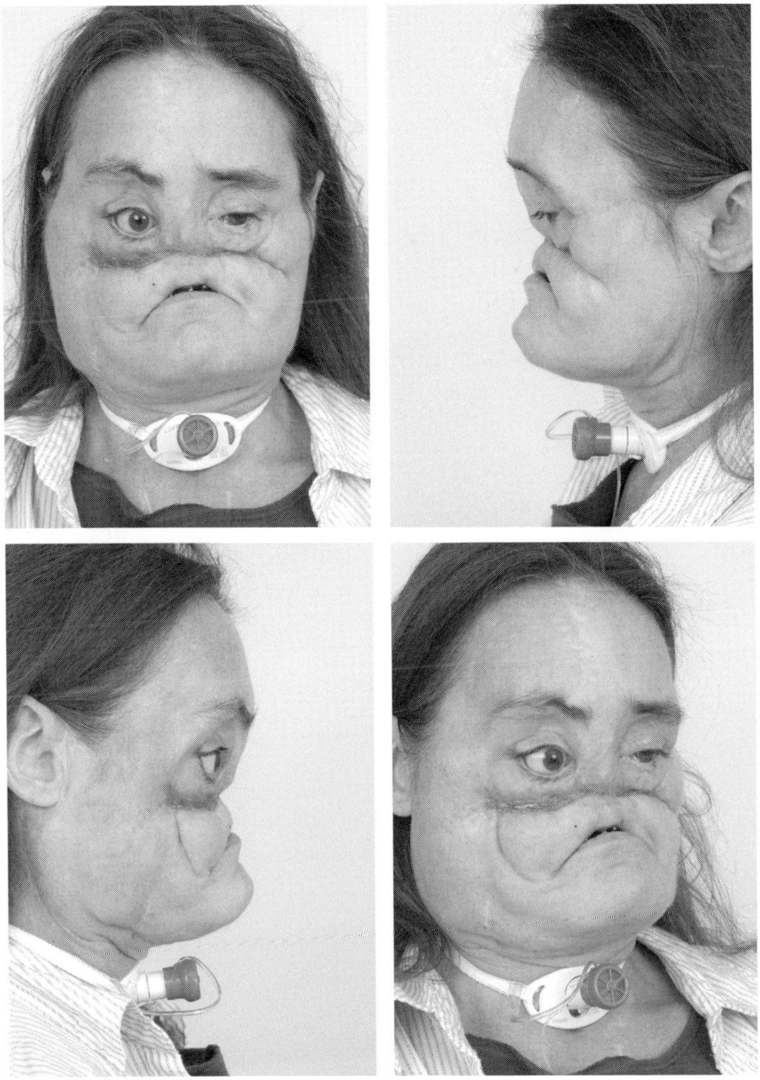

Figure 37.1 Patient prior to face transplant performed at Cleveland Clinic. Reproduced with permission from Siemionow MZ, Papay F, Djohan R, *et al.*, First U.S. near-total human face transplantation: A paradigm shift for massive complex injuries. *Plast Reconstr Surg* 2010; **125**: 111–22.

anti-microbial prophylaxis regimens have been reported. The most common regimen for face transplantation is based on kidney transplantation protocols and includes standard induction therapy with ATG followed by triple maintenance therapy. This maintenance therapy consists of TAC, MMF, and prednisolone. Additionally, the donor-derived bone marrow cell infusions aiming for chimerism and tolerance induction have been attempted.

Biopsy protocol

The protocol for monitoring facial allograft rejection includes punch biopsies of skin and oral mucosa every 72 hours for the first 2 weeks, then weekly for the first 3 months, twice a month during the first 6 months, and once a month thereafter during the first post-transplant year. The oral mucosa of the facial allograft may present with higher grades of graft rejections when compared with the skin component. Another method for monitoring graft rejection episodes is application of sentinel allografts such as radial forearm flap or skin graft from the face allograft donor. The presence of edema, skin blistering, scaling, erythema, hair weakness or loss, dermatitis, and papules of the allograft should alert the clinician for possible graft rejection. In these circumstances, the patient should be admitted and biopsies taken from the skin and mucosa

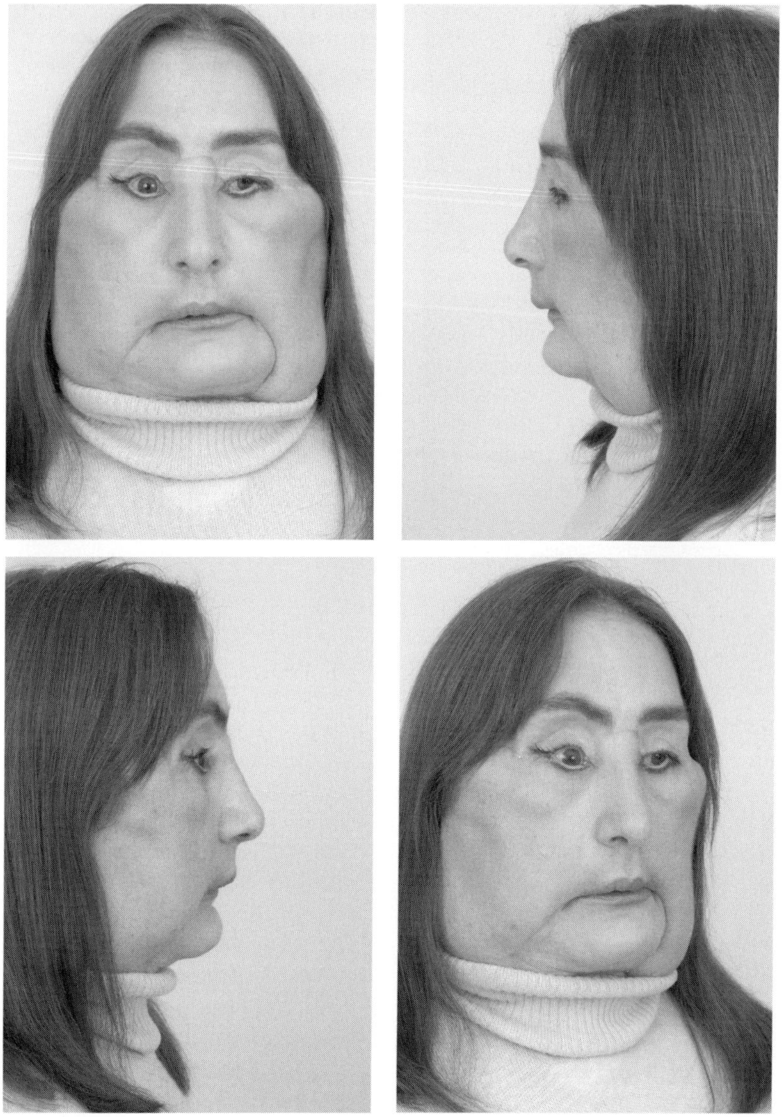

Figure 37.2 Patient after face transplant performed at Cleveland Clinic. Reproduced with permission from Siemionow MZ, Papay F, Djohan R, *et al.*, First U.S. near-total human face transplantation: A paradigm shift for massive complex injuries. *Plast Reconstr Surg* 2010; **125**: 111–22.

of the graft. The biopsy specimens must be reviewed by an experienced pathologist. A well-defined scale such as the Banff classification, developed for composite tissue allografts, should be used for grading of acute rejection.

Treatment for acute rejection depends on the clinical condition of each particular patient. The dose of immunosuppressants may be altered, a bolus of steroid given, or alternatively extracorporeal photo chemotherapy may be tried. Chronic rejection of the facial allotransplant has not yet been reported. This may be due to be relatively short follow-up of face transplant patients or early detection and reversal of acute graft rejection episodes.

Functional evaluation and physical rehabilitation

The comparison of functional outcomes for face transplant patients is difficult because each particular case presents with different facial defects and functional deficits. In addition, in contrast to aesthetic outcome, which can be seen immediately after transplantation, the final functional outcome depends on adequate motor recovery of facial nerves and muscles, which may take months or even years.

Professional rehabilitation teams should start facial re-education therapy and speech therapy in early post-transplant phase. Progression is measured by evaluation of facial muscle function (e.g., mimicry, smile, blinking, eyelid closing, nasal flaring, puckering), smell, swallowing, mastication, and speech. Functional MRI, electromyography studies, and volumetric analysis are objective measures of motor recovery of facial units, whereas temperature testing, two-point discrimination test, pressure-specified sensory device testing, and Semmes-Weinstein monofilament tests are used to monitor the sensory recovery of the facial allograft. According to the current literature, the motor recovery of facial nerves has been observed between 9 and 12 months post-transplant. In contrast, recovery of sensory nerves has been seen within 3–6 months. Additionally, serial photographic and video documentation is important for the comparative assessment of post-transplant function.

Ethical considerations

Due to the lack of long-term follow-up and outcomes, facial allotransplantation is still considered as an "experimental" procedure. This procedure currently carries a 14% death rate, as two of 14 patients have died (one due to non-compliance with immunosuppression and one due to infection). Because of the complexity of this procedure and the uncertain benefits and risks, it is important to carefully screen potential candidates. Further evaluation of outcomes is required, along with cooperation between different institutions performing these novel procedures.

Further reading

Cendales LC, Kanitakis J, Schneeberger S, *et al.* The Banff 2007 working classification of skin-containing composite tissue allograft pathology. *Am J Transplant* 2008; **8**: 1396–400.

Dubernard JM, Lengele B, Morelon E, *et al.* Outcomes 18 months after the first human partial face transplantation. *N Engl J Med* 2007; **357**: 2451–60.

Guo S, Han Y, Zhang X, *et al.* Human facial allotransplantation: a 2-year follow-up study. *Lancet* 2008; **372**: 631–8.

Siemionow M, Agaoglu G, Unal S. Mock facial allotransplantation: a cadaver study in facial allograft transplantation in humans – part II. *Plast Reconstr Surg* 2006; **117**: 876–85.

Siemionow M, Papay F, Alam D, *et al.* Near-total human face transplantation for a severely disfigured patient in the USA. *Lancet* 2009; **374**: 177–8.

Section 7 Other

Chapter 38

Hematopoietic stem cell transplantation

Charles Crawley and Thomas R. Spitzer

Key points

- Hematopoietic progenitor/stem cell transplantation remains an important treatment strategy for patients with marrow failure syndromes, inherited hematological disorders, and advanced hematological malignancies.
- Improvements in supportive care, the use of reduced-intensity conditioning regimens, and advances in human leukocyte antigen typing methodology have led to better outcomes.
- Cell sources have changed with an increasing utiliation of donors other than HLA matched siblings.
- It is likely that allogeneic transplantation and particularly cord blood as a stem cell source for transplantation will play an increasing role in the next 10 years.

Hematopoietic stem cell transplantation: principles and rationale

Hematopoietic stem cell (HSC) transplantation has expanded dramatically in its scope and range of indications over the past four decades. With the establishment of modern histocompatibility typing and improvements in graft-versus-host disease (GvHD) prophylaxis and supportive care, many patients without a human leukocyte antigen (HLA)-matched related donor are now able to receive a transplant, and less intensive preparative strategies have allowed older patients and patients with significant comorbidity to undergo transplantation.

As a rescue therapy, the infusion of HSCs can circumvent the myeloablative effects of many conditioning regimens, thereby permitting steep escalation of doses of chemotherapy and radiation therapy and overcoming the resistance that tumor cells may have developed to conventional doses of chemo/radiotherapy. As described next, multiple myeloma and non-Hodgkin's lymphoma are examples of hematologic malignancies for which myeloablative conditioning and autologous stem cell transplantation have improved survival outcomes compared with conventional-dose chemotherapy. The replacement aspect of stem cell transplantation relies on the engraftment of normal multi-potential progenitor cells in order to replace a diseased marrow or immune system. Many diseases, ranging from hematopoietic malignancies to acquired non-malignant blood dyscrasias such as severe aplastic anemia, to congenital disorders of the marrow or immune system such as sickle cell disease and severe combined immunodeficiency syndrome, have been cured by stem allogeneic cell transplants with the restoration of normal hematopoiesis and successful immune reconstitution. More recently, reduced-intensity conditioning regimens, based on elegant preclinical models that demonstrated that full hematopoietic chimerism can be reliably established as an immunological platform for adoptive cellular immunotherapy using donor lymphocyte infusions (DLI), have shown considerable potential as a strategy for reducing transplant-related complications and capturing potent graft versus malignancy effects of the transplant. The graft versus malignancy effect of this strategy is usually dependent on the the establishment of full donor hematopoiesis, either spontaneously or after DLI. Mixed chimerism alone may be sufficient for specific tolerance induction for organ transplantation and for the correction of

Organ Transplantation: A Clinical Guide, ed. A.A. Klein, C.J. Lewis, and J.C. Madsen. Published by Cambridge University Press.

certain non-malignant disorders of the marrow and immune system. The reduced intensity of the conditioning regimen has greatly expanded the application of stem cell transplantation by permitting transplants in patients who, by virtue of age or comorbidity, would not have previously been considered candidates for stem cell transplantation. The induction of mixed chimerism has recently been shown to be an important strategy for the induction of specific tolerance for solid organ transplantation. Sustained tolerance and anti-tumor responses have been observed in patients with multiple myeloma and end-stage renal disease who received an HLA-matched combined bone marrow and kidney transplant. This strategy has also been successfully performed in patients without an underlying malignancy who received an HLA-haploidentical bone marrow and kidney transplant. The demonstration of successful tolerance induction has great potential for avoiding the complications of long-term immunosuppression and for reconstituting normal immunity after transplant. These successful advances in stem cell transplantation have paved the way for future cell-based therapies involving either engineering of the stem cell graft or modulation of the cellular environment post-transplant to optimize the anti-tumor potential of the transplant while avoiding the deleterious effects of GvHD.

Hematopoietic stem cells: definition and sources

Stem cells are defined as a population of cells that retain the capacity for indefinite self-renewal and to generate progeny with the potential to differentiate into mature cells with a variety of functions. The therapeutic use of stem cells is frequently viewed as a very recent development. The use of HSCs, however, is not new, as these cells have been in regular and increasing clinical use for the last 50 years; indeed they remain the only adult somatic stem cell in routine use in 2011.

In adults, the only source of HSCs is the bone marrow. This is not true of the fetus, where HSCs may be found in the liver, spleen, and, more importantly, cord blood. Identification of HSCs in mouse and subsequently humans was initially through assays for clonogenic precursors in the form of long-term culture-initiating cells and colony-forming units. Subsequent phenotypic markers have been defined. Human HSCs are characterized by the absence of lineage markers (Lin−) and are negative for CD38 but express CD34, c-kit, and CD133. They represent approximately 0.1% of marrow cells, but the population is heterogeneous and may include c-kit and CD133-negative cells. Despite this, for practical purposes, $CD34^+$ and $CD38^-$ define a cell population of human progenitor cells (HPCs) that will re-establish hematopoiesis in the sublethally irradiated non-obese diabetic (NOD)/severe combined immunodeficiency (SCID) mouse and in humans.

Donors

The majority of HPC transplants undertaken worldwide use *autologous* cells, meaning the patient acts as his or her own donor. These cells are readily available and do not carry the same risks of GvHD or the risks of transmission of infection as allogeneic cells. Autologous transplantation allows for the delivery of high-dose chemotherapy where hematological toxicity would be dose-limiting. The use of autologous HPCs allows for marrow recovery and allows chemotherapy doses to be escalated to the next dose-limiting toxicity, which is usually gastrointestinal or lung. The benefit in terms of disease control relies on a beneficial dose response curve. The lack of a GvHD effect may also be a drawback. In addition, there is a risk of tumor contamination in the graft with an increased risk of disease relapse. This effect is seen most clearly in the lower relapse rate when syngeneic (identical twin) donors are used. The opportunity to use a syngeneic donor is rare, but these donors are analogous to the use of autologous cells with the certainty that the graft is tumor-free. *Allogeneic* HPCs are cells donated from a third party. Allogeneic donors (with the exception of syngeneic donors) carry the risk of causing GvHD, and this is strongly linked to HLA match; hence the preferred choice is usually an HLA-matched sibling. The majority of patients, however, do not have an HLA-matched sibling, and there is an increasing reliance on volunteer-unrelated donors. Bone Marrow Donors Worldwide is the central database to which most donor registries submit their data. It provides a searchable database of over 14 million donors, including over 400 000 cord blood units. Despite this, there remain patients for whom a donor cannot be found. One alternative in this situation is the use of haplo-identical donors. For almost all patients, a parent/child or sibling who has a 50% tissue type match is available. This requires the use of extensive T-cell depletion or post-transplant strategies to deplete alloreactive T cells to avoid GvHD. Recently, the importance of natural killer (NK) cell activation has become clear. Particularly in haploidentical transplants, NK cell activation is regulated by a balance of activating inhibitory and killer cell immunoglobulin-like receptors. The outcomes of transplantation with donors whose NK cells are alloreactive in a donor versus host direction are associated with substantially better outcomes.

Table 38.1 Cell dose

Cell source	Nucleated cells ($\times 10^8$/kg)	$CD34^+$ cells ($\times 10^6$/kg)	T cells ($\times 10^7$/kg)
Bone marrow	2.0	2.8	2.2
Peripheral blood	9.0	7.0	27.0
Cord blood	0.3	0.2	0.4

Sources of cells

During embryogenesis, hematopoiesis originates with primitive erythroblasts developing from mesodermal cells in the yolk sac. By 12 weeks gestation, the liver is the major hematopoietic organ and subsequently the spleen. Hematopoiesis starts within the bone marrow at 11 weeks of gestation and has become the major site of hematopoiesis from 20 weeks; by birth it is essentially the sole site. Under normal conditions, HPCs are relatively rare cells in the peripheral blood (approximately 100 per ml); however, much higher concentrations are found in the umbilical cord or in adults associated with factors driving proliferation with the marrow, such as recovery from chemotherapy or after exposure to cytokines.

In practical terms, there are three principal sources of HPCs for therapeutic use. Marrow may be harvested under general anesthesia in 5–10 ml aliquots from the posterior iliac crests. In general 15–20 ml/kg are collected. The advantages are that cytokines or chemotherapy are avoided, which is a consideration for allogeneic donors; however, collection volumes are limited and back pain and anemia are common. Peripheral blood collection is easier and does not require a general anesthetic. HPCs are mobilized from the marrow with cytokines, usually granulocyte colony-stimulating factor (G-CSF) with or without myelosuppressive chemotherapy. In general, the addition of chemotherapy increases the HPC yield, although it also increases toxicity. One additional benefit of chemotherapy is that it may also reduce tumor burden further; consequently, the choice of agent will be to a degree disease-specific. Typical drugs used include cyclophosphamide (CY) at doses of 1.5–4 g/m^2 or etoposide. Cells can also be mobilized with CXCR4 antagonists such as plerixafor, which triggers proliferation of CD34 stem cells and their release from their niche, the marrow microenvironment, into the peripheral blood. Cells are collected by leukapheresis: essentially blood is collected on a continuous sterile closed circuit, an anticoagulant added, and mononuclear cells separated by centrifugation. G-CSF mobilization of stem cells will typically take 5–6 days from start of G-CSF to completion of apheresis. If chemotherapy is used, then apheresis is usually started as the blood count is recovering to a level of approximately 1.0–3.0 $\times$ 10^9/l, and the whole mobilization procedure is approximately 10–14 days. In addition to ease of collection, peripheral blood collections result in higher cell doses and more rapid recovery of blood counts compared with marrow collection; consequently, for autologous transplantation, peripheral blood is the overwhelming source of cells. In Europe in 2008, bone marrow was used in less than 0.01% of autologous transplants.

Cord blood is an extremely rich source of stem cells, which, until recently, was simply discarded with the placenta after birth. Umbilical cord blood is either collected with the placenta still in utero by an obstetrician or midwife or after delivery of the placenta. The former results in higher cell doses and a lower risk of bacterial contamination but is clearly more disruptive to delivery. Cord blood HPCs have a high proliferate potential, low immunogenicity, and low risk of transmission of infection and this to a degree offsets the disadvantage of low cell doses (Table 38.1). Cord blood by its nature is used exclusively in allogeneic transplants, and with the establishment of cord blood banks (currently 31 registered with Netcord), these provide a source of cryopreserved stem cells that are rapidly available, avoiding the need for prolonged unrelated donor searches.

The first cord blood transplant was performed in 1988 for a child with Fanconi's anemia and resulted in full hematopoietic and immune reconstitution; the patient remains well some 15 years later. However, cell dose remains important and has delayed the use of cord blood in adults. A minimum cell dose of 3 $\times$ 10^7/kg is generally recommended, and frequently two cord units are combined in adults.

Principles of conditioning

Conditioning serves two key purposes during stem cell transplant. First, it is important in eradicating the underlying disease, which in most cases is a hematological malignancy. Indeed, for autologous (and syngeneic) transplants, it is the sole mechanism of disease control. For allogeneic transplants, there is the additional requirement to allow for effective engraftment of the donor cells. The initial concept, although probably incorrect, was that host HSCs needed to be eradicated from the marrow stroma to "create space" for the donor cells to engraft. A third function of pretransplant conditioning regimens, which is more important, is to suppress the host immune system sufficiently to prevent a host versus graft rejection of the donor cells. The degree to which the host immune system needs to be suppressed depends on factors such as the degree of HLA mismatch, prior sensitization, stem cell dose, and donor T-cell dose.

Historical conditioning regimes developed from the observation that radiation could eradicate leukemic cell populations at doses that did not result in irreversible organ toxicity. Hence the use of controlled total body irradiation (TBI) was developed. Subsequently CY was added, with reduction in leukemia or disease relapse, and this combination remains in routine use. Throughout the 1970s and 1980s, studies focused on attempts to find alternatives to radiotherapy and dose escalation; studies determined maximum-tolerated doses for drugs such as busulfan, melphalan, etoposide, and cytarabine. Studies addressing strategies to increase dose intensity further, with the aim of reducing the risk of leukemia relapse, demonstrate a fundamental problem, whereby increases in chemo/radiotherapy result in increasing organ toxicity. As a result, in all these studies, reductions in relapse were offset by increases in non-relapse mortality and did not translate into improvements in survival. There have been very limited phase III studies of these traditional conditioning regimens, with the exception of a number of studies comparing outcomes of CY and TBI with CY and busulfan. These show differences in toxicity but no real differences in survival, with the exception of acute lymphoblastic leukemia, where CY/TBI appears superior.

Reduced-intensity conditioning

It has been increasingly recognized that immune mechanisms, the graft versus malignancy effect, is an important factor in preventing disease relapse after allogeneic transplant. Indeed, this is probably the most important mechanism by which allogeneic transplant can cure hematological malignancies that are incurable with conventional chemotherapy. Given that much of the toxicity and non-relapse mortality is linked to intensive conditioning regimens, the focus of studies in the 1990s has been to develop conditioning regimens that allow for cell engraftment with minimal drug or radiation doses. The majority of these reduced-intensity conditioning (RIC) regimens focus on immunosuppressive rather than myelosuppressive drugs. Some of the seminal work was conducted by Storb and colleagues in Seattle. Using a dog model, they demonstrated that full donor engraftment could be obtained using a TBI dose of 2.0 Gy rather than the conventional dose of 14.4 Gy. A wide range of RIC regimens are now in clinical use, with an ever-increasing proportion of transplants being undertaken using this type of conditioning (Figure 38.1). Although in many cases there is no clear evidence of improved survival, there is a clear advantage in terms of reduction in non-relapse mortality (NRM). The increase in NRM seen with age had precluded the use of conventional transplants beyond the age of 50 years, whereas RIC has allowed the use of allogeneic transplants to be extended into patients in their seventh decade.

Early complications

The most common early complications occur as a consequence of the aplasia due to the conditioning regimen and gastrointestinal toxicity. Aplasia develops from approximately 5–7 days after the onset of the conditioning regimen and therefore often coincides at or after the time of cell infusion, customarily referred to as day 0. Engraftment occurs around day 12–16 for autologous transplants and a little later for allogeneic transplants. The timing of white cell count recovery is also dependent on cell source, being fastest with peripheral blood, followed by marrow, and slowest with cord blood. The gastrointestinal tract is also sensitive to chemotherapy. Nausea is an early complication, although it is relatively well controlled with 5HT3 antagonists or some of the newer anti-emetics. Mucositis develops from day 1–7 after transplant, usually reaching a maximum by day 10–12. Risk factors include poor dental hygiene, allogeneic transplantation, and particularly the use of methotrexate after transplant as GvHD prophylaxis. Despite widespread

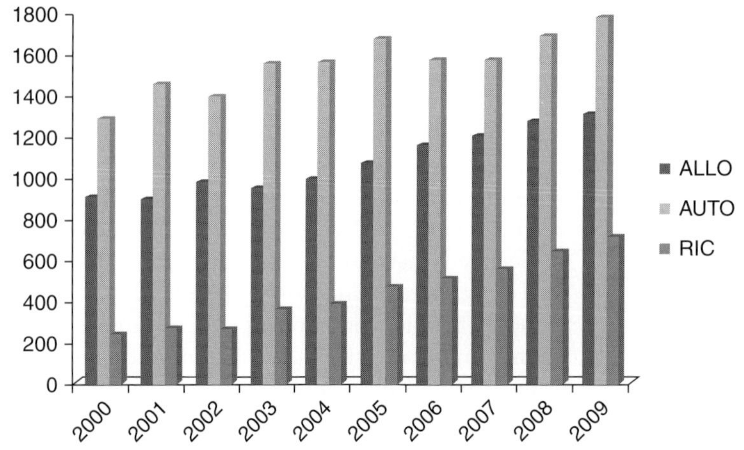

Figure 38.1 Transplant activity in the United Kingdom, 2000–2009. Allo: allogeneic; Auto: autologous; RIC: reduced-intensity conditioning. Provided by Keiren Kirkland, British Society of Blood and Marrow Transplantation.

use of interventions such as chlorhexidine or benzydamine mouth washes, there is little evidence of benefit over bland mouth washes such as saline or bicarbonate. Management is then focussed on analgesia and treatment of infection. Severe mucositis can result in a marked reduction in oral intake and even airway compromise. Nasogastric tubes are often poorly tolerated, and parenteral hydration and nutrition is often indicated. Lower gastrointestinal (GI) damage can result in dyspepsia and more commonly diarrhea. It is important to exclude infective causes, but in their absence, management is with anti-diarrheals.

Infections

Improvements in supportive care and particularly the management of infection have been an important factor in improving outcomes over the last 20 years; however, infections remain a major cause of mortality. The types of infections vary with time after transplant (Figure 38.2). During the aplastic phase (up to week 4), bacterial infections, fungal infections, and pneumonias are typical. Presentation is with neutropenic fever and the management is as for chemotherapy-induced neutropenic fever with the empiric use of broad-spectrum antibiotics. After engraftment for autologous transplants, the infection risk reduces very rapidly; however, for allogeneic transplants, months 1–4 are associated with a very marked impairment in cell-mediated immunity. In the 1980s and 1990s, cytomegalovirus (CMV) disease was a major cause of mortality. CMV reactivation and infection remains a problem; however, with the routine practice of screening by polymerase chain reaction or p65 antigenemia and the use of preemptive (or prophylactic) therapy, the mortality rate has fallen considerably. Other viral infections including adenovirus, Epstein Barr, and respiratory viruses are increasingly recognized during this period. From approximately 4 months, the presence and severity of GvHD has a major influence on immune reconstitution. Immunoglobulin deficiency is common, with susceptibility to pneumococcus and other encapsulated bacteria. Other complications are listed in Tables 38.2 and 38.4.

Hemorrhagic cystitis

Hemorrhagic cystitis is seen more frequently after allogeneic transplantation. BK virus also causes hemorrhagic cystitis. It is dormant in urothelium but can reactivate after allogeneic transplant, particularly with TBI-based conditioning regimens. Management of this can be problematic but involves intensive platelet support and bladder irrigation. The role of antiviral drugs such as cidofovir or leflunomide is unproven. Occasionally arterial embolization or even cystectomy is necessary. Anti-fibrinolytic drugs are contraindicated as they increase the risk of bladder and ureteric clot formation. Acrolein is a metabolite of CY and ifosfamide which is excreted in the urine and is toxic to urothelium. At high doses it causes hemorrhagic cystitis in up to 25% of patients. Mesna is an effective prevention, which binds and neutralizes acrolein in the bladder.

Veno-occlusive disease

Veno-occlusive disease (VOD) is a syndrome of hepatotoxicity due to the conditioning regimen. It usually occurs within the first 3 weeks after transplant

Table 38.2 Other early complications

Complication	Time of onset	Risk factors
Capillary leak syndrome	Weeks 0–3	Extensive prior chemotherapy; use of growth factors
Engraftment syndrome	Within 72 hours of neutrophil engraftment	Growth factors
Diffuse alveolar hemorrhage	Week 0–3	Age Radiation Conditioning intensity Allogeneic donor
Idiopathic pulmonary syndrome	Week 2–4	Conditioning intensity Age Radiation GvHD
Microangiopathic hemolytic anemia	Around 2 months	CNI Radiation Mismatched donors Developing GvHD infection

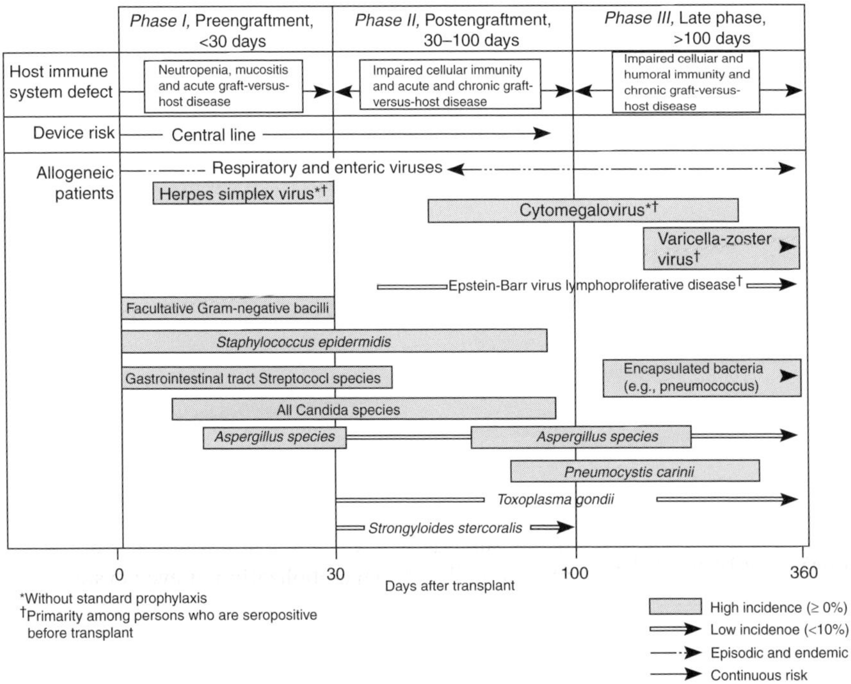

Figure 38.2 Patterns of infection after hemopoietic stem cell transplantation. With permission from Centers for Disease Control and Prevention guidelines.

and is characterized by jaundice, weight gain, tender hepatomegaly, and refractory thrombocytopenia. Risk factors include allogeneic transplantation, HLA match, stem cell source, and disease status. The intensity of conditioning is also important, as is previous hepatic damage (elevated alanine aminotransferase/aspartate aminotransferase pretransplant) or the use of hepatotoxic drugs. Specifically implicated drugs include gemtuzumab, busulfan, and CY. The incidence of severe disease varies but is approximately 8% and 3% in allogeneic and autologous transplants, respectively. Although there are diagnostic criteria

Table 38.3 Acute GvHD Organ Grading System – overall grade

Stage	Skin/rash	Bilirubin	Diarrhea
1	<25% body surface	34–50 μmol/l	500–1000 ml
2	25–50% body surface	51–102 μmol/	1000–1500 ml
3	Generalized erythema	103–255 μmol/	>1500 ml
4	Generalized erythema with bullae and or desquamation	>255 μmol/	Pain ± ileus

Adapted from Przepiorka D, Weisdorf D, Martin P, *et al.* Consensus Conference on Acute GVHD Grading. *Bone Marrow Transplant* 1995; **15**: 825–8.

(Seattle and Baltimore), the differential is wide. Prophylactic ursodeoxycholic acid reduces the risk, but the management of established VOD is difficult. Optimizing supportive care is crucial, and there are some data that the use of defibrotide reduces mortality even in critically ill patients.

Graft-versus-host disease

The host hematopoietic system is sufficiently suppressed by pretransplant conditioning to make graft rejection a rare occurrence. GvHD, however, is one of the commonest and most challenging complications arising after allogeneic stem cell transplant. It arises due to immune recognition between host antigen-presenting cells and mature donor T cells. It is subdivided into acute GvHD, which generally occurs within the first 3 months, and chronic GvHD, which occurs after 3 months, although it is categorized by the clinical features rather than the time of onset. The overall incidence varies and depends on factors such as the HLA match, sex mismatch (female donors for male recipients carrying a higher risk), prior alloimmunization of the donor, and source of stem cells. Recipient factors are also important, including age, type of conditioning, the use of T-cell depletion, and the prophylaxis strategy.

Acute GvHD

Acute GvHD presents with skin rashes, typically maculopapular and often starting on palms and soles, then developing into generalized erythema and desquamation (Table 38.3). GI symptoms start with anorexia and nausea leading to diarrhea and abdominal pain.

Table 38.4 Late complications

Complication	Time of onset	Risk factors	Intervention
Cataracts	3–10 years	TBI/steroids	Surgery
Keratoconjunctivitis sicca	Up to 20% at 15 years	Radiation Chronic GvHD Female	Topical lubricants Lacrimal plugs Topical steroid
Chronic obstructive pulmonary disease/obliterative bronchiolitis (OB)	Up to 20% OB 2–14%	Chronic GvHD Infection Smoking	Treatment of infection + GvHD
Restrictive lung disease	3–6 months	Radiation Chemotherapy	Fractionation of radiotherapy Lung shielding Steroids
Avascular necrosis	4–10% median time to inset 18 months	Steroid Radiation	Analgesia Surgery
Osteoporosis	10% at 12–18 months	Steroid Calcineurin exposure	
Hypothyroidism	months–years	TBI	Levothyroxine replacement
Gonadal failure/infertility		TBI/conditioning intensity	Sex hormone replacement
Atherosclerosis		GvHD Radiation CNI exposure	
Second malignancy	Median 5–6 years	TBI Chronic GvHD Autograft Myelodysplasia	
Psychological		Chronic GvHD	

Liver dysfunction is typically an obstructive picture with elevation of alkaline phosphatase and bilirubin earlier than transaminases. Other organ involvement and fever may be present but tends not to dominate the clinical picture.

Prevention of GvHD is problematic, as it is difficult to separate the detrimental effects of GvHD from the desirable graft versus leukemia/tumor effects. The standard prophylaxis is cyclosporine (CyA) and short-course methotrexate (10–15 mg/m^2 days 1, 3, 6, and 11), but other regimens using drugs such as tacrolimus (TAC), sirolimus (SRL), and mycophenolate mofetil (MMF) are used. The use of T-cell depletion, either ex vivo or in vivo with drugs such as alemtuzumab or anti-thymocyte globulin (ATG), is controversial. This is associated with a significant reduction of both acute and chronic GvHD, but this may be offset by an increase in relapse rate. Management of acute GvHD is with steroid (methylprednisolone 2mg/kg) plus a calcineurin inhibitor, reducing after 2 weeks if there is a complete response. Failure to control is usually defined as progression after 3 days, no change after 7 days, or incomplete response after 14 days. There is no consensus regarding best second-line therapy; a variety of agents show response rates of 30–70%. The prognosis of steroid-resistant acute GvHD is poor.

Chronic GvHD

Chronic GvHD usually develops within the first year after transplant. It may develop as a progression from or after resolution of acute GvHD. It may also develop de novo without prior acute GvHD. Risk factors include acute GvHD, the use of mismatched donors, patient age, the use of ATG or alemtuzumab in the conditioning phase, and the use of peripheral blood cells. Chronic GvHD typically affects the skin, liver, and gut. Skin features include depigmentation, lichen planus, and erythema and a maculopapular rash. Muscle cramps, myositis, and fasciitis can lead to joint contractures. In the GI tract, chronic diarrhea, pancreatic insufficiency, and esophageal strictures can develop. Oral ulceration is a common problem. Chronic GvHD is either classified as limited or extensive (revised Seattle classification) or graded as mild, moderate, or severe according to the National Institutes of Health Global Score, which combines severity of dysfunction with the number of organs involved.

Management of chronic GVHD is a major challenge, which as well as immunosuppression requires the input of a multi-disciplinary team that includes specialist medical services, physiotherapy, rehabilitation services, and psychological support. Immunosuppression is a combination of CyA and prednisolone (initial doses 1.0–1.5 mg/kg/d), and this may be continued for a number of years. As with acute GvHD, there is no consensus regarding second-line therapy, but agents used include TAC, MMF, SRL, psoralen and UVA therapy (PUVA), and extracorporeal photophoresis.

Both acute and chronic GvHD are major causes of mortality and morbidity. Mortality is in part related to organ damage but is also due to the profound immune deficiency associated with GvHD and intensive immunosuppressive medication, leading to life-threatening opportunistic infections. Supportive care is important, with prophylaxis for fungal and viral infections as well as encapsulated bacteria and *Pneumocystis carinii* pneumonia in chronic GvHD.

Donor lymphocyte infusions

The management of disease relapse is a difficult problem; however, in some circumstances, it may be possible to control disease by shifting the donor/host balance in favor of donor hematopoiesis. This can be achieved with an infusion of donor CD3-positive T cells. Further lymphapheresis from the donor is usually required, and cells given in escalating aliquots based on T-cell dose (e.g., $5 \times 10^6 - 1 \times 10^8$ CD3/kg). Donor lymphocyte infusions are also used when there is a fall in donor hematopoiesis in the absence of disease relapse (falling donor chimerism). The major risk of this approach is the risk of GvHD or aplasia, especially if donor hematopoiesis is low. A major component of the graft versus leukemia (GvL) effect is probably GvHD targeting the host hematopoietic system, and to date there is no reliable method for promoting GvL without promoting GvHD.

Indications and outcomes

The major indication for hematopoietic stem cell transplantation is for management of high risk or advanced hematological malignancy (Figures 38.3 and 38.4). For autologous transplantation, myeloma is the single most common indication. A meta-analysis of nine randomized studies has shown a clear benefit in terms of improvement in progression-free survival, and two studies have shown a benefit in

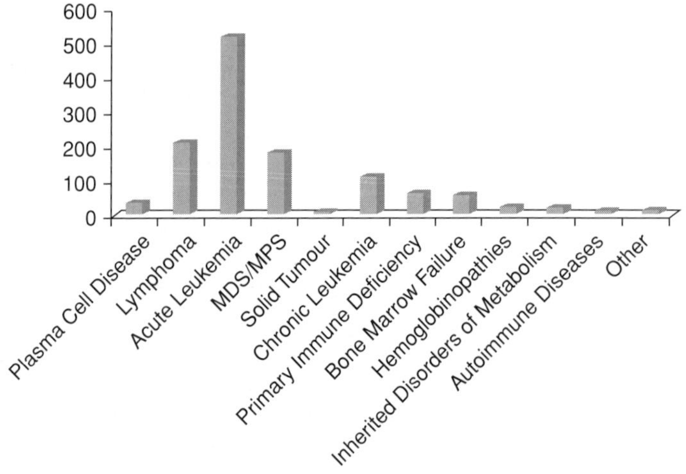

Figure 38.3 Indications for allogeneic hemopoietic stem cell transplant in the United Kingdom in 2009. MDS: myelodysplastic syndrome; MPS: myeloproliferative syndrome. Courtesy of Keiren Kirkland and British Society for Blood and Marrow Transplantation.

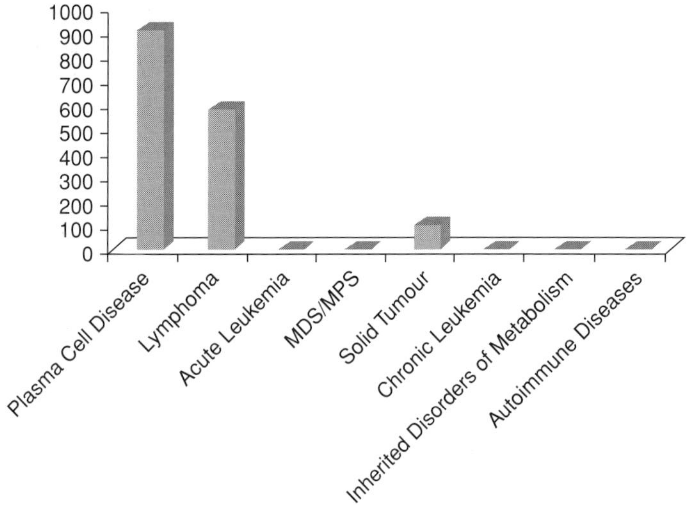

Figure 38.4 Indications for autologous hemopoietic stem cell transplant in the United Kingdom in 2009. MDS: myelodysplastic syndrome; MPS: myeloproliferative syndrome. Courtesy of Keiren Kirkland and British Society for Blood and Marrow Transplantation.

overall survival. As a consequence, an autologous transplant is considered a standard of care in first remission for myeloma, with a median survival of approximately 5 years. Lymphoma is the other major indication for autologous transplant; with the exception of some peripheral T-cell lymphomas and mantle cell lymphoma, it is generally used beyond remission. The PARMA study of relapse diffuse large B-cell lymphoma showed an improvement in 5-year survival from 32% to 53%. In Hodgkin's lymphoma, autologous transplant is widely recommended in relapsed disease, with the exception of late relapses. For refractory Hodgkin's, the outlook is very poor. Most series show a consistent long-term survival of 20–30% and autologous transplantation is widely offered, especially if there is some evidence of chemosensitivity. For the acute leukemias, the role of autologous transplantation is limited. The role of allogeneic transplantation for first remission acute myeloid leukemia is controversial. The risks of NRM outweigh the reduction in relapse risk for good-risk disease as determined by cytogenetics. Chronic myeloid leukemia is the disease in which the benefits of allogeneic transplantation were first and most clearly demonstrated, with survival in good-risk patients approaching 90%. Over the last 10 years, however, transplantation has almost ceased as a first-line treatment as superior results can be obtained with less toxicity with the tyrosine kinase inhibitors. Similarly, the goal posts are shifting for other diseases, with improvements in outcomes with unrelated and cord blood transplant as well as refinements in risk assessment, both largely driven by better molecular data.

Hematopoietic stem cell transplantation organizations

- British Society for Blood and Marrow Transplantation (bsbmt.org)
- European Group for Blood and Marrow Transplantation (ebmt.org)
- CIMBTR (cibmtr.org)
- JACIE (www.jacie.org)
- FACT (www.factwebsite.org)
- Netcord (www.netcord.org)
- ASBMT (www.asbmt.org)
- International Society for Cellular therapy (www.celltherapy.org)
- World Marrow Donor program (www.bmdw.org)

Further reading

Filipovich AH, Weisdorf D, Pavletic S, *et al.* National Institutes of Health consensus development project on criteria for clinical trials in chronic graft-versus-host disease: I. Diagnosis and staging working group report. *Biol Blood Marrow Transplant* 2005; **11**: 945–56.

Hughes WT, Armstrong D, Bodey GP, *et al.* Guidelines for the use of antimicrobial agents in neutropenic patients with cancer. *Clin Infect Dis* 2002; **34**: 730–51.

Koreth J, Cutler CS, Djulbegovic B, *et al.* High-dose therapy with single autologous transplantation versus chemotherapy for newly diagnosed multiple myeloma: A systematic review and meta-analysis of randomized controlled trials. *Biol Blood Marrow Transplant* 2007; **13**: 183–96.

Lee SJ, Vogelsang G, Flowers ME. Chronic graft-versus-host disease. *Biol Blood Marrow Transplant* 2003; **9**: 215–33.

Vogelsang GB, Pavletic SZ (eds). *Chronic Graft Verus Host Disease: Interdisciplinary Management.* Cambridge: Cambridge University Press, 2009.

Chapter 39

Corneal transplantation

Yvonne H. Luo and D. Frank P. Larkin

Key points

- In the United Kingdom and Europe, the availability of donor corneas for transplantation is almost sufficient for requirements.
- Most corneal transplants are performed as penetrating transplants in which a 7–8-mm diameter circle of full-thickness cornea is excised and replaced by donor cornea of similar diameter.
- Around one sixth of corneas undergo one or more rejection episodes; the first episode of acute onset rejection typically occurs between 6 and 12 months post-transplant.
- The key to successful treatment of corneal graft rejection is early recognition of the rejection episode by the patient and clinician.
- Corneal transplant survival in large published series is approximately 75% at 5 years, similar to that of vascularized organ grafts.

Cornea is by far the most commonly transplanted tissue worldwide, with nearly 40 000 procedures performed in the United States and 4000 in the United Kingdom annually. Corneal transplantation, or keratoplasty, is the surgical procedure most commonly used in the management of blinding opacification of the normally transparent cornea. In addition, it can be used in uncontrolled infection, pain, or perforation of the cornea. The first recorded corneal transplant in a human was in 1838, preceding by many years the invention even of anesthesia. The donor cornea in this procedure was from a pig, and this xenograft remained transparent for only a couple of weeks. Until the first reported successful lamellar, or partial-thickness, corneal transplant in 1888, almost all transplants were xenografts.

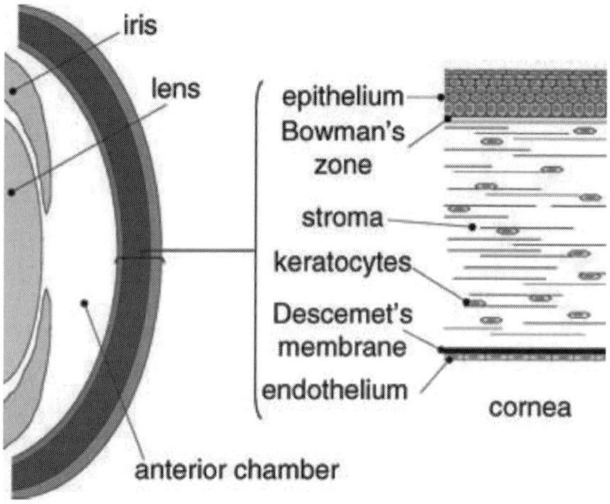

Figure 39.1 Diagrammatic cross section of the cornea. Reproduced with permission from American Society of Transplant Surgeons and American Society of Transplantation.

Corneal anatomy

Viewed from the exterior, adult human cornea is almost circular and approximately 11 mm in horizontal diameter, with an average central thickness of about 530 microns. It consists of three main layers: (1) epithelium, which regenerates rapidly; (2) stroma, which constitutes 90% of corneal thickness and is itself perfectly transparent on account of the parallel and evenly spaced ultrastructural arrangement of its collagen fibrils; and (3) endothelium. The monolayer of endothelial cells is critical for maintenance of stromal deturgescence by action of its ATPase pump to remove aqueous from the stroma. Endothelial cells in man do not have the capability to replace lost cells by mitosis,

Organ Transplantation: A Clinical Guide, ed. A.A. Klein, C.J. Lewis, and J.C. Madsen. Published by Cambridge University which is one reason why disease restricted to this monolayer is the indication for a high proportion of corneal transplants.

Processing of donor cornea prior to transplantation

In the United Kingdom and Europe, the availability of donor corneas for transplantation is almost sufficient for requirements. Satisfactory endothelial cell density is the quality parameter widely used in eye banks. Corneas of satisfactory quality can be obtained from postmortem donors of all ages, and in most countries there is no upper age restriction for corneal donation. Although some donor eyes are harvested at the time of multi-organ donation, most are removed postmortem. Endothelial cell density remains satisfactory up to 24 hours after death. When donor eyes are transported to eye banks, cornea is removed for storage at either 4°C for up to 10 days in chondroitin sulphate–based medium or 34°C in serum-based medium. This potential storage interval is a major difference between processing of donor cornea and other tissues. The feasibility of donor corneal storage allows quality assessment of donor corneas, testing for potential infective pathogens (including hepatitis, human immunodeficiency virus, and syphilis) and scheduling of transplant surgery. On account of current uncertainty about possible risk of prion disease transmission, neurological disorders of uncertain etiology such as dementia and Parkinson's disease are contraindications to corneal donation.

Techniques of corneal transplantation

Other than in children and young adults, most corneal transplants can be undertaken under local anesthesia. The majority are performed as penetrating transplants in which a 7–8-mm diameter circle of full-thickness cornea is excised and replaced by donor cornea of similar diameter. The proportion of partial thickness (lamellar) transplants has increased in recent years and involves replacement of either anterior (epithelium and most or all stroma) or posterior (endothelium and the underlying Descemet's membrane) cornea with donor tissue. Anterior lamellar surgery can be sufficient to restore transparency in those corneas with stromal opacity but healthy endothelium; conversely, posterior lamellar replacement may suffice in those with healthy stroma.

Table 39.1 Examples of indications for corneal transplantation with age at surgery

Diagnosis	Age at surgery (years)	Transplant technique
Keratoconus	18–40	ALK or PK
Fuchs endothelial disease	>60	PK or PLK
Post-cataract surgery endothelial decompensation	>60	PK or PLK
Stromal scarring Post-trauma/infection	20–35	ALK or PK
Rheumatoid disease Corneal melting	>40	PK
Peter's anomaly	2–5	PK
Transplant replacement	Any	PK

Keratoconus, Fuchs corneal endothelial disease, and corneal decompensation following cataract surgery are the commonest indications for transplantation in European centers. Transplant replacement is indicated in some patients following failure of a previous transplant. Case mix varies according to center. ALK: anterior lamellar keratoplasty; PLK: posterior lamellar keratoplasty; PK: penetrating keratoplasty.

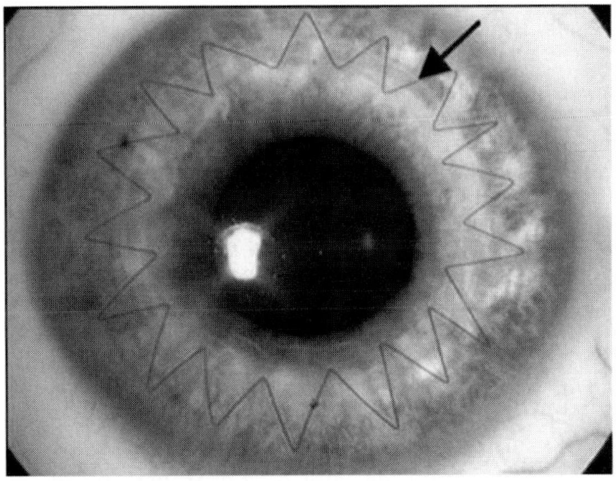

Figure 39.2 Full-thickness corneal transplant sutured to recipient eye with continuous 10/0 nylon suture. The edge of the donor cornea is indicated by the arrow.

Immune privilege in corneal transplantation

Both the (1) anterior chamber together with the peripheral recipient corneal bed and (2) allogeneic donor cornea itself enjoy relative immune privilege. Factors contributing to this privilege include the following:

1. Absence of blood and lymphatic vessels in normal cornea significantly reduces trafficking of immune cells and inflammatory mediators to/from the donor.
2. Expression of Fas ligand (FasL) on corneal cells. Many T-lymphocytes possess the surface molecule Fas. Binding of Fas+ alloreactive T lymphocytes by FasL on corneal surface cells induces lymphocyte apoptosis.
3. Low levels of major histocompatibility complex (MHC) class I and II molecule expression on the surface of corneal cells. Because graft proteins can only be recognized by host T lymphocytes after they are processed by antigen-presenting cells (APCs) and recombined with APC surface MHC molecules, low transplantation antigen expression by donor corneal cells reduces the chance of T-cell activation.
4. Paucity of professional APCs (particularly dendritic cells) in the cornea and anterior chamber. Lack of donor APCs within transplanted cornea implies that antigen presentation to host T lymphocytes by the direct pathway is negligible. Donor corneal allorecognition and rejection is therefore believed to occur in most patients via the indirect pathway, initiated by APCs of recipient origin that migrate into the transplant.
5. Anterior chamber–associated immune deviation (ACAID). In experimental studies it has been shown that prior introduction of alloantigens into the anterior chamber causes downregulation of systemic delayed-type hypersensitivity responses, a phenomenon known as ACAID. This downregulation of immune responses may contribute to graft acceptance in humans.
6. Presence of immunosuppressive proteins in aqueous humor. Proteins such as transforming growth factor β dampen the immune responses in the anterior chamber.

Corneal grafts at high risk of rejection are identified by several risk factors, most of which reflect breakdown of facets of immune privilege. Prospective clinical outcome studies identify the most significant of these to be recipient corneal vascularization, corneal inflammation at the time of transplantation, which induces APC infiltration in the recipient cornea prior to surgery, and a previously rejected ipsilateral graft.

Immunology of corneal allograft rejection

Some features of the immunobiology of corneal rejection differ from allogeneic rejection of other transplanted tissues. Also in contrast to other transplanted tissues, most information on mechanisms of rejection of cornea has come from experimental models rather than clinical biopsies. This is on account of the possibility of diagnosis of rejection by direct visualization of the transplant and the fact that tissue diagnosis is not required. As in all adaptive immune responses, afferent and efferent components can be identified and are described separately.

Afferent phase

Under circumstances that the immune-privileged features of the cornea are bypassed by the immune system, the first stage in rejection is recognition of the presence of non-self tissue. Of the two routes of allorecognition, the indirect pathway predominates in corneal rejection. Recipient-origin APCs enter the donor cornea to capture and process donor antigens and migrate to the neck lymph glands to present the antigen in context with self MHC class II molecules to T cells. From macrophage-depleting studies, evidence has been provided that these cells play a crucial role in the afferent phase of graft rejection. On account of the paucity of transplanted passenger donor APCs, it is assumed that corneal allorecognition by the direct pathway is insignificant in most patients, and this is an area of conceptual difference between the allorecognition of cornea and other tissues. Furthermore, the predominance of indirect allorecognition is believed to be the reason for the lack of benefit of human leukocyte antigen (HLA) class II matching in corneal transplantation: similarity between the MHC class II proteins expressed or upregulated on donor cells and the host would facilitate more effective presentation of graft alloantigens to host T lymphocytes by the host APCs.

Efferent phase

When T-helper cells have identified the presented antigen as non-self, effector mechanisms are generated against donor tissue. Cytokines, including particularly tumor necrosis factor, have been clearly identified in aqueous humor and the cornea prior to observed endothelial rejection onset. After corneal transplantation, it has been shown that alloantibody,

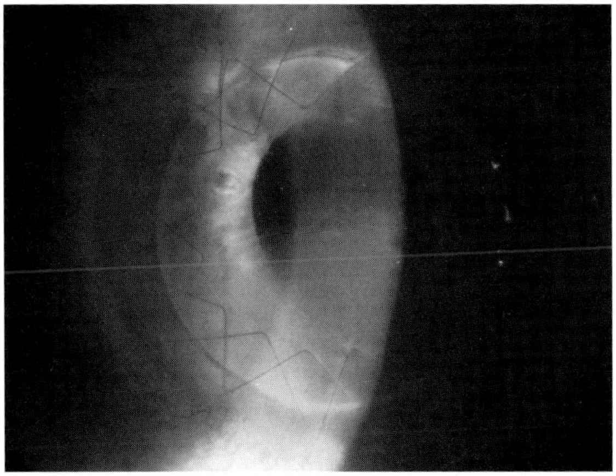

Figure 39.3 Endothelial corneal transplant rejection. Loss of transparency in the inferior cornea is indicated by poor visibility of the pupil margin.

Table 39.2 Corneal transplant survival rates and causes of failure

Corneal transplant survival rates	
1 year	86%
5 years	73%
10 years	62%
15 years	55%
Leading primary causes of transplant failure	
1	Allograft rejection 31%
2	Late endothelial failure 21%
3	Infection 13%
4	Glaucoma 8%

Data adapted from Australian Corneal Graft Register 2007 Report.

macrophages, cytotoxic T lymphocytes, and delayed-type hypersensitivity responses are components of the effector response.

Clinical features and treatment of corneal allograft rejection

Approximately one sixth of corneas undergo one or more rejection episodes. The first episode of acute onset rejection typically occurs between 6 and 12 months after transplant, but may occur much later. Signs of rejection can be directly visualized, may involve any of the three layers of cornea, and may progress from stroma to endothelium. Destruction of the epithelium is unimportant from a functional standpoint, as repopulation of the epithelium by recipient origin cells readily occurs. Stromal rejection is more frequently seen, typified by nummular transplant opacities in a patient presenting with moderate ocular discomfort. On account of the vital physiological importance of endothelial cells to donor corneal function and the incapability of repopulation by mitosis, endothelial rejection is of greatest importance. Rejection episodes irreversibly damage the endothelium to a degree, reducing cell density and the pumping function capability of the endothelium. Once the number of endothelial cells/mm^2 falls below the threshold level required to maintain cornea clarity, irreversible stromal swelling occurs and the cornea becomes cloudy. During an endothelial rejection episode, visual disturbance is caused by stromal edema; there are inflammatory aggregates on the donor endothelium and signs of inflammation in the anterior chamber.

Treatment is commenced as soon as possible with very frequent topical steroid (e.g., dexamethasone hourly), reducing in frequency with resolution of inflammatory signs. Addition of systemic to local steroid has no effect on outcomes of endothelial rejection treatment. In patients who do not present late, most episodes can be reversed. The key to successful treatment of corneal graft rejection is early recognition of the rejection episode by the patient and clinician.

Outcomes of corneal transplantation

Corneal transplant survival in large published series is approximately 75% at 5 years (Table 39.2), similar to that of vascularized organ grafts. The commonest reason for corneal transplant failure is allogeneic rejection, contrary to the standard belief in transplantation immunology that rejection of corneas does not occur. In transplants that are not identified prior to surgery to be at high risk of rejection, topical steroid alone for approximately 6 months is used as rejection prophylaxis, management that is very different from that of the cadaveric vascularized organ transplant recipient. For those with bilateral blinding corneal disease and also at high rejection risk (see above), systemic immunosuppression is used in some centers as prophylaxis. Published case series are the only evidence for drug selection. The only randomized trials in high rejection risk corneal transplants have been undertaken to examine the influence of HLA matching on outcome, which in summary show a weak benefit from matching class I antigens only. HLA matching is not routinely undertaken in patients who are not at high rejection risk.

Further reading

Chatel MA, Larkin DFP. Sirolimus and mycophenolate as combination prophylaxis in corneal transplant recipients at high rejection risk. *Am J Ophthalmol* 2010; **150**: 179–84.

George AJT, Larkin DFP. Corneal transplantation – the forgotten graft. *Am J Transplant* 2004; **4**: 678–85.

Gore SM, Vail A, Bradley BA, Rogers CA, Easty DL, Armitage WJ. HLA-DR matching in corneal transplantation. Systematic review of published evidence. Corneal Transplant Follow-up Study Collaborators. *Transplantation* 1995; **60**: 1033–9.

Niederkorn JY, Larkin DFP. Immune privilege of corneal allografts. *Ocul Immunol Inflamm* 2010; **18**: 162–71.

Williams KA, Coster DJ. The immunobiology of corneal transplantation. *Transplantation* 2007; **84**: 806–13.

Williams KA, Lowe MT, Bartlett CM, Kelly L, Coster DJ (eds). *The Australian Corneal Graft Registry 2007 Report*. Adelaide, Australia: Flinders University Press, 2007.

Chapter 40

UK and European service – legal and operational framework

Chris J. Rudge and Axel O. Rahmel

Key points

- The diagnosis and confirmation of death must be separated from anything to do with the issues surrounding organ donation and transplantation.
- In the UK, explicit consent/authorization must be given before organs are removed for transplantation.
- Living donors must be acting freely and voluntarily and no payment should be offered for the donation.
- A "usual not unusual" part of the care of dying patients should be to ensure that the option of donation is available to all suitable patients and their families.
- The organ allocation system should be open, transparent, fair, and equitable.

This chapter describes the legal and operational frameworks that are necessary at a national or supra-national level in order to support and regulate organ donation and transplantation. Although there are differences in detail between countries, all those with a well-established donation program have in place a legal framework, a national donation system, and processes to ensure quality and safety of organs. They also have a degree of regulation and oversight. Organ transplantation requires equitable organ allocation and measures to prevent organ or people trafficking, again with appropriate regulation and oversight. The role of a national or international transplant registry is critical.

Regulation and oversight are clearly essential, but there needs to be a constant effort to ensure that realistic risk–benefit decisions are made. There is a worldwide shortage of donated organs, with thousands of patients dying each year in the United Kingdom and Europe while waiting for the transplant that never comes. Regulation must accept that not all human organs donated for transplantation are ideal and that it is not possible to eliminate all risks.

In a single chapter it is not possible to document in detail the arrangements in every European country, but the authors have attempted to give a thorough review of the UK position and to describe the important similarities and differences across other European countries. Throughout, the terms donation after brain death (DBD) and donation after circulatory death (DCD) have been used rather than heart-beating and non–heart-beating donation.

Organ donation

Legal structures

Definition of death

United Kingdom

Traditionally in the United Kingdom, the law has not been used to define how the diagnosis or confirmation of death is to be performed, relying instead on the medical profession to produce a code of practice. The courts have, however, endorsed such professional guidance. Following the acceptance of the concept of brain death, the first such guidance was published in 1976. Several documents have been published since, the most recent and significant of which is "A Code of Practice for the Diagnosis and Confirmation of Death," produced under the auspices of the Academy of Medical Royal Colleges and endorsed by the Department of Health. This expands the basis on which death of the brainstem equates to death of the individual and clarifies the clinical steps that must be followed before death can be diagnosed. Moreover, it also, and for the first time, lays down clear clinical criteria for the

Organ Transplantation: A Clinical Guide, ed. A.A. Klein, C.J. Lewis, and J.C. Madsen. Published by Cambridge University Press.

diagnosis of death following irreversible cardiac and respiratory arrest. Of critical importance is the statement that the working party believes that it is important to separate completely the diagnosis and confirmation of death from anything to do with the issues surrounding organ donation and transplantation. This document deals solely with the diagnosis and confirmation of death, whatever the cause, allowing this to be carried out in a variety of circumstances where further intervention aimed at sustaining life can be of no further benefit to patients.

The UK Code of Practice is based on the essential prerequisite that the cause of the patient's deep coma must be known. Thereafter, in the majority of patients, a series of well-defined clinical bedside tests are used to demonstrate complete lack of any brainstem function, with the tests to be carried out twice by two medically qualified practitioners, of whom one must be a consultant. If the tests are unequivocal and can all be carried out, then no further confirmatory tests are required. These may, however, be helpful in certain circumstances such as severe facial trauma that preclude the ocular and corneal reflex testing.

Europe

In all European countries, organ transplantation is guided by the overarching ethical requirement known as the "dead donor rule," which states that patients must be declared dead before the removal of any vital organ for transplantation. Deceased donation can either take place after determination of brain death or of cardiac death. The determination of brain death is legally binding in all European countries prior to postmortem DBD. However, concerning the definition of brain death, two groups of countries can be distinguished: in the majority of European countries, brain death is defined as the complete and irreversible cessation of all cerebral and brainstem function. In Portugal and Switzerland, as in the United Kingdom, the verification of the complete and irreversible cessation of brainstem function is sufficient.

Although the need for brain (stem) death diagnosis as a prerequisite for organ donation is regulated by a parliamentary act in all countries, the medical and procedural details of the brain (stem) death diagnosis are typically laid down in guidelines by national medical associations or in specific decrees and thereby vary slightly from country to country.

The current situation with regard to regulations concerning DCD is much more heterogeneous in Europe. Four different categories of DCD donors are currently distinguished:

A. Uncontrolled
   - I. Dead on arrival at hospital
   - II. Unsuccessful resuscitation

B. Controlled
   - III. Awaiting cardiac arrest
   - IV. Cardiac arrest while brain dead

Category IV DCDs with a completed brain death diagnosis, if medically suitable, can obviously be used as organ donors in all countries, with the exception that DCD is legally not permitted at all in some countries (Croatia, Germany, Hungary, and Poland) because a completed brain death diagnosis according to the previously mentioned national regulations is required in all cases of deceased donation.

In other countries, DCD is not prohibited, but no respective programs are in place yet.

Active DCD transplant programs currently exist in nine European countries only (Austria, Belgium, Czech Republic, France, Italy, the Netherlands, Spain, Switzerland, United Kingdom). In some of these countries, only DCD of category I and II donors are legally approved (France, Spain), whereas in the other countries, all types of donors are permitted. In the latter, the category III donors typically represent the majority of all DCD donors.

Finally, there are substantial differences with regard to the DCD protocols used in the different countries and sometimes even between the different centers within one country. As an example, the "no-touch period" after cardiac arrest until the start of organ procurement varies between 2 and 20 minutes. Therefore, initiatives are underway aiming at harmonization of the DCD protocols.

Consent

United Kingdom

A legal framework for organ donation after death is an absolutely essential component of any transplant system. The Human Organ Transplant Act 1961 was replaced in England, Wales, and Northern Ireland by the Human Tissue Act 2004 (and in Scotland by the Human Tissue Act 2006). The principal activities covered by these acts are the removal from a deceased person of organs for the purpose of transplantation and, most importantly, the requirements for appropriate consent (or authorization in Scotland) before this can lawfully be carried out. Although there are small but relevant differences of detail between the acts, they are considered together, and the general term of "consent/authorization" will be used.

The fundamental import of the acts is that they require that explicit consent/authorization must be given before organs are removed for transplantation. This may be given by the donor themselves in life, for example, through registration on the National Health Service (NHS) Organ Donor Register. If the donor has not given consent/authorization, then it may be given by others on his or her behalf, and the two acts describe a hierarchy of individuals who may do so. The details differ slightly, but both place at the top of the order a nominated representative (if there is one) or the closest relatives of the donor and end with a friend of long standing. The issue of presumed consent, or opting-out legislation, was considered in detail in the United Kingdom, and a report in November 2008 concluded that although the decision was finely balanced, the recommendation was that there should be no change to the existing, explicit consent (or opting-in) legislation.

Europe

Consent to donation is the second prerequisite to postmortem organ donation, and details are laid down in national legislation in all European countries. In some countries, explicit consent by the donor is necessary (informed consent, opting-in). This consent can either be expressed by the donor already during lifetime in writing, for example, by a donor card or by registration in a respective national donor registry. If such a written statement does not exist, the relatives or other close persons to the donor are asked instead. The relatives are not asked about their opinion, but rather about the (presumed) opinion of the deceased person concerning organ donation, but of course, especially in the absence of an explicit statement, transition between the two is fluid. Informed consent systems exist for example in Germany, the Netherlands, Slovenia, Switzerland, and as already explained in detail in the previous section, in the United Kingdom.

In the majority of European countries, a presumed consent or opting-out system for achieving consent to donation is in place. Under this regulation, every deceased person is considered a donor if no objection was expressed during their lifetime. In most countries that have an opting-out system in place, a non-donor registry is established, the most prominent exception being Spain. But, as is the case in countries with informed consent systems, in countries with presumed consent, relatives or other close persons of the donor are involved when possible prior to transplantation: in all cases where there is no documented will of the donor, any objection from the family is respected. But even when the donor had consented but the family objects to donation, although legally a donation would be possible, in practice the wish of the family is respected and organ donation is not pursued.

So in summary, in spite of the formally different legal solutions to consent in the different European countries, family consent does in fact play a major role in every donation procedure. Therefore, it has been claimed that the varying donation rates that can be observed between European countries is only to a minor degree due to differences in legislation.

Living donation

United Kingdom

The two Human Tissue Acts mentioned above also set the legal framework for living donation. In principle they make several main provisions. First, that living donors must be acting freely and voluntarily, and that no payment is offered for the donation. The acts are clear that a criminal offense has been committed if any reward is given or is to be given to the donor. Second, the acts established the Human Tissue Authority (HTA), which is required to publish codes of practice that allow clinicians to work within the law. Most specifically, the HTA is required to give prior approval for all living donor transplants in the United Kingdom, regardless of the nature of the genetic or other relationship between the donor and recipient. In practice, the overwhelming majority of such transplants are between genetically related pairs or those with a long-standing and well-defined emotional relationship such as spouse or partner, and in these circumstances HTA approval is given on the basis of a written report from a trained and designated "Independent Assessor." However, if the circumstances are more complex, an HTA Panel is convened to consider the application and, if satisfied, to give approval for the transplant. This latter procedure is used, for example, in the case of the non-directed, altruistic, stranger donation when an individual wishes to donate a kidney anonymously to whichever patient on the national waiting list is the most appropriate recipient, and also in cases where there are increased risks to the donor and/or recipient, such as living donor liver transplantation.

Despite this apparently cumbersome requirement for HTA approval for all living donor transplants, the system has worked extremely well since its introduction in 2006, with approval being given within 2–3 days in the majority of occasions. Clinicians are supported in knowing that their judgment and decisions have been endorsed by an independent assessor, and the system provides a robust process to minimize the likelihood of organ trafficking from living donors. The legislation has also allowed the development of a paired-exchange program for incompatible living donor pairs, which is now well established, with a growing number of transplants, and "stranger" donations are also increasing in number.

Europe

In most European countries, living donation is regulated by law because the protection of the living donor has to be guaranteed, and any form of organ trade or trafficking is to be prevented. In order to achieve this, several restrictions to living donation are in place in the different European countries. In most countries, either a defined genetic relationship (typically first- or second-degree relatives) or another form of close relationship between donor and recipient is required. In several countries, an exception to this rule is allowed in case of cross-over (paired exchange) living donation, as long as the relation of each donor/recipient couple fulfills the above-mentioned prerequisites. In a few countries altruistic donation is allowed, typically as non-directed donation to the recipient pool, because in the case of directed, altruistic donation, it is considered difficult to prevent abuse leading to organ trading. In all countries, informed consent to donation is required. As a consequence, donation by minors is in most countries not possible. In only a few countries, e.g., Slovenia, Switzerland, and the United Kingdom, are exceptions to this general rule possible under clearly defined, narrow preconditions.

The majority of European countries have established specific ethics committees that check whether living donation is in fact voluntary by the donor and, in case of genetically unrelated donor–recipient pairs, whether in fact a close relationship between donor and recipient exists to prevent exploitation of the donor and possible organ trafficking. These committees are also involved in all cases of altruistic donation.

In some countries, living donor transplantation is considered subsidiary to deceased donor transplantation, so that living donor transplantation is only allowed if no deceased donor can be identified. In practice this rule has only minor implications, because in general the time between the decision to perform a living donor transplant and the transplantation is so short that a suitable deceased donor organ for the recipient does not become available in time.

In all European countries, living donation has to be unpaid, organ trafficking is prohibited, and violations will be prosecuted, focusing on vendors and any medical personnel involved.

Organ donation organization

Donor coordination

United Kingdom

In January 2008, the UK Health Departments published the report from the Organ Donation Task Force "Organs for Transplants." This report identified the obstacles to donation after death in the United Kingdom and made 14 recommendations. One overarching principle runs throughout the report: the ambition to make donation "usual, not unusual." Central to this is the aim to transform the approach of those working in the care of potential organ donors and to develop a collaborative of clinicians and donor coordinators within every hospital. This has involved a complete reorganization of the donor transplant coordinator (DTC) network in the United Kingdom. Prior to 2008, DTCs were employed in a variety of ways around the country, with the majority, but not all, based within transplant units. Funding arrangements also varied. A key task force recommendation was that NHS Blood and Transplant (NHSBT) should take over the direct employment of DTCs, that their numbers should increase from approximately 100 to well over 200, and that their working arrangements should change significantly. Most of these changes have taken place over the past 18 months and are expected to be complete early in 2011. There are currently over 185 DTCs, and the majority of them are nurses from an intensive care background. Their focus is entirely on organ donation; they have no responsibility for transplant recipients. The intention is that in due course they will all be "embedded" within the individual hospital in which they are based, as part of the intensive care and end-of-life teams. Their role is to raise awareness, ensure that local training needs are met, and to encourage the identification of all potential donors. Typically they will work in their hospital for

3–4 days/week, but (on a regional basis) they will all participate in a 24/7 on-call rota to facilitate actual donors.

Europe

Historically, donor coordination was taken care of in most countries by local coordinators associated with or even employed by the transplant centers. Such a model still exists, for example, in Belgium and until recently in Switzerland. In most countries, organ donation is now centrally organized, and national coordination offices have been set up. These are responsible for the training, accreditation, and often also the employment of the donor coordinators. As a result of this centralization process, in some countries such as Germany and the Netherlands, local coordinators are no longer directly linked to the donor hospital but are located outside the hospitals. The Spanish experience with central management of in-hospital coordinators has resulted in substantial increase in organ donation and is considered to be a central element in successful transplantation. Therefore, most countries are strengthening in-house coordination, of course taking into account organizational and structural differences in their national health care systems.

The tasks of the transplant coordinators vary from country to country. In some countries they are already involved in the identification of possible donors, whereas in other countries their tasks start with the assessment of identified potential donors. In all countries they are responsible for the organization of the whole donation process. If necessary they take care that brain death diagnosis can be performed by trained experts, they support the local hospital staff in maintaining the donor on the intensive care unit (ICU), and they cooperate with the retrieval teams prior to and during organ procurement.

In some countries transplant coordinators are responsible for most or all of the communication with the donor family, whereas in others they only talk to the donor's family when requested by the local hospital team. Recent data concerning the achieved consent rates suggest that specifically trained coordinators are more successful in this regard than ICU personnel. This is another argument in favor of the establishment of local in-house donor coordinators. The directive on organ transplantation and the accompanying action plan therefore explicitly support the introduction of in-house coordination in Europe.

The role of critical care and emergency medicine

United Kingdom

The task force recognized that one of the key elements in a successful donation program is the need for those working in critical care (intensive care and emergency medicine) to believe that a "usual not unusual" part of their care of dying patients should be to ensure that the option of donation is available to all suitable patients and their families. This approach, which is building considerable momentum in the United Kingdom, can only be sustained when all clinicians are supported and are able to work within a clear and unambiguous framework of good practice based on legal, ethical, and professional guidelines. To this end, the Department of Health published guidance on the legal framework for DCD in November 2009, which is based on an understanding of the Mental Capacity Act 2005 in England and Wales (and similar guidance was published in May 2010 on The Adults with Incapacity Act 2000 in Scotland). The main legal concerns relate to the management of a patient who is dying but not dead and who lacks capacity to give consent for treatment. The thrust of the advice is that if a person's wishes were to be a donor, then certain actions that facilitate donation may be considered to be in his or her best interests (and thus lawful) if they do not cause the person harm or distress. Furthermore, an independent, high-profile UK Donation Ethics Committee has been established under the auspices of the Academy of Medical Royal Colleges, which met for the first time in January 2010.

The second component of the "collaborative" mentioned above, which is to be established in every acute hospital, is a Clinical Lead for organ donation. More than 95% of hospitals have now made an appointment, and the overwhelming majority are consultants from a clinical background in intensive care. They are paid (by NHSBT) for approximately half a day to 1 day per week. Their role is to act as a local "Lead" for donation through raising local awareness, establishing training, and ensuring that protocols for donation are in place based on national guidelines. The task force described minimal notification criteria that would ensure that all potential donors would be referred to the DTC network, at the appropriate time, and this will not only help to maximize actual donation, but will also provide an accurate and consistent measurement of the performance of every hospital toward maximizing donation.

Table 40.1 Definitions of brain death and cardiac death donors

	Donation after brain death (DBD)	Donation after cardiac death (DCD)
Potential donor	A person whose clinical condition is suspected to fulfill brain death criteria.	A person in whom the cessation of circulatory and respiratory functions is anticipated to occur within a time frame that will enable organ recovery.
Eligible donor	A medically suitable person who has been declared dead based on neurological criteria as stipulated by the law of the relevant jurisdiction.	A medically suitable person who has been declared dead based on the irreversible absence of circulatory and respiratory functions as stipulated by the law of the relevant jurisdiction, within a time frame that enables organ recovery.
Actual donor	A consented eligible donor: In whom an operative incision was made with the intent of organ recovery for the purpose of transplantation and/or From whom at least one organ was recovered for the purpose of transplantation.	
Utilized donor	An actual donor from whom at least one organ was transplanted.	

Europe

The crucial role of intensive care nurses and doctors in the identification and maintenance of potential donors has already been noted and is acknowledged in all European countries. In some countries, intensive care personnel are legally obliged to report potential donors to the national donor coordination organizations. In day-to-day practice, the effect of such legislation has been limited: raising the awareness around organ donation and continuous training of ICU personnel on the other hand is of pivotal importance.

The potential for donation

United Kingdom

The UK Potential Donor Audit (PDA) was established in 2003 and collects data on every patient who dies in every intensive care unit in the country. The hierarchical structure of the PDA allows the reasons for which a potential donor failed to become an actual donor to be identified, and the data can be used both nationally and locally. The most recent data (UK Transplant Registry, unpublished) shows that for potential donors after brain death, 25% of patients were not subjected to brainstem tests, 11% of patients certified dead were not referred to the DTC network, and the refusal rate for donation was 39%. Thus the overall conversion rate in 2008/2009 was only 51%. There are many reasons for these figures, not all of which represent a failure of the system, but the availability of such data allows focused efforts, both nationally and locally, on areas for improvement. At a local level, a further recommendation of the task force was that every hospital should have a "non-clinical champion," and in practice this is being achieved through the establishment of a hospital Donation Committee, and the chairs of these committees. The chair will typically come from a non-clinical background and have a high local profile within the hospital or the local community. The members of the committee will include clinicians, nurses, faith leaders, ethics, management, and others. The committee will receive (every 6 months) the donation activity for their hospital based on the PDA, assess progress, identify local obstacles and solutions, and report to the management board of the hospital.

Europe

Data on donor potential is not collected in Europe; part of the problem is that generally agreed definitions are not established. Recently the World Health Organization (WHO) suggested a set of definitions for DBD and DCD. Although data on actual and on utilized donors are typically available, information on eligible and especially potential donors is lacking in almost all countries so far.

In Spain, a systematic retrospective review of all ICU deaths is performed; this allows clear identification of all potential donors and helps to increase awareness of potential donors among the ICU personnel in the future.

The Donor Action program works in a similar manner. One of the steps of this initiative to increase organ donation is a systematic medical record review (MRR). The MRR uses specially designed forms to collect retrospective and prospective data on critical care unit mortalities. These data are used to establish the unit's donor potential and to pinpoint where and when potential donors failed to convert into actual donors. A recent comparison of the conversion rates in countries with an opting-out versus an opting-in system showed

Table 40.2 Donor and transplant rates per million population (2008)

	Deceased donors	Kidneys	Livers	Hearts	Lungs
UK	14.7	23.0	11.9	2.1	2.3
Spain	34.2	44.9	24.0	6.3	4.2
Germany	14.6	26.6	13.7	4.7	3.3
France	25.3	41.9	15.9	6.0	3.4
Netherlands	12.8	21.5	8.0	1.6	3.4
Italy	21.1	26.9	17.8	5.7	1.6
Norway	20.5	37.6	16.5	8.1	6.3
Sweden	16.5	30.7	15.8	4.9	5.6

a significantly higher conversion rate in the countries with presumed consent, related to a lower number of refusals in these countries.

Donor and transplant rates in the United Kingdom and Europe

The United Kingdom has, for many years, had one of the lower deceased donation rates in Europe while moving in recent years to achieve one of the higher living donor rates. There are many reasons for this, and it is important to recognize that a wide range of factors influence both the number of possible or potential deceased donors and the proportion of those that progress to become actual donors (the conversion rate). Although every country must endeavor to maximize the conversion rate, it is not realistic to expect every country to achieve the same actual deceased donor rate. Factors likely to have an impact include the mortality rates from head injuries (particularly road traffic accidents) and various forms of intracerebral hemorrhage, the number of intensive care beds, and the donation infrastructure. Of note in the United Kingdom are two important observations. First, the PDA shows that the number of patients in ICU in whom brainstem death is a possible diagnosis has fallen by almost a third in the last 5 years, as has the number of patients in whom death is diagnosed by these tests. Thus there has been a marked fall in the number of patients from whom organ donation (DBD) is possible. Second, the number of DCD donors has risen from 128 to 335 in the same time period. There is considerable speculation (but little evidence) that increasingly a decision is being made at a relatively early stage that further active treatment of patients with severe brain injury is futile and/or inappropriate and that as a result treatment is withdrawn before the patient reaches the stage of brainstem death. There is also the likelihood that changes in the clinical management of such patients, such as decompressive craniectomy and stenting/coiling of intracerebral arteriovenous malformations, are changing the outcome for such patients. Finally, there is also anecdotal evidence that critical management decisions about patients are being made at an even earlier stage, i.e., in the Department of Emergency Medicine, with the result that patients who are thought to have untreatable or unsurvivable injuries are not being admitted to critical care facilities. Any developments that reduce mortality from major brain injury are clearly welcome, but it is important to understand these changing patterns of clinical care in order to focus efforts on optimizing donation in the most appropriate ways.

The demographics of deceased organ donors are changing in the United Kingdom as elsewhere, with more donors being older and obese and fewer dying from trauma. As a result, an increasing proportion of donated organs are "marginal," but the proportion of "offered" organs that are in fact retrieved and transplanted has stayed remarkably constant, implying that a greater proportion of transplanted organs are also increasingly marginal. There is an interesting (but unanswered) question regarding the appropriate "discard rate" of donated organs; too low suggests that the criteria for donation/transplantation may be too rigid, whereas too high suggests inappropriate retrieval of organs from some possible donors. There are considerable differences between the main European countries: although the donor rate in Spain is 2.36 times that of

Table 40.3 Risk levels for donor organs

Category	Definition
Standard risk	Evaluation process did not identify any transmittable disease
Calculated risk	Evaluation identified a transmissible disease, but recipient has same disease or protective serology
Increased but acceptable risk	Evaluation identified a transmissible disease, but organ utilization is justified by the recipient-specific health situation
Unacceptable risk (absolute contraindication)	In these cases the donor is not suitable for transplantation. Typically this category includes: • HIV 1 or 2 seropositivity • HBsAg and HDV contemporaneous seropositivity • Current neoplastic conditions (some exceptions apply) • Systemic infections caused by agents for which treatments are not feasible • Documented prion diseases
Not assessable risk	Evaluation process does not allow an appropriate risk assessment for transmittable diseases

HBsAg: Hepatitis B virus surface antigen; HDV: hepatitis D virus; HIV: human immunodeficiency virus.

the United Kingdom, the kidney transplant rate is only 1.95 times greater, still a very significant advantage, but suggesting a higher discard rate in Spain.

Safety and quality of donors

United Kingdom

All human organs donated after death for transplantation potentially carry a risk of disease transmission from the donor to the recipient. The main risks are of transmission of an infectious agent or of malignant cells from a primary tumor elsewhere in the donor. Although all possible steps are taken to minimize the risk of any such transmission, transplantation differs fundamentally from many forms of tissue transplantation and blood transfusion. The interval between donation and transplantation is measured in hours rather than days or weeks (thus limiting the testing that can be performed), and many forms of organ transplantation are life-saving, with the alternative to use of an available organ likely to be the death of the recipient within days or weeks in some circumstances. A sensible approach therefore should allow some discretion for informed decision making about a possible transplant by the patient, his or her family, and the clinicians responsible for the patient's care.

Guidance on the testing of organ donors and decision making about the use of organs with known risk factors comes from the Advisory Committee on the Safety of Blood, Tissues and Organs, the committee established by the Department of Health in 2008 to succeed the Advisory Committee on the Microbiological Safety of Blood, Tissues and Organs for Transplantation, which had previously been responsible for publishing guidance. Updated guidance was published in 2011 and emphasizes the importance of counseling and consenting potential recipients about specific risk factors for imparied outcome of organ transplantation.

Europe

Currently there are neither common binding European rules on donor evaluation nor on possible contraindications to transplantation. As indicated earlier in this chapter, the process of evaluation of donor suitability is influenced by the limited availability of organs. In every case the individual balance between risks and expected benefits for the recipient have to be taken into account prior to acceptance of an organ for transplantation. In addition, time constraints surrounding the donation process and due to the limited ischemic tolerance of the donor organs may preclude performing certain screening procedures. In the past, the Council of Europe has published several documents on this subject. In the course of the Alliance O project, in which representatives from several European organ procurement and organ exchange organizations participated, the following recommendations were developed: the evaluation of the suitability of the donor has to be based on medical history, physical examination, instrumental as well as laboratory tests, and histological examination and/or postmortem examination with the aim to clarify issues that have emerged during the previous evaluation steps or still to be investigated. Based on the findings gathered during the donor evaluation, the donor (organs) can be attributed to a risk level (Table 40.3).

The final decision of organ suitability has to be taken by the clinician caring for the potential recipient. In cases in which a patient becomes a potential recipient of an organ with an increased risk, a transplant team member must explain the specific risks and informed consent should be obtained from the recipient or his or her family. Later in 2010, an EU Directive on Organs was published that could harmonize donor evaluation in the EU member countries.

Regulation and Oversight in the United Kingdom and Europe

The EU Directive on the Standards of Quality and Safety of Human Organs intended for Transplantation has now been adopted, and it will require implementation by 2012. While it is not possible to describe the details of the directive, it is clear that every member state is to be required to establish a competent authority that will have considerable regulatory and oversight responsibilities. In a number of countries, many of these functions are already in place through the various established authorities as described earlier in this chapter, and at present it would appear that the directive is unlikely to add a significant bureaucratic burden. Harmonization of minimum safety and quality standards will allow easier and safer cross-border organ sharing where this is desirable.

Organ allocation and transplantation

Allocation – principles and practice

United Kingdom

Open, *transparent*, *fair*, and *equitable* are the terms frequently used to describe the requirements of any organ allocation system. These are clearly spelled out in the WHO Guiding Principles that were adopted in May 2010 (Guiding Principle 9). The key question for any organization responsible for devising and implementing allocation rules is "What do we want to achieve?" and in the United Kingdom, this responsibility rests primarily with the organ-specific Advisory Groups of NHSBT.

There are numerous, often conflicting, possible principles for organ allocation, of which the most frequently proposed include:

- Need: Give priority to the sickest patient
- Outcome: Maximize the health benefit from every donated organ
- Program driven: Good survival results, either for the transplant center or the overall national transplant program
- Public policy: Cost effectiveness
- Lobby groups: Appeals to the media by individual patients or groups representing patients with a particular disease
- Willing to pay: With money or with organ donation
- Social worth: Status, job, children or other dependants, lifestyle ("good" or "bad")
- Queuing: First come, first served
- Random selection

In practice, the over-riding principle is that of national equity of access to transplantation, such that similar patients with similar severity of disease should have an equal chance of receiving a transplant regardless of where they live, their race or gender, and, as far as possible, the biological determinants such as blood group and human leukocyte antigen (HLA) phenotype. However, a number of other factors are also taken into account, such as waiting time, the ideal of offering well-matched organs to younger patients, and the specific needs of individual patients such as those with multiple anti-HLA antibodies or with fulminant organ failure for whom death may be expected within days or weeks without transplantation. Added to this must be the different safe storage (cold ischemic) times for different organs and the need to minimize transport times within safe limits.

It is not possible to describe in detail in this chapter the different allocation schemes for the different organs, and indeed they are all subject to regular review and revision. However, several key steps toward the development of a satisfactory scheme can be described. First, they should be based on as much information as is available, on donor and recipient factors that influence outcome and on the demographics of both donor and recipient pools. Second, they should be based on patient needs and outcomes rather than on the perceived interests of individual centers. Third, the advisory groups have available to them sophisticated computer simulation tools that, although not necessarily predicting the exact outcome of any proposed scheme, are invaluable in comparing the benefits and disadvantages of a number of proposed alternatives to inform a balanced judgment regarding the optimal scheme. These tools have, in fact, proved to be remarkably accurate in predicting the observed outcomes of changes that have been introduced.

To summarize the various schemes very briefly:

National Kidney Allocation Scheme

1. Introduced in 2006, this allocates all kidneys from DBDs nationally, whereas kidneys from DCDs are allocated by the local retrieval center.
2. There are five hierarchical tiers, the highest being pediatric recipients who are highly sensitized and for whom the kidney is a zero-mismatch, the lowest being adult patients who are not highly sensitized and for whom the kidney is more than a zero-mismatch.
3. Within each tier, the selected recipient is chosen on a points score that includes waiting time, HLA match, and age points combined: age difference between the donor and recipient, additional points for HLA homozygous patients, and blood group points that allocate a certain proportion of blood group O kidneys to blood group B recipients.

National Liver, Heart and Lung Allocation Schemes

These schemes are broadly similar in that each transplant center is allocated a number of local donor hospitals and is able to choose a recipient from their own waiting list for an organ from a local donor. This is over-ridden by the Super-Urgent Liver scheme and the Urgent Heart scheme, whereby patients meeting defined urgency criteria are listed nationally and take priority over local allocation if the organ is suitable.

National Pancreas Allocation Scheme

A national patient-based allocation scheme for kidney–pancreas and pancreas-alone transplants, incorporating the need for islet transplantation, has been developed and recently introduced.

Europe

Organ allocation rules vary substantially between the different European countries. Some basic ethical principles apply for all countries: equity and justice are considered important, priority is given to urgent patients, and outcome after transplantation is taken into account. The largest differences exist concerning the relative weight assigned to local allocation in the different countries. This can be explained based on the historical development of organ transplantation. Similar to the situation described for organ procurement, organ allocation was in the early days of transplantation taken care of by the transplant centers, and the organs were allocated locally. Quickly, (mandatory) exchange with other centers was introduced to address the needs of specific patients, with this allocation being patient-oriented. On the other hand, regional allocation was typically center-oriented, giving the transplant team the choice to select the most suitable patient from the waiting list at their center. Organs for which no suitable recipient could be found in the donor center or region were offered to other transplant centers or regions within the donor country. Some countries established multi-national cooperation: the largest is Eurotransplant (Austria, Belgium, Croatia, Germany, Luxemburg, the Netherlands, Slovenia), but there is also Scandiatransplant (Denmark [including Greenland], Finland, Iceland, Norway, and Sweden) and the United Kingdom, with mandatory exchange rules between the participating countries.

Some of the historical elements persist in most European countries to a certain extent. For example mandatory exchange for specific patient groups such as high urgent, highly immunized, or pediatric recipients is in place in most countries. In some cases, this mandatory exchange is combined with a regional balancing or pay-back system. Besides the rules for mandatory exchange criteria, organ-specific allocation rules have been developed in most countries based on the above-mentioned ethical and medical criteria. In general, medical expert groups are responsible for the establishment of these rules; in some countries, other stakeholders such as patient groups and legal experts are also involved in the process. In many countries (e.g., France [kidneys], Hungary, Portugal, and Spain), the resulting match list is in case of regional allocation not binding, but is rather considered as a recommendation.

In some countries (Switzerland, Eurotransplant countries [with the exception of non-renal organs in Austria], France [non-renal organs], and the UK [see above]), a strict patient-oriented allocation system has been developed. Due to the expected shorter ischemic time and the therefore expected better result of local and regional allocation, some preference to regional allocation is also given in these patient-oriented systems. Independent of the allocation rules, the final decision concerning acceptance of an organ offer and the transplantation of a specific patient always remains with the transplant center.

Organ tracking

United Kingdom

It is clearly necessary to be able to track all organs (and tissues) from an individual donor to the several recipients of different organs and tissues. One of the main reasons for this is the possibility of potential or actual disease transmission from the donor to one or more of the recipients. This possibility may be apparent very early after transplantation if relevant results become available from microbiological screening tests or postmortem examination of the donor after the organs have been transplanted. It may also occur many years later, for example, if a recipient sero-converts for any of the relevant viruses (in particular, hepatitis and human immunodeficiency virus) or develops a tumor, where suspicion arises that the donor may have been the source of the disease. A mechanism must be in place that allows clinicians caring for the other recipients to receive notification of such a possibility and to respond appropriately. The UK Transplant Registry performs this function in the United Kingdom, and the procedures that are in place are currently being strengthened.

Europe

In order to both maintain public trust and to increase recipient safety, it is mandatory that the final use of any donor organ offered for transplantation can be identified. The complete system of tracing and linkage has to be achieved with strict adherence to the relevant data safety regulations established both on the European and the sometimes even more strict national level. In general, this task is the responsibility of the organ procurement and/or allocation organization. Typically, donor and recipient information is stored after pseudonymization using unique donor and recipient identification numbers.

In the case of cross-border allocation involving multiple (European) organ exchange organizations, organ tracing is a little more complex. Currently every organ exchange organization has its own donor coding system as described above. Therefore, it is necessary that in case of organ exchange between organizations, both the donor number of the procuring organ exchange organization and the donor number of the transplanting organization is stored. In the course of the implementation of the new EU Directive of the European Parliament and of the Council on Standards of Quality and Safety of Human Organs Intended for Transplantation, a common European donor identification number is planned that will allow easier communication.

Transplant registry

United Kingdom

In organ donation and transplantation, comprehensive and accurate data are essential. The UK Transplant Registry (part of NHSBT, and formerly known as UK Transplant) and the transplant database serve a number of functions:

1. Maintain data on all patients waiting for an organ transplant
2. Record data on all organ donors (living and deceased)
3. Document organ allocation
4. Record data on all transplant operations
5. Collect follow-up data on all recipients until transplant failure or death
6. Collect follow-up data on all living donors
7. Collect data submitted to the Potential Donor Audit

There are several specific databases in the United Kingdom, such as that on antibody-incompatible transplants and the paired-exchange living donor program. It is not possible to provide detailed examples of all these activities, but the Annual Activity Report and the references quoted below give an indication of the ways in which the UK Transplant Registry is used.

Europe

Currently there exists no comprehensive overview of how the collection of transplant-related data are organized and structured in the different European countries. However, in April 2008, the European Parliament endorsed a resolution on organ donation and transplantation asking for monitoring of post-transplant and post-donation results. For this purpose, a common method of data analysis is required in order to allow optimal comparability of results across member states. The aim is to ensure the quality and safety of organ donation and transplantation to reduce transplant risks. To achieve this, the Commission and the member states have been asked to launch a pan-European database and communication network to interconnect the national databases and provide them with a platform for exchange of comprehensive data on organ donation and transplantations: The European Framework for the Evaluation of Organ Transplants.

Further reading

Collett D, Sibanda N, Pioli S, Bradley JA, Rudge C. The UK scheme for mandatory continuous monitoring of early transplant outcome in all kidney transplant centers. *Transplantation* 2009; **88**: 970–5.

Johnson RJ, Fuggle SV, Mumford L, Bradley JA, Forsythe JL, Rudge CJ, Kidney Advisory Group of NHS Blood and Transplant. A New UK 2006 National Kidney Allocation Scheme for deceased heart-beating donor kidneys. *Transplantation* 2010; **89**: 387–94.

UK Department of Health. Legal issues relevant to non-heart beating organ donation. Available at: http://www.dh.gov.uk/en/Publicationsandstatistics/Publications/PublicationsPolicyAndGuidance/DH_108825

UK Department of Health. Organs for transplants: a report from the Organ Donation Taskforce. Available at: http://www.dh.gov.uk/en/Publicationsandstatistics/Publications/PublicationsPolicyAndGuidance/DH_082122

UK Department of Health. The potential impact of an opt out system for organ donation in the UK: an independent report from the Organ Donation Taskforce. Available at: http://www.dh.gov.uk/en/Publicationsandstatistics/Publications/PublicationsPolicyAndGuidance/DH_090312

Chapter 41

US transplant service – legal and operational framework

Walter K. Graham, Richard S. Luskin, and Francis L. Delmonico

Key points

- The Organ Procurement and Transplantation Network (OPTN) includes all hospitals that provide solid organ transplantation as well as all organ procurement organizations (OPOs) and tissue-typing laboratories.
- The OPTN provides support and oversight for every organ transplant in the country for both living donor and deceased donor transplants.
- United Network for Organ Sharing (UNOS) is a private membership corporation that is also a non-profit, charitable organization that under federal contract established and continues to operate the OPTN.
- UNOS collects and maintains all data for the Scientific Registry of Transplant Recipients (SRTR), which maintains data on every organ transplant recipient in the United States, including annual follow-up data for the life of the recipient and/or graft.
- UNOS maintains a centralized computer network linking all organ procurement organizations and transplant centers. When a donated organ from a deceased donor is available, that program will rank order the candidates on the waiting list and then offer the donated organ according to the rank order of the match.

The first successful human organ transplant took place at the Peter Bent Brigham Hospital in Boston, Massachusetts, in 1954. The living kidney donor was the identical twin brother of the recipient. Although subsequent transplants were limited initially to other closely related donors and recipients, it quickly became clear that it would be necessary to use organs from deceased donors if there was to be significant application of transplant therapy. In these early years, the surgeons responsible for performing the transplants also took responsibility for recovering the organs from deceased donors. However, there were severe limitations on the process. There was no formal system for identifying potential donors. Organs had to be removed very rapidly once the patient became asystolic and could not be preserved ex vivo for any extended period of time. This severely limited the availability of organs and meant that most organs were recovered at the transplant center itself. There was very limited sharing of organs among transplant centers, and all recovery-related activities were carried out by physicians and surgeons.

In 1968, the first independent (i.e., non–transplant center based) organ recovery organization, the Inter Hospital Organ Bank, was formed by transplant hospitals in the Boston area. Similar organizations followed in other metropolitan areas with multiple transplant programs as a way to streamline and improve the quality of the recovery process. At about the same time, development of the concept of brain death, and thus the ability to maintain the heart beat and respirations of potential donors on a ventilator, expanded the pool of potential donors significantly. With the 1972 passage of the End-Stage Renal Disease Program and initiation of Medicare payment for kidney transplants of end-stage renal disease patients of all ages, demand for kidneys increased significantly. To meet this demand, deceased organ recovery needed to expand to include donors at non-transplant centers. The logistics of the recovery process made it imperative that a new kind of transplant professional, the donation and transplant coordinator, needed to be created. These new coordinators, whether based at a transplant

Organ Transplantation: A Clinical Guide, ed. A.A. Klein, C.J. Lewis, and J.C. Madsen. Published by Cambridge University Press.

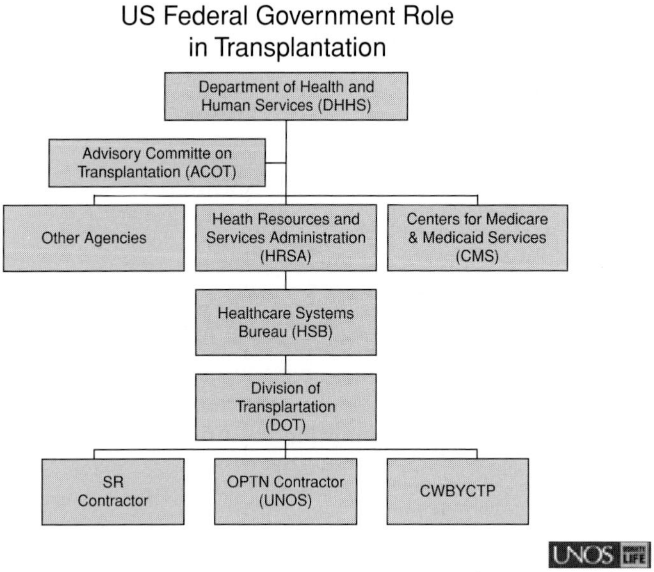

Figure 41.1 Organization of US National Transplantation Support.

center or at an independent organ procurement organization, assumed responsibility for public and professional education about donation; assistance with the pre-recovery and intraoperative clinical management of the donor; assisting the surgeon with the recovery procedure; and organ packaging, preservation, and transportation.

The National Organ Procurement and Transplantation Network

In 1984, spurred by the shortage of organs and the lack of oversight and coordination in the organ procurement system, the United States Congress passed legislation that prescribed the establishment and operation of a national network to coordinate organ transplantation for the country. That network is known as the Organ Procurement and Transplantation Network (OPTN). The network includes all hospitals that provide solid organ transplantation as well as all organ procurement organizations (OPOs) and tissue-typing laboratories. It also includes other organizations and individuals interested in organ transplantation. It provides support and oversight for every organ transplant in the country for both living donor and deceased donor transplants. Although many OPOs procure tissue and corneas, the network itself does not provide oversight or support of tissue, cornea, or bone marrow/cellular transplants. There is a separate network for bone marrow and cellular transplants, the CW "Bill" Young Cellular Transplant Program. There is not a single national network for either tissue or cornea transplantation.

The OPTN history and its current working authority

The National Organ Transplant Act (NOTA) of 1984 specified that the Secretary of the US Department of Health and Human Services was to provide for the establishment and operation of an Organ Procurement and Transplantation Network in the private sector. United Network for Organ Sharing (UNOS) is a private membership corporation that is also a non-profit, charitable organization (Figure 41.1). It is located in Richmond, Virginia, and was established in 1984 by the American Society of Transplant Surgeons and the South Eastern Organ Procurement Foundation. UNOS was awarded the initial federal contract on September 30, 1986, to establish the OPTN. In 1987, the Health Resources and Services Administration (HRSA) and agency of the US Department of Health and Human Services (HHS) awarded a contract to UNOS to begin operating the network that UNOS had established. UNOS has been awarded successive contracts to continue operations since that time, is the only organization to ever manage the OPTN, and has continued to administer the contract for more than 22 years and five successive contract renewals.

As the contractor for operating the OPTN, UNOS collects and maintains all data for the Scientific Registry of Transplant Recipients (SRTR). This registry, established in 1987, maintains data on every organ transplant recipient in the United States, including annual follow-up data for the life of the recipient and/or graft. HRSA awards a separate contract for the analysis of SRTR data and producing reports to support the work of OPTN committees and for the public (not currently held by UNOS).

NOTA requires that the OPTN be a private, non-profit entity (i.e., not a government agency) with a Board of Directors to govern the network. The law stated that the OPTN should establish a list of all persons who need organ transplants as well as a national system to match organs with patients waiting for them, maintain a 24-hour telephone service to facilitate matching, assist OPOs in the distribution of organs, and coordinate transportation of organs. It also required the OPTN to collect, analyze, and publish data about organ donation and work to increase the supply of donated organs.

In 1987, Congress enacted additional legislation stating that in order for a hospital that transplanted organs or an OPO to be eligible to receive Medicare and Medicaid funds, such hospital or OPO must belong to and abide by the rules and requirements of the OPTN. Since that time, all transplant hospitals and organ procurement organizations in the U.S. have been members of the OPTN.

HHS has determined that OPTN actions may be regarded as such "rules and requirements" once they have been adopted as federal regulations, and only HHS is empowered to deny membership in the OPTN or participation in the Medicare program. HHS cannot delegate this power to the OPTN as a private body. Because adoption of OPTN policies as a federal regulation is a rare occurrence, each member hospital and OPO has agreed by private contract to abide by the policies and bylaws of the OPTN. This contractual agreement gives the OPTN the ability to take certain consequential adverse actions designed to bring members into compliance when they fail to follow the policies and bylaws.

Effective March 16, 2000, HHS issued federal regulations (the OPTN Final Rule) establishing a regulatory framework for the structure and operation of the OPTN. Under the terms of those regulations, the OPTN should develop policies governing the network's operation through the OPTN committees with approval by the OPTN Board of Directors. Should the OPTN Board desire that any such policy be made binding upon OPTN members as one of the OPTN rules and requirements for the purposes of Medicare eligibility as defined in the Social Security Act, the Board would then submit that policy to the Secretary of HHS for final approval as a federal regulation. Because OPTN policies need to be updated frequently to stay abreast of changes in the field, and federal regulations sometimes require long periods of time to amend, no policy has ever been referred to the Secretary for adoption. Rather, as a way of ensuring policy compliance, the OPTN has relied on the contractual agreement of its members. However, because submission of data to the OPTN is required by the OPTN Final Rule, which is a federal regulation, failure to submit the data to the OPTN, which are required on data forms approved by the federal Office of Management and Budget, would be considered by HHS to be a violation of the requirements of Section 1138 of the Social Security Act.

The OPTN evaluates member compliance through routine monitoring of data submission and transplant activity, as well as confidential medical peer review of member complaints. If a member is found to be consistently substandard in performance or is in violation of OPTN requirements, the OPTN provides notice to the offending member that they are planning to take an adverse action against the member as provided in the OPTN bylaws, which gives the member the opportunity to appeal. If the offense is serious enough, the OPTN Board of Directors makes recommendations to the Secretary of HHS regarding adverse actions that may be taken against the member. As a result of these enforcement measures, compliance with OPTN policies continues to be very high.

The OPTN Final Rule

The federal regulations that govern the OPTN are comprehensive. They specify the organization and governance of the network, including detailed requirements for the composition of the OPTN Board of Directors. In 2010, the OPTN included all 249 US hospitals that perform organ transplantation, all 58 OPOs, all 59 independent histocompatibility laboratories, 17 medical/scientific organizations or societies, 2 business members, and 10 individuals.

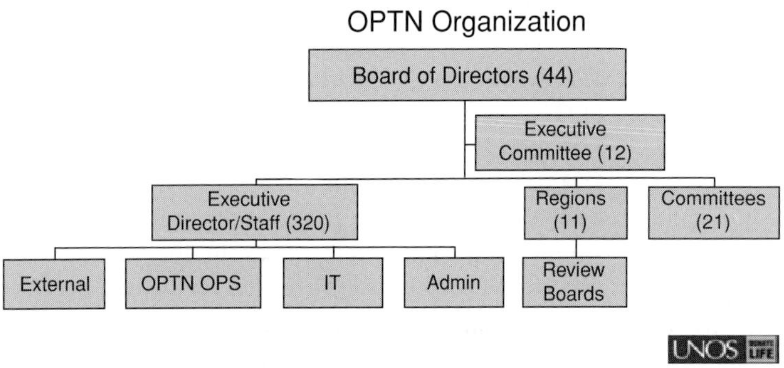

Figure 41.2 Organization of the US Organ Procurement and Transplantation Network.

Policy development

The OPTN Final Rule gives the OPTN Board of Directors responsibility for developing policies for the OPTN in specific areas:

- Equitable allocation of cadaveric organs
- Testing of organ donors and follow-up of transplant recipients to prevent the spread of infectious diseases
- Reducing inequities resulting from socioeconomic status
- The training and experience of transplant surgeons and transplant physicians in designated transplant programs
- Nomination of officers and members of the Board of Directors
- Policies on such other matters as the Secretary may direct

OPTN policies and bylaws govern the procedural aspects of policy development, allocation of donated organs, and collection of transplant data nationwide. Members and the public are included in the process through solicitation of feedback via the public comment process. UNOS maintains an extensive number of committees made up of transplant professionals, patients, donors, donor family members, and others interested in the OPTN's issues (Figure 41.2). The committees are responsible for developing policy proposals. Once a proposal is developed, UNOS' staff prepares a written rationale for the proposed policy, including the scientific data analysis and any other background considered by the committee in developing the proposal. That proposal and rationale are then published for a 90-day period when anyone in the membership or general public may submit comments to UNOS regarding the proposal.

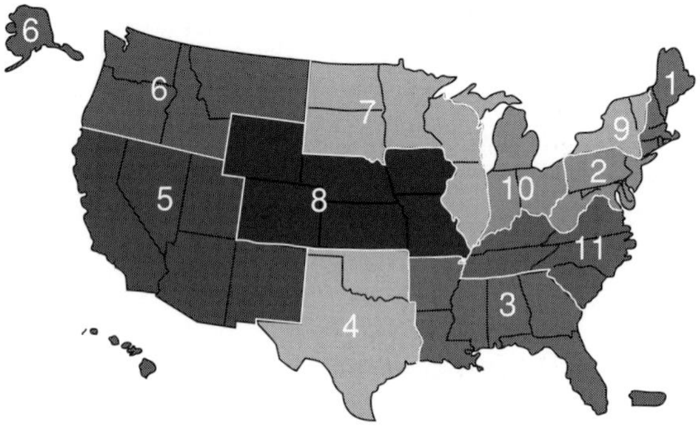

Figure 41.3 UNOS and OPTN Regions.

During the public comment period, the proposal is reviewed by all of the other OPTN committees, which may submit comments to the originating committee. UNOS and the OPTN are divided into 11 geographic regions of the United States, and each region will conduct a meeting of its members twice a year for the purpose of reviewing policy proposals and providing feedback to the originating committee and the Board of Directors (see below and Figure 41.3). The timing of the publication of policy proposals is coordinated with these regional meetings so that all regions have an opportunity to comment on all proposals. Each region has members representing each committee and a regional councilor who conducts the meeting and represents the region on the Board of Directors. This provides an opportunity for members in a region to give direct input to their representatives.

At the end of the public comment period, the originating OPTN committee considers and responds to each comment received and finalizes the policy proposal for consideration by the Board of Directors. The Board then decides whether to approve the policy, amend it, return it to the committee, or reject it.

The development of UNOS regions

As the OPTN contractor, UNOS uses its 11 geographic regions as the OPTN's regions. This regional structure was developed to facilitate organ allocation and provide individuals with the opportunity to identify concerns regarding organ procurement, allocation, and transplantation that are unique to their particular geographic area.

The basis for the regions is historical organ sharing relationships. Prior to the creation of the OPTN, there were seven regional organ banks that were funded by grants from HHS. The original UNOS regions were based on the territories covered by those seven regional organizations. Over time, several of the regions were split into more workable sizes. For example, the territory covered by the South Eastern Organ Procurement Foundation, one of the original seven grantees, was divided into regions 3 and 11. The state of New York was split off of the New England region so that it became region 9, and so on.

Listing requirements

A potential transplant candidate is referred by his or her doctor to a transplant center for evaluation. The transplant center runs a number of tests and considers the patient's mental and physical health, as well as his or her social support system. If the center decides to accept this person as a transplant candidate, they will add his or her medical profile to the OPTN's national patient waiting list for organ transplant. The candidate is not placed on a ranked list at that time. Rather, his or her information is kept in a constantly updated, computerized database. Whichever OPTN member places the patient on the waiting list must pay a "patient registration fee" to the OPTN.

OPTN policies permit a patient to be listed at multiple transplant hospitals. Organs are to be offered and transplanted only for patients who are on the OPTN waiting list. Should a patient be unable to receive a transplant, the program may indicate the patient's status on the waiting list as being inactive. Once the patient has undergone transplantation, the program is required to remove the patient from the list within 24 hours.

Organ allocation

Specific direction is given by the OPTN Final Rule for the principles to be included in policies for the equitable allocation of organs. Those policies meet certain criteria:

- Based on sound medical judgment
- Seek to achieve the best use of donated organs
- Preserve the ability of a transplant program to decline an offer of an organ or not to use the organ for the potential recipient
- Be specific for each organ type or combination of organ types
- Be designed to avoid wasting organs, to avoid futile transplants, to promote patient access to transplantation, and to promote the efficient management of organ placement
- Not be based on the candidate's place of residence or place of listing, except to the extent required by consideration of the foregoing principles

An important factor for the OPTN in its policy development deliberations is the fact that NOTA limits the policy considerations for organ allocation policy to medical criteria. The final rule amplifies this restriction by requiring that the patient rankings resulting from the allocation policy be based on objective and measurable medical criteria. Therefore, allocation policies do not take into account social criteria such as social worth or economic criteria. Thus organ allocation policy does not consider, for example, whether a patient is an unemployed vagrant as opposed to the CEO of a major corporation. Likewise, the underlying cause of a disease such as drug or alcohol addiction is not considered by the allocation policies. An individual transplant program may consider whether a patient has maintained a suitable period of abstinence as part of its evaluation of whether the patient is an acceptable candidate, but once a patient is on the OPTN waiting list, whether the patient's disease was caused by substance abuse may not be considered because it is understood to be "social criteria."

The OPTN Final Rule includes performance goals for allocation policies. In addition to the use of objective and measurable medical criteria, the policies are to provide for candidate rankings that give priority to patients based on medical urgency with patients having the most urgent need receiving highest priority. Also, organs are to be allocated over as broad a geographic area as feasible, considering the principles for allocation included in the Final Rule, and the amount of inter-program variance among performance measures is to be reduced to as low a level as can reasonably be achieved.

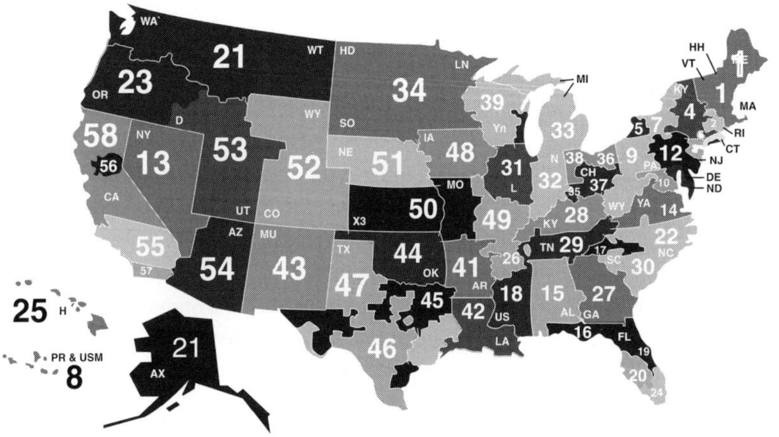

Figure 41.4 Donation service areas in the US (58 total areas).

Prior to NOTA there were more than 120 OPOs, some independent and some transplant-hospital based. However, each operated independently and there was no effective system for sharing organs among recovery regions. As part of NOTA's implementation, in 1987 HRSA solicited proposals from organizations to become the designated OPO for a specific geographic region of the United States. In 1988, 74 organizations were selected and given exclusive responsibility for all activities related to the procurement of organs from deceased donors. These newly designated OPOs, all non-profit, were a mix of previously existing OPOs and new organizations formed by the merger of OPOs that had served overlapping geographic regions. By 2010, the number of OPOs was reduced to 58 through mergers of geographically adjacent OPOs (Figure 41.4). Some consolidations were voluntary, whereas others were the result of HHS enforcement of standards of performance.

Identification of the organ recipient

Under its OPTN contract with HRSA, UNOS maintains a centralized computer network linking all organ procurement organizations and transplant centers. This computer network is accessible 24 hours a day, 7 days a week, with organ placement specialists in the UNOS Organ Center always available to answer questions. When a donated organ from a deceased donor is available, the OPO procuring the organ must enter information about the donor into the OPTN contractor's computer system and execute the computer match program. That program will rank order the candidates on the OPTN waiting list according to the organ allocation policies that have been adopted by the Board of Directors. The OPO then offers the organ to designated transplant programs in according to the rank order of the match. The transplant program may accept or refuse the offer. The match is patient-specific as required by NOTA. The organ may not simply be offered to a transplant program for the program to use at its discretion. If an organ is offered to a transplant program for a certain patient, but the program decides to decline the offer, the organ is then offered to the next patient on the ranked OPTN match list, even if the patient is at another institution. Exceptions can be made in certain circumstances, but those are not the norm. The match for each donor organ will be different and unique to the circumstances of the donor and the patients waiting. Factors affecting ranking may include tissue match, blood type, length of time on the waiting list, immune status, and the distance between the potential recipient and the donor. For heart, liver, lung, and intestines, the potential recipient's degree of medical urgency is also considered. The organ is offered to the transplant team for the first person on the match list. Often, the top-ranked patient will not get the organ for one of several reasons. When a patient is selected, he or she must be available, healthy enough to undergo major surgery, and willing to undergo transplantation immediately. Also, a laboratory test to measure compatibility between the donor and recipient may be necessary. For example, patients with high antibody levels often prove incompatible to the donor organ and cannot receive the organ because the patient's immune system would reject it. Once a patient is selected and contacted and all testing is complete, the transplant procedure is scheduled.

Transplant program requirements and evaluation

The OPTN Final Rule states that organs may only be offered to transplant programs that are "designated programs." In order to become designated, a transplant program must be approved as a Medicare transplant program or be part of a federal government hospital (e.g., Veterans Administration hospitals) or meet certain requirements defined by the OPTN. Those criteria include minimum standards for the education, training, and experience of a primary surgeon and a primary physician for the transplant program. OPTN Bylaws require that all programs meet the criteria for a primary surgeon and physician regardless of Medicare certification, and OPTN membership approval may include a site review designed to ensure that the necessary resources and personnel are available to provide transplantation services.

The OPTN oversees transplant center performance by monitoring center-specific reports provided by the SRTR contractor on a quarterly basis. In these reports, center-specific data are compared with expected risk-adjusted outcomes using three well-defined criteria adopted by the OPTN for quality assurance. If a program has results that meet all three criteria, the OPTN Membership and Professional Standards Committee (MPSC) commissions a group of reviewers who investigate potential causes for inferior outcomes and then report back to the MPSC. Based on their findings, the MPSC makes recommendations regarding the necessary steps required to improve outcomes. The OPTN continues to monitor performance until outcomes are improved. If serious deficiencies persist and are not corrected, the OPTN may take actions against the transplant center, including a letter of warning, a letter of reprimand, declare the transplant center to be on probation, or declare it to be a "member not in good standing." If the problem is serious enough, the OPTN may recommend that HHS remove the transplant program's "designated" status, which will deny the transplant center access to deceased donor organs for transplant.

Living donor organ transplantation

Neither NOTA nor the OPTN Final Rule issued in 2000 included living donor transplantation as part of the OPTN's charge. The Advisory Committee on Transplantation (ACOT) issued its first set of recommendations to the Secretary of HHS in 2002 after a year's deliberations. Included among those recommendations were several regarding the need for protections for living donors. Specifically, the ACOT recommended that qualifications of programs performing living donor transplants be verified, that ethical principles and informed consent standards be implemented for all living donors, and that certain informed consent practices be instituted, including the requirement of an independent donor advocate at each transplant center performing living donor transplantation. In June 2006, HRSA issued a directive to the OPTN to develop and enforce policies regarding living donors and living donor transplant recipients.

In response, UNOS, together with the American Society of Transplant Surgeons and the American Society of Transplantation, convened a consensus conference to develop guidelines for the psychosocial evaluation of prospective living kidney donors who have neither a biological nor longstanding emotional relationship with the transplant candidate (i.e., unrelated donors). Those recommendations were adopted by the OPTN, which also developed membership criteria for transplant programs that perform living donor transplantation and a series of guidelines/policies for providing informed consent to potential donors as well as the medical evaluation of potential living donors.

Transplant centers are required to submit reports to the OPTN on all transplants, including living donor transplants, even when both donor and recipient are from another country and in the United States only for the transplant. Transplant programs are also required to report all instances of living donor deaths and failure of the living donor's native organ function to the OPTN within 72 hours after the program becomes aware of such an event. In 2005, HRSA determined that failure by a transplant center to report required data to the OPTN would be a violation of the OPTN Final Rule, and as such would be a violation of OPTN "rules and requirements," which could lead to the entire hospital being made ineligible to receive Medicare or Medicaid payments.

Success and ongoing challenges of the US system

Organ transplantation is different from any other medical service because transplantation practice does not rely solely on professional expertise. The success of transplantation necessitates either a willing living donor or suitable deceased organ donor. Society has an oversight responsibility to assure a just distribution of deceased organs and the proper care of the live donor. The OPTN system fulfills that societal responsibility in that every provider of organ transplantation participates in the network under a model of self-governance with federal oversight. The practitioners who provide the medical and surgical services also develop and implement the standards and policies by which the field is governed with federal oversight. One of the greatest strengths of the system is the fact that data for every organ, every transplant, every organ donor, and every transplant recipient are collected and maintained in the OPTN databases for analyses and publication. These data are widely available to researchers, enabling the field to continually improve. The data are assessed for performance of individual institutions, and through a process of confidential medical peer review, efforts are made to improve those institutions that are not performing at an acceptable level. No other part of medicine and surgery in the United States can claim such successes for its entire field.

Further reading

Luskin RS, Glazier AK, Delmonico FL. Organ donation and dual advocacy. *N Engl J Med* 2008; **358**: 1297–8.

McDiarmid SV, Pruett TL, Graham WK. The oversight of solid organ transplantation in the United States. *Am J Transplant* 2008; **8**: 739–44.

Organ Procurement and Transplantation Network. Available at: http://optn.transplant.hrsa.gov

Pretagostini R, Gabbrielli F, Fiaschetti P, *et al.* Risk management systems for health care and safety development on transplantation: a review and a proposal. *Transplant Proc* 2010; **42**: 1014–6.

Tuttle-Newhall JE, Krishnan SM, Levy MF, McBride V, Orlowski JP, Sung RS. Organ donation and utilization in the United States: 1998–2007. *Am J Transplant*2009; **9**: 879–93.

United Network for Organ Sharing. Available at: http://www.unos.org

Chapter 42

Conclusions

Clive J. Lewis

Key points

- Transplant medicine has more Nobel Prize winners than any other field.
- Uterus and ovary transplant may allow successful pregnancy.
- Biological heart valves are an essential part of the cardiac surgeon's armamentarium.
- Thymus transplant is an important therapeutic option for infants with Di George syndrome.
- Cell transplant and tissue engineering is a significant area of research and may provide great strides in future treatment for a wide variety of diseases.

Transplantation has evolved enormously over the last 50 years, with many significant milestones and with the contribution of many individuals of all disciplines to make transplant medicine an exciting and research-focused area with more Nobel prizes than any other field! Every conceivable cell, tissue, and organ has been transplanted either in an experimental model or full clinical transplant program. This book has considered the most commonly transplanted tissues and solid organs, yet much research continues in the cell laboratory, in animal models, and in early human clinical studies. This chapter briefly outlines a number of these areas that have not already been discussed.

Uterus transplantation

Human uterus transplant may have a role as a future method to treat uterine causes of infertility. However, there remain significant barriers, including surgical and ethical factors. The first human uterus transplant occurred in 1931 as part of gender reassignment surgery, but the patient died from acute rejection. Partial success was seen with a functioning uterus for approximately 3 months in 2000. Potential recipients include those with congenital absence of a uterus (e.g., Mayer-Rokitansky-Kuster-Hauser syndrome) or hysterectomy due to a number of causes, including obstetric complication (e.g., postpartum hemorrhage), pelvic inflammatory disease, fibroids, and cervical or ovarian malignancies. Experimental animal studies have established the feasibility of uterus transplant, including donor retrieval techniques, cold ischemic tolerance of greater than 24 hours, and the surgical implant procedure, although problems remain with vascular anastomosis and thrombosis. Pregnancies have been reported in syngenic animal models. Other remaining issues include ethical concerns and immunosuppression regimes with their inherent complications. Human uterine transplant remains experimental but may soon reach a stage for further attempts.

Ovary transplantation

The objective of ovarian transplantation is similar to that of uterus transplantation in that successful engraftment would result in fertility. Research in this area was largely taken over by the successes of in vitro fertilization and uterine implantation. However, in select situations (e.g., following chemo/radiotherapy for childhood cancers), implantation of autotransplanted previously frozen ovary (partial or total) has been reported to give rise to successful pregnancies. Syngeneic ovary transplantation has also been reported. Both of these methods have the advantages of avoiding immunosuppression and providing long-term benefits of endogenous estrogen.

Organ Transplantation: A Clinical Guide, ed. A.A. Klein, C.J. Lewis, and J.C. Madsen. Published by Cambridge University Press.

Cardiac valves and vessels

When hearts are not procured for human transplantation, the valves and vessels may be harvested for use in conventional cardiac surgery. Aortic and pulmonary valves may be taken together with a length of artery (homograft) or excised alone and placed in valve support structure or conduits for ventriculoarterial valve replacement. These have the advantage of immune privilege and therefore do not require immunosuppression. Homograft tissue is likely to lead to the development of human leukocyte antigen sensitization, which may be important in patients who may require organ transplant in the future. The use of animal tissue (xenograft) for transplantation has been long considered one answer to the shortage of donor organs. Primate to human organ transplants have failed due to rapid immune recognition and rejection. Significant advances in immunobiology will be needed before xenotransplantation becomes a reality. However, animal valves (particularly porcine and bovine) have been successfully used in human cardiac valve replacement for many years without the problem of rejection.

Thymus

Thymus transplantation has been used to treat the rare condition of complete athymia in Di George syndrome. Di George anomaly is characterized by varying defects of the heart, thymus, and parathyroid glands. Infants may present with very low T-cell counts or develop oligoclonal T cells that produce a rash and adenopathy and are at increased risk of infection. Thymus for transplant is obtained from donor infants undergoing cardiac surgery and, following culture, is usually placed ectopically (e.g., into quadriceps muscle). Approximately 50% require immunosuppression. Reported mortality rates are 25% at 1 year, although thereafter, survival is excellent with minimal subsequent mortality over many years. Recipients also appear to develop stable immunoconstitution and responses. Complications include graft-versus-host disease and long-term immunosuppression.

Cell-based therapies

Transplanting cells derived from fetal tissue (embryonic stem cells; ESCs) have the potential to improve a wide variety of human disease because they can differentiate and replace damaged tissues without the need for immunosuppression and their inherent complications. This area of research is likely to make the biggest ever impact on human disease. A number of stem cell therapeutics exist, but most are at experimental stages. Only bone marrow transplantation is in current clinical use. Potential areas of treatment include spinal cord injury (neural ESC – oligodendrocyte progenitor cells; the subject of a clinical trial), diabetes mellitus (insulin-producing ESC-derived beta cells), heart failure (ESC-derived cardiac stem cells), and degenerative disease, such as juvenile macular degeneration (subretinal transplantation of ESC-derived retinal stem cells), Parkinson's disease (substantia nigra–grafted ESC-derived dopaminergic cells), and Huntington's disease (striatum-grafted ESC-derived striatal cells). This is likely to be a very exciting area of development in the next decade.

Index

Note: Page numbers followed by **f** refer to figures; page numbers followed by **t** refer to tables.